Radiation Therapy for Cancer

Radiation Therapy for Cancer

Editor: Karolina Sturm

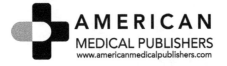

AMERICAN
MEDICAL PUBLISHERS
www.americanmedicalpublishers.com

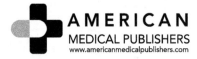

AMERICAN
MEDICAL PUBLISHERS
www.americanmedicalpublishers.com

Cataloging-in-Publication Data

Radiation therapy for cancer / edited by Karolina Sturm.
     p. cm.
Includes bibliographical references and index.
ISBN 979-8-88740-417-2
1. Cancer--Radiotherapy. 2. Tumors--Radiography. 3. Radiography. 4. Cancer--Treatment.
5. Diagnostic imaging. 6. Imaging systems in medicine. I. Sturm, Karolina.
RC271.R3 R333 2023
616.994 064 2--dc23

American Medical Publishers,
41 Flatbush Avenue,
1st Floor, New York,
NY 11217, USA

ISBN 979-8-88740-417-2 (Hardback)

Contents

Preface

Radiation therapy refers to a technique used for treating cancer with the help of high energy charged particles. It is one of the three major modalities utilized for the treatment of malignant diseases, the other two modalities being chemotherapy and surgery. Radiotherapy utilizes ionizing radiation to treat cancer and is significantly reliant on modern technology. It is also dependent on the joint efforts of a number of medical specialties, such as radiation oncology and medical physics, whose coordinated team approach has a significant impact on the outcome of the treatment. Radiation therapy for cancer requires an understanding of radiation physics along with the interaction of ionizing radiation with human tissue. It is utilised as a primary treatment for cancer, and can be given individually or in combination with other treatments like medications or chemotherapy. This book explores all the important aspects of radiation therapy in the present day scenario. It is a valuable compilation of topics, ranging from the basic to the most complex advancements in this form of cancer therapy. This book is appropriate for students seeking detailed information in this area as well as for experts.

This book is a comprehensive compilation of works of different researchers from varied parts of the world. It includes valuable experiences of the researchers with the sole objective of providing the readers (learners) with a proper knowledge of the concerned field. This book will be beneficial in evoking inspiration and enhancing the knowledge of the interested readers.

In the end, I would like to extend my heartiest thanks to the authors who worked with great determination on their chapters. I also appreciate the publisher's support in the course of the book. I would also like to deeply acknowledge my family who stood by me as a source of inspiration during the project.

Editor

Differential Superiority of Heavy Charged-Particle Irradiation to X-Rays: Studies on Biological Effectiveness and Side Effect Mechanisms in Multicellular Tumor and Normal Tissue Models

Stefan Walenta and Wolfgang Mueller-Klieser*

Institute of Pathophysiology, University Medical Center, University of Mainz, Mainz, Germany

Correspondence:
Wolfgang Mueller-Klieser
mue-kli@uni-mainz.de

This review is focused on the radiobiology of carbon ions compared to X-rays using multicellular models of tumors and normal mucosa. The first part summarizes basic radiobiological effects, as observed in cancer cells. The second, more clinically oriented part of the review, deals with radiation-induced cell migration and mucositis. Multicellular spheroids from V79 hamster cells were irradiated with X-rays or carbon ions under ambient or restricted oxygen supply conditions. Reliable oxygen enhancement ratios could be derived to be 2.9, 2.8, and 1.4 for irradiation with photons, $^{12}C^{+6}$ in the plateau region, and $^{12}C^{+6}$ in the Bragg peak, respectively. Similarly, a relative biological effectiveness of 4.3 and 2.1 for ambient pO_2 and hypoxia was obtained, respectively. The high effectiveness of carbon ions was reflected by an enhanced accumulation of cells in G_2/M and a dose-dependent massive induction of apoptosis. These data clearly show that heavy charged particles are more efficient in sterilizing tumor cells than conventional irradiation even under hypoxic conditions. Clinically relevant doses (3 Gy) of X-rays induced an increase in migratory activity of U87 but not of LN229 or HCT116 tumor cells. Such an increase in cell motility following irradiation *in situ* could be the source of recurrence. In contrast, carbon ion treatment was associated with a dose-dependent decrease in migration with all cell lines and under all conditions investigated. The radiation-induced loss of cell motility was correlated, in most cases, with corresponding changes in β_1 integrin expression. The photon-induced increase in cell migration was paralleled by an elevated phosphorylation status of the epidermal growth factor receptor and AKT-ERK1/2 pathway. Such a hyperphosphorylation did not occur during $^{12}C^{+6}$ irradiation under all conditions registered. Comparing the gene toxicity of X-rays with that of particles using the γH2AX technique in organotypic cultures of the oral mucosa, the superior effectiveness of heavy ions was confirmed by a twofold higher number of foci per nucleus. However, proinflammatory signs were similar for both treatment modalities, e.g., the activation of NFκB and the release of IL6 and IL8. The presence of peripheral blood mononuclear cell increased the radiation-induced release of the proinflammatory cytokines by factors of

2–3. Carbon ions are part of the cosmic radiation. Long-term exposure to such particles during extended space flights, as planned by international space agencies, may thus impose a medical and safety risk on the astronauts by a potential induction of mucositis. In summary, particle irradiation is superior to gamma-rays due to a higher radiobiological effectiveness, a reduced hypoxia-induced radioresistance, a multicellular radiosensitization, and the absence of a radiation-induced cell motility. However, the potential of inducing mucositis is similar for both radiation types.

Keywords: radiobiology, particle irradiation, oxygen enhancement ratio, relative biological effectiveness, organotypic tumor and mucosa cultures, mucositis, cell migration

INTRODUCTION

This article summarizes data which we have acquired in close collaboration with a number of scientists at the Gesellschaft fuer Schwerionenforschung (GSI) Darmstadt, Germany, for more than one decade. At the beginning of this collaboration, little was known about the basic radiobiology of particle irradiation, although there was emerging evidence already at that time for the usefulness of a carbon ion radiotherapy in clinical oncology (1). Consequently, the ultimate goal of the interactive work at the GSI accelerator was to augment our knowledge on biological effects of heavy charged particles in malignant tumors and in healthy tissue in comparison to the effect of conventional X-rays under equivalent conditions.

In most of the experiments, a carbon-12 ($^{12}C^{6+}$) beam was applied in the scanning mode either in the extended Bragg peak or in the plateau region at 227 MeV/nucleon. Conventional X-rays served as a reference, and X-ray equivalent doses were derived for heavy charged particle irradiation. Since beam-time is highly cost-intensive and since there is a pronounced competition among scientists for the acquisition of beam-time, design and performance of experiments with heavy charged particles are subjected to practical limitations by the restricted availability of the particle beam. This reduces the number of experiments within a given time frame and consequently restricts statistical corroboration of findings by multiple approaches. This has to be kept in mind, when data from particle irradiation are compared with those from other assays.

All irradiation experiments were carried out on cultured cells using various tumor and normal cell models. Besides conventional single cell cultures, complex three-dimensional (3D) cell cultures were used; these included organotypic cultures of the human oral mucosa with or without immune cells, planar cell multilayers of WiDr colon adenocarcinoma cells or of SiHa cervix carcinoma cells, and multicellular spheroids (MCS) from V79 cells. With a few exceptions, irradiation was routinely performed under standardized cell culture conditions at 37°C and ambient (20% O_2) or reduced (pO$_2$ close to 0 mmHg) oxygen supply conditions.

"Classical" radiobiological endpoints, such as clonogenic cell survival, spheroid volume growth, or cell cycle effects as a function of radiation dose, were used to quantify the efficiency of particle versus conventional radiation. Furthermore, the relative biological effectiveness (RBE) and the oxygen enhancement ratio (OER) for the two radiation modalities were derived. One specific endpoint was cell migration and motility in 2D and 3D conditions under the impact of irradiation. The gene toxicity of both radiation types in normal tissue was quantified using the γH2AX technique in organotypic mucosa cultures. In this multicellular model, assays for early events of a radiation-induced mucositis, such as activation of the transcription factor NFκB or release of cytokines IL6 and IL8, were applied. The cocultivation of the mucosa model with human peripheral blood mononuclear cells (PBMCs) revealed a significant role of immune cells in the emergence of radiation-related mucositis.

Following the introduction, the experimental part of this review article is subdivided into three major chapters. The first chapter deals with our data related to the basic radiobiology of carbon ion irradiation compared to that of conventional gamma-radiation. This includes the relative biological effectiveness, the oxygen effect, and the multicellular radioresistance. The second chapter is focused on our findings regarding clinical aspects of undesirable side effects of the two radiation types considered. These aspects refer to radiation-induced cell motility and to radiation-associated mucositis. The third chapter of this review links our own data to findings from the literature. For many years, radiobiological studies on heavy charged particles have remained sparse, but very recently, there is a tremendous increase in the number of reports on radiobiology of heavy ions, on their clinical use, as well as on a combination of their radiobiological and clinical aspects. Consequently, the intention of the third chapter of this review is by no means to give a comprehensive review of the literature on particle irradiation, but rather to present a selection of very recent reports that are closely related to the data presented here. The final paragraph of this review presents a brief resume of the article.

BASIC RADIOBIOLOGY OF HEAVY CHARGED PARTICLES

RBE and OER Values for Carbon Ion Irradiation of Multicellular V79 Spheroids

Ever since the pioneering work of Robert Sutherland and colleagues (2), reviewed in Ref. (3), MCS represent classical 3D cell models in radiation research. Based on a sabbatical in Sutherland's laboratory (4) and on the pioneer's personal assistance as a Humboldt awardee at the University of Mainz (5), one of us set up a state-of-the-art spheroid laboratory at our research institute.

Within the frame of a number of different research projects, we collected a large amount of data on 3D versus 2D growth characteristics, on 3D interaction between tumor and immune cells, or on tumor microenvironment with regard to hypoxia, hypoglycemia, acidosis, and other factors (6).

Occasionally, these data sparked the interest of scientists at the GSI in using our expertise with the spheroid technology for the exploration of heavy charged particle radiobiology. Spheroids from immortalized and tumorigenic V79 hamster cells have been frequently used in radiobiological investigations, and we decided to initiate our studies on heavy ion radiobiology with this spheroid type having an abundance of comparative data from X-ray experiments.

Multicellular spheroids from V79 cells with 200 μm in diameter were irradiated with X-rays or carbon $^{12}C^{6+}$ ions under elevated, ambient, or restricted oxygen supply conditions. From previous microelectrode measurements, the oxygen tension distribution within the MCS as a function of the external oxygen tension was known, which made it possible to exactly relate the local oxygen to the radiation effects. For reasons of simplicity, average numbers for the environmental oxygen tension (pO_2) in mm Hg are given for characterizing the experimental conditions. **Figure 1** shows clonogenic cell survival curves for V79 MCS irradiated with X-rays (**Figure 1A**) in environmental pO_2 values of 144 mmHg (circles), 35 mmHg (squares), and 0 mmHg (diamonds) or irradiated with $^{12}C^{6+}$ ions in the extended Bragg peak (**Figure 1B**) in environmental pO_2 values of 690 mmHg (circles) and 0 mmHg (diamonds). It is obvious that (i) survival curves after particle irradiation are close to being linear with almost no shoulder compared to the X-ray data and (ii) the oxygen effect is much less pronounced with particle compared to photon irradiation. Survival curves of V79 single cells were almost identical with that

of V79 spheroids with no indication of a multicellular resistance or contact effect (data not shown). Irradiation of V79 MCS with carbon ions in the plateau region (227 MeV/nucleon $^{12}C^{6+}$) in the same oxygen atmospheres as used with X-ray treatment produced survival curves that were almost identical with those from photon irradiation (data not shown).

The survival curves of V79 MCS displayed in **Figure 1** were fitted with the linear quadratic model. This was used for deriving reliable OER and relative biological effectiveness (RBE values). OER values at several survival levels S (=37, 10, 1, and 0.1%) were calculated as the ratio of doses to achieve a given survival under hypoxia compared to normoxia. Averages were derived from the individual values, which varied with S by around 5%. A corresponding procedure was used for the derivation of RBE, which was defined as the ratio of X-ray dose to that of particle radiation to reach a given S. These data are compiled in **Table 1**. Besides the very low OER value of 1.40 for particle irradiation, the RBE value of heavy charged particles is remarkably high at 4.31. Further details on the data evaluation were published earlier (7).

Furthermore, the high effectiveness of heavy charged particles in the extended Bragg peak compared to conventional radiation was reflected by a massive, dose-dependent induction of apoptosis [quantified by the TUNEL assay (7)], as shown in **Figure 2**. Although a respective curve for the extended Bragg peak induction of apoptosis under ambient oxygen conditions could not be assessed in this set of experiments for technical reasons, explorative data were indicative of an absence of an oxygen effect with regard to apoptotic cell kill [for further details, see Ref. (7)]. All data obtained in this spheroid study clearly show that heavy charged particles are more efficient in sterilizing tumor cells than conventional irradiation even under hypoxic conditions.

Unexpected Multicellular Radiosensitization in Human Colon Adenocarcinoma-Derived Multilayer Cells

Planar cell multilayers in comparison with monolayer cultures of WiDr and SiHa human colon adenocarcinoma-derived cells were used for investigations on the role of cell cycle effects in the treatment with photon or particle irradiation. Development of a special cryostat sectioning technique made it possible to assess histology and growth characteristics of the planar 3D model (8). This is exemplified by **Figure 3**, with **Figure 3A** displaying cryostat sections that were cut perpendicular to the multilayer

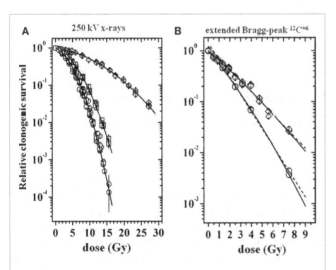

FIGURE 1 | Relative clonogenic survival of cells from V79 MCS as a function of dose [modified according to Ref. (7)]. **(A)** Following X-ray irradiation at external pO_2 values of 144 mmHg (circles), 35 mmHg (squares), and 0 mmHg (diamonds), **(B)** following $^{12}C^{6+}$ irradiation in the extended Bragg peak at external pO_2 values of 690 mmHg (circles) and 0 mmHg (diamonds); dose values represent X-ray equivalent dose.

TABLE 1 | Oxygen enhancement ratio (OER) and relative biological effectiveness (RBE) values derived from the clonogenic survival curves shown in Figure 1 after irradiation in atmospheres with a pO_2 of 690 mmHg or 145 mmHg (aerobic) or 0 mmHg (hypoxic).

Radiation type	OER	RBE	
		Aerobic	Hypoxic
X-rays	2.87	1.00	1.00
Ext. Bragg peak	1.40	2.11	4.31

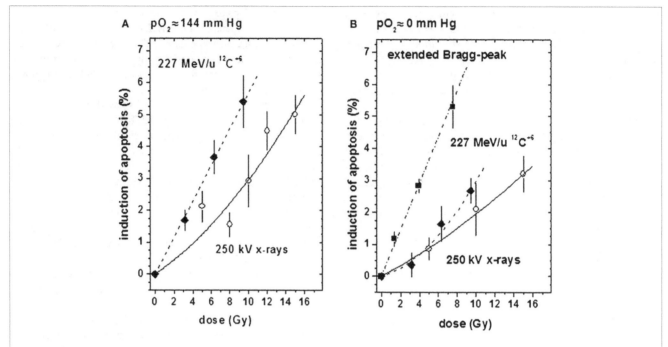

FIGURE 2 | Induction of apoptosis (relative to untreated controls) by X-ray (open circles) or ¹²C⁶⁺ irradiation in the plateau region (filled diamonds) or in the extended Bragg peak (filled squares) under ambient or hypoxic oxygen supply conditions [modified according to Ref. (7)]. (A) At an external pO₂ of 144 mm Hg and **(B)** at an external pO₂ of 0 mm Hg.

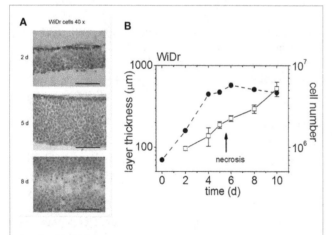

FIGURE 3 | Multilayers of WiDr cells at various days in culture [modified according to Ref. (7, 8)]. (A) H&E-stained cryosections of multilayers on three different days (d) in culture (scale bar: 100 μm), **(B)** multilayer thickness and cell content as a function of days in culture (the arrow indicates the emergence of a central necrotic layer).

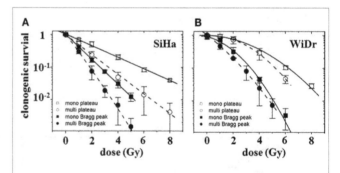

FIGURE 4 | Clonogenic survival of cells in monolayer (squares) or multilayer (circles) culture as a function of dose after carbon-ion irradiation in the plateau region (370 MeV/nucleon; open symbols) or in the extended Bragg peak [closed symbols; modified according to Ref. (8)]. (A) SiHa cells (n = 4) and **(B)** WiDr cells (n = 2–3).

plane at three different times of growth for both cell lines considered. **Figure 3B** shows the multilayer thickness and viable cell content as a function of time in culture. Obviously, the total layer thickness is expanding continuously after the emergence and expansion of a central necrotic layer, whereas the total number of viable cells is stagnating. As such, planar cellular multilayers grow in a way, which is very similar to that of MCS despite the different diffusion geometries.

Unexpectedly, there was a multicellular radiosensitization of multi- versus monolayers under all treatments considered, as demonstrated by standardized clonogenic survival curves for ¹²C⁶⁺ ion irradiation in the plateau region and the Bragg peak (**Figure 4**). This is in contrast to the generally detected multicellular radioresistance. The phenomenon was attributable, at least in parts, to a difference in the proportion of cells in the G_0/G_1 phase between the two culture types used. Furthermore, **Figure 4** illustrates cell line-dependent differences in the type of cell survival curves: whereas WiDr cells exhibit "classical" shoulder curves except for Bragg peak particle irradiation, SiHa cell survival curves are very close to linearity with all treatments considered.

Differential Superiority of Heavy Charged-Particle Irradiation to X-Rays: Studies on Biological Effectiveness...

5

This difference may indicate a different extent of DNA repair in these two cell lines due to either a different intensity/quality of DNA damage or different repair capacities.

Flow cytometric studies showed that X-rays induced a G_2/M arrest, which was considerably prolonged in multi- compared to monolayers (**Figure 5A**). After Bragg peak irradiation of monolayers, the arrest time was increased compared to X-rays by 12–24 h, and more cells were arrested than with X-rays (**Figures 5A,B**). However, in multilayers, both radiation modalities lead to similar growth arrests (see **Figures 5A,B**).

In essence, our data obtained in the multilayer project contribute to accumulating results in the literature regarding differences in biological properties and molecular mechanisms between 2D and 3D culture systems. Under many aspects, 3D planar cellular multilayers and 3D spherical cellular aggregates share common properties and behave in similar ways. On the other hand, multilayers tend to show a small but reproducible multicellular radiosensitization, whereas most spheroids exhibit a multicellular resistance. It is worth noting that this effect is even more pronounced with heavy charged particles than with photons [for further details on planar multilayers, see Ref. (8)].

CLINICAL ASPECTS OF POTENTIAL SIDE EFFECTS OF HEAVY CHARGED PARTICLE IRRADIATION

Differential Effects of Radiation on Cell Migration Depending on Radiation Type and Cell Line

When we initiated this project, there was an ongoing controversy within the science community about radiation-related modulation of tumor cell migration, mainly with regard to irradiation of glioblastomas (GBMs). The cellular motility of certain tumor cell lines is enhanced under *in vitro* conditions by sublethal doses of photon irradiation, as we and others have previously reported (9–11). In contrast, several other studies demonstrated that either similar sublethal or slightly higher doses impair GBM cell migration and invasion (12) or fail to modify these cell functions (13). The clarification of the respective controversy is clinically highly relevant: if therapeutic irradiation would enhance cell motility, tumor cells may leave the therapeutic field without receiving a cytotoxic dose and may thus be a source of recurrence. Some

recent data were suggestive of heavy charged particle irradiation to consistently reduce the migratory potential of tumor cells, but the respective study was lacking parallel evaluation of radiation-induced cell killing (14).

Recent therapeutic strategies target the epidermal growth factor receptor (EGFR), which is overexpressed in about 40–50% of GBMs (15). There is evidence in the literature for such anti-EGFR therapeutics to improve the efficacy of conventional radiotherapy (16). EGFR is a member of the cell-surface receptor family ErbB and functions as an oncogene. Activation of EGFR by binding of its specific ligands, including epidermal growth factor (EGF), leads to dimerization of the receptor and subsequently to autophosphorylation of its tyrosine-kinase domain. Following activation, the EGFR kinase stimulates a number of cellular signaling cascades, such as the phosphatidylinositol-3-kinase (PI3K)/AKT or the mitogen-activated protein kinase (MAPK) pathway (17). Thereby, numerous cellular responses are precisely regulated, such as proliferation, cell survival, and cell migration. EGF-induced EGFR activation has been shown to promote tumor cell migration (18). In addition to auto- and paracrine stimulation, it remains to be clarified whether therapies, such as radiotherapy, induce EGFR activation and pro-proliferative signaling directly or indirectly *via* production of radicals. Before starting our research in this field, no data existed with respect to EGFR activation by heavy charged particle irradiation.

Considering this background information, we initiated investigations on the impact of carbon ion irradiation on GBM cell motility and EGFR-related cell signaling *in vitro*. Most cell migration data were generated in "classical" Boyden (or transwell) chamber assays. Core proteins and phospho-proteins were analyzed with Western Blotting.

Investigations on U87 and LN229 glioma cells (with overexpression of EGFR[++]) showed that the migratory response of cancer cells to radiation is dependent on radiation dose, as well as on cell and radiation type. Clinically relevant doses (2 or 3 Gy) of X-rays induced a small, but consistent and significant, increase in migratory activity of U87, but not of LN229, as illustrated in **Figure 6A**. [12]C[6+] ion treatment was associated with a dose-dependent decrease in migration with all cell lines and under all conditions investigated (**Figure 6B**). The radiation-induced loss of cell motility was correlated, in most cases, with corresponding changes in β_1 integrin expression (9, 14). The photon-induced increase in cell migration in U87 glioma cells was paralleled by an elevated phosphorylation status of the EGFR and AKT–ERK1/2 pathway (see **Figures 7** and **8**). Such a hyperphosphorylation did not occur during [12]C[6+] irradiation under all conditions registered (see **Figures 7** and **8**). Using a 3D collagen type I invasion and migration model, glioma cell migration remained unaffected by irradiation with either photon or particles, despite the induction of massive gene toxicity as determined by the γH2AX technique (13).

On the one hand, with a few exceptions, our *in vitro* findings on the interrelationship between irradiation and tumor cell migration are in accordance with data from the literature (14, 20, 21). On the other hand, *in vivo* studies are warranted for the evaluation of the clinical significance of this issue.

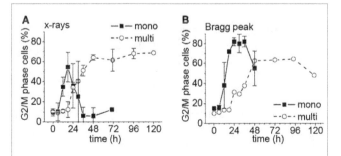

FIGURE 5 | Percentage of WiDr cells from mono- or multilayers in G_2/M phase as a function of time after irradiation [modified according to Ref. (8)] with (A) X-rays and (B) carbon ions.

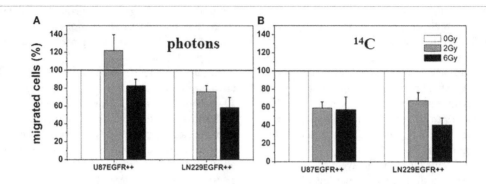

FIGURE 6 | Relative cell migration 24 h after photon and ¹²C heavy ion irradiation. U87 EGFR⁺⁺ and LN229 EGFR⁺⁺ were irradiated with single doses of 2 and 6 Gy of photon radiation, respectively **(A)** and ¹²C heavy ions **(B)** and migrated cells were counted after Boyden Chamber assay. The relative mean numbers of migrated cells ± SD of at least three independent experiments are plotted with the migration of untreated cells set to 100%. All differences between treated and untreated cells are significant ($p < 0.05$, t-test). There was no significant change in cell viability under all conditions investigated (data not shown) [modified according to Ref. (19)].

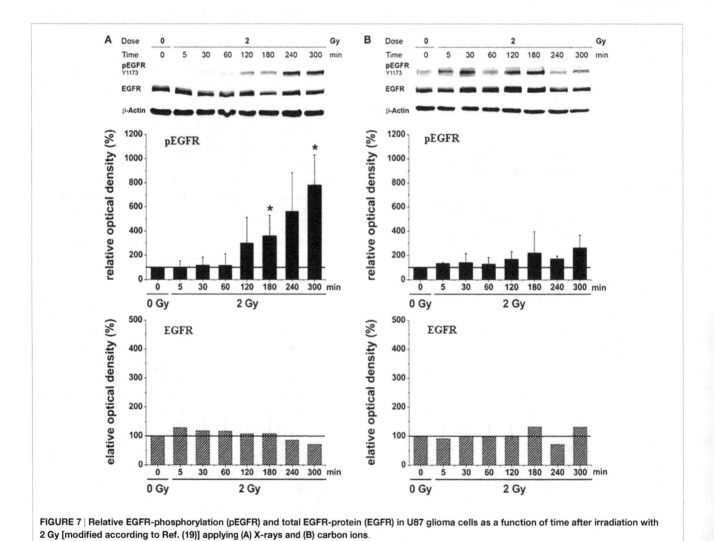

FIGURE 7 | Relative EGFR-phosphorylation (pEGFR) and total EGFR-protein (EGFR) in U87 glioma cells as a function of time after irradiation with 2 Gy [modified according to Ref. (19)] applying (A) X-rays and (B) carbon ions.

Four major conclusions were derived from the *in vitro* migration studies on glioma cells: (i) the impact of radiation on glioma cell migration depends on the migration assay used with both X-rays and carbon ions; (ii) under certain conditions and in a few glioma cell lines, clinically relevant doses of photons but not particles consistently increases cell migration; (iii) under a wide

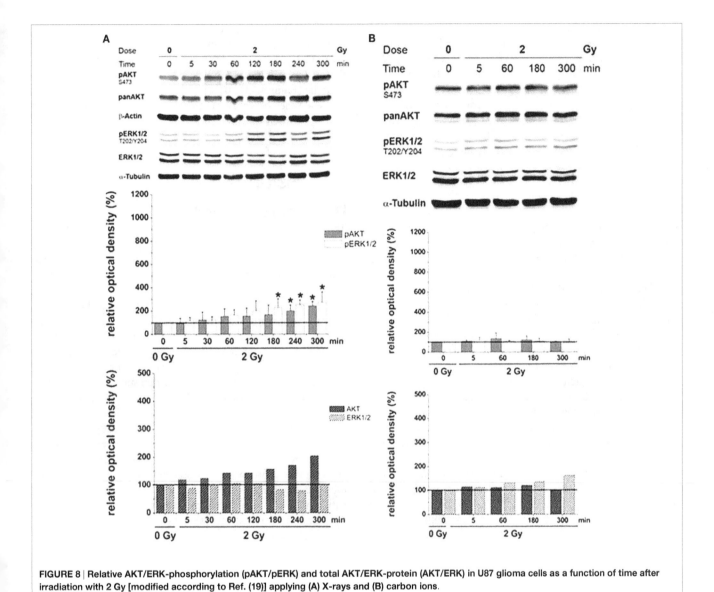

FIGURE 8 | Relative AKT/ERK-phosphorylation (pAKT/pERK) and total AKT/ERK-protein (AKT/ERK) in U87 glioma cells as a function of time after irradiation with 2 Gy [modified according to Ref. (19)] applying (A) X-rays and (B) carbon ions.

spectrum of conditions, glioma cell migration *in vitro* was either unaffected or reduced by $^{12}C^{6+}$ irradiation; and (iv) this differential between photon and particle irradiation may contribute to a higher efficiency of a local carbon ion treatment compared to X-rays with regard to tumor recurrence.

Studies on Early Events in Radiation-Induced Mucositis Using Organotypic Cultures of the Oral Mucosa Including Immune Cells

Oral mucositis is a frequent complication of standardized radiotherapy in the clinic. There is an abundance of literature regarding preclinical and clinical research in this field, as reviewed recently, among others, by Mallick and colleagues (22). Much less is known, in this regard, about the side effects of particle irradiation, although the induction of mucositis by carbon ions has been clearly documented in patients already in 2002 (23). Although the

number of centers for treatment with heavy charged particle is still undesirably low, the successful application of this technology in radiation oncology for the past two decades confers clinical relevance to particle treatment-associated mucositis (24).

A relatively novel aspect of radiation-associated mucositis results from the ambitious plans of several space agencies, in particular of the NASA and the ESA, for manned missions to the Mars. During such a mission which would last around 3 years, astronauts would be chronically exposed to cosmic radiation due to the absence of a protecting magnetic field. Space radiation consists of protons (87%), α-particles (12%), and heavy ions (1%) in solar particle events and galactic cosmic rays (25). In particular, highly ionizing heavy ions can be hardly shielded exposing the crew members to a serious medical safety risk (26), since the probability of getting a hit by heavy charged particles increases with time in space. It is obvious that the occurrence of oral or intestinal mucositis during a prolonged space flight would lead to hazardous situations.

Oral mucositis as a result of X-ray exposure has been studied in numerous animal models, the advantages and limitations of which have been reviewed recently by Viet and co-workers (27). One major cutback of animal models that has been reported earlier is their unsuitability for the assessment of early molecular and pathophysiological events following irradiation (28).

Based on this background knowledge, we initiated a project, which was supported mainly by the GSI Darmstadt and the ESA, with investigations on early inflammatory events induced by heavy charged particle irradiation in organotypic cultures of the human oral mucosa. We re-activated a 3D culture model, previously established in our laboratory (29). The artificial mucosa, which was cultured at the liquid–gas interface, consisted of immortalized human gingival keratinocytes (IHGK) and immortalized human dermal fibroblasts (HH4ded), grown with or without PBMCs. The organotypic mucosa culture exhibited many features of the human oral mucosa, such as the formation of a basal membrane, a papillary shape of the epithelium-connective tissue boundary, or the differentiation status of the keratinocytes with regard to expression of keratins. A special technology was designed making it possible to irradiate the 3D cultures in the extended Bragg peak of the heavy ion beam including an appropriate dosimetry. Further details are described in Ref. (30).

Comparing the gene toxicity of X-rays with that of particles using the γH2AX technique, the superior effectiveness of heavy ions was confirmed by a roughly twofold higher number of foci per nucleus 4 and 48 h after treatment. This is shown in **Figure 9** for X-rays (**Figure 9A**) and $^{12}C^{6+}$ irradiation (**Figure 9B**).

Proinflammatory signs were quantitatively similar for both treatment modalities. For example, confocal microscopy made it possible to quantify the activation of NFκB by the assessment of the nuclear location of NFκB p50. The corresponding results are depicted in **Figures 10A,B** for photons and particles, respectively. The release rates of the proinflammatory cytokines IL6 and IL8

from the organotypic cultures into the culture medium was registered using commercial ELISA assays [further details in Ref. (30)]. **Figure 11** demonstrates a consistent and significant elevation of the release of both cytokines upon irradiation for both photons (**Figures 11A,B**) and particles (**Figures 11C,D**), albeit in the absence of a consistent dose dependency. **Figures 12A,B** illustrate for X-rays and carbon ions, respectively, that the addition of PBMC increases the radiation-induced release of IL6 and IL8 by factors of 2–3.

DISCUSSION AND RESUME

Data from the Literature

The very recent literature on heavy charged particle research clearly emphasizes the advantages of particle versus X-ray irradiation in a meanwhile broad spectrum of tumor entities as shown in a large number of patients mainly in Japan (more than 8,000 patients) and Germany (31, 32). Whereas different ions, such as carbon, helium, or protons (33), may be used in different treatment scenarios, carbon and helium appear to be superior to protons in the majority of cases (34). One review lately points out the importance of combining radiobiological and clinical research with carbon ion therapy (35–37). There is a common optimism among these authors with regard to further spread of charged particle treatment facilities world-wide (31, 32, 34, 38). Besides these clinical aspects, the already-mentioned significance of charged particle radiobiology for long-term exposition to space radiation during extended space flights has been detailed explicitly by an international consortium of experts in a recent article (39).

Several actual reports on cell and animal studies using carbon ions present RBE values, which are in a fairly good agreement with our data from multicell spheroid studies (35, 40, 41). At the same time, data are presented that show a multitude of parameters to impact on RBE values, such as radiation dose, linear energy transfer (LET), and the model used for the derivation of RBE

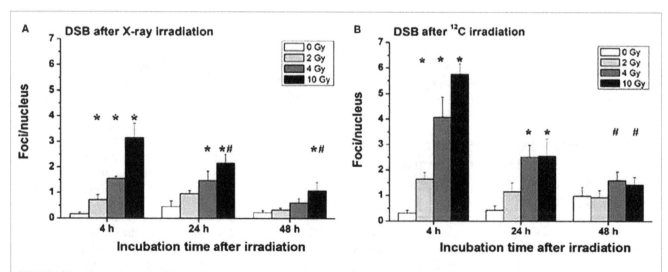

FIGURE 9 | Double-strand breaks (DSB) in organotypic cultures of oral mucosa, determined by evaluation of γH2AX stainings in immune fluorescence microscopy, as a function of radiation dose and time after radiation [modified according to Ref. (19)] applying (A) X-rays and (B) carbon ions.

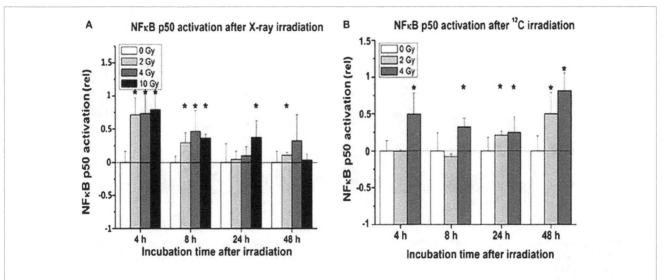

FIGURE 10 | Activation of NFκB in organotypic cultures of oral mucosa, determined by evaluation of nuclear translocation of NFκB p50 stainings in immune fluorescence confocal microscopy, as a function of radiation dose and time after radiation [modified according to Ref. (19)] applying (A) X-rays and (B) carbon ions.

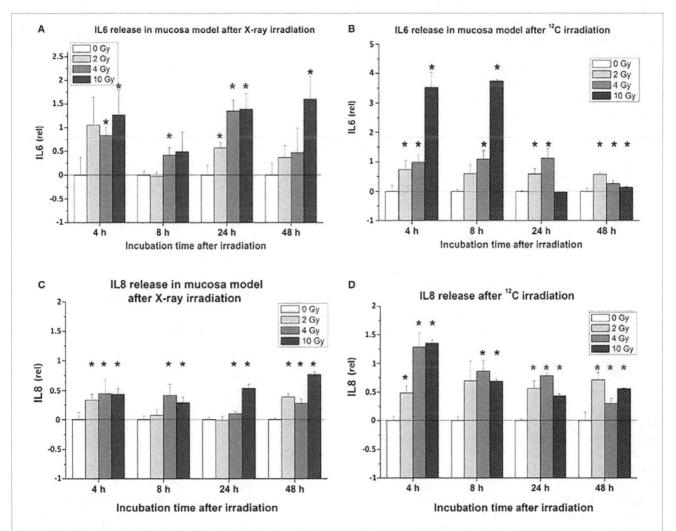

FIGURE 11 | Cytokine release [IL6: (A,B); IL8: (C,D)] in organotypic cultures of oral mucosa, determined by commercial ELISA test, as a function of radiation dose and time after radiation [modified according to Ref. (19)] applying (A,C) X-rays and (B,D) carbon ions.

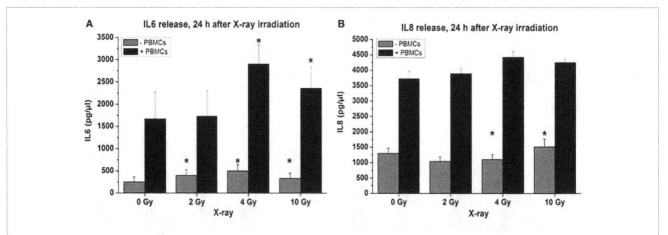

FIGURE 12 | Cytokine release following X-ray treatment of organotypic cultures of oral mucosa, determined by commercial ELISA test, as a function of radiation dose and time after radiation with or without coculturing of peripheral blood mononuclear cells [PBMCs; modified according to Ref. (19)]. (A) IL6 and (B) IL8.

(35, 37). Taking this into account, the derivation of RBE values for clinical dosimetry is still a matter of debate (37). In a recent simulation study on hypoxia in clinical tumors treated with carbon ions, OER were found that corresponded well to our data from MCS (42). The authors also point to the existence of a non-negligible oxygen effect that can influence the outcome of carbon ion therapy at low LET in the spread-out Bragg peak. A recent investigation using a carbon ion beam or X-rays for irradiating neuro-spheres of human GBM cells documents the occurrence of a multicellular resistance that was much less pronounced – but still detectable – with particle radiation compared to photons (43). As many studies with X-rays before, this investigation demonstrates a multicellular radioresistance, eventually termed contact effect, to exist for carbon ions as well. This is in contrast to the multicellular radiosensitization, which we have shown for charged particle irradiation of planar tumor cell multilayers compared to corresponding single cells [(8); see above].

There are two recent reports confirming our observation on charged particle effects on cell migration and related signaling pathways. Simon et al. (44) were able to show that migration of meningioma cells was promoted by photon but not by carbon ion irradiation. Our results on an increased cell migration associated with an elevated phosphorylation status of the EGFR and AKT–ERK1/2 pathway following X-ray but not carbon irradiation was partially confirmed by corresponding findings of Jin and colleagues (45). These data are in accordance with previous observations regarding the inhibitory influence of heavy charged particle irradiation on tumor cell migration and formation of metastasis (21, 46). Recent reviews, such as the article by Fujita (47), mirror a still ongoing and partially controversial debate with regard to the impact of radiation on cancer cell motility, invasiveness, and metastatic potential. Interestingly, a recent experimental study using carbon ion irradiation in a rat prostate carcinoma has demonstrated an increase in the metastatic rate upon treatment (48).

As a brief resume, the experimental therapeutics part of the data compiled clearly demonstrates the efficiency of $^{12}C^{6+}$ irradiation to be consistently higher than that of conventional X-rays;

this is mirrored by RBE values for particles versus photons of >1.0 and up to 4.3 under hypoxic conditions. Since hypoxia occurs in 50–60% of all human solid tumors (49), it is of high clinical relevance that $^{12}C^{6+}$ irradiation is much more efficient than conventional radiation under these conditions. Whereas OER values are close to 3 for X-rays, an OER value of 1.4 was derived for carbon ions. Here, multicellular tumor spheroids proved themselves as useful models for quantitative studies on the radiobiology of heavy charged particles. In the experimental inflammation part of the data compilation, organotypic cultures of the oral mucosa were shown to be useful for investigations on immediate and early inflammatory events, i.e., within a few hours up to 2 days following $^{12}C^{6+}$ radiation treatment. Besides the quantification of gene toxicity and proinflammatory cytokine release, the consistent, immediate, and early, as well as dose-dependent activation of NFκB by $^{12}C^{6+}$ irradiation of oral mucosa cultures is one of the core results of this part of the studies.

AUTHOR CONTRIBUTIONS

Both the authors listed have made substantial, direct, and intellectual contribution to the work and approved it for publication.

ACKNOWLEDGMENTS

Special thanks are given to Nicole Averbeck, Gerhard Kraft, Michael Scholz, and Gisela Taucher-Scholz at the GSI Darmstadt and to Nils Cordes at Oncoray, University of Dresden, for many helpful discussions and for their professional support of the projects.

FUNDING

This work was supported by the Gesellschaft für Schwerionenforschung (GSI) Darmstadt, Germany, the European Space Agency (ESA)/German Aerospace Center (DLR)/Federal Ministry of Economics and Technology (BMWi): 50 WB 0926 and by the Deutsche Forschungsgemeinschaft (DFG; MU 576/17-1).

REFERENCES

1. Schulz-Ertner D, Nikoghosyan A, Didinger B, Debus J. Carbon ion radiation therapy for chordomas and low grade chondrosarcomas – current status of the clinical trials at GSI. *Radiother Oncol* (2004) **73**(Suppl 2):S53–6. doi:10.1016/S0167-8140(04)80014-8

2. Sutherland RM, McCredie JA, Inch WR. Growth of multicell spheroids in tissue culture as a model of nodular carcinomas. *J Natl Cancer Inst* (1971) **46**(1):113–20.

3. Sutherland RM. Cell and environment interactions in tumor microregions: the multicell spheroid model. *Science* (1988) **240**(4849):177–84. doi:10.1126/science.2451290

4. Mueller-Klieser WF, Sutherland RM. Influence of convection in the growth medium on oxygen tensions in multicellular tumor spheroids. *Cancer Res* (1982) **42**(1):237–42.

5. Sutherland RM, Sordat B, Bamat J, Gabbert H, Bourrat B, Mueller-Klieser W. Oxygenation and differentiation in multicellular spheroids of human colon carcinoma. *Cancer Res* (1986) **46**(10):5320–9.

6. Hirschhaeuser F, Menne H, Dittfeld C, West J, Mueller-Klieser W, Kunz-Schughart LA. Multicellular tumor spheroids: an underestimated tool is catching up again. *J Biotechnol* (2010) **148**(1):3–15. doi:10.1016/j.jbiotec.2010.01.012

7. Staab A, Zukowski D, Walenta S, Scholz M, Mueller-Klieser W. Response of Chinese hamster v79 multicellular spheroids exposed to high-energy carbon ions. *Radiat Res* (2004) **161**(2):219–27. doi:10.1667/RR3113

8. Topsch J, Scholz M, Mueller-Klieser W. Radiobiological characterization of human tumor cell multilayers after conventional and particle irradiation. *Radiat Res* (2007) **167**(6):645–54. doi:10.1667/RR0775.1

9. Goetze K, Scholz M, Taucher-Scholz G, Mueller-Klieser W. The impact of conventional and heavy ion irradiation on tumor cell migration in vitro. *Int J Radiat Biol* (2007) **83**(11–12):889–96. doi:10.1080/09553000701753826

10. Rieken S, Habermehl D, Mohr A, Wuerth L, Lindel K, Weber K, et al. Targeting alphanubeta3 and alphanubeta5 inhibits photon-induced hypermigration of malignant glioma cells. *Radiat Oncol* (2011) **6**:132. doi:10.1186/1748-717X-6-132

11. Wild-Bode C, Weller M, Rimner A, Dichgans J, Wick W. Sublethal irradiation promotes migration and invasiveness of glioma cells: implications for radiotherapy of human glioblastoma. *Cancer Res* (2001) **61**(6):2744–50.

12. Cordes N, Hansmeier B, Beinke C, Meineke V, van Beuningen D. Irradiation differentially affects substratum-dependent survival, adhesion, and invasion of glioblastoma cell lines. *Br J Cancer* (2003) **89**(11):2122–32. doi:10.1038/sj.bjc.6601429

13. Eke I, Storch K, Kastner I, Vehlow A, Faethe C, Mueller-Klieser W, et al. Three-dimensional invasion of human glioblastoma cells remains unchanged by X-ray and carbon ion irradiation in vitro. *Int J Radiat Oncol Biol Phys* (2012) **84**(4):e515–23. doi:10.1016/j.ijrobp.2012.06.012

14. Rieken S, Habermehl D, Wuerth L, Brons S, Mohr A, Lindel K, et al. Carbon ion irradiation inhibits glioma cell migration through downregulation of integrin expression. *Int J Radiat Oncol Biol Phys* (2012) **83**(1):394–9. doi:10.1016/j.ijrobp.2011.06.2004

15. Schlegel J, Stumm G, Brandle K, Merdes A, Mechtersheimer G, Hynes NE, et al. Amplification and differential expression of members of the erbB-gene family in human glioblastoma. *J Neurooncol* (1994) **22**(3):201–7. doi:10.1007/BF01052920

16. Nieder C, Pawinski A, Dalhaug A, Andratschke N. A review of clinical trials of cetuximab combined with radiotherapy for non-small cell lung cancer. *Radiat Oncol* (2012) **7**(1):3. doi:10.1186/1748-717X-7-3

17. Eppenberger U, Mueller H. Growth factor receptors and their ligands. *J Neurooncol* (1994) **22**(3):249–54. doi:10.1007/BF01052929

18. Dittmar T, Husemann A, Schewe Y, Nofer JR, Niggemann B, Zanker KS, et al. Induction of cancer cell migration by epidermal growth factor is initiated by specific phosphorylation of tyrosine 1248 of c-erbB-2 receptor via EGFR. *FASEB J* (2002) **16**(13):1823–5. doi:10.1096/fj.02-0096fje

19. Stahler C, Roth J, Cordes N, Taucher-Scholz G, Mueller-Klieser W. Impact of carbon ion irradiation on epidermal growth factor receptor signaling and glioma cell migration in comparison to conventional photon irradiation. *Int J Radiat Biol* (2013) **89**(6):454–61. doi:10.3109/09553002.2013.766769

20. Mukherjee B, McEllin B, Camacho CV, Tomimatsu N, Sirasanagandala S, Nannepaga S, et al. EGFRvIII and DNA double-strand break repair: a molecular mechanism for radioresistance in glioblastoma. *Cancer Res* (2009) **69**(10):4252–9. doi:10.1158/0008-5472.CAN-08-4853

21. Ogata T, Teshima T, Inaoka M, Minami K, Tsuchiya T, Isono M, et al. Carbon ion irradiation suppresses metastatic potential of human non-small cell lung cancer A549 cells through the phosphatidylinositol-3-kinase/Akt signaling pathway. *J Radiat Res* (2011) **52**(3):374–9. doi:10.1269/jrr.10102

22. Mallick S, Benson R, Rath GK. Radiation induced oral mucositis: a review of current literature on prevention and management. *Eur Arch Otorhinolaryngol* (2015). doi:10.1007/s00405-015-3694-6

23. Schulz-Ertner D, Haberer T, Scholz M, Thilmann C, Wenz F, Jakel O, et al. Acute radiation-induced toxicity of heavy ion radiotherapy delivered with intensity modulated pencil beam scanning in patients with base of skull tumors. *Radiother Oncol* (2002) **64**(2):189–95. doi:10.1016/S0167-8140(02)00153-6

24. Loeffler JS, Durante M. Charged particle therapy – optimization, challenges and future directions. *Nat Rev Clin Oncol* (2013) **10**(7):411–24. doi:10.1038/nrclinonc.2013.79

25. Maalouf M, Durante M, Foray N. Biological effects of space radiation on human cells: history, advances and outcomes. *J Radiat Res* (2011) **52**(2):126–46. doi:10.1269/jrr.10128

26. Durante M, Cucinotta FA. Heavy ion carcinogenesis and human space exploration. *Nat Rev Cancer* (2008) **8**(6):465–72. doi:10.1038/nrc2391

27. Viet CT, Corby PM, Akinwande A, Schmidt BL. Review of preclinical studies on treatment of mucositis and associated pain. *J Dent Res* (2014) **93**(9):868–75. doi:10.1177/0022034514540174

28. Yeoh A, Gibson R, Yeoh E, Bowen J, Stringer A, Giam K, et al. Radiation therapy-induced mucositis: relationships between fractionated radiation, NF-kappaB, COX-1, and COX-2. *Cancer Treat Rev* (2006) **32**(8):645–51. doi:10.1016/j.ctrv.2006.08.005

29. Kunz-Schughart LA, Mueller-Klieser W. Three-dimensional culture. 3rd ed. In: Masters JRW, editor. *Animal Cell Culture: A Practical Approach*. Oxford; New York; Tokyo: IRL Press at Oxford University Press (2000). p. 123–48.

30. Tschachojan V, Schroer H, Averbeck N, Mueller-Klieser W. Carbon ions and X rays induce proinflammatory effects in 3D oral mucosa models with and without PBMCs. *Oncol Rep* (2014) **32**(5):1820–8. doi:10.3892/or.2014.3441

31. Kamada T, Tsujii H, Blakely EA, Debus J, De NW, Durante M, et al. Carbon ion radiotherapy in Japan: an assessment of 20 years of clinical experience. *Lancet Oncol* (2015) **16**(2):e93–100. doi:10.1016/S1470-2045(14)70412-7

32. Marx V. Cancer treatment: sharp shooters. *Nature* (2014) **508**(7494):133–8. doi:10.1038/508133a

33. Tommasino F, Durante M. Proton radiobiology. *Cancers (Basel)* (2015) **7**(1):353–81. doi:10.3390/cancers7010353

34. Grun R, Friedrich T, Kramer M, Zink K, Durante M, Engenhart-Cabillic R, et al. Assessment of potential advantages of relevant ions for particle therapy: a model based study. *Med Phys* (2015) **42**(2):1037–47. doi:10.1118/1.4905374

35. Saager M, Glowa C, Peschke P, Brons S, Grun R, Scholz M, et al. Split dose carbon ion irradiation of the rat spinal cord: dependence of the relative biological effectiveness on dose and linear energy transfer. *Radiother Oncol* (2015) **117**(2):358–63. doi:10.1016/j.radonc.2015.07.006

36. Schlaff CD, Krauze A, Belard A, O'Connell JJ, Camphausen KA. Bringing the heavy: carbon ion therapy in the radiobiological and clinical context. *Radiat Oncol* (2014) **9**(1):88. doi:10.1186/1748-717X-9-88

37. Steinstrater O, Scholz U, Friedrich T, Kramer M, Grun R, Durante M, et al. Integration of a model-independent interface for RBE predictions in a treatment planning system for active particle beam scanning. *Phys Med Biol* (2015) **60**(17):6811–31. doi:10.1088/0031-9155/60/17/6811

38. Tomlinson DC, Baldo O, Harnden P, Knowles MA. FGFR3 protein expression and its relationship to mutation status and prognostic variables in bladder cancer. *J Pathol* (2007) **213**(1):91–8. doi:10.1002/path.2207

39. Barcellos-Hoff MH, Blakely EA, Burma S, Fornace AJ Jr, Gerson S, Hlatky L, et al. Concepts and challenges in cancer risk prediction for the space radiation environment. *Life Sci Space Res (Amst)* (2015) **6**:92–103. doi:10.1016/j.lssr.2015.07.006

40. Ferrandon S, Magne N, Battiston-Montagne P, Hau-Desbat NH, Diaz O, Beuve M, et al. Cellular and molecular portrait of eleven human glioblastoma cell lines under photon and carbon ion irradiation. *Cancer Lett* (2015) **360**(1):10–6. doi:10.1016/j.canlet.2015.01.025

41. Sorensen BS, Horsman MR, Alsner J, Overgaard J, Durante M, Scholz M, et al. Relative biological effectiveness of carbon ions for tumor control, acute skin damage and late radiation-induced fibrosis in a mouse model. *Acta Oncol* (2015) **54**(9):1623–30. doi:10.3109/0284186X.2015.1069890

42. Antonovic L, Lindblom E, Dasu A, Bassler N, Furusawa Y, Toma-Dasu I. Clinical oxygen enhancement ratio of tumors in carbon ion radiotherapy: the influence of local oxygenation changes. *J Radiat Res* (2014) **55**(5):902–11. doi:10.1093/jrr/rru020

43. Takahashi M, Hirakawa H, Yajima H, Izumi-Nakajima N, Okayasu R, Fujimori A. Carbon ion beam is more effective to induce cell death in sphere-type A172 human glioblastoma cells compared with X-rays. *Int J Radiat Biol* (2014) **90**(12):1125–32. doi:10.3109/09553002.2014.927933

44. Simon F, Dittmar JO, Brons S, Orschiedt L, Urbschat S, Weber KJ, et al. Integrin-based meningioma cell migration is promoted by photon but not by carbon-ion irradiation. *Strahlenther Onkol* (2015) **191**(4):347–55. doi:10.1007/s00066-014-0778-y

45. Jin X, Li F, Zheng X, Liu Y, Hirayama R, Liu X, et al. Carbon ions induce autophagy effectively through stimulating the unfolded protein response and subsequent inhibiting Akt phosphorylation in tumor cells. *Sci Rep* (2015) **5**:13815. doi:10.1038/srep13815

46. Ogata T, Teshima T, Kagawa K, Hishikawa Y, Takahashi Y, Kawaguchi A, et al. Particle irradiation suppresses metastatic potential of cancer cells. *Cancer Res* (2005) **65**(1):113–20.

47. Fujita M, Yamada S, Imai T. Irradiation induces diverse changes in invasive potential in cancer lines. *Semin Cancer Biol* (2015) **35**:45–52. doi:10.1016/j.semcancer.2015.09.003

48. Karger CP, Scholz M, Huber PE, Debus J, Peschke P. Photon and carbon ion irradiation of a rat prostate carcinoma: does a higher fraction number increase the metastatic rate? *Radiat Res* (2014) **181**(6):623–8. doi:10.1667/RR13611.1

49. Harrison L, Blackwell K. Hypoxia and anemia: factors in decreased sensitivity to radiation therapy and chemotherapy? *Oncologist* (2004) **9**(Suppl 5):31–40. doi:10.1634/theoncologist.9-90005-31

2

Impact of Charged Particle Exposure on Homologous DNA Double-Strand Break Repair in Human Blood-Derived Cells

Melanie Rall[1†], Daniela Kraft[2†], Meta Volcic[1], Aljona Cucu[2], Elena Nasonova[2‡],
Gisela Taucher-Scholz[2], Halvard Bönig[3], Lisa Wiesmüller[1†]* and Claudia Fournier[2†]*

[1] Department of Obstetrics and Gynaecology, Ulm University, Ulm, Germany, [2] Department of Biophysics, GSI Helmholtz Center for Heavy Ion Research, Darmstadt, Germany, [3] German Red Cross Blood Service Baden-Wuerttemberg – Hessen, Institute for Transfusion Medicine and Immunohematology, Johann Wolfgang Goethe-University Hospital, Frankfurt, Germany

*Correspondence:
Lisa Wiesmüller
lisa.wiesmueller@uni-ulm.de;
Claudia Fournier
c.fournier@gsi.de

†Shared co-authorship;
these authors contributed equally to
this work.

Ionizing radiation generates DNA double-strand breaks (DSB) which, unless faithfully repaired, can generate chromosomal rearrangements in hematopoietic stem and/or progenitor cells (HSPC), potentially priming the cells towards a leukemic phenotype. Using an enhanced green fluorescent protein (EGFP)-based reporter system, we recently identified differences in the removal of enzyme-mediated DSB in human HSPC versus mature peripheral blood lymphocytes (PBL), particularly regarding homologous DSB repair (HR). Assessment of chromosomal breaks via premature chromosome condensation or γH2AX foci indicated similar efficiency and kinetics of radiation-induced DSB formation and rejoining in PBL and HSPC. Prolonged persistence of chromosomal breaks was observed for higher LET charged particles which are known to induce more complex DNA damage compared to X-rays. Consistent with HR deficiency in HSPC observed in our previous study, we noticed here pronounced focal accumulation of 53BP1 after X-ray and carbon ion exposure (intermediate LET) in HSPC versus PBL. For higher LET, 53BP1 foci kinetics was similarly delayed in PBL and HSPC suggesting similar failure to repair complex DNA damage. Data obtained with plasmid reporter systems revealed a dose- and LET-dependent HR increase after X-ray, carbon ion and higher LET exposure, particularly in HR-proficient immortalized and primary lymphocytes, confirming preferential use of conservative HR in PBL for intermediate LET damage repair. HR measured adjacent to the leukemia-associated *MLL* breakpoint cluster sequence in reporter lines revealed dose dependency of potentially leukemogenic rearrangements underscoring the risk of leukemia-induction by radiation treatment.

Keywords: breakpoint cluster region, charged particles, chromosomal breaks, radiation damage response, DNA double-strand break repair, hematopoietic stem and progenitor cells, radiation-induced leukemia

INTRODUCTION

Radiation exposure increases the risk for acute myeloid leukemia (AML), as observed in atomic bomb survivors (1), occupational radiation workers (2, 3), and cancer survivors treated with radiotherapy (4). This is important especially in light of the increasing use of charged particles in cancer therapy (5, 6). Furthermore, a long-term leukemia risk for astronauts exposed to protons and high-energy charged particles during extended space travel is expected (7–9). As for all of these radiation scenarios densely ionizing radiation, such as charged particles or neutrons, contribute to the delivered dose, we need to understand whether densely ionizing radiation and photons differ in their impact on AML development.

Densely ionizing charged particles differ from sparsely ionizing photons in both physical characteristics and biological effectiveness (10). The greater effectiveness of densely ionizing charged particles is reflected in the severity of DNA lesions, which manifests both at the nanometer and the micrometer scale: DNA lesions are more complex and hence, more difficult to repair, as well as the complexity of chromosomal aberrations is higher (11, 12). In consequence, the number of unrepaired or misrepaired lesions and their transmission to the affected cell's progeny, considered to be the basis for cancer induction, is greater for charged particles than for photons.

In the context of radiation exposure, induction of hematological malignancies, in particular of AML, was discussed to originate from error-prone repair of radiation-induced double-strand breaks (DSB) causing chromosomal rearrangements (13–16). Especially precarious targets for leukemic transformation are hematopoietic stem and/or progenitor cells (HSPC). HSPC are long-lived, self-renewed, and give rise to all types of mature blood cells and therefore are an ideal model system to study consequences of radiation exposure and the fate changes associated there with. On the other hand, mature peripheral blood lymphocytes (PBL) represent an extensively studied system in which cytogenetic damage has been established as a reliable biomarker of radiation late effects (17–19).

In our previous work, we studied the repair of DSB induced by photon radiation in the hematopoietic system (20, 21). We comparatively analyzed the capacity and quality of DSB repair in cycling human HSPC and PBL cultures mimicking exit from quiescence in response to stress conditions, such as infection or irradiation (22). Even though γH2AX signals and cytogenetic analysis suggested quantitatively similar DSB formation and removal after irradiation, we found substantial qualitative differences in DNA damage responses, i.e., differential use of DNA repair pathways. To dissect DSB repair mechanisms, we used our fluorescence-based assay system for extrachromosomal DSB repair (23), which has proven a valuable tool in various cell types including lymphoblastoid cell lines (LCL) derived from patients with genomic instability syndromes (24–26). Using this system, recombination of DSB can be detected after I-SceI-endonuclease-mediated cleavage, but also independently of targeted cleavage by I-SceI after various carcinogenic treatments including ionizing radiation (27–29). Application of this enhanced green fluorescent protein (EGFP)-based

reporter system revealed a relative preference of error-prone non-homologous end joining (NHEJ), such as microhomology-mediated end joining (MMEJ) and single-strand annealing (SSA) in HSPC, as opposed to conservative NHEJ and high-fidelity homologous DSB repair (HR) in PBL. Furthermore, differential recruitment of repair proteins suggested a delay in the progress of the repair steps toward HR. We could identify differential NF-κB signaling as a critical molecular component underlying the observed differences: while in PBL, active NF-κB promotes HR and prevents compensatory accumulation of radiation-induced 53BP1 foci, in HSPCs, significantly reduced NF-κB activity and hence NF-κB target genes impedes accurate DSB repair.

To assess the effect of different radiation qualities in this study, we used the substrates HR-EGFP/3′EGFP or HR-EGFP/5′EGFP which detect both conservative and non-conservative HR or solely conservative HR, respectively, i.e., the very repair pathways which markedly differ in HSPC compared to PBL (20). Since radiation not only causes clean DSB but also generates base damage, single-strand breaks and complex DSB (12, 30), recombinative rearrangements, as monitored in our assay system, are ideal readouts to sense all these types of DNA lesions (29). The usage of differentially designed repair substrate plasmids allows discrimination between different repair mechanisms and repair qualities which is of major interest with regard to the repair of complex DNA lesions, such as are induced by charged particle radiation (11, 18, 31).

A refined repair assay variant integrates a highly fragile region within the mixed lineage leukemia breakpoint cluster region (MLLbcr), where cancer treatment-induced translocation sites predisposing to secondary leukemia have been found to cluster (29, 32, 33). Rearrangements involving the MLL gene are found in ~40% of therapy-related acute leukemias (33). Both chemotherapy and radiotherapy increase the risk factor for secondary malignancies of the hematopoietic system (34). Moreover, MLL rearrangements were identified after radiation exposure following the Chernobyl accident (35). Our own published data confirm preferential MLLbcr breakage compared to other sequences within the genome by γ-rays in both human HSPC and human PBL (20). In the current study, MLLbcr-based reporter cell lines were employed for the detection of radiation-induced chromosomal rearrangements. To this end, a 0.4 kb fragment of the MLLbcr sequence was introduced between the differentially mutated EGFP genes in the HR-EGFP/3′EGFP substrate. MLLbcr-based reporter cell clones were generated by stably integrating the substrate into the genome of the human myeloid leukemia cell line K562 and the human LCL WTK1 (29). The resulting K562(HR-EGFP/3′EFP-MLL) and WTK1(HR-EGFP/3′EFP-MLL) reporter cell lines represent more sensitive systems to study genotoxic treatment-induced (and thus likely also radiation-inducible) rearrangements.

The work presented here focuses on the impact of high LET compared to photon exposure on the induction and removal of DNA damage in immature and mature hematopoietic cells. Extra- and intrachromosomal reporter systems as described above were applied to compare maturity-dependent HR pathway usage and to analyze leukemia-associated rearrangements in reporter cell lines as a function of radiation quality.

MATERIALS AND METHODS

Primary Cells

Hematopoietic stem and/or progenitor cells and PBL were isolated from peripheral blood samples of healthy donors, provided by one of us (HB). Donors provided written informed consent. The study was approved by the local advisory boards (approvals #329/10; #157/10; and #155/13). Donor treatment was performed with 10 μg/kg G-CSF per day for five consecutive days as described (36). HSPC were enriched by immuno-magnetically isolating CD34$^+$ cells (MicroBead Kit, Miltenyi Biotech, Bergisch Gladbach, Germany) from G-CSF-mobilized donor blood as described (31). PBL were isolated from healthy donor buffy coats by Ficoll density-gradient centrifugation as described in Ref. (26).

Quiescent (G$_0$-phase) HSPC and PBL were recruited into cell cycle prior to irradiation experiments by culturing in expansion media for 72 h at 37°C in a humidified atmosphere (95%). HSPC were kept in serum-free StemSpan SFEM medium supplemented with 100 ng/ml Flt-3 ligand (Flt3L), 100 ng/ml stem cell factor (SCF), 20 ng/ml Interleukin-3 (IL3), and 20 ng/ml Interleukin-6 (IL6) (Cytokine Cocktail CC100, both from StemCell Technologies Inc., Cologne, Germany). PBL were cultured in RPMI 1640 medium supplemented with 20% fetal calf serum (FCS), 3 mM L-glutamine, and 2% phytohemagglutinin (PHA) (components from Biochrom AG, Berlin, Germany).

Cell Lines

In parallel to primary cells and as internal standards, we used the LCL 416MI and TK6, cultured in RPMI 1640 medium supplemented with 10% FBS, 1% penicillin/streptomycin, and 1% L-glutamine, as described before (25).

The human myeloid leukemia cell line K562(HR-EGFP/3'EFP-MLL) and the human B-LCL WTK1(HR-EGFP/3'EFP-MLL) were grown in suspension culture in RPMI 1640 medium supplemented with 10 and 12% FCS, respectively, and 100 U/ml penicillin and 100 μg/ml streptomycin (all reagents from Biochrom AG).

Irradiation with Photons and Heavy Ions

Actively cycling cells were exposed to X-rays (16 mA, 250 kV, Seifert Isovolt DSI X-ray tube) or to γ rays (gamma irradiator, GSR D1, Gamma-Service Medical GmbH). Exposure of cells to heavy ions was performed at the heavy ion synchrotron ("Schwerionensynchroton," SIS, GSI Helmholtzzentrum für Schwerionenforschung GmbH, Darmstadt, Germany).

At the time of photon exposure, cells were kept in medium in 5 ml tubes or 24-well plates with a dose rate of ~1 Gy/min. For heavy ion irradiation, the exposure with a monoenergetic beam or spread-out Bragg peak (SOBP) was performed, as described in Ref. (31). The parameters of the radiation exposure for the heavy ions used in this study are listed in **Table 1**.

Premature Chromosome Condensation

At different time points after irradiation (0–9 h) radiation-induced breaks were measured in G$_2$-phase cells by premature chromosome condensation (PCC) technique, as described elsewhere (38). Briefly, PCC was chemically induced by Calyculin A. Samples were processed as for metaphase analysis and stained with Giemsa, as described in Becker et al. (31). At least 50 G$_2$-phase cells were analyzed per data point. In G$_2$-phase cells, the total number of breaks was counted; chromatid and isochromatid breaks were scored as one and two breaks, respectively. In the following, we refer to the sum of both as "chromatid breaks." A minor number of exchanges ($\leq$5% of the breaks and comparable for both cell types), which appeared some hours after exposure, were scored as two breaks. The type of exchanges and the low fraction are comparable to previously reported ones (38).

Quantitative Immunofluorescence Microscopy

At different time points after irradiation (1–24 h), cells were spun on cover slips, fixed with 3.7% PFA and permeabilized with 0.5% Triton followed by washing and blocking steps with PBS and 5% goat serum in PBS. Cells on cover slips were immunostained with primary antibodies anti-γH2AX (Ser139, clone JBW301, Millipore), anti-53BP1 rabbit NB100-304 (Novus Biologicals, Littleton, CO, USA) and with Alexa Fluo®555-conjugated secondary antibodies (Invitrogen). Nuclear counter staining was performed with DAPI and cover slips were mounted with VectaShield mounting media (Vector Labs, Burlingame, CA, USA). Immunofluorescence signals were visualized by an Olympus BX51 epifluorescence microscope equipped with an Olympus XC10 camera and acquired images automatically analyzed by CellF2.5_analysis software including the mFIP software (Olympus Soft Imaging System, Münster, Germany) or by Keyence BZ-II Analyzer software (Keyence, Neu-Isenburg, Germany).

DSB Repair by HR in HSPC and PBL

Pathway-specific DSB repair analysis in HSPC and PBL was performed as described in Ref. (23, 26, 39). Briefly, actively cycling cells were transiently nucleofected with the DSB repair substrate HR-EGFP/5'EGFP (long homologies), detecting conservative HR, according to an Amaxa® protocol (Human B Cell Nucleofector Kit; Human CD34$^+$ Cell Nucleofector Kit; Lonza, Cologne, Germany) via electroporation (Bio-Rad Laboratories, Hercules, CA, USA). While DSB formation within the substrate is usually induced by co-nucleofection of the I-SceI meganuclease expression plasmid pCMV-I-SceI, in the present study, the nucleofection mixture did not contain the expression plasmid. Instead, DSB were induced by exposing the cells 2–4 h after nucleofection to X-rays or heavy ions (carbon and calcium ions).

The assay monitors reconstitution of wild-type EGFP, so that EGFP-positive cells were quantified 24 h post-irradiation by the diagonal gating method in the FL1/FL2 dot plot (FACS Calibur® FACScan, Becton Dickinson, Heidelberg, Germany), as described in Ref. (40). All nucleofections were performed in triplicates. The transfection controls additionally contained pBS filler plasmid (pBlueScriptII KS, Stratagene, Heidelberg, Germany) and wild-type EGFP expression plasmid for normalization of repair frequencies.

TABLE 1 | Parameters for the heavy ions used.

Ion	Energy (MeV/u)	LET (keV/μm)	Track radius (μm)[a]	Dose	Fluence[b] (particles/cm²)	Hits per nucleus[c]
Nitrogen	130	40–65	243	2 Gy	2.4×10^7	14 (HSPC) 12 (PBL)
Carbon	114–158	60–85	262	2 Gy	1.72×10^7	10 (HSPC) 9 (PBL)
Titanium	1000	150	310	2 Gy	8.3×10^6	5 (HSPC) 4 (PBL)
Iron	1000	155	328	2 Gy	8.1×10^6	5 (HSPC) 4 (PBL)
Calcium	200	180	505	2 Gy	7×10^6	4 (HSPC) 3,5 (PBL)

[a]The maximum range of delta electrons/track radius was calculated according to Ref. (37): R_{max} (μm) = 0.062 × E (MeV/u)$^{1.7}$.

[b]The fluence was calculated according to the formula: $D[Gy] = 1.6 \times 10^{-9} \times L_\Delta \left[\frac{keV}{\mu m} \right] \times \varphi \left[\frac{1}{cm^2} \right]$.

If SOBP irradiation was performed, the fluence of particles mostly contributing to dose deposition was calculated from the mean of the dose averaged LET.

[c]The hits per nucleus were calculated based on the geometric cross section, i.e., area of the cell nuclei (HSPC: 60 μm²; PBL: 50 μm²) and the fluence.

Cell Lines (K562 and WTK1) with Stably Integrated *MLL*bcr Repair Substrate

Clones containing a single stably integrated copy of HR-EGFP/3′EGFP-MLL repair substrate were established from K562 and WTK1 cell lines, as described in detail in Ref. (29, 41). Briefly, cells were stably transfected with the *Xmn*I-linearized recombination vector pHR-EGFP/3′EGFP-MLLbcr.fwd. This DNA recombination substrate contains a 0.4-kb sequence of the genomic breakpoint cluster region (bcr) from the human *MLL* gene, which undergoes carcinogenic rearrangements in response to genotoxic treatment (42, 43). The cells were irradiated with X-rays or carbon ions. The reconstitution of wild-type EGFP (via conservative HR and SSA) was measured 24–48 h post-irradiation, as described in the previous section (see DSB Repair by HR in HSPC and PBL).

RESULTS

Induction, Rejoining, and Manifestation of Radiation-Induced Chromatid Breaks

Induction and rejoining of radiation-induced breaks in PBL and HSPC were investigated with the PCC technique. Following *ex vivo* cultivation for 72 h, cells were irradiated with X-rays or charged particles (nitrogen, carbon, titanium, and calcium) in the LET range 45–180 keV/μm.

Regarding the induction level, it has to be taken into account that the number of chromatid breaks at 0 h (referred to as "initial breaks") corresponds to the number of chromatid breaks detectable 5–15 min after exposure during which Calyculin A reaches the cells and prevents further repair. As shown in Figure S1 in Supplementary Material, the number of initial chromatid breaks increased in a linear dose-dependent fashion for both PBL and HSPC and also depended on radiation quality. For both cell types, the yield of chromatid breaks was similar. At the same physical dose (2 Gy), around 60–70 versus 40 chromatid breaks after irradiation with the different ions versus after X-ray exposure were measured in G₂-phase cells, respectively.

Rejoining of radiation-induced chromatid breaks was observed for 9 h after exposure (**Figure 1**). The number of chromatid breaks decreased with culture time with similar kinetics in both cell types. For X-ray irradiation, 1–2 h after irradiation more than half of the initial chromatid breaks had already been repaired. The time course of rejoining was similar for carbon ions (intermediate LET, 60–85 keV/μm, assessed in PBL) (**Figure 1A**), although the level of initial damage was higher compared to photons. However, following high LET exposure (calcium and titanium ions, 180 and 150 keV/μm, respectively), rejoining of chromatid breaks was slower. A major difference between the repair kinetics following exposure to X-rays and ions was that the number of chromatid breaks dropped to the level of controls, i.e., rejoining was finished almost completely within 9 h after irradiation (10% residual chromatid breaks, **Figures 1A,B**). In contrast, following irradiation with carbon ions a significant fraction of breaks remained unrejoined (23% residual chromatid breaks in PBL, **Figure 1A**), and after high LET calcium and titanium exposure, the level of residual damage was even higher (40–48% residual chromatid breaks, **Figures 1A,B**).

Immunofluorescence Analysis of DSB Processing

To monitor DSB processing in response to treatment with ionizing radiation, we performed quantitative immunofluorescence microscopy of discrete nuclear foci, indicative of DNA lesions and in time course experiments of the accumulation and their removal (44). As shown in **Figure 2**, we measured γH2AX and 53BP1 foci in PBL and HSPC up to 24 h after radiation exposure with 2 Gy of X-rays, carbon (60–85 keV/μm), and iron ions (155 keV/μm). The different data sets were normalized to maximum foci values reached after X-ray irradiation to facilitate comparison with our recently published results (20). Using γH2AX as a DSB marker, formation and disappearance of foci was similar in both cell types for X-rays (**Figure 2A**), in agreement with our previous observations (20). Similar γH2AX curves for both cell types were also obtained following high LET iron ion exposure, but approximately threefold elevated levels

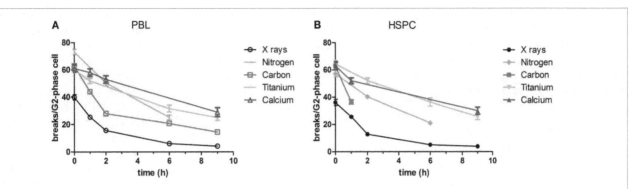

FIGURE 1 | Rejoining of radiation-induced chromatid breaks. PBL and HSPC were stimulated for 72 h prior to irradiation with a dose of 2 Gy X-rays or charged particles. After irradiation, the cells were cultivated during the indicated periods of time. Charged particle exposure: nitrogen (45–65 keV/μm), carbon (60–85 keV/μm), titanium (150 keV/μm), or calcium (180 keV/μm). Premature chromosome condensation (PCC) was induced by Calyculin A. Slides were stained with Giemsa and at least 50 G_2-phase cells were scored per data point. Numbers of independent experiments were for X-rays: $n = 3$; nitrogen, carbon, titanium, and calcium: $n = 1$. Mean values and SEM are indicated. For X-rays, SEM was calculated from mean values derived from independent experiments. For nitrogen, carbon, titanium, and calcium, SEM was calculated from values attributed to individual nuclei (>50). Connecting lines serve to guide the eye. Data for X-ray exposure are plotted from Kraft et al. (20). **(A)** PBL and **(B)** HSPC.

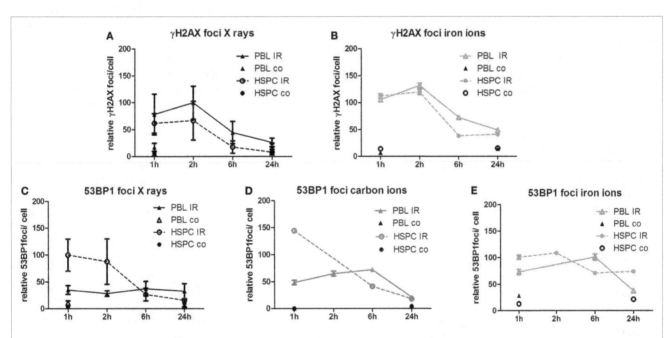

FIGURE 2 | Immunofluorescence analysis of DSB induction and repair after irradiation. PBL and HSPC were stimulated for 72 h prior to irradiation without (co) or with (IR) a dose of 2 Gy of **(A,C)** X-rays, **(D)** carbon ions (60–85 keV/μm), or **(B,E)** iron ions (155 keV/μm). After irradiation, the cells were re-cultivated, fixed at the indicated time points, and immunolabeled for detection of **(A,B)** γH2AX or **(C–E)** 53BP1. Foci were scored by automated quantification from ~250 nuclei at each time point. Each number of foci per cell was normalized to the maximum mean value from the X-ray exposure time course data from the same experimental day. The 100% relative foci represent the following mean scores after X-ray exposure for γH2AX: 8 foci/cell (PBL/2 h) and 53BP1: 8 foci/cell (HSPC/1 h). Mean normalized values attributed to individual nuclei are shown with SEM (number of independent experiments for X-rays, PBL: $n = 5$; HSPC: $n = 4$; and heavy ions PBL and HSPC: $n = 1$).

of persisting DNA damage were detectable 24 h post-iron ion versus X-ray exposure (**Figure 2B**). Recently, we reported more pronounced accumulation of X-ray-induced nuclear 53BP1 foci in HSPC relative to PBL (20), which was confirmed here for X-ray and newly demonstrated for carbon ion exposure with intermediate LET (**Figures 2C,D**). However, with high LET iron

ions, this striking difference between 53BP1 foci peak levels in HSPC and PBL disappeared (**Figure 2E**), mostly due to an increase of 53BP1 foci numbers in PBL 1 h post-irradiation with iron ions versus X-ray (**Figures 2C,E**). Concomitantly, the level of persisting 53BP1 foci 24 h post-irradiation was fivefold greater in HSPC following iron ion compared with X-ray exposure resulting in aggregate in very similar 53BP1 foci numbers 1–24 h post-irradiation. We obtained similar results as for iron ions with cells irradiated with high LET calcium ions (180 keV/μm, Figure S2 in Supplementary Material), i.e., 53BP1 foci curves for PBL and HSPC were comparable and the level of 53BP1 foci diminished only slightly over the time.

Extrachromosomal DSB Repair Analysis Using Plasmid Reporter Systems

In order to detect HR after exposure to X-rays and charged particles in PBL and HSPC, we used the EGFP-based plasmid reporter system described elsewhere (20, 23). In difference from our previous analyses engaging I-SceI meganuclease for targeted cleavage, we tested if DSB formation within the substrate and subsequent repair can be induced by ionizing radiation. For this purpose, we transfected first the LCL 416MI and TK6 (25) either with the substrate HR-EGFP/3′EGFP (which supports both conservative and non-conservative HR) or HR-EGFP/5′EGFP (which detects conservative HR only), as these repair mechanisms were previously shown to be differentially active in PBL and HSPC (20). As demonstrated in **Figure 3**, in all LCL, exposure to photons (2 and 5 Gy) induced a significant dose-dependent HR increase. A dose-dependent effect was only detectable for the substrate HR-EGFP/5′EGFP, whereas for substrate HR-EGFP/3′EGFP, a general increase was observed (data not shown).

Based on these results, we investigated HR focusing on substrate HR-EGFP/5′EGFP in PBL and HSPC after photon or charged particle exposure by applying doses of 2 and 5 Gy (**Figure 4**). We observed a twofold higher 5 Gy radiation-induced HR frequency in PBL versus HSPC (0.2×10^{-2} versus 0.1×10^{-2}), consistent with previous results for enzymatic cleavage (20). Interestingly, as can be seen in **Figure 4A**, X-ray irradiation led to relative increases in

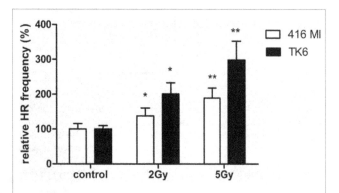

FIGURE 3 | Extrachromosomal DSB repair analysis in LCL following photon exposure. The LCL 416MI and TK6 were transfected with HR-EGFP/5′EGFP, a DSB repair substrate which supports HR. Irradiation was performed with 2 or 5 Gy of photons (γ or X-rays). After subsequent incubation for 24–48 h, the fraction of EGFP-positive cells was quantified by flow cytometric measurement. Data were normalized to the non-irradiated control each. Mean values and SEM were calculated (416MI: n = 9–15 and TK6: n = 15–18). Statistically significant of differences between non-irradiated control and irradiated cells were calculated with the Wilcoxon matched-pairs signed rank test with *p < 0.05 and **p < 0.01.

HR frequencies particularly in PBL even though in contrast to the LCL data (**Figure 3**), not reaching statistical significance with the limited number of experiments performed. Comparing radiation qualities at a single physical dose (2 Gy) revealed moderately, albeit statistically not significantly increased HR frequencies with higher LET (intermediate carbon ions and high LET calcium ions) (**Figure 4B**). Reminiscent of 53BP1 foci data, differences between HR frequencies were smaller in PBL and HSPC after calcium compared with carbon ion exposure.

In order to rule out that HR frequencies were influenced by potentially confounding factors in PBL and HSPC, the fraction of apoptotic cells and the cell cycle distribution were determined for X-ray and 60–85 keV/μm carbon ion exposures (Figure S3 in Supplementary Material). These radiation treatments increased the fraction of apoptotic cells (Figure S3A in Supplementary Material) and G₂-phase cells (Figure S3B in Supplementary Material) in PBL and HSPC to a similar extent excluding a major role in cell type-specific HR activities.

Radiation-Induced Intrachromosomal Recombination at the *MLL*bcr Sequence

The observed differences in extrachromosomal HR when comparing radiation qualities or cell types were mostly not statistically significant, which can be explained by the low probability of inducing a DSB in the target sequence of the reporter plasmid. The fraction of cells with one DSB was estimated at around 0.3%, taking into account the transfection efficiency, copy numbers, the size of the target sequence, and the estimated number of DSB per gray. As the fraction of cells with DSB is small and not all DSB are repaired by HR, we pursued an additional experimental strategy, using leukemia K562(HR-EGFP/3′EFP-MLL) and lymphoblastoid WTK1(HR-EGFP/3′EFP-MLL) cell lines (29) stably transfected with plasmid reporter comprising the highly fragile *MLL*bcr sequence (33). Exposure to different doses of X-rays or charged particles was performed. Highest doses (10 and 15 Gy X-rays, 5 Gy carbon and calcium ions) were excluded from the analyses because of associated cytotoxic effects as indicated by apoptosis-induction from sub G₁ analysis (data not shown).

Results from recombination measurements 24 and 48 h post-irradiation, indicating intrachromosomal rearrangements adjacent to the *MLL*bcr sequence, are shown in **Figure 5**. In general, radiation-induced stimulation of intrachromosomal HR was detectable in both cell lines (**Figures 5A,B**). Thus, we observed increased HR frequencies at least 48 h after X-ray exposure, except for one data point [0.5 Gy X-rays; WTK1(HR-EGFP/3′EFP-MLL)], displaying dose dependency and reaching statistical significance for 5 Gy in WTK1(HR-EGFP/3′EFP-MLL) cells. When comparing the same physical dose of 2 Gy in K562(HR-EGFP/3′EFP-MLL) cells applying X-ray versus ion exposure (**Figure 5C**), for carbon ions, more pronounced HR stimulation was observed after 48 h and for calcium, a trend toward enhancement was detectable after 24 h (48 h was not assessed). These data suggest that stably integrated *MLL*bcr sequences in a cell-based reporter assay can be useful for assessment of biological radiation effects.

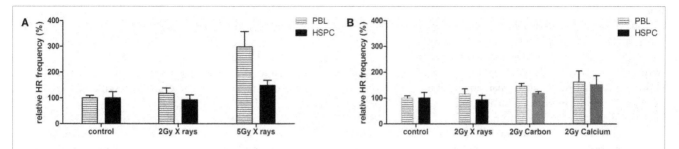

FIGURE 4 | Extrachromosomal DSB repair analysis in PBL and HSPC after irradiation with X-rays or charged particles. PBL and HSPC were cultivated for 72 h, transfected with the DSB repair substrate HR-EGFP/5'EGFP which supports HR prior to irradiation with 2 or 5 Gy of **(A)** X-rays or **(B)** X-rays and charged particles (carbon ions, 60–85 keV/μm and calcium ions, 180 keV/μm). After incubation for 24 h, the fraction of EGFP-positive cells was quantified. HR data were individually normalized to the non-irradiated control representing 100% (PBL: 0.043 × 10⁻² and HSPC: 0.048 × 10⁻²). Mean values and SEM are indicated (X-rays: $n = 3$ from one to three independent experiments, and carbon and calcium ions: $n = 3$ from one experiment). Mean values for non-irradiated controls and irradiated cells were compared with the Wilcoxon matched-pairs signed rank test; however, none of the differences reached statistical significance with *$p < 0.05$.

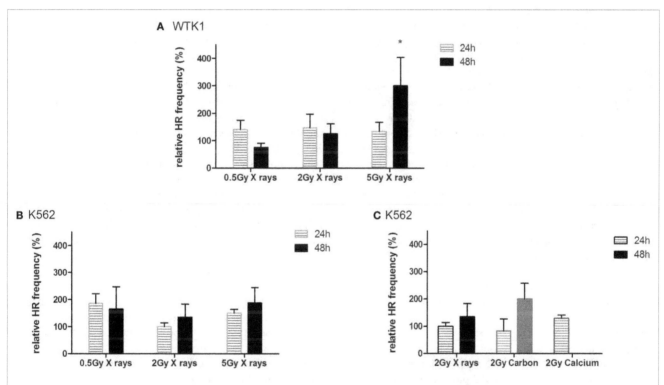

FIGURE 5 | Intrachromosomal DSB repair in WTK1(HR-EGFP/3'EFP-MLL) and K562(HR-EGFP/3'EFP-MLL) cells after irradiation. Stably transfected WTK1(HR-EGFP/3'EFP-MLL) and K562(HR-EGFP/3'EFP-MLL) reporter cells were irradiated with **(A,B)** X-rays or **(C)** X-rays and charged particles (carbon ions, 60–85 keV/μm and calcium ions, 180 keV/μm). Radiation-induced breakage in the *MLL*bcr sequence within the chromosomally integrated HR reporter (HR-EGFP/3'EGFP-MLL) initiated HR events. After subsequent incubation for 24 or 48 h, EGFP-positive viable cells were analyzed within the total cell population by flow cytometric measurement. HR measurements were individually normalized to the unirradiated control representing 100%. Mean values and SEM are indicated (X-rays, WTK1 cells: $n = 12$ from four independent experiments; X-rays, K562 cells: $n = 18$ from six independent experiments; exposure to calcium and carbon ions: $n = 3$ from one independent experiment). Values for non-irradiated control and irradiated cells were compared with the Wilcoxon matched-pairs signed rank test with *$p < 0.05$.

DISCUSSION

Development of AML can be induced by ionizing radiation exposure (2, 3) and is contingent on the induction of specific chromosomal rearrangements and instability (45–47). For some time, we have known that chromosomal aberrations are mainly the result of DSB, which remain unrepaired or are not correctly repaired (48, 49). The frequency of misrepair depends on the type of damage, which can be simple or complex, and on the fidelity of the repair pathway chosen by the damaged cells.

The induction of complex DNA lesions is characteristic of ionizing irradiation; DNA and chromosomal damage induced by heavy ion irradiation is of higher complexity than photon induced damage due to the densely ionizing events occurring along the track of heavy ions. This leads to the occurrence of clustered lesions, i.e., closely spaced single-strand breaks or DSB that are frequently associated with additional types of lesions (50). These clustered lesions are difficult to repair and the level of unrepaired, persisting damage increases with ionizing density. Unrepaired lesions remain detectable as chromosome breakage (12), i.e., for terminal deletions, or lead to complex exchanges involving more than three chromosome breaks and multiple chromosomes (51, 52). Incorrect repair after high LET irradiation can cause point mutations (53) or enhance formation of intra- and interchromosomal exchanges (54–57). If the aberrations are lethal, these result in cell death or reduced clonogenic survival (58).

In our current study, we show a dose-dependent induction of chromatid breaks by X-ray irradiation (Figure S1 in Supplementary Material), and a more pronounced break induction and incomplete rejoining in response to high LET radiation qualities in PBL. We irradiated with five different ions (nitrogen, carbon, calcium, titanium, and iron ions) covering a LET range from 45 to 180 keV/μm (**Figure 1A**; Figure S1A in Supplementary Material). The level of residual damage at 9 h increased with LET, indicating a larger fraction of initial chromatid breaks refractory to rejoining after high LET compared to photon irradiation. This is in accordance with studies performed in different cell types (PBL, fibroblasts, epithelial cells) measuring residual chromosomal damage in mitotic or interphase cells (38, 52, 59–61). Of note, when comparing our results to reported data, one has to take into account that the absolute number of breaks depends on the protocol used for PCC technique (fusion with mitotic cells or Calyculin induced chromosome condensation) (62), the cell type (63), and the cell cycle stage of the irradiated and analyzed cells.

Up to now, rejoining of DSB in terms of chromosomal breaks by PCC has not been investigated for hematopoietic progenitor cells, i.e., HSPC. We demonstrate here similar, dose-dependent induction of chromatid breaks as for PBL and similarly decelerated rejoining after high LET exposure (**Figure 1B**; Figure S1B in Supplementary Material). Cytogenetic changes are considered a valid biomarker for cancer risk assessment (64), and have as such mostly been investigated in PBL isolated from blood of exposed individuals. The observed equivalent induction and repair of chromatid breaks in PBL and HSPC provides useful information because the cell of origin of leukemia is believed to be a transformed HSPC (65) and PBL are a commonly used model for assessment of chromosomal breakage and rejoining.

In good agreement with the cytogenetic data, using phosphorylation of H2AX as a DSB marker, we show that formation and removal of γH2AX foci is similar in both cell types for low and high LET radiation qualities (X-rays, iron ions). Based on the observed enhanced biological efficiency of titanium ions for the induction of chromatid breaks (**Figure 1B**), a higher induction of γH2AX foci by iron ions compared to photons might have been expected but was not observed (**Figures 2A,B**). We posit that this was most likely due to the limited resolution of γH2AX foci formed along a particle track (66, 67), although it is difficult to assess to what extent irradiation geometry would impact the irradiation of suspension cells.

As observed in the cytogenetic analyses, we also measured a higher level of persisting DNA damage after exposure to high LET iron ions compared to X-ray (**Figures 2A,B**). This characteristic of the high LET response, i.e., enhanced levels of γH2AX foci persisting after 24 h, was previously reported mainly in human fibroblasts, epithelial cells, and organotypic cultures (12, 68–72), while data for HSPC were not available.

Having identified an NF-κB-mediated decrease of HR in HSPC versus PBL in our preceding work (20), we assessed how this pathway is affected by radiation and damage quality in the different cell types. Using an EGFP-based reporter plasmid without expression of the cleaving enzyme, we found that extrachromosomal HR frequencies increased in immortalized lymphocytes (LCL 416MI and TK6) with X-ray dose (**Figure 3**). Consistent with previous results from enzyme-mediated cleavage, HR frequencies increased in X-ray-treated PBL and, less so, in HSPC (**Figure 4**). Interestingly, the difference between PBL and HSPC, best observed for 5 Gy X-ray, was not detectable for high LET calcium ions at 2 Gy despite a trend toward HR stimulation by 2 Gy heavy ion versus 2 Gy X-ray exposure.

Higher HR frequencies in PBL after irradiation were indeed expected from the previously obtained results for enzyme mediated cleavage. Comparing the same physical dose of 2 Gy X-ray and heavy ion irradiation, we further noticed a trend toward HR stimulation by heavy ion versus X-ray exposure. Interestingly, the difference between PBL and HSPC observed best for 5 Gy X-ray (**Figure 4A**) was no longer visible for high LET calcium ions (**Figure 4B**). This observation is likely not attributable to differences in cell cycle distribution between PBL and HSPC, because of a comparable radiation-induced cell cycle delay in G_2 phase (Figure S3B in Supplementary Material).

In addition, we recently reported that the more pronounced formation of 53BP1 foci after X-ray-induced DSB in HSPC was a consequence of reduced NF-κB activity (20). Compromised NF-κB-mediated BRCA1-CtIP activation (73) can explain the observed relative shift to error-prone repair pathways in HSPC, possibly under participation of EXO1 nuclease as a resection factor (74, 75). This might also be relevant for particle radiation-induced DSB because we similarly found accumulation of 53BP1 foci after X-ray and carbon ion exposure (intermediate LET) of HSPC. However, this difference between immature and mature cells was lost after higher LET exposure (**Figure 2E**), consistent with similar HR frequencies after calcium ion irradiation (**Figure 4B**). Neutralization of the differences in 53BP1 foci numbers between PBL and HSPC was mostly due to elevated 53BP1 signals in PBL, suggesting incomplete HR repair of higher LET damage not only in HSPC but also in PBL. Results using LCL with stably integrated *MLL*bcr sequences further supported the impression of a dose and LET-dependent increase in HR frequencies (**Figure 5**). Even though further experiments are needed to generate a robust assay system to monitor the effects of different radiation qualities, our results provided clues for future directions (e.g., lentivirus-based integration of the reporter into primary cells of the hematopoietic system). Moreover, it underscored the detrimental potential of radiation-induced breaks to induce AML-related genome rearrangements at the *MLL*bcr in particular. Notably, HR was identified as a DNA repair pathway involved in *MLL*bcr rearrangements in response to replication stress, which can be induced in HSPC by stimuli, such as infection or irradiation (33).

Similarly, elevated 53BP1 damage levels and HR frequencies induced by high LET in PBL and HSPC match the concept that heavy ion-induced complex DSBs are predominantly repaired by HR and thus may exhaust the cellular HR machinery in both cell types (76). Conservative HR is limited to S/G_2-phase cells (77–79) representing 40–60% of the primary cell populations in our study (Figure S3B in Supplementary Material). Other resection-dependent pathways, which are error-prone, have been suggested to contribute to the repair of complex damage (80). However, errors in repair can lead to chromosomal aberrations, in particular translocations (81, 82). Consistent with error-prone pathway usage in HSPC (20, 21), HSPC show a higher level of translocations compared to PBL at moderately enhanced LET (21, 31, 83). An additional explanation for similar HR frequencies in PBL and HSPC after high LET versus X-ray and carbon ion exposure could be earlier activation of NF-κB with increasing LET (84), which could compensate for the low intrinsic NF-κB activity in HSPC. In addition, activation of ATM, a prerequisite for NF-κB signaling, is also more pronounced with increasing LET (67).

Taken together, we could show that overall removal of radiation-induced DNA damage and chromosomal breaks is comparable for mature and immature cells of the hematopoietic system (PBL and HSPC). However, exposure to low and moderate LET reveals higher conservative HR in PBL versus HSPC, consistent with increased usage of low fidelity pathways during repair of enzyme-mediated DSB by HSPC. However, after exposure to high LET HR frequencies of PBL and HSPC are comparable, underlining the importance of HR for the repair of complex DNA damage for the outcome of the damaged cells (85, 86).

ACKNOWLEDGMENTS

We would like to thank P. Partscht, Darmstadt, L. Bauer Darmstadt, and Andreea I. Stahl, Ulm, for dedicated help in the experiments. We also thank Michael Scholz and Thomas Friedrich and the dosimetry team for excellent technical support during the experimental runs. Furthermore, we are grateful to Marco Durante for his continuous support.

FUNDING

This work was partly supported by the German Ministry of Economy (BMWi), grant no. 50WB1225; A0-10 IBER from Federal Ministry of Economics and Technology provided by ESA, German Aerospace Center; grant no. 02NUK017A (GREWIS) from German Federal Ministry of Research and Education; German Research Foundation (DFG, PA3 in Research Training Group 1789 "Cellular and Molecular Mechanisms in aging," CEMMA). MR is a member of the International Graduate School in Molecular Medicine Ulm. AC is a member of DFG-funded Graduate College 1657 and the Helmholtz Graduate School for Hadron and Ion Research. HB is a member of the LOEWE Cell and Gene Therapy Frankfurt faculty funded by Hessian Ministry of Higher Education, Research and the Arts ref. no.: III L 4-518/17.004 (2010). The authors thank the Helmholtz Association for funding of this work through Helmholtz-Portfolio Topic "Technology and Medicine."

REFERENCES

1. Hsu W-L, Preston DL, Soda M, Sugiyama H, Funamoto S, Kodama K, et al. The incidence of leukemia, lymphoma and multiple myeloma among atomic bomb survivors: 1950-2001. *Radiat Res* (2013) **179**(3):361–82.

2. Muirhead CR, O'Hagan JA, Haylock RGE, Phillipson MA, Willcock T, Berridge GLC, et al. Mortality and cancer incidence following occupational radiation exposure: third analysis of the national registry for radiation workers. *Br J Cancer* (2009) **100**(1):206–12. doi:10.1038/sj.bjc.6604825

3. Linet MS, Kim KP, Miller DL, Kleinerman RA, Simon SL, Berrington de Gonzalez A. Historical review of occupational exposures and cancer risks in medical radiation workers. *Radiat Res* (2010) **174**(6):793–808. doi:10.1667/RR2014.1

4. Newhauser WD, Durante M. Assessing the risk of second malignancies after modern radiotherapy. *Nat Rev Cancer* (2011) **11**(6):438–48. doi:10.1038/nrc3069

5. Schulz-Ertner D, Tsujii H. Particle radiation therapy using proton and heavier ion beams. *J Clin Oncol* (2007) **25**(8):953–64. doi:10.1200/JCO.2006.09.7816

6. Durante M. New challenges in high-energy particle radiobiology. *Br J Radiol* (2014) **87**(1035):20130626. doi:10.1259/bjr.20130626

7. Cucinotta FA, Durante M. Cancer risk from exposure to galactic cosmic rays: implications for space exploration by human beings. *Lancet Oncol* (2006) **7**(5):431–5. doi:10.1016/S1470-2045(06)70695-7

8. Durante M, Cucinotta FA. Heavy ion carcinogenesis and human space exploration. *Nat Rev Cancer* (2008) **8**(6):465–72. doi:10.1038/nrc2391

9. Barcellos-Hoff MH, Blakely EA, Burma S, Fornace AJ, Gerson S, Hlatky L, et al. Concepts and challenges in cancer risk prediction for the space radiation environment. *Life Sci Space Res* (2015) **6**:92–103. doi:10.1016/j.lssr.2015.07.006

10. Durante M, Loeffler JS. Charged particles in radiation oncology. *Nat Rev Clin Oncol* (2010) **7**(1):37–43. doi:10.1038/nrclinonc.2009.183

11. Anderson RM, Stevens DL, Sumption ND, Townsend KMS, Goodhead DT, Hill MA. Effect of linear energy transfer (LET) on the complexity of alpha-particle-induced chromosome aberrations in human CD34+ cells. *Radiat Res* (2007) **167**(5):541–50. doi:10.1667/RR0813.1

12. Asaithamby A, Hu B, Chen DJ. Unrepaired clustered DNA lesions induce chromosome breakage in human cells. *Proc Natl Acad Sci U S A* (2011) **108**(20):8293–8. doi:10.1073/pnas.1016045108

13. Pedersen-Djergaard J, Christiansen DH, Desta F, Andersen MK. Alternative genetic pathways and cooperating genetic abnormalities in the pathogenesis of therapy-related myelodysplasia and acute myeloid leukemia. *Leukemia* (2006) **20**(11):1943–9. doi:10.1038/sj.leu.2404381

14. Francis R, Richardson C. Multipotent hematopoietic cells susceptible to alternative double-strand break repair pathways that promote genome rearrangements. *Genes Dev* (2007) **21**(9):1064–74. doi:10.1101/gad.1522807

15. Mohrin M, Bourke E, Alexander D, Warr MR, Barry-Holson K, Le Beau MM, et al. Hematopoietic stem cell quiescence promotes error-prone DNA repair and mutagenesis. *Cell Stem Cell* (2010) **7**(2):174–85. doi:10.1016/j.stem.2010.06.014

16. Zhang L, Wang SA. A focused review of hematopoietic neoplasms occurring in the therapy-related setting. *Int J Clin Exp Pathol* (2014) **7**(7):3512–23.

17. IAEA. *Cytogenetic Analysis for Radiation Dose Assessment a Manual [Internet]* (2015) [cited 2015 Aug 23]. Available from: http://www-pub.iaea.org/books/IAEABooks/6303/Cytogenetic-Analysis-for-Radiation-Dose-Assessment-A-Manual

18. Durante M, Bonassi S, George K, Cucinotta FA. Risk estimation based on chromosomal aberrations induced by radiation. *Radiat Res* (2001) **156**(5 Pt 2):662–7. doi:10.1667/0033-7587(2001)156[0662:REBOCA]2.0.CO;2

19. Tucker JD. Low-dose ionizing radiation and chromosome translocations: a review of the major considerations for human biological dosimetry. *Mutat Res* (2008) 659(3):211–20. doi:10.1016/j.mrrev.2008.04.001

20. Kraft D, Rall M, Volcic M, Metzler E, Groo A, Stahl A, et al. NF-κB-dependent DNA damage-signaling differentially regulates DNA double-strand break repair mechanisms in immature and mature human hematopoietic cells. *Leukemia* (2015) 29(7):1543–54. doi:10.1038/leu.2015.28

21. Kraft D, Ritter S, Durante M, Seifried E, Fournier C, Tonn T. Transmission of clonal chromosomal abnormalities in human hematopoietic stem and progenitor cells surviving radiation exposure. *Mutat Res* (2015) 777:43–51. doi:10.1016/j.mrfmmm.2015.04.007

22. Walter D, Lier A, Geiselhart A, Thalheimer FB, Huntscha S, Sobotta MC, et al. Exit from dormancy provokes DNA-damage-induced attrition in haematopoietic stem cells. *Nature* (2015) 520(7548):549–52. doi:10.1038/nature14131

23. Akyüz N, Boehden GS, Süsse S, Rimek A, Preuss U, Scheidtmann K-H, et al. DNA substrate dependence of p53-mediated regulation of double-strand break repair. *Mol Cell Biol* (2002) 22(17):6306–17. doi:10.1128/MCB.22.17.6306-6317.2002

24. Keimling M, Kaur J, Bagadi SAR, Kreienberg R, Wiesmüller L, Ralhan R. A sensitive test for the detection of specific DSB repair defects in primary cells from breast cancer specimens. *Int J Cancer* (2008) 123(3):730–6. doi:10.1002/ijc.23551

25. Keimling M, Volcic M, Csernok A, Wieland B, Dörk T, Wiesmüller L. Functional characterization connects individual patient mutations in ataxia telangiectasia mutated (ATM) with dysfunction of specific DNA double-strand break-repair signaling pathways. *FASEB J* (2011) 25(11):3849–60. doi:10.1096/fj.11-185546

26. Keimling M, Deniz M, Varga D, Stahl A, Schrezenmeier H, Kreienberg R, et al. The power of DNA double-strand break (DSB) repair testing to predict breast cancer susceptibility. *FASEB J* (2012) 26(5):2094–104. doi:10.1096/fj.11-200790

27. Akyüz N, Wiesmüller L. Proof of principle: detection of genotoxicity by a fluorescence-based recombination test in mammalian cells. *ALTEX* (2003) 20(2):77–84.

28. Siehler SY, Schrauder M, Gerischer U, Cantor S, Marra G, Wiesmüller L. Human MutL-complexes monitor homologous recombination independently of mismatch repair. *DNA Repair* (2009) 8(2):242–52. doi:10.1016/j.dnarep.2008.10.011

29. Ireno IC, Baumann C, Stöber R, Hengstler JG, Wiesmüller L. Fluorescence-based recombination assay for sensitive and specific detection of genotoxic carcinogens in human cells. *Arch Toxicol* (2014) 88(5):1141–59. doi:10.1007/s00204-014-1229-3

30. Fernández JL, Vázquez-Gundín F, Rivero MT, Genescá A, Gosálvez J, Goyanes V. DBD-fish on neutral comets: simultaneous analysis of DNA single- and double-strand breaks in individual cells. *Exp Cell Res* (2001) 270(1):102–9. doi:10.1006/excr.2001.5328

31. Becker D, Elsässer T, Tonn T, Seifried E, Durante M, Ritter S, et al. Response of human hematopoietic stem and progenitor cells to energetic carbon ions. *Int J Radiat Biol* (2009) 85(11):1051–9. doi:10.3109/09553000903232850

32. Boehden GS, Restle A, Marschalek R, Stocking C, Wiesmüller L. Recombination at chromosomal sequences involved in leukaemogenic rearrangements is differentially regulated by p53. *Carcinogenesis* (2004) 25(8):1305–13. doi:10.1093/carcin/bgh092

33. Gole B, Wiesmüller L. Leukemogenic rearrangements at the mixed lineage leukemia gene (MLL)-multiple rather than a single mechanism. *Front Cell Dev Biol* (2015) 3:41. doi:10.3389/fcell.2015.00041

34. Allan JM, Travis LB. Mechanisms of therapy-related carcinogenesis. *Nat Rev Cancer* (2005) 5(12):943–55. doi:10.1038/nrc1749

35. Klymenko SV, Bink K, Trott KR, Bebeshko VG, Bazyka DA, Dmytrenko IV, et al. MLL gene alterations in radiation-associated acute myeloid leukemia. *Exp Oncol* (2005) 27(1):71–5.

36. Mueller MM, Bialleck H, Bomke B, Brauninger S, Varga C, Seidl C, et al. Safety and efficacy of healthy volunteer stem cell mobilization with filgrastim G-CSF and mobilized stem cell apheresis: results of a prospective longitudinal 5-year follow-up study. *Vox Sang* (2013) 104(1):46–54. doi:10.1111/j.1423-0410.2012.01632.x

37. Kiefer J, Straaten H. A model of ion track structure based on classical collision dynamics. *Phys Med Biol* (1986) 31(11):1201–9. doi:10.1088/0031-9155/31/11/002

38. Kawata T, Gotoh E, Durante M, Wu H, George K, Furusawa Y, et al. High-LET radiation-induced aberrations in prematurely condensed G2 chromosomes of human fibroblasts. *Int J Radiat Biol* (2000) 76(7):929–37. doi:10.1080/09553000050050945

39. Bennardo N, Cheng A, Huang N, Stark JM. Alternative-NHEJ is a mechanistically distinct pathway of mammalian chromosome break repair. *PLoS Genet* (2008) 4(6):e1000110. doi:10.1371/journal.pgen.1000110

40. Böhringer M, Wiesmüller L. Fluorescence-based quantification of pathway-specific DNA double-strand break repair activities: a powerful method for the analysis of genome destabilizing mechanisms. *Subcell Biochem* (2010) 50:297–306. doi:10.1007/978-90-481-3471-7_15

41. Restle A, Färber M, Baumann C, Böhringer M, Scheidtmann KH, Müller-Tidow C, et al. Dissecting the role of p53 phosphorylation in homologous recombination provides new clues for gain-of-function mutants. *Nucleic Acids Res* (2008) 36(16):5362–75. doi:10.1093/nar/gkn503

42. Mirault M-E, Boucher P, Tremblay A. Nucleotide-resolution mapping of topoisomerase-mediated and apoptotic DNA strand scissions at or near an MLL translocation hotspot. *Am J Hum Genet* (2006) 79(5):779–91. doi:10.1086/507791

43. Meyer C, Hofmann J, Burmeister T, Gröger D, Park TS, Emerenciano M, et al. The MLL recombinome of acute leukemias in 2013. *Leukemia* (2013) 27(11):2165–76. doi:10.1038/leu.2013.135

44. Löbrich M, Rief N, Kühne M, Heckmann M, Fleckenstein J, Rübe C, et al. In vivo formation and repair of DNA double-strand breaks after computed tomography examinations. *Proc Natl Acad Sci U S A* (2005) 102(25):8984–9. doi:10.1073/pnas.0501895102

45. Mitelman Database. *Mitelman Database of Chromosome Aberrations and Gene Fusions in Cancer [Internet]* (2015) [cited 2015 Aug 23]. Available from: http://cgap.nci.nih.gov/Chromosomes/Mitelman

46. Rassool FV, Gaymes TJ, Omidvar N, Brady N, Beurlet S, Pla M, et al. Reactive oxygen species, DNA damage, and error-prone repair: a model for genomic instability with progression in myeloid leukemia? *Cancer Res* (2007) 67(18):8762–71. doi:10.1158/0008-5472.CAN-06-4807

47. Negrini S, Gorgoulis VG, Halazonetis TD. Genomic instability – an evolving hallmark of cancer. *Nat Rev Mol Cell Biol* (2010) 11(3):220–8. doi:10.1038/nrm2858

48. Bender MA, Griggs HG, Bedford JS. Mechanisms of chromosomal aberration production. 3. Chemicals and ionizing radiation. *Mutat Res* (1974) 23(2):197–212. doi:10.1016/0027-5107(74)90140-7

49. Obe G, Pfeiffer P, Savage JRK, Johannes C, Goedecke W, Jeppesen P, et al. Chromosomal aberrations: formation, identification and distribution. *Mutat Res* (2002) 504(1–2):17–36. doi:10.1016/S0027-5107(02)00076-3

50. Asaithamby A, Chen DJ. Mechanism of cluster DNA damage repair in response to high-atomic number and energy particles radiation. *Mutat Res* (2011) 711(1–2):87–99. doi:10.1016/j.mrfmmm.2010.11.002

51. Savage JR, Simpson PJ. FISH "painting" patterns resulting from complex exchanges. *Mutat Res* (1994) 312(1):51–60. doi:10.1016/0165-1161(94)90008-6

52. Loucas BD, Durante M, Bailey SM, Cornforth MN. Chromosome damage in human cells by γ rays, α particles and heavy ions: track interactions in basic dose-response relationships. *Radiat Res* (2013) 179(1):9–20. doi:10.1667/RR3089.1

53. Hall EJ, Hei TK. Genomic instability and bystander effects induced by high-LET radiation. *Oncogene* (2003) 22(45):7034–42. doi:10.1038/sj.onc.1206900

54. Lee R, Sommer S, Hartel C, Nasonova E, Durante M, Ritter S. Complex exchanges are responsible for the increased effectiveness of C-ions compared to X-rays at the first post-irradiation mitosis. *Mutat Res* (2010) 701(1):52–9. doi:10.1016/j.mrgentox.2010.03.004

55. Ritter S, Durante M. Heavy-ion induced chromosomal aberrations: a review. *Mutat Res* (2010) 701(1):38–46. doi:10.1016/j.mrgentox.2010.04.007

56. Durante M, Bedford JS, Chen DJ, Conrad S, Cornforth MN, Natarajan AT, et al. From DNA damage to chromosome aberrations: joining the break. *Mutat Res* (2013) 756(1–2):5–13. doi:10.1016/j.mrgentox.2013.05.014

57. Ray FA, Robinson E, McKenna M, Hada M, George K, Cucinotta F, et al. Directional genomic hybridization: inversions as a potential biodosimeter for retrospective radiation exposure. *Radiat Environ Biophys* (2014) 53(2):255–63. doi:10.1007/s00411-014-0513-1

58. Franken NAP, Oei AL, Kok HP, Rodermond HM, Sminia P, Crezee J, et al. Cell survival and radiosensitisation: modulation of the linear and quadratic

parameters of the LQ model (review). *Int J Oncol* (2013) **42**(5):1501–15. doi:10.3892/ijo.2013.1857

59. Nasonova E, Ritter S. Cytogenetic effects of densely ionising radiation in human lymphocytes: impact of cell cycle delays. *Cytogenet Genome Res* (2004) **104**(1–4):216–20. doi:10.1159/000077492

60. Hada M, Cucinotta FA, Gonda SR, Wu H. mBAND analysis of chromosomal aberrations in human epithelial cells exposed to low- and high-LET radiation. *Radiat Res* (2007) **168**(1):98–105. doi:10.1667/RR0759.1

61. Okayasu R. Repair of DNA damage induced by accelerated heavy ions – a mini review. *Int J Cancer* (2012) **130**(5):991–1000. doi:10.1002/ijc.26445

62. Deperas-Standylo J, Lee R, Nasonova E, Ritter S, Gudowska-Nowak E. Production and distribution of aberrations in resting or cycling human lymphocytes following Fe-ion or Cr-ion irradiation: emphasis on single track effects. *Adv Space Res* (2012) **50**(5):584–97. doi:10.1016/j.asr.2012.05.007

63. Themis M, Garimberti E, Hill MA, Anderson RM. Reduced chromosome aberration complexity in normal human bronchial epithelial cells exposed to low-LET γ-rays and high-LET α-particles. *Int J Radiat Biol* (2013) **89**(11):934–43. doi:10.3109/09553002.2013.805889

64. Bonassi S, Norppa H, Ceppi M, Strömberg U, Vermeulen R, Znaor A, et al. Chromosomal aberration frequency in lymphocytes predicts the risk of cancer: results from a pooled cohort study of 22 358 subjects in 11 countries. *Carcinogenesis* (2008) **29**(6):1178–83. doi:10.1093/carcin/bgn075

65. Brendel C, Neubauer A. Characteristics and analysis of normal and leukemic stem cells: current concepts and future directions. *Leukemia* (2000) **14**(10):1711–7. doi:10.1038/sj.leu.2401907

66. Jakob B, Scholz M, Taucher-Scholz G. Biological imaging of heavy charged-particle tracks. *Radiat Res* (2003) **159**(5):676–84. doi:10.1667/0033-7587(2003)159[0676:BIOHCT]2.0.CO;2

67. Costes SV, Boissière A, Ravani S, Romano R, Parvin B, Barcellos-Hoff MH. Imaging features that discriminate between foci induced by high- and low-LET radiation in human fibroblasts. *Radiat Res* (2006) **165**(5):505–15. doi:10.1667/RR3538.1

68. Asaithamby A, Uematsu N, Chatterjee A, Story MD, Burma S, Chen DJ. Repair of HZE-particle-induced DNA double-strand breaks in normal human fibroblasts. *Radiat Res* (2008) **169**(4):437–46. doi:10.1667/RR1165.1

69. Asaithamby A, Hu B, Delgado O, Ding L-H, Story MD, Minna JD, et al. Irreparable complex DNA double-strand breaks induce chromosome breakage in organotypic three-dimensional human lung epithelial cell culture. *Nucleic Acids Res* (2011) **39**(13):5474–88. doi:10.1093/nar/gkr149

70. Groesser T, Chang H, Fontenay G, Chen J, Costes SV, Helen Barcellos-Hoff M, et al. Persistence of γ-H2AX and 53BP1 foci in proliferating and non-proliferating human mammary epithelial cells after exposure to γ-rays or iron ions. *Int J Radiat Biol* (2011) **87**(7):696–710. doi:10.3109/09553002.2010.549535

71. Saha J, Wilson P, Thieberger P, Lowenstein D, Wang M, Cucinotta FA. Biological characterization of low-energy ions with high-energy deposition on human cells. *Radiat Res* (2014) **182**(3):282–91. doi:10.1667/RR13747.1

72. Sridharan DM, Chappell LJ, Whalen MK, Cucinotta FA, Pluth JM. Defining the biological effectiveness of components of high-LET track structure. *Radiat Res* (2015) **184**(1):105–19. doi:10.1667/RR13684.1

73. Volcic M, Karl S, Baumann B, Salles D, Daniel P, Fulda S, et al. NF-κB regulates DNA double-strand break repair in conjunction with BRCA1-CtIP complexes. *Nucleic Acids Res* (2012) **40**(1):181–95. doi:10.1093/nar/gkr687

74. Tomimatsu N, Mukherjee B, Deland K, Kurimasa A, Bolderson E, Khanna KK, et al. Exo1 plays a major role in DNA end resection in

humans and influences double-strand break repair and damage signaling decisions. *DNA Repair* (2012) **11**(4):441–8. doi:10.1016/j.dnarep.2012.01.006

75. Desai A, Gerson S. Exo1 independent DNA mismatch repair involves multiple compensatory nucleases. *DNA Repair* (2014) **21**:55–64. doi:10.1016/j.dnarep.2014.06.005

76. Shibata A, Conrad S, Birraux J, Geuting V, Barton O, Ismail A, et al. Factors determining DNA double-strand break repair pathway choice in G2 phase. *EMBO J* (2011) **30**(6):1079–92. doi:10.1038/emboj.2011.27

77. Tamulevicius P, Wang M, Iliakis G. Homology-directed repair is required for the development of radioresistance during S phase: interplay between double-strand break repair and checkpoint response. *Radiat Res* (2007) **167**(1):1–11. doi:10.1667/RR0751.1

78. Daley JM, Sung P. 53BP1, BRCA1, and the choice between recombination and end joining at DNA double-strand breaks. *Mol Cell Biol* (2014) **34**(8):1380–8. doi:10.1128/MCB.01639-13

79. Mjelle R, Hegre SA, Aas PA, Slupphaug G, Drabløs F, Saetrom P, et al. Cell cycle regulation of human DNA repair and chromatin remodeling genes. *DNA Repair* (2015) **30**:53–67. doi:10.1016/j.dnarep.2015.03.007

80. Averbeck NB, Ringel O, Herrlitz M, Jakob B, Durante M, Taucher-Scholz G. DNA end resection is needed for the repair of complex lesions in G1-phase human cells. *Cell Cycle* (2014) **13**(16):2509–16. doi:10.4161/15384101.2015.941743

81. Hlatky L, Sachs RK, Vazquez M, Cornforth MN. Radiation-induced chromosome aberrations: insights gained from biophysical modeling. *Bioessays* (2002) **24**(8):714–23. doi:10.1002/bies.10126

82. Roukos V, Misteli T. The biogenesis of chromosome translocations. *Nat Cell Biol* (2014) **16**(4):293–300. doi:10.1038/ncb2941

83. Hartel C, Nikoghosyan A, Durante M, Sommer S, Nasonova E, Fournier C, et al. Chromosomal aberrations in peripheral blood lymphocytes of prostate cancer patients treated with IMRT and carbon ions. *Radiother Oncol* (2010) **95**(1):73–8. doi:10.1016/j.radonc.2009.08.031

84. Hellweg CE, Baumstark-Khan C, Schmitz C, Lau P, Meier MM, Testard I, et al. Carbon-ion-induced activation of the NF-κB pathway. *Radiat Res* (2011) **175**(4):424–31. doi:10.1667/RR2423.1

85. Zafar F, Seidler SB, Kronenberg A, Schild D, Wiese C. Homologous recombination contributes to the repair of DNA double-strand breaks induced by high-energy iron ions. *Radiat Res* (2010) **173**(1):27–39. doi:10.1667/RR1910.1

86. Gerelchuluun A, Manabe E, Ishikawa T, Sun L, Itoh K, Sakae T, et al. The major DNA repair pathway after both proton and carbon-ion radiation is NHEJ, but the HR pathway is more relevant in carbon ions. *Radiat Res* (2015) **183**(3):345–56. doi:10.1667/RR13904.1

3

Short DNA Fragments are a Hallmark of Heavy Charged-Particle Irradiation and may Underlie their Greater Therapeutic Efficacy

Dalong Pang[1]*, Sergey Chasovskikh[1], James E. Rodgers[2] and Anatoly Dritschilo[1]

[1] Radiation Medicine, Georgetown University Medical Center, Washington, DC, USA, [2] Radiation Oncology, Medstar Franklin Square Medical Center, Rosedale, MD, USA

*Correspondence:
Dalong Pang
dalong.pang@gunet.georgetown.edu

Growing interest in proton and heavy ion therapy has reinvigorated research into the fundamental biological mechanisms underlying the therapeutic efficacy of charged-particle radiation. To improve our understanding of the greater biological effectiveness of high-LET radiations, we have investigated DNA double-strand breaks (DSBs) following exposure of plasmid DNA to low-LET Co-60 gamma photon and electron irradiation and to high-LET Beryllium and Argon ions with atomic force microscopy. The sizes of DNA fragments following radiation exposure were individually measured to construct fragment size distributions from which the DSB per DNA molecule and DSB spatial distributions were derived. We report that heavy charged particles induce a significantly larger proportion of short DNA fragments in irradiated DNA molecules, reflecting densely and clustered damage patterns of high-LET energy depositions. We attribute the enhanced short DNA fragmentation following high-LET radiations as an important determinant of the observed, enhanced biological effectiveness of high-LET irradiations.

Keywords: short DNA fragments, radiation, AFM, low-LET, charged particle

INTRODUCTION

DNA is the critical target of ionizing radiation-induced cellular damage, and DNA double-strand breaks (DSBs) are the most lethal of more than 100 various DNA lesions induced by ionizing radiation (1–3). Biological observations implicate DNA DSBs resulting from high-LET radiation in cell death and carcinogenesis to a greater extent than that observed following low-LET radiations (4–6). Mechanisms underlying such observations have focused on dense and complex ionization events resulting in clustered DNA DSBs that are more difficult to repair (7, 8).

Established methods for measurements of DSBs include sucrose gradient sedimentation (9), neutral filter elusion (10), continuous or pulsed-field gel electrophoresis (PFGE) (11–13), the comet assay (14, 15), and, more recently, the γ-H2AX foci quantification (16, 17). DSBs induced in cellular environment and in denatured DNA have been determined (18–23); however, measured DSBs following high-LET radiations were reported equal to or only marginally greater than that observed following low-LET radiations (6, 24, 25). This is in contradiction to the observed greater relative biological effectiveness (RBE) by several fold for cell survival following high-LET radiation exposures (26, 27). However, a better correlation between RBE survival and DSB induction was found with assays of unrepaired DSBs (28–31).

This apparent discrepancy between RBE for cell survival as compared to DSB induction contradicted the accepted thesis of DSB as the primary lesion for cell killing. Subsequently, detailed examination of the techniques used for DSB measurements has revealed that they were reliable only for DNA fragments in the kilobase-pair region and possible shorter DNA fragments were potentially unaccounted for (32–34).

In addition to experimental investigation of DSB induction by ionizing radiation, theoretical modeling employing individual particle track structures has also been pursued (35–38). Ionizing events by individual particles based on established physics principles have shown that heavy charged-particle radiations produce a much greater clustered energy depositions (within a few base pairs) imparting sufficient energy to generate free radicals, which can lead to DNA DSBs or directly cause DSBs when occurring on the opposite strand within a certain distance (39–41). Such Monte Carlo simulations have revealed induction of short DNA fragments less than a few hundred base pairs by both low- and high-LET radiations, which were not quantified in experimental measurements (41, 42).

As a single molecule imaging instrument, the atomic force microscopy (AFM) offers the resolution to image individual atoms of solid state materials and nanometer resolution to visualize biological molecules, e.g., DNA molecules (43–46). Unlike Electron Microscopy or Scanning Tunneling Microscopy, AFM requires minimum sample preparation, reducing or eliminating potential distortions attributable to sample preparation (47, 48). In addition, its ability to measure biomolecules in aqueous solutions, similar to the native environment, offers the possibility for examining *in vitro* behaviors and interactions of biomolecules of interest (49–51).

We have previously reported the presence of short DNA fragments in neutron irradiated plasmid DNA, reflecting the high-LET energy deposition of neutrons (52). Here, we address the effectiveness of high-LET charged-particle irradiation in producing short DNA fragments in plasmid DNA. Use of plasmid DNA molecules as the targets allows for high-resolution imaging and easy identification of DNA fragmentation in sizes of a few to a few hundred nanometers in lengths. We investigated DNA fragmentation following radiations of the low-LET Co-60 photon and electron, and the high-LET Beryllium and Argon ions.

MATERIALS AND METHODS

DNA Samples
Plasmid DNA (pUC19, 2686 bp in length) was purchased from New England Biolab at a concentration of 1000 μg/ml in HEPES buffer (Beverley, MA, USA). The samples were diluted to a concentration of 5 μg/ml in buffer containing 10 mM HEPES and 1 mM $MgCl_2$ and aliquoted into vials containing 250 μl DNA solution each.

Irradiation
Irradiation of the aliquots of DNA solutions was performed at the following sites.

Electron irradiations were performed at the Georgetown University Medical Center in Washington, DC, USA on a medical linear accelerator with 6 MV energy (Varian 2100 C/D, Varian, Palo Alto, CA, USA) to doses of 1000–8000 Gy in 1000 Gy increment. The dose was calibrated using a NIST traceable ionization chamber.

Co-60 photon irradiations were performed at Neutron Products in Dickerson, MD, USA using an industrial Co-60 irradiator at a dose rate of 20 kGy/h in the same dose range as that for electrons.

Beryllium ion irradiations were performed at the Oak Ridge National Laboratory in Oak Ridge, TN, USA. The energy of the Beryllium particle beam was 100 MeV/n, and the LET was 11.6 keV/μm. The doses delivered ranged from 3 to 12 kGy, calculated as the product of the particle fluence rate and the LET of the ion multiplied by the time the beam was on.

Argon ion irradiations were performed on the HIMAC charged-particle accelerator at the National Institute of Radiological Science in Chiba, Japan. The energy of the Argon ion beam was 390 MeV/n, and the LET was 99.5 keV/μm. The doses delivered were 3–12 kGy, using a similar way for dose determination as that for Beryllium irradiation.

As a control, a set of three un-irradiated DNA samples was prepared for each experiment.

AFM Imaging
A Bruker Nano Scope IIIa AFM (Bruker, Santa Barbara, CA, USA) was used for DNA imaging in tapping mode in air. The AFM cantilevers were commercially available from Bruker with a tip radius of approximately 10 nm. Sample preparation for imaging consisted of deposition of 2 μl of the DNA solution on freshly cleaved mica surface, followed by a gentle rinse with 1 ml of distilled water and subsequent drying in the gentle flow of Nitrogen gas. The Scanning frequency was 1 Hz and typical scanning size was 2 μm × 2 μm.

The sizes of the DNA fragments in each image were measured individually using the NanoScope IIIa software. Over a thousand DNA fragments were measured for each irradiated DNA sample to ensure a statistical uncertainty of <5%. Fragment size distribution profiles relating the numbers of DNA fragments to their sizes were constructed. The average numbers of DSBs per DNA, per broken DNA, and DSB distributions as a function of spatial distance were derived from the constructed size distribution profiles. For details on the technique and data analysis, the reader is referred to our previous paper (52).

RESULTS

Figures 1A–E show representative AFM images of the plasmid DNA of un-irradiated controls and following irradiation by Co-60 photon, electron, Beryllium, and Argon ions to doses of 6 kGy. As shown in **Figure 1A**, the majority of the control DNA molecules were in relaxed circular conformation with occasional super coiling of one or two twists. In **Figures 1B,C**, the amount of DNA fragmentation and sizes appear similar, demonstrating similar physical characteristics of low-LET energy deposition patterns following Co-60 photon and electron irradiations.

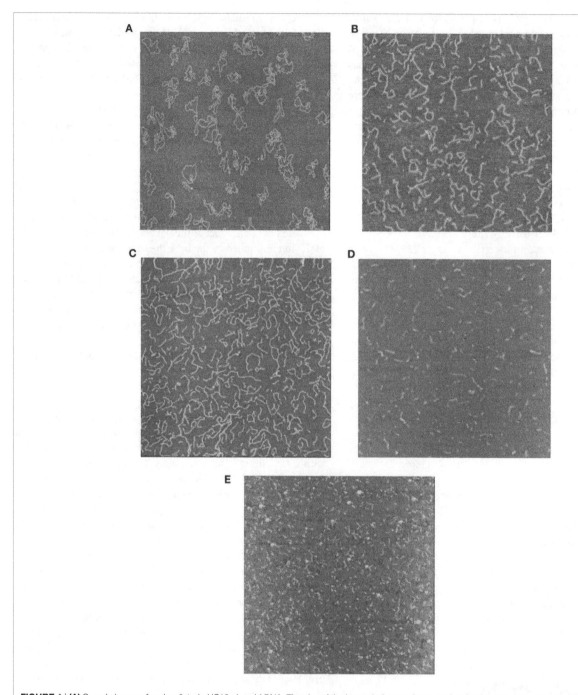

FIGURE 1 | (A) Sample image of un-irradiated pUC19 plasmid DNA. The size of the image is 2 μm × 2 μm, as that for the rest of the images. **(B)** Sample image of Co-60 photon irradiated pUC19 plasmid DNA. The radiation dose is 6 kGy. **(C)** Sample image of electron irradiated pUC19 plasmid DNA. The radiation dose is 6 kGy. **(D)** Sample image of Beryllium ion irradiated pUC19 plasmid DNA. The radiation dose is 6 kGy. **(E)** Sample image of Argon ion irradiated pUC19 plasmid DNA. The radiation dose is 6 kGy.

Examination of **Figures 1D,E** shows that DNA fragmentation is markedly greater than that shown in **Figures 1B,C**. Furthermore, the average sizes of DNA fragments are shorter, demonstrating the enhanced capability of the high-LET Beryllium and Argon ions to fragment DNA to a much greater extent.

Figures 2A–E show the corresponding reconstructed DNA fragment size distributions based on individually measured

DNA fragment sizes for each irradiated samples. The size of the original, un-fragmented pUC19 plasmid DNA is 850 nm and is evenly divided into 50 nm bins in the range of 0–850 nm. Size profile of the un-irradiated DNA was marked by a near 100% uni-spike at the 850 nm bin, represented by the unbroken and occasional DNA molecules with one break only. Mirroring images shown in **Figures 1B,C**, the DNA fragment size distributions in **Figures 2B,C** are essentially identical, and approximating an exponential distribution as a function of the fragment sizes. However, the size distributions shown in **Figures 2D,E** are quite different from that in **Figures 2B,C**, marked by pronounced spikes of fragments in the shortest bin of 50 nm. This demonstrates a much enhanced induction of short DNA fragments by the Beryllium and Argon ions. Size distributions in bins longer than 50 nm follow a similar exponential-like distribution as that in **Figures 2B,C**, but at a more accelerated drop off with increasing fragment size.

Based on the measured DNA fragment sizes, the average numbers of DNA DSB per DNA molecule are derived for DNA molecules including both fragmented and intact DNA. In addition, DSBs per DNA for fragmented DNA molecules only are also derived to further illustrate the DNA fragmentation capability by different types of radiation. Derivation of these quantities is based on the following considerations. If a plasmid DNA contains only

one DSB, it becomes linearized as a single linear DNA fragment of the original length of 850 nm; if it contains two DSBs, a plasmid is broken into two pieces and the combined lengths of the two fragments add up to the original DNA length and this pattern holds for DNA containing N DSBs. Therefore, the number of fragments equals the number of DSBs, and consequently, the number of DSBs per DNA molecule simply equals to the number of fragments divided by the total number of DNA molecules from which the fragments are originated, which can be calculated as the sum of all the fragment lengths divided by the length of an intact DNA.

In addition to the average number of DSB per DNA, which provides a general indication of the DNA breaking capability by ionizing radiation, information on the spatial correlation of the DSBs on a DNA molecule can be further derived from the size distributions. As an illustrative example, we calculate the number of DSBs distributed within a distance of 50 nm on a DNA

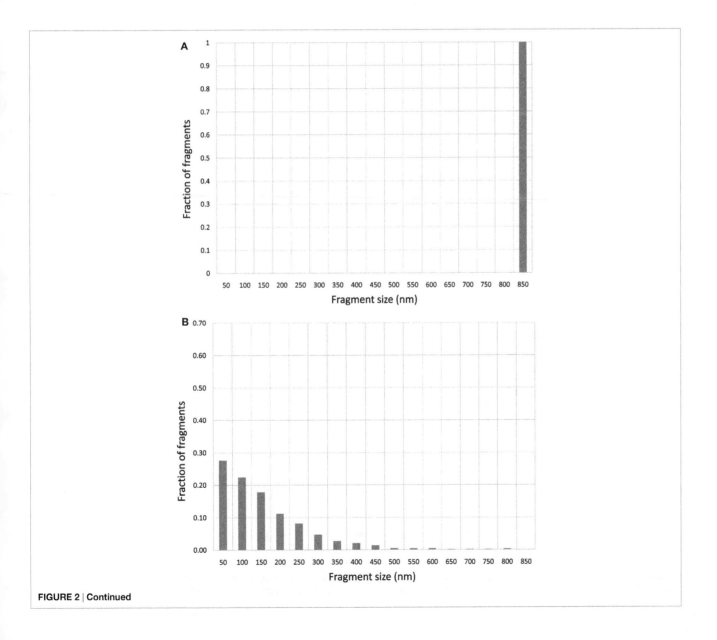

FIGURE 2 | Continued

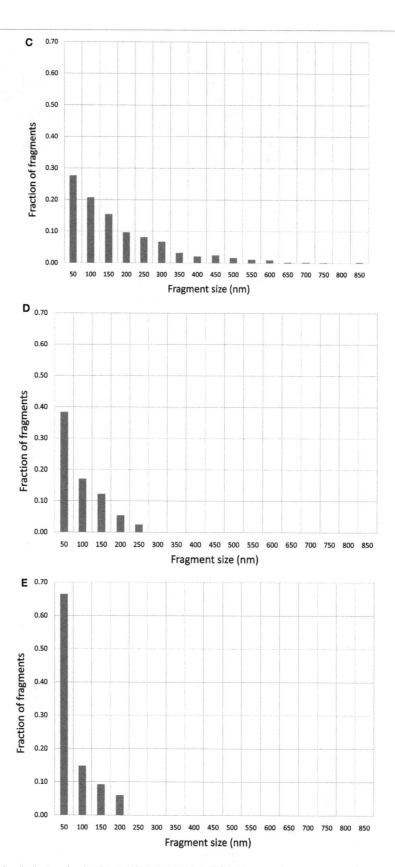

FIGURE 2 | (A) DNA fragment size distribution of un-irradiated pUC19 plasmid DNA. **(B)** DNA fragment size distribution of 6 kGy Co-60 photon irradiated DNA. **(C)** DNA fragment size distribution of 6 kGy electron irradiated DNA. **(D)** DNA fragment size distribution of 6 kGy Beryllium ion irradiated DNA. **(E)** DNA fragment size distribution of 6 kGy Argon ion irradiated DNA.

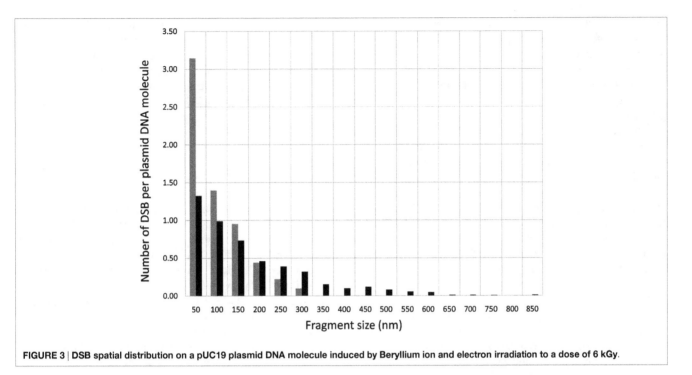

FIGURE 3 | DSB spatial distribution on a pUC19 plasmid DNA molecule induced by Beryllium ion and electron irradiation to a dose of 6 kGy.

TABLE 1 | Measured DSB per DNA molecule and corresponding RBE for radiations investigated in this and a previous report (52).

Radiation	DSB/DNA	STD	RBE	STD	LET (keV/um)
Electron	4.77	0.4	0.82	0.08	0.2
Co-60	5.83	0.33	1.00	0.08	0.2
Neutron	7.36	0.78	1.26	0.15	55
Be	6.24	0.71	1.07	0.14	11.6
Argon	26.09	5.69	4.48	1.01	99.5

The comparison was made for the radiation dose of 6 kGy. RBE was calculated with Co-60 as the reference. The LET value for neutron is the average LET of the recoil protons generated by the primary neutrons, and the LET for Co-60 photon is the average LET of the secondary electrons produced by the primary photon through Compton effects.

molecule. This is derived by counting the number of fragments in the length interval from 0 to 50 nm, which is then divided by the total number of DNA molecules as determined in the previous paragraph. This calculation can be extended to determine DSBs distributed in other longer length intervals. By this information, we obtain a clear indication of whether DSBS are distributed in a confined small spatial region or more spread out on a DNA molecule. Correlation of this DSB distribution pattern with the type of radiation provides a simple measure for the assessment of ionization clustering. In **Figure 3**, we construct the number of DSBs per DNA for electron and Beryllium irradiated DNA samples to a dose of 6 kGy in relation to the fragment sizes to demonstrate the DSB spatial distribution on a DNA molecule. Clearly, Beryllium ions induce more dense and localized DSBs, whereas electrons generate more uniformly distributed DSBs on a DNA molecule, demonstrating the high degree of DNA damage clustering by high-LET irradiations.

We further calculated the RBE for DSB induction as a function of radiation quality. The RBE calculated in this report is defined

as the ratio of the number of DSBs per unit DNA molecule of a given type of radiation to that by Co-60 photon. **Table 1** gives the DSB per DNA molecule for the radiations investigated and the corresponding RBEs determined at 6 kGy. For comparison purposes, we also have included the RBE for neutron studied in a previous publication (52).

DISCUSSION

In this report, we employ AFM for the measurement of DNA fragmentation by the charged particles of Beryllium and Argon in comparison to that by the low-LET photon and electron to demonstrate the enhanced DNA fragmentation capability of high-LET radiations. As shown in the AFM images, short DNA fragments are produced after plasmid DNA exposure to both low- and high-LET radiations. However, the relative amounts of short DNA fragments are substantially greater after high-LET irradiations, with Beryllium and Argon ions, demonstrating a prevalence of clustered DNA DSBs produced by high-LET radiations not previously quantified due to limitations in the conventional biological techniques.

As discussed in the Section "Introduction," the RBE for cell killing reported in the literature are generally a few fold higher for high-LET radiations (4, 5), but the DSB induction as measured using gel electrophoresis or other biological techniques are approximately unity or only slightly higher (25), presenting a contradiction to the fundamental concept of lethality of DSBs. Using Monte Carlo modeling of radiation-induced DNA damage, the groups led by Paretzke and Goodhead have reported clustered DNA lesions after exposure of modeled DNA molecules to high-LET radiations (38, 41, 53, 54). Campa and coauthors have further calculated the frequency of short DNA fragments generation by high energy protons and ions (42). The prominence of short DNA fragments induced by high-LET radiations presented in this and our previous publications, as well as reports by other investigators, provide experimental validation of the model-predicted short DNA fragments (52, 55, 56). It is apparent that short DNA fragments were undetected by techniques exploiting the migratory property of DNA fragments in gels, leaving accounted the DSBs corresponding to short DNA fragments, in particular, DSBs induced by high-LET radiations. It appears likely that with short DNA fragments included, the DSB induction by high-LET radiations should correlate better to RBE for cell survival.

To evaluate the capacity for DNA strand breakage by radiations of different quality, we calculated the RBE for DSB induction by the radiations investigated in this report together with that by neutrons for which the DNA fragment size distributions have been reported before (52). As shown in **Table 1**, the RBE increases as the LET of radiation increases, demonstrating the greater capacity of DNA damage by high-LET radiations. The ability of AFM to image short DNA fragments has permitted measurement of DSBs produced in close proximity resulting from clustered DSBs by high-LET radiations, and therefore offers a sensitive technique to quantify clustered DSBs not easily measurable using conventional biological methods.

In a previous report, we investigated the biological significance of short DNA fragments in DNA damage and repair and their potentially important roles in cell survival and carcinogenesis (57). We evaluated DNA binding and rejoining by Ku and DNA-PK, two major DNA repair proteins involved in the non-homologous end-joining (NHEJ) pathway and confirmed reports by other investigators on the minimum DNA length requirements for protein binding and activation (58, 59). When DNA fragments are short, the challenge to rejoin and repair them by the cell's repair mechanisms becomes greater. Furthermore, the presence of un-rejoined and repaired short DNA fragments in cells can trigger genomic instability, leading to mutation or cell death by way of apoptosis (57, 60). Compared to longer DNA fragments, which are more frequently produced by low-LET radiations, short DNA fragments present a more lethal challenge to cellular repair mechanisms and survivability after exposure to high-LET radiations.

The fragment size distribution data for Co-60 photon and Argon ion at 10 kGy presented in this paper were for illustrative purpose only to show the greater capacity of high-LET radiations in generating short fragments. That data, as well as the data at 6 kGy presented in this report, are a subset of the range explored in our experiments. Naturally, it would be desirable to construct a complete dose–response for DSB induction for all the doses and radiation types investigated. However, contamination of certain samples has precluded AFM image acquisition of sufficient quality for more extensive analysis as we performed in our previous study of neutron and electron irradiations (55). Nonetheless, the DSB data at 6 kGy clearly show a radiation quality dependence of RBE for DSB induction.

The RBE for DSB induction has been measured for both cells and in aqueous solutions. Prise et al. summarized the DSB induction data for radiations of varying quality for various cell line (25). It was shown that the RBE generally remained approximately close to 1 for a wide range of LET values from 10.9 to 998 keV/μm. In a subsequent report, Prise et al. presented additional DSB induction data for a few additional ions in the LET range of 40–225 keV/μm obtained with the PFGE either using the fraction of activity released (FAR) or fragmentation method and showed a substantial difference in RBE values obtained with these two techniques (61). Again, the RBE values obtained with the FAR method remained close to 1 or less, but varied from 1.1 to 1.5 when measured using the fragmentation method. They concluded that the fragmentation method permitted quantification of shorter DNA fragments that were not measured with the FAR method and thus resulted in increased DSB collection.

The RBE values determined in this report were based on AFM measurement of individual DNA fragments induced in aqueous solution that were orders of magnitude shorter than what measured using the gel electrophoresis fragmentation method. The much larger RBE values obtained here reflect a much enhanced capability of AFM to measure short DNA fragments. It is, however, difficult to make a direct comparison of these RBE values to what Prise and coauthors have summarized, as our DNA model system is plasmid DNA in aqueous solution, while that in Prise's report were DNA in cellular environments. The different DNA configuration and the substantially greater scavenging capacity of cells influence greatly the induction of DSB. Nevertheless, the techniques employed for DSB measurement have much greater impact on the accuracy of RBE values determined.

Therapeutic application of proton and heavy charged-particle irradiation has been gaining increasing acceptance, recognition, and popularity in the radiation oncology community worldwide (62–64). Heavy charged particles possess highly desired dosimetric advantages over photon or electron irradiations, exemplified by their finite range in tissue and Bragg peak in energy deposition (65). Furthermore, the biological advantage, as represented by their greater RBE for cell survival, adds another important dimension to the medical application of charged-particle irradiation. As presented in this and previous studies, heavy charged-particle radiations produce significantly more short DNA fragments than do low-LET radiations. We propose that the greater RBE of high-LET radiations is a result of the increased production of short DNA fragments by high-LET radiations.

CONCLUSION

Atomic force microscopy imaging of plasmid DNA molecules as the DNA targets of irradiation demonstrates that heavy charged particles induce a significantly greater proportion of short DNA fragments than observed following low-LET irradiations. The increased short DNA fragment generation is attributed to clustered DNA DSB generation following high-LET irradiations. The increased short DNA fragment production may be a critical factor underlying the greater biological effectiveness of heavy charged-particle radiation.

AUTHOR CONTRIBUTIONS

DP designed, performed the experiments, data analyses, and wrote the manuscript; SC performed AFM imaging of the DNA samples; JR participated in electron and Co-60 irradiation experiments and reviewed the manuscript; AD participated in design of the experiments, reviewed, and edited the manuscript.

ACKNOWLEDGMENTS

The authors gratefully acknowledge the important contributions made by Barry L. Berman and Seldon Datz in arranging and participating in the irradiations performed at Oak Ridge National Laboratory and at HIMAC in Chiba, Japan. The authors are saddened that both Professors Berman and Datz have since passed away. The authors also gratefully acknowledge the technical and scientific staff at Oak Ridge and Chiba for their expertise in assisting performance of the irradiation experiments. Finally, the authors acknowledge the numerous hours Max Goldberg, a high school intern from Witmann High School in Bethesda, MD, USA, had spent on measuring the DNA fragment sizes.

REFERENCES

1. Curtis SB. Lethal and potentially lethal lesions induced by radiation – a unified repair model. *Radiat Res* (1986) 106(2):252–70. doi:10.2307/3576798

2. Frankenberg D, Frankenberg-Schwager M, Blöcher D, Harbich R. Evidence for DNA double-strand breaks as the critical lesions in yeast cells irradiated with sparsely or densely ionizing radiation under oxic or anoxic conditions. *Radiat Res* (1981) 88(3):524–32. doi:10.2307/3575641

3. Radford IR. The level of induced DNA double-strand breakage correlates with cell killing after X-irradiation. *Int J Radiat Biol Relat Stud Phys Chem Med* (1985) 48(1):45–54. doi:10.1080/09553008514551051

4. Barendsen G. RBE-LET relationships for different types of lethal radiation damage in mammalian cells: comparison with DNA DSB and an interpretation of differences in radiosensitivity. *Int J Radiat Biol* (1994) 66(5):433–6. doi:10.1080/09553009414551411

5. Blakely EA. Cell inactivation by heavy charged particles. *Radiat Environ Biophys* (1992) 31(3):181–96. doi:10.1007/BF01214826

6. Weber K, Flentje M. Lethality of heavy ion-induced DNA double-strand breaks in mammalian cells. *Int J Radiat Biol* (1993) 64(2):169–78. doi:10.1080/09553009314551261

7. Ward JF. The complexity of DNA damage: relevance to biological consequences. *Int J Radiat Biol* (1994) 66(5):427–32. doi:10.1080/09553009414551401

8. Prise KM, Folkard M, Newman HC, Michael BD. Effect of radiation quality on lesion complexity in cellular DNA. *Int J Radiat Biol* (1994) 66(5):537–42. doi:10.1080/09553009414551581

9. Martin RG, Ames BN. A method for determining the sedimentation behavior of enzymes: application to protein mixtures. *J Biol Chem* (1961) 236(5):1372–9.

10. Bradley MO, Kohn KW. X-ray induced DNA double strand break production and repair in mammalian cells as measured by neutral filter elution. *Nucleic Acids Res* (1979) 7(3):793–804. doi:10.1093/nar/7.3.793

11. Schwartz DC, Cantor CR. Separation of yeast chromosome-sized DNAs by pulsed field gradient gel electrophoresis. *Cell* (1984) 37(1):67–75. doi:10.1016/0092-8674(84)90301-5

12. Olive PL, Wlodek D, Banáth JP. DNA double-strand breaks measured in individual cells subjected to gel electrophoresis. *Cancer Res* (1991) 51(17):4671–6.

13. Smith CL, Klco SR, Cantor CR. Pulsed-field gel electrophoresis and the technology of large DNA molecules. In: Davies K, editor. *Genome Analysis: A Practical Approach*. Oxford, England: IRL Press (1988). p. 41–72.

14. Fairbairn DW, Olive PL, O'Neill KL. The comet assay: a comprehensive review. *Mutat Res* (1995) 339(1):37–59. doi:10.1016/0165-1110(94)00013-3

15. Collins AR. The comet assay for DNA damage and repair. *Mol Biotechnol* (2004) 26(3):249–61. doi:10.1385/MB:26:3:249

16. Pilch DR, Sedelnikova OA, Redon C, Celeste A, Nussenzweig A, Bonner WM. Characteristics of γ-H2AX foci at DNA double-strand breaks sites. *Biochem Cell Biol* (2003) 81(3):123–9. doi:10.1139/o03-042

17. Sedelnikova OA, Rogakou EP, Panyutin IG, Bonner WM. Quantitative detection of 125IdU-induced DNA double-strand breaks with γ-H2AX antibody. *Radiat Res* (2002) 158(4):486–92. doi:10.1667/0033-7587(2002)158[0486:QDOIID]2.0.CO;2

18. Kraxenberger F, Weber KJ, Friedl AA, Eckardt-Schupp F, Flentje M, Quicken P, et al. DNA double-strand breaks in mammalian cells exposed to Á-rays and very heavy ions. *Radiat Environ Biophys* (1998) 37(2):107–15. doi:10.1007/s004110050102

19. Ikpeme S, Löbrich M, Akpa T, Schneider E, Kiefer J. Heavy ion-induced DNA double-strand breaks with yeast as a model system. *Radiat Environ Biophys* (1995) 34(2):95–9. doi:10.1007/BF01275213

20. Obe G, Johannes C, Schulte-Frohlinde D. DNA double-strand breaks induced by sparsely ionizing radiation and endonucleases as critical lesions foe cell death, chromosomal aberrations, mutations and oncogenic transformation. *Mutagenesis* (1992) 7(1):3–12. doi:10.1093/mutage/7.1.3

21. Schulte-Frohlinde D. Biological consequences of strand breaks in plasmid and viral DNA. *Br J Cancer Suppl* (1987) 8:129.

22. Siddiqi MA, Bothe E. Single-and double-strand break formation in DNA irradiated in aqueous solution: dependence on dose and OH radical scavenger concentration. *Radiat Res* (1987) 112(3):449–63. doi:10.2307/3577098

23. Spotheim-Maurizot M, Charlier M, Sabattier R. DNA radiolysis by fast neutrons. *Int J Radiat Biol* (1990) 57(2):301–13. doi:10.1080/09553009014552421

24. Sutherland BM, Bennett PV, Sidorkina O, Laval J. Clustered DNA damages induced in isolated DNA and in human cells by low doses of ionizing radiation. *Proc Natl Acad Sci U S A* (2000) 97(1):103–8. doi:10.1073/pnas.97.1.103

25. Prise K, Ahnström G, Belli M, Carlsson J, Frankenberg D, Kiefer J, et al. A review of DSB induction data for varying quality radiations. *Int J Radiat Biol* (1998) 74(2):173–84. doi:10.1080/095530098141564

26. Prise KM, Davies S, Michael BD. The relationship between radiation-induced DNA double-strand breaks and cell kill in hamster V79 fibroblasts irradiated with 250 kVp X-rays, 2·3 MeV neutrons or 238Pu α-particles. *Int J Radiat Biol Relat Stud Phys Chem Med* (1987) 52(6):893–902. doi:10.1080/09553008714552481

27. Barendsen G. The relationships between RBE and LET for different types of lethal damage in mammalian cells: biophysical and molecular mechanisms. *Radiat Res* (1994) 139(3):257–70. doi:10.2307/3578823

28. Blöcher D. DNA double-strand break repair determines the RBE of α-particles. *Int J Radiat Biol* (1988) 54(5):761–71. doi:10.1080/09553008814552201

29. Frankenberg D, Frankenberg-Schwager M, Harbich R. Interpretation of the shape of survival curves in terms of induction and repair/misrepair of DNA double-strand breaks. *Br J Cancer Suppl* (1984) 6:233.

30. Frankenberg-Schwager M. Induction, repair and biological relevance of radiation-induced DNA lesions in eukaryotic cells. *Radiat Environ Biophys* (1990) 29(4):273–92. doi:10.1007/BF01210408

31. Frankenberg-Schwager M, Frankenberg D, Harbich R. Repair of DNA double-strand breaks as a determinant of RBE of alpha particles. *Br J Cancer Suppl* (1984) 6:169.

32. Hada M, Georgakilas AG. Formation of clustered DNA damage after high-LET irradiation: a review. *J Radiat Res* (2008) 49(3):203–10. doi:10.1269/jrr.07123

33. Holley WR, Chatterjee A. Clusters of DNA damage induced by ionizing radiation: formation of short DNA fragments. I. Theoretical modeling. *Radiat Res* (1996) 145(2):188–99. doi:10.2307/3579174

34. Löbrich PC, Cooper PK, Rydberg MB. Non-random distribution of DNA double-strand breaks induced by particle irradiation. *Int J Radiat Biol* (1996) 70(5):493–503. doi:10.1080/095530096144680

35. Friedland W, Dingfelder M, Kundrát P, Jacob P. Track structures, DNA targets and radiation effects in the biophysical Monte Carlo simulation code PARTRAC. *Mutat Res* (2011) 711(1):28–40. doi:10.1016/j.mrfmmm.2011.01.003

36. Friedland W, Jacob P, Paretzke HG, Merzagora M, Ottolenghi A. Simulation of DNA fragment distributions after irradiation with photons. *Radiat Environ Biophys* (1999) 38(1):39–47. doi:10.1007/s004110050136

37. Goodhead D. Molecular and cell models of biological effects of heavy ion radiation. *Radiat Environ Biophys* (1995) 34(2):67–72. doi:10.1007/BF01275208

38. Goodhead DT. Initial events in the cellular effects of ionizing radiations: clustered damage in DNA. *Int J Radiat Biol* (1994) 65(1):7–17. doi:10.1080/09553009414550021

39. Nikjoo H, O'Neill P, Terrissol M, Goodhead DT. Quantitative modelling of DNA damage using Monte Carlo track structure method. *Radiat Environ Biophys* (1999) 38(1):31–8. doi:10.1007/s004110050135

40. Semenenko V, Stewart R. Fast Monte Carlo simulation of DNA damage formed by electrons and light ions. *Phys Med Biol* (2006) 51(7):1693. doi:10.1088/0031-9155/51/7/004

41. Friedland W, Jacob P, Paretzke HG, Stork T. Monte Carlo simulation of the production of short DNA fragments by low-linear energy transfer radiation using higher-order DNA models. *Radiat Res* (1998) 150(2):170–82. doi:10.2307/3579852

42. Campa A, Ballarini F, Belli M, Cherubini R, Dini V, Esposito G, et al. DNA DSB induced in human cells by charged particles and gamma rays: experimental results and theoretical approaches. *Int J Radiat Biol* (2005) 81(11):841–54. doi:10.1080/09553000500530888

43. Binnig G, Quate CF, Gerber C. Atomic force microscope. *Phys Rev Lett* (1986) 56(9):930. doi:10.1103/PhysRevLett.56.930

44. Hansma HG, Vesenka J, Siegerist C, Kelderman G, Morrett H, Sinsheimer RL, et al. Reproducible imaging and dissection of plasmid DNA under liquid with the atomic force microscope. *Science* (1992) 256(5060):1180–4. doi:10.1126/science.256.5060.1180

45. Lyubchenko YL, Shlyakhtenko LS. AFM for analysis of structure and dynamics of DNA and protein-DNA complexes. *Methods* (2009) 47(3):206–13. doi:10.1016/j.ymeth.2008.09.002

46. Binnig G, Gerber CH, Stoll E, Albrecht TR, Quate CF. Atomic resolution with atomic force microscope. *EPL Europhys Lett* (1987) 3(12):1281. doi:10.1209/0295-5075/3/12/006

47. Williams DB, Carter CB. *The Transmission Electron Microscope*. New York: Springer (1996).

48. Tersoff J, Hamann D. *Theory of the Scanning Tunneling Microscope, in Scanning Tunneling Microscopy*. Netherlands: Springer (1985). p. 59–67.

49. Drake B, Prater CB, Weisenhorn AL, Gould SA, Albrecht TR, Quate CF, et al. Imaging crystals, polymers, and processes in water with the atomic force microscope. *Science* (1989) 243(4898):1586–9. doi:10.1126/science.2928794

50. Hansma HG, Bezanilla M, Zenhausern F, Adrian M, Sinsheimer RL. Atomic force microscopy of DNA in aqueous solutions. *Nucleic Acids Res* (1993) 21(3):505–12. doi:10.1093/nar/21.3.505

51. Hinterdorfer P, Baumgartner W, Gruber HJ, Schilcher K, Schindler H. Detection and localization of individual antibody-antigen recognition events by atomic force microscopy. *Proc Natl Acad Sci U S A* (1996) 93(8):3477–81. doi:10.1073/pnas.93.8.3477

52. Pang D, Berman BL, Chasovskikh S, Rodgers JE, Dritschilo A. Investigation of neutron-induced damage in DNA by atomic force microscopy: experimental evidence of clustered DNA lesions. *Radiat Res* (1998) 150(6):612–8. doi:10.2307/3579883

53. Ottolenghi A, Merzagora M, Tallone L, Durante M, Paretzke HG, Wilson WE. The quality of DNA double-strand breaks: a Monte Carlo simulation of the end-structure of strand breaks produced by protons and alpha particles. *Radiat Environ Biophys* (1995) 34(4):239–44. doi:10.1007/BF01209749

54. Goodhead DT. Mechanisms for the biological effectiveness of high-LET radiations. *J Radiat Res* (1999) 40(Suppl):S1–13. doi:10.1269/jrr.40.S1

55. Pang D, Rodgers JE, Berman BL, Chasovskikh S, Dritschilo A. Spatial distribution of radiation-induced double-strand breaks in plasmid DNA as resolved by atomic force microscopy. *Radiat Res* (2005) 164(6):755–65. doi:10.1667/RR3425.1

56. Psonka K, Gudowska-Nowaka E, Bronsb S, Elsässerb TH, Heissb M, Taucher-Scholz G. Ionizing radiation-induced fragmentation of plasmid DNA – atomic force microscopy and biophysical modeling. *Adv Space Res* (2007) 39(6):1043–9. doi:10.1016/j.asr.2007.02.089

57. Pang D, Winters TA, Jung M, Purkayastha S, Cavalli LR, Chasovkikh S, et al. Radiation-generated short DNA fragments may perturb non-homologous end-joining and induce genomic instability. *J Radiat Res* (2011) 52(3):309–19. doi:10.1269/jrr.10147

58. Ma Y, Lieber MR. DNA length-dependent cooperative interactions in the binding of Ku to DNA. *Biochemistry* (2001) 40(32):9638–46. doi:10.1021/bi010932v

59. Blier PR, Griffith AJ, Craft J, Hardin JA. Binding of Ku protein to DNA. Measurement of affinity for ends and demonstration of binding to nicks. *J Biol Chem* (1993) 268(10):7594–601.

60. Wang H, Wang X, Zhang P, Wang Y. The Ku-dependent non-homologous end-joining but not other repair pathway is inhibited by high linear energy transfer ionizing radiation. *DNA Repair* (2008) 7(5):725–33. doi:10.1016/j.dnarep.2008.01.010

61. Prise KM, Pinto M, Newman HC, Michael BD. A review of studies of ionizing radiation-induced double-strand break clustering. *Radiat Res* (2001) 156(5):572–6. doi:10.1667/0033-7587(2001)156[0572:AROSOI]2.0.CO;2

62. Levin WP, Kooy H, Loeffler JS, DeLaney TF. Proton beam therapy. *Br J Cancer* (2005) 93(8):849–54. doi:10.1038/sj.bjc.6602754

63. Hug EB, Loredo LN, Slater JD, DeVries A, Grove RI, Schaefer RA, et al. Proton radiation therapy for chordomas and chondrosarcomas of the skull base. *J Neurosurg* (1999) 91(3):432–9. doi:10.3171/jns.1999.91.3.0432

64. Schulz-Ertner D, Tsujii H. Particle radiation therapy using proton and heavier ion beams. *J Clin Oncol* (2007) 25(8):953–64. doi:10.1200/JCO.2006.09.7816

65. Kjellberg RN, Hanamura T, Davis KR, Lyons SL, Adams RD. Bragg-peak proton-beam therapy for arteriovenous malformations of the brain. *N Engl J Med* (1983) 309(5):269–74. doi:10.1056/NEJM198308043090503

4

Effects of Charged Particles on Human Tumor Cells

Kathryn D. Held[1]*, Hidemasa Kawamura[2,3], Takuya Kaminuma[1,2,3], Athena Evalour S. Paz[2], Yukari Yoshida[2], Qi Liu[1], Henning Willers[1] and Akihisa Takahashi[2]

[1] Department of Radiation Oncology, Massachusetts General Hospital, Harvard Medical School, Boston, MA, USA, [2] Gunma University Heavy Ion Medical Center, Gunma, Japan, [3] Department of Radiation Oncology, Gunma University Graduate School of Medicine, Gunma, Japan

*Correspondence:
Kathryn D. Held
kheld@mgh.harvard.edu

The use of charged particle therapy in cancer treatment is growing rapidly, in large part because the exquisite dose localization of charged particles allows for higher radiation doses to be given to tumor tissue while normal tissues are exposed to lower doses and decreased volumes of normal tissues are irradiated. In addition, charged particles heavier than protons have substantial potential clinical advantages because of their additional biological effects, including greater cell killing effectiveness, decreased radiation resistance of hypoxic cells in tumors, and reduced cell cycle dependence of radiation response. These biological advantages depend on many factors, such as endpoint, cell or tissue type, dose, dose rate or fractionation, charged particle type and energy, and oxygen concentration. This review summarizes the unique biological advantages of charged particle therapy and highlights recent research and areas of particular research needs, such as quantification of relative biological effectiveness (RBE) for various tumor types and radiation qualities, role of genetic background of tumor cells in determining response to charged particles, sensitivity of cancer stem-like cells to charged particles, role of charged particles in tumors with hypoxic fractions, and importance of fractionation, including use of hypofractionation, with charged particles.

Keywords: charged particles, proton therapy, carbon-ion therapy, relative biological effectiveness, clustered DNA damage, cancer stem cells, hypoxic radioresistance, altered fractionation

INTRODUCTION

Radiation therapy is a mainstay of cancer treatment, being a common and effective therapy for both curative and palliative treatment of cancer patients. In the last few decades, there has been increasing use of charged particles in radiation therapy. Protons were first proposed for use in cancer therapy by Robert R. Wilson (1), and the number of patients treated with protons has increased dramatically in recent years to a total of over 100,000 patients now treated worldwide (http://www.ptcog.ch/index.php/facilities-in-operation). Radiation treatment of cancer with helium ions began at Berkeley in the late 1950s and was expanded to heavier ions in the 1970s [see a review of the history of charged particles by Skarsgard (2)]. Much of the emphasis has been on carbon ions, with most patients treated in Japan and now totaling over 10,000 patients treated worldwide. The major clinical advantage of protons and heavier charged particles, such as carbon, comes from physics: the Bragg curve provides excellent radiation dose distributions [see reviews in Ref. (3, 4)]. In addition, heavier ions, e.g., carbon, offer the potential of additional biological gains such as increased relative biological effectiveness (RBE) and decreased oxygen enhancement ratio (OER) due to their higher linear energy transfer (LET) in the Bragg peak region, where the tumor is located [reviewed, e.g., in Ref. (3, 5, 6)].

Despite the often-made assumption that the RBE for tumor cells is higher than that for normal cells irradiated under identical conditions, there is only a limited amount of experimental *in vitro* data that support that assertion (3). However, there have been interesting recent research findings on the differential DNA repair pathways of cancer cells after particle versus photon irradiation, new studies on the effects of charged particles on cancer stem cells, and increasing questions about different responses of tumor and normal cells to hypofractionation, especially with charged particle irradiations, suggest that there may be novel ways to take advantage of differences in characteristics of tumor cells from normal cells to improve or better tailor the use of charged particles in cancer therapy. This review will discuss these issues, with emphasis on data on responses of human tumor cells, largely based on *in vitro* findings. As discussed in more detail below, RBE is a complex quantity, depending on physical parameters, such as particle type and energy, dose and LET, and biological parameters, including cell/tissue type, cell cycle phase, oxygen level, and endpoint. *In vitro* assays have limitations compared to *in vivo* studies and the clinical situation due to lack of 3D architecture and microenvironmental context, including interactions among various cell types, vasculature, and immune system influences. Nevertheless, for studies of RBE, *in vitro* assays are critical for systematic testing and characterization of effects of various ions, elucidation of DNA damage pathways, and the importance of DNA repair processes and other genetic factors. Furthermore, *in vitro* studies provide experimental tests for validation of biophysical models, e.g., the local effects model (LEM), prior to clinical application (7), and yield insight on systematic variations in RBE relevant to clinical use (8, 9).

In this review, we start with brief overview sections on the unique biological advantages of charged particle therapy and DNA damage responses that may be important for particle therapy. That introduction is followed by consideration of recent findings on RBEs in human tumor cells, including discussion of the possible roles of genetic factors on RBE, then discussions of new findings on cancer stem cells, hypoxia, and fractionation. In particular, we stress approaches to use the increasing knowledge of the properties of tumors and tumor cells to better advantage when using charged particles in cancer therapy.

AN OVERVIEW OF THE UNIQUE BIOLOGICAL ADVANTAGES OF CHARGED PARTICLE THERAPY

A number of reviews [e.g., in Ref. (3–5)] have discussed the substantial dose distribution advantages of charged particles where, as a result of the Bragg peak, normal tissues can be spared by limiting dose to them, while maximum dose is deposited in the tumor. Heavier ions, such as carbon, have an additional dose distribution advantage over protons because of their reduced lateral scattering compared to protons. However, the major potential advantage of heavier ions in tumor irradiations is their enhanced biological effects, which include increased cell killing, decreased protection

by hypoxia, decreased effect of fractionation, and decreased cell cycle dependence. The biological effectiveness of cell killing by higher LET radiations is usually quantified by use of RBE, the ratio of the dose of low-LET radiation (usually X-rays or gamma-rays) to dose of high-LET radiation (e.g., charged particle) for the same biological effect. Many *in vitro* studies over the years have shown the bell-shaped dependence of RBE for cell killing on LET (6, 10–12) wherein RBE increases with LET to a maximum at about 30–150 keV/μm, then decreases at higher LET. The LET value at which the RBE is maximal depends on the individual ion species, with the peak at higher LET with increasing atomic number of the ions (2). Furthermore, it has also long been recognized that there is great variation in the absolute values of RBE because RBE depends on numerous factors, including particle type and energy, cell type, experimental endpoint, cell cycle phase, dose and dose rate, oxygenation status, culture conditions, etc. (6, 7, 11).

The increased biological effectiveness of radiations with increasing LET lies in the physical dose distribution of the energy of the particles on the micro, and even nano, scale as they traverse matter, the clustering of DNA damages that results from the particle tracks and the increased difficulty cells have in accurately repairing the clustered damage (13–16). As energetic charged particles traverse matter, e.g., cells and tissues of organisms, their electronic interactions with atoms and molecules, mostly through inelastic collisions with atomic electrons, create a path, or track of ionizations before they run out of energy at a finite range, the Bragg peak. The tracks of heavy charged particles are fairly straight, but the electrons ejected from atoms along the track, being much lighter, follow paths that are quite tortuous, with their ranges depend on the energy they acquired when ejected. LET is a measure of the energy imparted to matter by the passage of an ionizing particle. Along the path of a charged particle, the three-dimensional distribution of energy depositions, which cause ionizations and excitations, is called the track structure. For low-LET sparsely ionizing radiations, there are relatively long distances between the energy depositions except at track ends, but with increasing LET, the ionizations along the track become denser and there is lateral spread of the track due to delta-ray electrons, the spectrum of which is determined by the velocity of the heavy charged particle.

If the ionizations from radiation were randomly distributed in cells, the consequences of those energy depositions would likely be minimal, but the non-randomness of the energy depositions accounts for the increased effectiveness of ionizing radiation (14, 17, 18). The clustering of ionizations along radiation tracks occurs on the same scale as the diameter of a DNA molecule and nucleosomes such that if a track traverses DNA it can effectively create clustered DNA damages, such as double-strand breaks (DSBs), clusters of two or more base damages, or clusters of single-strand breaks with base damages. As LET of radiation increases, the clustering becomes more complex, creating, for example, a complex DSB where the break is associated with additional damages, such as base changes or single-strand breaks. Both the proportion and degree of complexity increase with high-LET radiations (19). A number of studies have shown that the complex DNA damages produced by high-LET radiations are repaired less rapidly, less accurately, and less completely than damages from low-LET photons [reviewed recently in Ref. (20, 21)]. Additionally, it is important to bear in mind that track structure has biological relevance not only at the level of DNA damage but also at higher levels of chromatin organization (17): a single high-LET particle track passing through a cell nucleus may cause correlated damages through chromatin structures, such as chromatin fibers, or in adjacent chromosome territories *via* a string of DSBs along its path, and these correlated damages may result in complex chromosome aberrations. Altogether, the net effect is that complex DNA damages resulting from the greater clustering of ionizations with increasing LET of radiation increases the production of all chromosome aberrations, simple as well as complex.

The increased DNA damage complexity and decreased repair accuracy with radiations of increasing LET not only cause increased cell killing but also result in decreased cell cycle dependence of that killing and play a factor in the decrease in OER. Cells exposed to low-LET radiation show increased resistance when irradiated in late S-phase and increased sensitivity when irradiated in M-phase (22). This fluctuation through the cell cycle decreases with higher LET radiations. However, since in many tumors, the majority of cells are not in the radiation-resistant phases, this effect on treatment outcome in irradiated tumors is likely to be modest (3). The importance of the decreased OER with high LET is discussed below.

Although there has been increasing interest in recent years in the so-called "non-targeted" effects of radiation, including bystander effects and genomic instability in progeny of irradiated cells [for recent reviews, see Ref. (23, 24)], it remains far from clear whether non-targeted effects are similar or different after irradiation with photons versus charged particles (25–27). Furthermore, the role of non-targeted effects or intercellular signaling in response of tumors to radiation remains under investigation (28, 29), with very little work having been done with charged particles. This review is limited to discussion of targeted effects of charge particles.

OVERVIEW OF DNA DAMAGE RESPONSES RELEVANT TO CHARGED PARTICLE BIOLOGY

Central to any consideration of the effects of charged particles on cells and tissues must be DNA damage response processes. Cells have two main pathways for the repair of radiation-induced DSBs: non-homologous end-joining (NHEJ) and homologous recombination (HR) (30–32). NHEJ is active throughout the cell cycle and is responsible for the repair of most DSBs in cells. NHEJ involves the initial binding of the Ku70/Ku80 heterodimer, recruitment of DNA–PKcs and eventual ligation of the DNA ends by XRCC4–DNA Ligase IV. However, NHEJ is an error-prone repair, and the quality of its repair processes can decrease with increasing levels of DNA damage. HR is active primarily during the S/G2 phases of the cell cycle, when a homologous DNA region is available, and generally results in the preservation of the original DNA sequence. HR involves DSB recognition by the MRN complex (Mre11, Rad50, Nbs1), 3′–5′ DNA resection, DNA stabilization by replication protein A (RPA), Rad51-mediated

formation of Holliday junctions, and ultimately resolution of the Holliday junction (31, 33). HR is also involved in the repair and restart of collapsed DNA replication forks (34). At the forks, the BRCA1/2-dependent HR pathway converges with the Fanconi anemia (FA) pathway to resolve the damage (35). It has been suggested that unrepaired clustered DNA damages that collide with replication forks in cells in S-phase require HR for DNA repair and replication restart (36, 37).

It also has been reported that the end-resection activity in cells in the G1 phase may promote micro-homology-mediated end joining (MMEJ) to repair DSBs that cannot be repaired efficiently by NHEJ (38). However, it is unknown how much the activation of HR and MMEJ pathways contribute to escaping cell death in high-LET-irradiated cells. Recently, we showed that targeting and suppressing NHEJ repair yields a high radiosensitivity in cells exposed to carbon-ion beams when compared to the suppression of HR repair (39).

RBEs OF CHARGED PARTICLES IN HUMAN TUMOR CELLS

Experimental studies to determine RBEs have been conducted for many years, with the majority using clonogenic cell survival as the endpoint. It has been felt that lack of clonogenicity is a highly relevant indicator of the efficacy of radiation and its modification because eradication of tumor cells is needed to cure tumors (22). In fact, the shape of curves of tumor control probability, as detected in a clinical context, can be explained from the random nature of tumor cell killing by radiation and the need to kill every cell, as a single cell may give rise to tumor regrowth (22). Furthermore, RBE values, measured or predicted by computer models, are used in clinical treatment planning approaches, which are continually being updated [e.g., Ref. (40, 41)].

It has been argued recently that further studies measuring RBE values may be of limited usefulness because they will have little impact on reducing the uncertainties in ion beam therapy (4, 6). However, determinations of RBEs can help guide understanding of mechanistic underpinnings to the increased effectiveness of higher LET radiations and, thus, may lead to better identification, based on genetic profiles or biomarker evaluation, of patients' tumors that may benefit most from charged particle therapy.

Shifting the Paradigm of a Generic RBE for Clinical Proton Beam Therapy

Clinical proton beam therapy has been based on the use of a generic RBE of ~1.1 at the center of the spread-out Bragg peak (SOBP) for cancer as well as for normal tissues (8). This RBE value represents an average of a wide range of experimental data *in vitro* and *in vivo* and has been intended to be a conservative estimate (8, 42). However, there is now a growing appreciation that the use of a generic value ignores RBE variations that may result, for example, from the heterogeneity of human cancers, LET variations along the SOBP, or the particular clinical endpoint under consideration (42–46). In this section, we will focus primarily on recent data that indicate a dependence of RBE on certain DNA repair defects, with the implication being that proton therapy may have a biological advantage in human tumors that harbor such defects.

There exists very little experimental data on RBE variations in human cancers. In a 2002 review by Paganetti and colleagues (8), the average RBE at the mid-SOBP was estimated as ~1.2 in vitro and ~1.1 in vivo. However, most of the 20 cell lines considered in that analysis were of rodent origin resulting in a somewhat higher in vitro RBE. Only seven human cancer cell lines were included. There is growing evidence for considerable genomic heterogeneity across cancers even of the same type and histology, and it is increasingly appreciated that much of the variations in treatment sensitivity observed clinically are due to genomic heterogeneity, which may include alterations of DNA repair pathways (47–49). Therefore, it is highly doubtful that small numbers of non-representative cell lines are adequate pre-clinical models for assessing clinically relevant variations in RBE values in human cancers. In a recent screen of 17 lung cancer cell lines, RBE estimates at the mid-SOBP of a clinical beam relative to Co60 photons [Co60 equivalent (Eq)] ranged from 0.93 to 1.77 and 1.09 to 1.48 for clonogenic survival fractions of 0.5 and 0.1, respectively (44). In five cell lines (29%), the RBE increase was statistically different from 1.1. Furthermore, in at least three of these cell lines, the RBE increase correlated with defects in the so-called FA/BRCA pathway of DNA repair, and this observation was confirmed in several isogenic cell line models. The FA/BRCA pathway is critical for the maintenance and repair of DNA replication forks [reviewed in Ref. (34, 50)]. Inactivation of any of the FA/BRCA genes has been known to result in hypersensitivity to a variety of anti-cancer agents. However, apart from an involvement of the RAD51 recombinase (FANCR) in the cellular response to proton radiation (43, 51), the importance of the FA/BRCA genes for the repair of proton damage to DNA had been unknown. These observations are clinically significant because genetic or epigenetic defects in the FA/BRCA pathway have been found in large subsets of human cancers (34).

What are the mechanisms through which the FA/BRCA pathway acts on proton damage? For low-LET radiation, which includes X-rays and protons, it has been estimated that 20–40% of the initial damage is clustered, and the majority of clustered damage is present as non-DSB damage (52, 53). Proton radiation causes slightly more complex clustered DNA damages than photons, which is a reflection of the different LET values, i.e., ~2.5 keV/µm for protons at mid-SOBP versus ~0.3–2.0 keV/µm for different photon radiations. DNA repair-proficient tumor cells and normal cells remove these damages almost equally well, consistent with a proton RBE of 1.1 (Co60Eq). Because the FA genes are specifically involved in replication fork maintenance and repair, it can be inferred that the RBE increase that is seen with defects in this pathway results from impaired repair of forks that collide with clustered proton damages. The requirement for the FA/BRCA pathway is greater for proton damage compared to damage caused by, for example, X-rays, even though the RBE (Co60Eq) and LET of these two radiation modalities are almost identical [RBE(Co60) ~1.1 and LET = 2.0–2.5 keV/µm]. This is illustrated in **Figure 1A**. Proton-irradiated FA/BRCA-defective cells will accumulate greater numbers of DNA DSB in S-phase and subsequently G2-phase than X-irradiated cells, as has been shown

experimentally (44) (Willers et al., unpublished). Interestingly, an increase in the size of DSB-associated foci persisting after proton irradiation has been observed (44), likely signifying unrepaired clustered damages (**Figure 1A**). It has been proposed that these DSB foci could serve as predictive biomarkers to identify cancers that may be more susceptible to proton beam therapy (44). Alternatively, genetic or epigenetic defects in the FA/BRCA pathway could be detected through genomics techniques in order to identify patients for proton therapy. This approach will require a more detailed knowledge of the genes involved in the cellular response to clustered proton damages. The available data indicate that functional loss of any of several key genes in the FA/BRCA pathway will increase the RBE, with the best current estimate being an average RBE of 1.33 (95% confidence limits, 1.25–1.41) at mid-SOBP as shown in **Figure 1B**. This is a conservative estimate derived at a surviving fraction of 0.1. For 0.5 survival fraction, which is more applicable to fraction sizes of 2 Gy as used in the clinic and which overlaps with the shoulder of the survival curves, the RBE values of the most proton-sensitive cell lines tended to be even higher than for 0.1 survival fraction. For example, the five most sensitive lung cancer cell lines in the report by Liu et al. (44) had an average RBE of 1.30 (range, 1.22–1.48) and 1.46 (range, 1.31–1.77) at survival fractions of 0.1 and 0.5, respectively.

In conclusion, these recent pre-clinical data strongly suggest inter-tumoral heterogeneity of proton RBE that may yield opportunities to identify proton susceptible tumors in the clinic within the next few years. This "New Biology" of protons in cancer coupled with the increasing knowledge of RBE variations as a function of physical proton beam parameters in both cancers and normal tissues is expected to shift the paradigm of a generic proton RBE to a variable RBE.

RBE Determinations with Heavy Charged Particles

The proton studies just described provide a possible DNA repair capacity-based explanation for some of the variation seen in proton RBE values at a given LET. Could a similar finding apply to human tumors exposed to high-LET charged particles? Unfortunately, no single study with a substantial number of cell lines has yet been done for any heavy ion, although many small studies with a few cell lines each have been performed. Some large compilations of cell survival RBE values for many cell types, endpoints and radiation qualities have been published recently (7, 54, 55), and the composite data clearly show that RBEs depend on LET, endpoint, ion, etc. In this section, we focus on analysis of RBE values for human tumor cells exposed to ions heavier than protons. Published papers that describe the cell survival RBE of human tumor cells have been searched by using PubMed; many of these papers are included in the compilations mentioned. A total of 430 RBE values were collected from 36 published papers (56–91). When authors provided RBE values along with dose–response data, those values were used. In cases where authors showed dose–response curves but did not cite any RBE value, an isoeffect line was drawn in the dose–response curves to read corresponding doses of ions and reference photons. As reference beam, 30 papers used X-rays and 6 papers used gamma-rays.

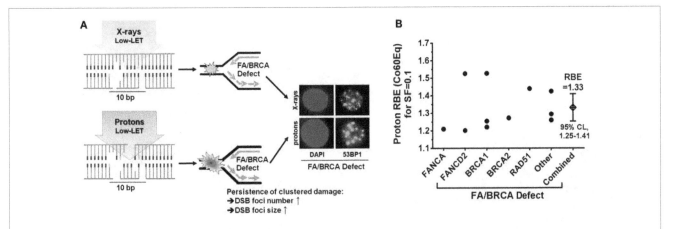

FIGURE 1 | A "New Biology" of proton beam therapy. (A) Illustration of how FA/BRCA defects may sensitize cells to proton irradiation. Left, clustered DNA damages after equal physical doses of X-rays and mid-SOBP protons are slightly different despite similar LET (2–2.5 keV/μm) and identical RBE in repair-proficient cells (~1.1). In the presence of a FA/BRCA defect that affects the repair of replication forks encountering clustered damages, there will be greater unrepaired damage after proton-irradiation, as marked by an increased number and relative size of repair-related protein accumulations of DNA double-strand break markers. Representative immunofluorescence microscopy images showing nucleus (DAPI) and 53BP1 foci (green) in FANCD2-mutant cells are shown on the right.
(B) Summary of RBE estimates relative to Co60 photons as a function of defects in the FA/BRCA pathway (44, 45). Other, taken from unpublished data (Willers et al.); CoEq, Co60 equivalent; SF, surviving fraction; CL, confidence limits.

For the analyses here, the biological differences in effect between X-rays and gamma-rays were not considered.

Endpoint

Endpoint is one of the major factors, which affects the values of RBE (7, 54, 55, 92). The RBE data as a function of LET sorted by endpoint are shown in **Figures 2** and **3**. All papers included in **Figure 2** presented RBE values for colony formation after exposure to a range of single doses. Within a total of 363 RBE values, 295 values in 31 papers were calculated using an isoeffect dose of 10% survival (D10). The other values that were calculated included D0, D30, D50, D75, ratio of alpha parameters, or isodose effectiveness. The RBE values for D10 ranged from 1.03 to 4.99, showing the "classic" increase in RBE with LET followed by a decrease at higher LET (22) although the range in RBE values at any given LET is substantial in many cases. The RBE values based on D0, D30, D50, and D75 also showed considerable variation at any given LET, but, as expected, there was a trend for higher RBE values at higher levels of survival (22). Some of the highest RBE values were derived using the alpha ratio; this, too, is consistent with higher RBEs at higher survival, since alpha ratios would tend to be derived based on high survival data.

The other endpoint that tends to show high RBE values is apoptosis (**Figure 3B**). This is consistent with the observations that most solid tumor cell lines are resistant to X-ray-induced apoptosis (93) and that apoptosis may be characterized by the alpha-component of the cell survival curve [reviewed, e.g., in Ref. (94)]. In a recent review on proton radiobiology, Tommasino and Durante (95) pointed out that there is a general tendency for an increased apoptotic response with increasing LET and that tumor cells resistant to photon-induced apoptosis may have apoptosis triggered by an alternative pathway by protons, a suggestion that could likely extend to heavier charged particles. However, it should also be pointed out that several groups, including Brown

and colleagues (96), have demonstrated that apoptosis induction can be markedly affected by tumor cell genetics and the overall level of cell killing as determined in a clonogenic assay *in vitro* may not correlate well with apoptosis induction [also reviewed in Ref. (94)].

Two papers reported RBE values calculated for residual unrepaired chromatin breaks using premature chromosome condensation (PCC) (**Figure 3A**), with the paper by Suzuki et al. using primary cells obtained by biopsy from patients (67, 72). Authors of both studies noted the good correlation between their data on residual chromatin breaks as measured using the PCC technique and colony formation, and concluded that the PCC technique was a potential predictive assay of tumor response to ion therapy. Information on correlation of chromatin breaks using PCC with DNA repair protein foci formation and/or FA/BRCA pathway status, as discussed above for potential use with proton therapy patients, would be helpful for assessment of possible predictive assays.

Ion

The data on RBE values calculated using D10 and sorted by ions are shown in **Figure 4**. A total of 29 papers reported 247 RBE values for carbon-ion beam, whereas there were 21 RBE values for helium ions in 3 papers, 24 values for neon ion in 2 papers, 6 values for boron ions in 1 paper, 6 values for silicon beam in 2 papers, 5 values for iron beam in 3 papers, 2 values for nitrogen beam in one paper, and 3 values for argon beam in 2 papers. The RBE values showed substantial variation at any given LET, independent of ion species used, but in all cases the RBE increased with LET to a maximum then decreased at high-LET levels. It is well known that the RBE values of carbon ions peak around an LET of 100 keV/μm (7, 54, 55, 92). The other ion beams had peaks between LETs of 100 and 200 keV/μm, with a trend toward a maximum at higher LET with heavier ions.

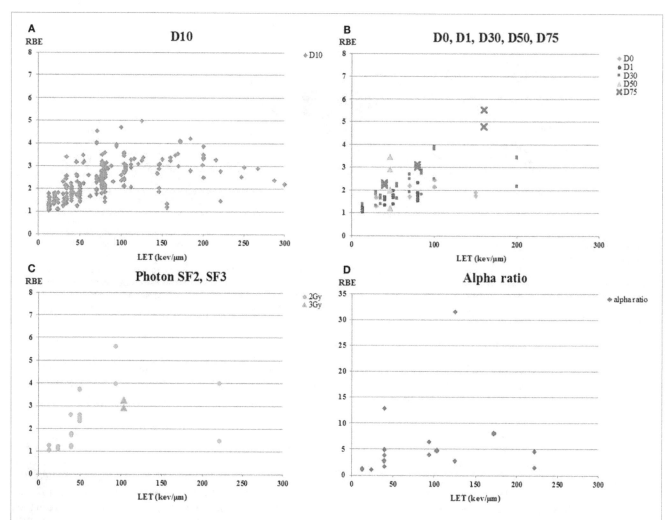

FIGURE 2 | RBE versus LET for human tumor cell lines for various endpoints. RBE values are all based on colony formation assays. (A) RBE values calculated as the ratio of isoeffect doses at 10% survival (D10). (B) RBE values calculated as ratios of doses for D0, D30, D50, and D75. D0 was calculated by fitting the survival curve to the single-hit multi-target (SHMT) model: $S/S0 = 1 - (1 - e^{-D/D0})^n$. (C) RBE values calculated as the ratio of doses at the level of photon doses of 2 Gy (SF2) or 3 Gy (SF3). (D) RBE values calculated as the ratios of the alpha parameters of survival curves.

Furusawa et al. (59) exposed human salivary gland tumor cells to carbon, neon, and helium ion beams and calculated the RBE values of each beam. They showed that the RBE values for helium ions were higher than those for the other ions, which seems unexpected. This finding deserves more investigation as there is some interest in development of helium ion beams for cancer therapy since they have less lateral dose than protons (i.e., a better dose distribution) (97), which might make their use particularly relevant in children. Furthermore, in their report, Furusawa et al. show that the peaks of the RBE values shifted to higher LET values with increasing atomic number, an observation that had been made earlier on the basis of work by a number of authors [e.g., Ref. (11, 98, 99)] as reviewed by Skarsgard (2). Such findings deserve emphasis as they highlight the fact that LET is not adequate as the sole descriptor of energy deposition in cells and tissues, but that ion track structure, the nanometer scale distribution of energy, must be considered when evaluating biological effects. In this context, it is interesting to note that NASA's

model for calculating risk of radiation-induced cancer from space radiation takes into account track structure of heavy ions rather than simply LET (100). In a clinical context in heavy ion therapy, the LEM, which is used for RBE prediction, also provides particle species and LET-specific RBE values that are then propagated, using a treatment planning system, to a representative RBE value at each position in the irradiated field (9, 101), a process needed because ion fragmentation produces a mixed radiation field.

With regard to ions, it is worth pointing out that we did not include data with oxygen ions in **Figure 4** because we found only one study using oxygen ions, and that work used only a single LET (87). That work reported that for four human hepatocellular carcinoma cell lines irradiated in the SOPB of oxygen ions with a mean energy of 154 MeV/u (LET of 146 keV/µm), the clonogenic RBE_{10} values ranged from 1.9 to 3.1, with the values not being significantly different from those obtained in the same study using 130 MeV/u carbon ions (LET of 112 keV/µm). However, this study is noteworthy because of the current interest in using

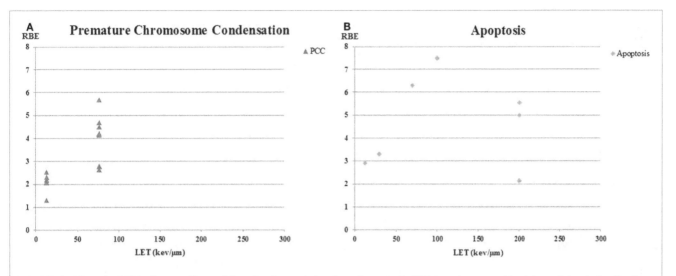

FIGURE 3 | **RBE versus LET for human tumor cell lines for chromatin breaks and apoptosis**. **(A)** is from data on unrejoined chromatin breaks in cells after premature chromosome condensation (PCC). Residual unrejoined chromatin breaks were detected using Giemsa staining in cells after chromatin condensation. **(B)** is RBE values for apoptosis.

oxygen ions, with their lower OER, in treating tumors with large hypoxic fractions (102).

Type of Tumor Cells

The data on RBE values as a function of LET for carbon-ion beam only, calculated using D10 and sorted by tumor type, are shown in **Figure 5**. **Figure 6** shows a subset of the data separated out by adenocarcinoma and squamous cell carcinoma. The graphs show data only for LET < 100 keV/µm. The number of data points, or cell lines, varies greatly with tumor type. Generally, the brain tumors (composite slope of 0.018) and adenocarcinomas (composite slope of 0.018) appear to have lower slopes for the RBE versus LET curves than do squamous cell carcinomas (composite slope of 0.024 or higher). It should be noted, however, that data from Suzuki et al. (71) for cervical cancer included in the squamous cell carcinoma graph were derived from primary cultured cells from biopsies from patients, the only data from primary cultures included in this analysis. These primary culture data appear to have lower slopes than the other squamous cell data, although it should also be noted that the steeper slopes for the established squamous carcinoma cell lines are determined by only four data points at high-LET values. Thus, it is not possible to determine whether there is a systematic difference between primary squamous cell cultures compared to established tumor cell lines or between squamous cell carcinomas and adenocarcinomas. It is not clear from clinical data with carbon ions whether a difference exists between sensitivity of squamous tumors and adenocarcinomas, suggesting an area for further *in vitro*, *in vivo*, and/or clinical study. For comparison, it can be pointed out that in a similar analysis approach, Ando (54) found that the RBE versus LET plot for cultured human fibroblasts had a slope of 0.027, which the author noted was steeper than the composite slope for the human tumor data he analyzed.

The RBE values for the pancreas cancer cells are the lowest in all the data (64). The slope of the graph of pancreas is 0.0084, which is gentler than the others. This might suggest that pancreatic cancer would not be a good candidate for carbon-ion therapy, yet clinical trials of carbon ions for pancreas cancer in Japan have shown promising results (4, 103). The clinical results may reflect properties of the human tumors *in situ*, such as high hypoxia, radioresistance (high cancer stem cell component?), and anatomic location, that might not be evident in studies of isolated tumor cells.

It is noteworthy that there are few tumor cell data on RBE values with charged particles for prostate cancer or bone and soft tissue cancers, which are the two cancer types with the most patients treated to-date with carbon ions at NIRS in Japan (103). Furthermore, we found no experimental RBE data for human cell lines of mucosal malignant melanoma, adenoid cystic carcinoma, or rectal carcinoma, which are all being treated with carbon ions at NIRS with favorable outcomes (103).

D10 has been used as the parameter for calculating RBE values in this analysis by tumor type (**Figures 5** and **6**) because that is the parameter most frequently reported in the literature. However, the use of D10 may have minimized the ability to see differences between tumor cell types, resulting in the relatively similar values of the slopes of the RBE versus LET curves for the various tumor cells. Generally, inherent photon radiosensitivity differences between cell types become most evident at high and low cell survival levels, and it has long been recognized that RBE values are larger at high survival levels than at low ones because of the "shoulder" on photon survival curves (22). For example, this is consistent with the data shown in **Figure 2** where RBEs based on alpha ratio (generally reflecting high survival, low dose results) tend to be higher than those based on D10. Since it has been shown that photon dose–response curves for different tumor cell types have significant differences [e.g., Ref. (104, 105)], one might expect that the RBE

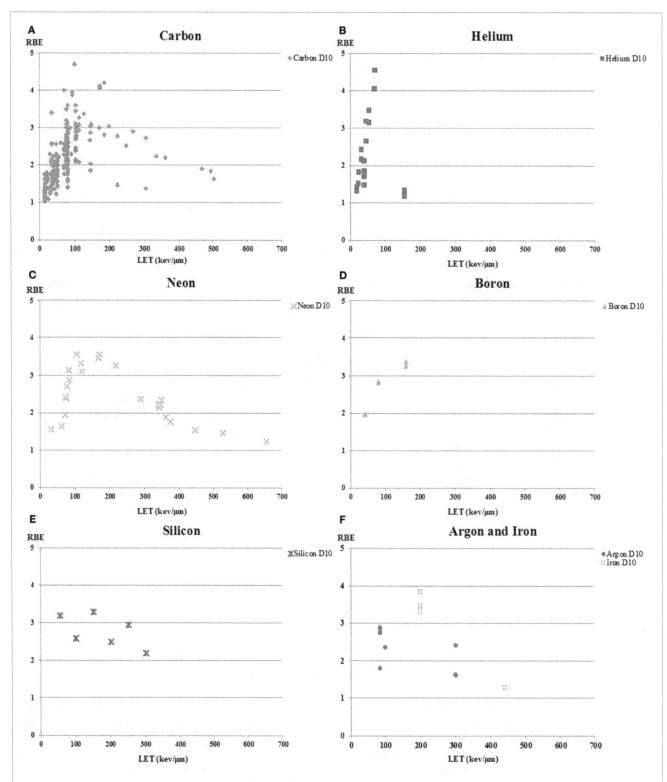

FIGURE 4 | RBE at 10% survival (D10) versus LET for human tumor cell lines exposed to various charged particles heavier than protons. RBE values derived at 10% survival from clonogenic survival curves from all available literature are shown as a function of LET for human tumor cells exposed to **(A)** carbon ions; **(B)** helium ions; **(C)** neon ions; **(D)** boron ions; **(E)** silicon ions; and **(F)** argon and iron ions. The RBE values showed substantial variation at any given LET, independent of ion species, but in all cases the RBE increased with LET to a maximum, then decreased at high-LET levels.

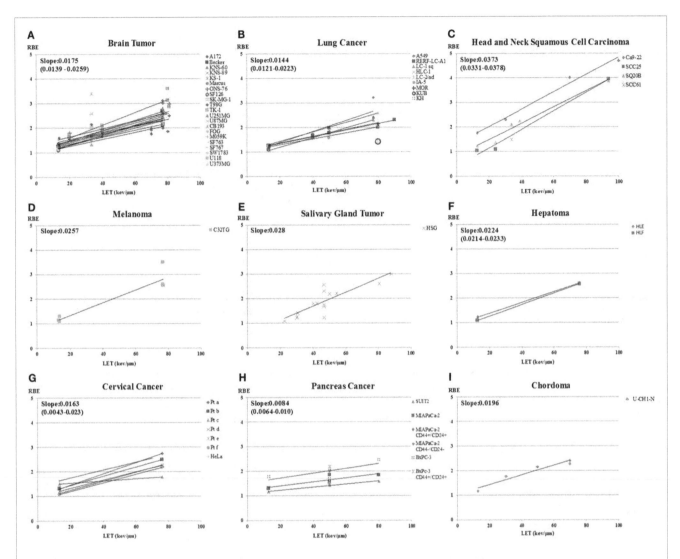

FIGURE 5 | RBE at 10% survival versus LET for cells from various types of human tumors exposed to carbon ions. RBE values as a function of LET for carbon-ion beam only, calculated using D10 and sorted by tumor type, are shown. Tumor types included are: **(A)** brain tumor; **(B)** lung cancer; **(C)** head and neck squamous cell carcinoma; **(D)** melanoma; **(E)** salivary gland tumor; **(F)** hepatoma; **(G)** cervical cancer; **(H)** pancreatic cancer and **(I)** chordoma. The graphs include data only for LET < 100 keV/μm. The number of data points, or cell lines, varies greatly with tumor type. The slopes of the RBE versus LET curves are calculated for each cell line and tumor type.

versus LET curves would also differ in a manner consistent with the photon sensitivity. The finding here (**Figures 5** and **6**) that the differences seem small may reflect the use of the less discriminating parameter, D10. If sufficient data existed to do this analysis with a parameter more weighted toward lower or, especially, higher survival levels, e.g., alpha ratio, greater differences in dependence of RBE on LET for various cell types might be seen.

Role of Genetic Background of Tumor Cells in Response to Charged Particles

In light of the proton data, discussed above, indicating a correlation between cell lines with higher proton RBE values and defects in DNA repair, specifically in HR repair, we wondered whether the same finding would extend to heavier ions, notably carbon ions. Although the literature data on RBEs for human tumor cell lines shows substantial variations at any given LET, even just for

carbon ions (**Figures 2**–**6**), we could not find any information in the literature on possible DNA repair deficiencies, particularly in HR repair, for the cell lines with the highest RBEs after carbon-ion irradiation, e.g., TK-1 brain tumor, Ca9–22 gingival squamous cell carcinoma, SQ20B head-and-neck cancer. Therefore, experiments to ascertain carbon RBE values for human tumor cell lines known to be defective in the FA/BRCA DNA repair pathway are warranted. Furthermore, both the proton data of Liu et al. (44) and the carbon-ion data of Suzuki et al. (70) on residual unrepaired DNA damage (assays of 53BP1 foci and DNA damage revealed by PCC, respectively) suggest that such assays may be useful biodosimeters to select patients for charged particle therapy.

What would be the clinical application of increased tumor RBE values in subsets of patients? Identifying patients with proton- and/or heavy ion-sensitive tumors may allow us to: (a) de-escalate the physical dose of charged particles if normal tissue

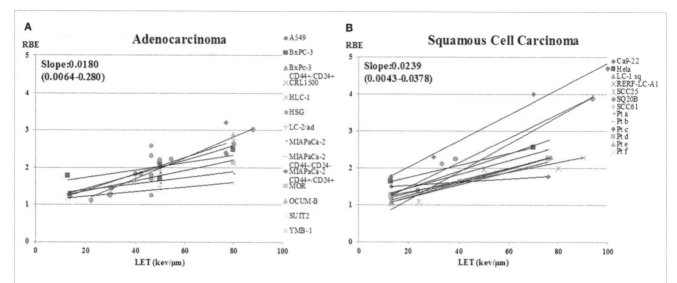

FIGURE 6 | RBE at 10% survival versus LET for cells from human adenocarcinomas and squamous cell carcinomas exposed to carbon ions. RBE values as a function of LET for carbon ion beam only, calculated using D10 for **(A)** adenocarcinomas and **(B)** squamous cell carcinomas. The graphs show data only for LET < 100 keV/μm. The slopes of the curves are shown for each cell line.

damage is a particular concern; (b) select patients for proton or heavy ion treatment slots who would have not otherwise had the opportunity to be treated with such radiations, thereby increasing the odds of local tumor control; or (c) biologically optimize tumor-directed therapy, for example, by employing intensity-modulated ion therapy algorithms to superimpose an LET increase on the already pre-existing RBE advantage, thereby further improving local tumor control. Because RBE values tend to increase with increasing fractionation sensitivity of tumors (i.e., decreasing alpha/beta values) (42), there exists additional opportunity to improve the outcome of ion beam therapy in tumors with low alpha/beta values, such as prostate or breast cancer. However, this approach will require better knowledge of the inter-tumoral variation of alpha/beta values and the development of predictive biomarkers to identify appropriate tumors.

SENSITIVITY OF CANCER STEM-LIKE CELLS TO CHARGED PARTICLES

In recent years, considerable interest has developed in the possibility that cancer stem-like cells (CSCs) in human tumors could be major contributors to resistance of tumors to conventional photon radiotherapy (RT) (106–108). However, intriguing data also suggest that the presence of CSCs might be overcome by carbon-ion therapy (89, 109). In this section, we discuss such a potential from a radiobiological perspective.

Cancer stem-like cells, also called cancer-initiating cells (CICs), are tumorigenic and have the potential to give rise to all cell types identified in hematological cancers and in several types of solid tumors (110). CSCs are regarded as "roots of cancer," analogous to normal stem cells in hierarchical tissues, although the origin of CSCs is still not clear and various theories have been proposed to explain their origin (111). It is believed that

tumor growth is driven by a discrete subpopulation of CSCs that are defined by their capacity for self-renewal and their ability to generate heterogeneous lineages of cancer cells (110). The CSCs can survive and usually persist in tumors for a substantial length of time as a distinct population and can eventually cause cancer recurrence after treatment and tumor metastasis. It seems reasonable to suggest that cancer cure can be achieved only if this population is eliminated.

There is growing evidence that CSCs are inherently resistant to conventional fractionated RT. This radioresistant phenomenon of CSCs has been described within the framework of the four Rs of radiobiology: (i) repair, (ii) redistribution, (iii) reoxygenation, and (iv) repopulation (112).

(i) Regarding DNA repair, CSCs exhibit fewer DNA DSBs after exposure to ionizing radiation than non-tumorigenic cancer cells, which has been correlated with efficient DNA repair machinery due to constitutive hyperphosphorylation of the DNA checkpoint kinases Chk1 and Chk2 (106).

(ii) Regarding redistribution, quiescent or slowly cycling cells, normal or cancer stem cells, generally are radioresistant, although dose fractionation can cause redistribution of radioresistant S-phase cells into a more sensitive phase of the cell cycle. If this happens only in tumor cells, it could result in a therapeutic benefit for slowly cycling normal cells, sparing late responding normal tissues during fractionation. However, if tumors also have a significant proportion of CSCs that are slowly cycling, any benefit from redistribution may not apply (112).

(iii) Regarding reoxygenation, if the niche in which CSCs reside is hypoxic, during radiation fractionation the quiescent CSCs may be exposed to increasing oxygen levels causing increasing radiosensitivity due to transition of cells into an activated, proliferative state. It appears that in some cases, the CSC niche may be in perivascular regions (113, 114) where they may be exposed to rapidly changing cycles of hypoxia-reoxygenation (112). During reoxygenation, the cells would become more radiosensitive, and reoxygenation triggers metabolic processes that generate damaging reactive oxygen species (ROS). However, CSCs manifest enhanced protection against ROS (107, 108). It was reported that expression of the CSC marker CD44, in particular that of a variant isoform (CD44v), contributes to ROS defense by promoting the synthesis of glutathione (GSH), a primary intracellular antioxidant radical scavenger (115). Hence, the roles of hypoxia, reoxygenation, and ROS defenses in CSCs appear quite complex, and more research is required to elucidate their roles in radiation response.

(iv) Regarding repopulation, it was reported that developmental signaling pathways, such as TGF-β, Notch, Wnt/B-catenin, and Sonic hedgehog pathways greatly contribute to maintenance of CSCs, as they do with normal tissue stem cells (112). Intrinsic inter-conversion and dynamic equilibrium between CSCs and non-stem cancer cells (NSCCs) exist under normal and irradiation conditions, and TGF-β might have important roles in the equilibrium (116).

In addition to the four Rs of radiobiology, it has been shown that CSCs can acquire radioresistance through activation of anti-apoptotic Bcl-2 (117) and serine/threonine protein kinase B (PKB, also known as AKT) survival signaling (118, 119). Hence, there is substantial reason to believe that CSCs are a radiation-resistant cell population in at least some tumors exposed to photon irradiation.

On the other hand, intriguing studies have reported that CSCs may be more effectively killed by carbon ions compared to photons in colon and pancreas cancers both *in vitro* and *in vivo* (89, 109, 120), and CSCs from colon and breast cancers may be more efficiently eliminated by proton irradiation than photon treatment, at least *in vitro* (121, 122). One or more of several processes may explain the observations that ion beams have biological advantages for killing CSCs compared to photons. These include the diminished capacity for NHEJ repair, which may play an important role in the quiescent G0 cell cycle phase, after heavy ion exposure (39); a decreased OER with heavy ions (59, 123), and an efficacy in dealing with radioresistant tumor cells (*TP53*-mutated and BCL2-overexpressing cells) (124) compared with results produced by photon beams. We demonstrated that heavy ion beams depress AKT-related survival signaling (125). Therefore, we speculate that heavy ion beams may target CSCs *via* depression of AKT survival signaling. Indeed, we demonstrated that the population of CSCs is only slightly increased or unchanged after carbon-ion irradiation because carbon ions may simultaneously kill CSCs and non-CSCs, while X-rays have less effect on CSCs than on the bulk cancer cells (126). These results suggest that carbon ions may enhance apoptosis and autophagy through activation of death signaling and may target CSCs *via* the depression of AKT survival signaling (**Figure 7**). However, it should be noted that the observations of CSCs being preferentially more sensitive to charged particles is not universal as it has been reported that head-and-neck cancer CSCs are resistant

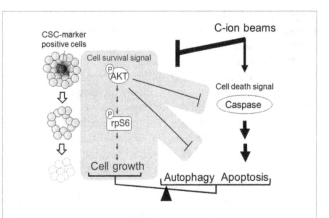

FIGURE 7 | A model for carbon ion-induced apoptosis and autophagy through the enhancement of death signals and the depression of survival signals. The model is based on AKT survival signaling as shown in our work (126). An arrow "→" indicates enhancement; a sidewise "⊣" indicates depression.

to both photon and carbon-ion irradiation (127). Clearly, more detailed studies are necessary, for example, using tumor samples from carbon- and photon-irradiated patients, to understand the potential significant therapeutic benefit of heavier charged particles on CSCs. It is also worth investigating whether, or how, the enhanced DNA repair advantages in CSCs might relate to the potential for development of biomarkers based on residual DNA damage for identifying patients whose cancers might be treated more efficaciously using charged particles, as discussed in the section above.

SENSITIVITY OF HYPOXIC TUMOR CELLS TO CHARGED PARTICLES

A long-recognized property of tumors is their development of hypoxic regions. It has also been documented, for many years, that hypoxic cells are resistant to photons, but that resistance is reduced when hypoxic cells are irradiated with higher LET particles (22). Suit et al. (3) postulated that the potential gain from high-LET radiations in the clinic may be due principally to the lower OER (ratio of doses for a given endpoint in hypoxic to well-aerated cells). This section discusses the reduced hypoxic protection with carbon-ion therapy and how that might be exploited in cancer therapy.

Cellular sensitivity to low-LET radiations (photons, clinical energy protons) depends on the degree of hypoxia at the time of irradiation, increasing in a sigmoid fashion from an OER = 1.0 (no difference between anoxic and well-aerated cells) at very low oxygen levels to a maximum (OER ~ 3.0) usually obtained by about 2–3% oxygen (22, 128). Sensitivity also depends on the duration of exposure to the hypoxic conditions. There are two distinct mechanisms that promote oxygen deficiency in tumor cells; each exposes cells to different periods of hypoxia. Acute or perfusion-limited hypoxia is caused by poorly formed or dysfunctional vasculature that can cause transient closing of blood vessels that deprives the surrounding cells of an appropriate oxygen supply (129). On the other hand, in chronic or diffusion-limited hypoxia, the imbalance of oxygen supply and consumption in actively proliferating tumor cells causes cells far from blood vessels to experience a deficiency in oxygenation for long periods of time (130). Historically, most studies of hypoxic radioresistance have dealt with chronic hypoxia, but experiments investigating the influence of acute and chronic oxygenation conditions on cell response have shown increased radioresistance for the acute case (131–133). Ma and colleagues demonstrated that for both X-ray and carbon-ion irradiation, cells under acute anoxia were more radioresistant than those under chronic anoxia, whereas cells subjected to acute and chronic hypoxia (0.5% O_2) exhibited no significant difference in sensitivity (131, 132). They argued that prolonged exposure to anoxia induced a breakdown in cellular energy metabolism, which led to delays in cell cycle progression. They found that cells were arrested in the G1 phase of the cell cycle with a significant decrease in the number of active S-phase cells after 24 h of hypoxia. However, abrupt changes in the oxygenation status did not result in changes in the cell cycle distribution. The energy deficiency of cells also has been associated with the reduction of DNA damage repair (133). Therefore, chronically hypoxic cells were found to be more vulnerable to radiation damage.

The poor performance of photons in curing hypoxic tumor cells has prompted researchers to turn to high-LET radiation, such as ion beams that have lower OERs [reviewed, e.g., in Ref. (22, 128, 134, 135)]. Radiation damage from low-LET beams is mostly mediated by free radicals (indirect effects), i.e., secondary electrons generated from the ionizations interact with molecules, such as water, to produce free radicals which in turn damage the DNA. In contrast to their low-LET counterparts, the contribution of radiation damage by direct ionizations in DNA is higher for high-LET beams. Here, the secondary electrons directly interact with the critical target, thus producing, at least in part, different damage. Hence, the oxygen effect can be explained, at least in part, by differences in induction and repair of DNA damage. Hirayama et al. reported that the rejoining kinetics of DNA DSBs incurred from carbon-ion irradiation were the same for cells in oxic and hypoxic conditions (136). This led them to postulate that DNA DSBs produced by carbon ions are the same for the two oxygenation conditions. However, their results for X-ray irradiation showed a dependence of the repair dynamics on the oxygen level, with DSBs generated under oxic conditions rejoined more efficiently than those produced under hypoxia. They postulated that this resulted from different mechanisms for DNA damage depending on oxygenation, namely, that in the presence of oxygen, oxygen-reacting radicals could cause additional DNA DSBs but in hypoxia more damage is produced by direct ionizations or by radicals irrelevant to oxygen. Furthermore, the repair times were longer after carbon-ion irradiation and more unrepaired DNA DSBs remained after 5 h while for X-rays almost all DSBs were efficiently rejoined. This can be explained by the high ionization density generated along the track of heavy charged particles that produces complex DNA damages, making repair more difficult. Therefore, the OER decreases with increasing LET values, with the OER of carbon ions about half that with X-rays. Typical survival curves obtained using carbon-ion and X-ray irradiation under oxic and

hypoxic conditions are illustrated in **Figure 8**. The difference with oxygenation status is diminished with the high-LET carbon ions and the survival curves tend to converge. By contrast, the larger variation in the cell response seen for X-ray irradiation is reflected by the higher OER value. A consequence of the enhanced radioresistance observed in X-ray survival curves under hypoxia is that $RBE_{hypoxic}$ generally exceeds RBE_{oxic}. In vitro studies have also shown that OER approaches unity at dose-averaged LETs of ~300 keV/μm (59, 134). Oxygen ions, with their high-LET values within therapeutic fields, might be advantageous for tumors with significant hypoxic fractions. Scifoni et al. (135) compared computed OER values in a tumor irradiated with oxygen or carbon ions, and showed that, assuming the same dose in the entrance region, there was a dramatic decrease in OER for the oxygen ions.

The advantage of high-LET carbon ions over photons in treating tumor hypoxia has been confirmed in the clinical setting by Nakano et al. (137). They measured the intratumor oxygen partial pressure of uterine cervical cancer patients prior to and at the fifth day of treatment with either photons or carbon ions using a polarographic electrode. The 4-year local control rates were found to be independent of the oxygenation condition for carbon-ion treatment, whereas the control rate for photon therapy of patients with high pO_2 status was more than twice that with low pO_2.

It has been suggested that further improvements in treatment outcome with carbon therapy can be achieved by considering the time course of reoxygenation of hypoxic areas in the tumor. According to Antonovic et al. (138), the number of fractions and the dose per fraction for carbon therapy can be optimized by taking into account the effect of local oxygenation changes on tumor control probability. In the future, more detailed studies are necessary to take into account the OER and rates of reoxygenation in treatment planning for carbon-ion RT, as are underway (134, 135).

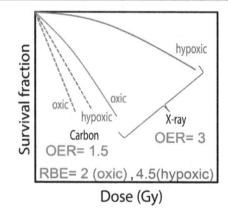

FIGURE 8 | The dependence of survival curves on oxygen concentration typically observed after exposure to X-rays and carbon ions. The importance of the oxygen effect is reduced with high-LET carbon-ion irradiation as is apparent in the small separation of the survival curves compared to that seen with X-rays. The large difference between the cell response in air and hypoxia for X-rays results in a $RBE_{hypoxic}$ that is greater than RBE_{oxic}.

DOSE FRACTIONATION WITH CHARGED PARTICLES

Fractionated irradiation is a valuable tool in conventional RT to reduce early and late effects in normal tissue by allowing repair of sublethal damage or increase tumor response due to reoxygenation of a hypoxic tumor. The linear quadratic (LQ) model describes cell killing using single-hit and double-hit components (22). The shape of the curve is determined by:

$$SF(D) = e^{-\left(\alpha D + \beta D^2\right)}. \tag{1}$$

The α parameter describes the linear component of the curve, while the β component describes the quadratic portion of the curve. The α/β ratio, the point at which linear cell killing is equivalent to quadratic cell killing, is an important parameter used to model cell killing by radiation. Presently, this ratio is used as a staple for predicting the clinical effects in response to RT despite various limitations. A high α/β ratio, seen in many human tumors, suggests a predominance of the α component, implying a decreased response to fractionation and, therefore, clinical benefit from hypofractionation (decreased number of fractions of larger dose per fraction). A lower α/β ratio is usually associated with late responding normal tissue and is the basis for the therapeutic gain achieved using hyperfractionation (increased number of fractions of small dose per fraction), which allows for greater repair/recovery of normal tissues (139). However, some human tumors, e.g., prostate cancer, melanoma, and some sarcomas, may have α/β values similar to late responding tissues (140–142).

In image-guided RT, intensity-modulated RT, and X-ray stereotactic body RT (SBRT), there are tendencies to reduce the number of fractions and increase the dose per fraction (i.e., hypofractionation) (143, 144). With carbon-ion RT, superiority of the physical dose distribution can lead to a reduction in the number of fractions (145), allowing hypofractionation. There are few relevant experimental data using human tumor cells on hypofractionation effects with high-LET charged particles. Experiments involving high-LET fast neutron beams demonstrated that increasing the dose per fraction tended to decrease the RBE for both tumor and normal tissues (146). However, the dose-dependent decrease in the RBE for the tumor was less pronounced than that for normal tissues, such as skin and lung (147). These experiments led to the assumption that the therapeutic gain of carbon-ion RT would increase when the dose per fraction increased. This assumption was confirmed in animal experiments that compared RBE for carbon ions between tumor and skin (148). In additional studies with high-LET radiation, RBE depends on dose and dose per fraction: dose-dependent decrease of RBE was reported after fast neutrons to normal skin, intestine, growing cartilage, and hematopoietic tissues (149), and after Ne-ions to the skin of mice and hamsters (150). The change in dose dependence is caused by the higher α/β ratio of target cells after high-LET radiation than after photons (151).

The value of the α term increases with increasing LET in both tumor and normal tissue, while the issue of whether the value of the β term changes with LET remains controversial (148, 152). In our study (153) by evaluating the therapeutic gain of carbon-ion fractionation using intestinal crypt survival and tumor growth delay (TGD) assays, the values of the α and β terms for the mouse fibrosarcoma (NFSa) tumor are close to those reported by Ando et al. (148), while those for normal tissues are different (**Figure 9**). In addition, the LET-dependent increase (e.g., slope of the regression line) of the α term for NFSa is similar to that for human salivary gland tumor cells (148, 154). LET-dependent increase of α terms for crypt is greater than that for the early skin reaction after daily fractionated doses to leg skin (148), whereas it is similar to that for the late skin reaction after 4-h interval fractionations to foot skin (154). These results indicate that therapeutic gain for carbon-ion RT depends on the normal tissue and fractionation schedule. Further studies with mouse skin and rat spinal cord where the normal tissues were exposed to varying numbers of fractions and doses per fraction of γ-rays and carbon ions have shown that the magnitude of damage repair depends on both the number of fractions and the size of dose per fraction for high-LET radiation (155, 156). It was concluded that repair of radiation injury is much reduced with dose per fraction, especially with 125 keV/μm carbon ions. Unfortunately, few studies of fractionation effects with carbon ions have been performed with tumors, especially human tumors.

As discussed above, hypoxia is one of the main factors reducing local control in some solid tumors, and fractionation in RT may have an advantage because of reoxygenation of the hypoxic areas. It has been reported that reoxygenation in several tumors irradiated with carbon ions occurs earlier than that in those irradiated with photons (157, 158). Reoxygenation in the NFSa fibrosarcoma was observed at 4 days, 1 day, and within 0.5 days after irradiation with photons, low-LET carbon ions (14 and 18 keV/μm) and high-LET carbon ions (43, 58, and 74 keV/μm), respectively (157). Thus, short-term fractionated irradiation with carbon ions may be effective in the treatment of tumors, at least in part, because of altered reoxygenation.

The clinical RBE is replaced by an LET-dependent RBE for *in vitro* cell killing data determined in single-dose experiments and is employed to design the SOBP and in the Japanese treatment planning system for carbon-ion RT (159, 160). A question remains as to whether the biological effects with fractionated doses are also uniform within the SOBP. Uzawa et al. evaluated uniformity of a new ridge filter that was designed based on α and β values for various LETs to cause mouse foot skin reaction by carbon-ion fractionated irradiation (154). The physical dose distribution of the new ridge filter was almost identical to the ridge filter designed based on *in vitro* cell kill. While the LQ model is useful for conversion between relatively low radiation doses as used in conventional RT, it has been suggested that it is not applicable to higher fractional doses or smaller fraction numbers (6, 161). It has been questioned whether the LQ model is applicable to hypofractionated carbon-ion RT. For establishment of the optimal fractionation strategy in carbon-ion RT, applicability of the LQ model should be investigated in future studies.

With photon RT, the rapidly expanding use of hypofractionation even to the extreme of single fractions as used in stereotactic radiosurgery (SRS) and SBRT has lead to recent discussion about whether "new" biology should be advanced to explain the greater than expected anti-tumor efficacy of some hypofractionation

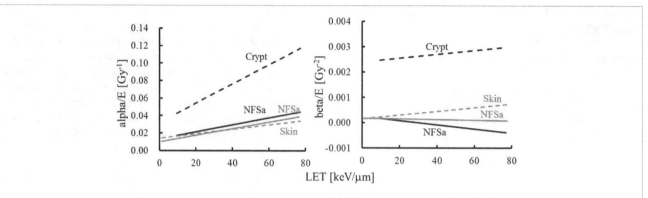

FIGURE 9 | α and β terms for mouse normal tissues and tumors plotted against LET. The comparison of survival parameters of Ando et al. (red) (148) and our study (153) using crypt survival and tumor growth delay assays (black). The solid lines show NFSa tumor and broken lines show the normal tissues (crypt or skin).

regimens. Some have proposed that consideration of only the clonogenic survival of only the tumor cells is not sufficient to account for the observed responses [e.g., Ref. (162, 163)], although not all agree [e.g., Ref. (164–166)]. Brown et al. reviewed the clinical data for early-stage NSCLC and suggested that radiobiological modeling with the LQ model is adequate to explain the efficacy of SRS and SBRT (166). Fowler showed the potential advantages of hypofractionation for prostate cancer by using the LQ model and concluded that use of the LQ model can yield consistent results, for example, the remarkable agreement for tumor effects of some of the best schedules in regular use (167). It is likely that the same considerations apply to carbon-ion therapy, although few data exist, especially for human tumors in experimental situations. Here, we briefly review some aspects that may pertain.

In some situations, vascular damage may be a dominant pathway for tumor suppression. Irradiation of human tumor xenografts or rodent tumors with 5–10 Gy in a single dose causes relatively mild vascular damages. On the other hand, numerous studies with experimental tumors indicate that irradiation with doses higher than 10 Gy in a single fraction or 20–60 Gy in limited numbers of fractions causes severe vascular damage, including endothelial cell apoptosis, leading to the deterioration of the intratumor microenvironment and indirect death of tumor cells (163, 168, 169). Little is known about the vascular changes in human tumors treated with high-dose hypofractionation, particularly with heavy ions, but experimentation is indicated to address whether radiation-induced vascular damage and the resulting indirect death of tumor cells may play important roles in the response of tumors to high-dose hypofractionation with charged particles.

In addition to potential vascular effects, it has been suggested that high-dose irradiation evokes immune reactions and thereby eradicates tumor cells that escaped radiation-induced death (170, 171). In support of such notion, a recent report showed that ablative RT dramatically increased T-cell priming in lymphoid tissues, leading to reduction/eradication of the primary tumor or distant metastasis in a CD8+ T-cell dependent fashion (170). Several studies have shown that carbon ions induce anti-tumor immunity (172–176), although the effects of high-LET radiation on immune

function have not been studied in detail. Hence, enhanced immune reactions might be involved in the response of tumors to high-dose hypofractionation, especially with charged particles (177).

It is also noteworthy that, unlike photon irradiation, particle irradiation may suppress the metastatic potential of cancer cells (172, 178), and a recent paper has shown that there is a decrease in metastasis with decreasing fraction number of carbon ions (179). Clearly, further studies are warranted to gain better insights into the effects of high-dose hypofractionation with heavy ions on tumor vasculature, immune system, and metastasis, and how such biology might impact human tumor RBE values and therapeutic gain.

CONCLUSION

In a recent review of charged particle therapy, Loeffler and Durante (4) stated that "Considering the current uncertainties in clinical results [with charged particles] and the difficulties in performing clinical trials, research in physics and radiobiology should reduce the cost/benefit ratio." In this review, we have focused on discussion of selected aspects of radiobiological data with human tumors exposed to protons and heavier charged particles, raising specific instances where further laboratory research may contribute to improving particle therapy. With increasing understanding of the genetic heterogeneity in human tumors, particularly with regard to alterations in DNA repair pathways, a fruitful research area appears to be elucidation of DNA repair pathways selectively involved in repair of the unique clustered DNA damages caused by charged particles. With increases in such knowledge, the differences can be exploited to identify patients who may be better treated with particles because of characteristics of their tumors and to develop novel pharmacologic approaches that capitalize on the differences in DNA damage and repair. Another area ripe for charged particle biology study with implications to clinical advances is in cancer stem cells. The intriguing observations that cancer stem cells from human tumors may be more effectively killed by carbon ions than by photons begs for further study on mechanisms involved – altered DNA repair? location in a hypoxic niche? – and consideration of how to exploit such a difference to the advantage of ion therapy. Finally, the biology underlying the notable clinical effectiveness of high dose, hypofractionated charged particles, which may be explained by radiosensitivity of tumor cells themselves at high doses or may involve vasculature and/or immune system responses, requires further elucidation.

This article has focused on data from *in vitro* studies of human tumor cells, for reasons described in the Section "Introduction" and recognizing that there are limitations when applying *in vitro* findings to the *in vivo* and clinical situations. However, it is also clear that because of the stochastic natures of radiation-induced cell killing and tumor cure and the, albeit simplistic, relationship of the two endpoints *via* $\text{TCP} = e^{-(\text{SF} \times \text{M})}$ (where TCP is tumor control probability, SF is surviving fraction, and M is number of clonogens), understanding effects of radiations of varying qualities on the tumor cells themselves can be informative. The questions and issues raised herein require follow-up *in vivo* studies leading to transfer of knowledge to the clinic, but guidance from the *in vitro* work, e.g., on use of DNA damage assays and exploiting DNA repair as biomarkers for patient selection or using *in vitro* survival α/β information to help guide design of hypofractionation protocols *in vivo* and in the clinic, is critical.

AUTHOR CONTRIBUTIONS

KH, HK, TK, AP, YY, QL, HW, and AT contributed to the conception, drafting, and revising of the review article.

ACKNOWLEDGMENTS

This work was supported by the National Cancer Institute of the National Institutes of Health under Award Number R21CA182259 (KH), the Gunma University Initiative for Advanced Research (KH), Federal Share of program income earned by Massachusetts General Hospital on C06 CA059267, Proton Therapy Research and Treatment Center (HW and KH), Ministry of Education, Culture, Sports, Science and Technology of Japan (MEXT) Number 15H05945 (AT), Gunma University Program for Cultivating Global Leaders in Heavy Ion Therapeutics and Engineering of the MEXT (AP), Research Project with heavy ions at the Gunma University Heavy Ion Medical Center (HK, TK, AP, YY, and AT). The content is solely the responsibility of the authors and does not necessarily represent the official views of the National Institutes of Health.

REFERENCES

1. Wilson RR. Radiological use of fast protons. *Radiology* (1946) **47**:487–91. doi:10.1148/47.5.487
2. Skarsgard LD. Radiobiology with heavy charged particles: a historical review. *Phys Med* (1998) **14**(Suppl. 1):1–19.
3. Suit H, DeLaney T, Goldberg S, Paganetti H, Clasie B, Gerweck L, et al. Proton vs carbon ion beams in the definitive radiation treatment of cancer patients. *Radiother Oncol* (2010) **95**:3–22. doi:10.1016/j.radonc.2010.01.015
4. Loeffler JS, Durante M. Charged particle therapy – optimization, challenges and future directions. *Nat Rev Clin Oncol* (2013) **10**:411–24. doi:10.1038/nrclinonc.2013.79
5. Durante M, Loeffler JS. Charged particles in radiation oncology. *Nat Rev Clin Oncol* (2010) **7**:37–43. doi:10.1038/nrclinonc.2009.183
6. Durante M. New challenges in high-energy particle radiobiology. *Br J Radiol* (2014) **87**(1035):20130626. doi:10.1259/bjr.20130626
7. Friedrich T, Scholz U, Elsasser T, Durante M, Scholz M. Systematic analysis of RBE and related quantities using a database of cell survival experiments with ion beam irradiation. *J Radiat Res* (2013) **54**(4):494–514. doi:10.1093/jrr/rrs114
8. Paganetti H, Niemierko A, Ancukiewicz M, Gerweck LE, Goitein M, Loeffler JS, et al. Relative biological effectiveness (RBE) values for proton beam therapy. *Int J Radiat Oncol Biol Phys* (2002) **53**:407–21. doi:10.1016/S0360-3016(02)02754-2
9. Friedrich T, Grun R, Scholz U, Elsasser T, Durante M, Scholz M. Sensitivity analysis of the relative biological effectiveness predicted by the local effect model. *Phys Med Biol* (2013) **58**(19):6827–49. doi:10.1088/0031-9155/58/19/6827
10. Barendsen GW. Responses of cultured cells, tumors, and normal tissues to radiation of different linear energy transfer. *Curr Top Radiat Res Q* (1968) **4**:293–356.
11. Blakely EA, Ngo FQH, Curtis SB, Tobias CA. Heavy-ion radiobiology: cellular studies. *Adv Radiat Biol* (1984) **11**:295–389. doi:10.1016/B978-0-12-035411-5.50013-7
12. Sorensen BS, Overgaard J, Bassler N. In vitro RBE-LET dependence for multiple particle types. *Acta Oncol* (2011) **50**:757–62. doi:10.3109/02841 86X.2011.582518
13. Kraft G, Kramer M, Scholz M. LET, track structure and models. A review. *Radiat Environ Biophys* (1992) **31**:161–80. doi:10.1007/BF01214825
14. Goodhead DT. Initial events in the cellular effects of ionizing radiations: clustered damage in DNA. *Int J Radiat Biol* (1994) **65**:7–17. doi:10.1080/09553009414550021

15. Ward JF. The complexity of DNA damage: relevance to biological consequences. *Int J Radiat Biol* (1994) **66**:427–32. doi:10.1080/09553009414551401
16. Hada M, Sutherland BM. Spectrum of complex DNA damages depends on the incident radiation. *Radiat Res* (2006) **165**:223–30. doi:10.1667/RR3498.1
17. Goodhead DT. Mechanisms for the biological effectiveness of high-LET radiations. *J Radiat Res* (1999) **40**(Suppl):1–13. doi:10.1269/jrr.40.S1
18. Goodhead DT. Fifth Warren K. Sinclair keynote address: issues in quantifying the effects of low-level radiation. *Health Phys* (2009) **97**(5):394–406. doi:10.1097/HP.0b013e3181ae8acf
19. Nikjoo H, O'Neill P, Wilson WE, Goodhead DT. Computational approach for determining the spectrum of DNA damage induced by ionizing radiation. *Radiat Res* (2001) **156**:577–83. doi:10.1667/0033-7587(2001)156[0577:CAFDTS]2.0.CO;2
20. Georgakilas AG, O'Neill P, Stewart RD. Induction and repair of clustered DNA lesions: what do we know so far? *Radiat Res* (2013) **180**(1):100–9. doi:10.1667/RR3041.1
21. Sridharan DM, Asaithamby A, Bailey SM, Costes SV, Doetsch PW, Dynan WS, et al. Understanding cancer development processes after HZE-particle exposure: roles of ROS, DNA damage repair and inflammation. *Radiat Res* (2015) **183**(1):1–26. doi:10.1667/RR13804.1
22. Hall EJ, Giaccia A. *Radiobiology for the Radiologist*. Philadelphia, PA: Lippincott Williams & Wilkins Publishers (2012).
23. Morgan WF, Sowa MB. Non-targeted effects induced by ionizing radiation: mechanisms and potential impact on radiation induced health effects. *Cancer Lett* (2015) **356**(1):17–21. doi:10.1016/j.canlet.2013.09.009
24. Kadhim MA, Hill MA. Non-targeted effects of radiation exposure: recent advances and implications. *Radiat Prot Dosimetry* (2015) **166**(1–4):118–24. doi:10.1093/rpd/ncv167
25. Sowa MB, Goetz W, Baulch JE, Pyles DN, Dziegielewski J, Yovino S, et al. Lack of evidence for low-LET radiation induced bystander response in normal human fibroblasts and colon carcinoma cells. *Int J Radiat Biol* (2010) **86**(2):102–13. doi:10.3109/09553000903419957
26. Yang H, Asaad N, Held KD. Medium-mediated intercellular communication is involved in bystander responses of X-irradiated normal human fibroblasts. *Oncogene* (2005) **24**:2096–103. doi:10.1038/sj.onc.1208439
27. de Toledo SM, Buonanno M, Li M, Asaad N, Qin Y, Gonon G, et al. The impact of adaptive and non-targeted effects in the biological responses to low dose/low fluence ionizing radiation: the modulating effect of linear energy transfer. *Health Phys* (2011) **100**(3):290–2. doi:10.1097/HP.0b013e31820832d8
28. McMahon SJ, McGarry CK, Butterworth KT, Jain S, O'Sullivan JM, Hounsell AR, et al. Cellular signalling effects in high precision radiotherapy. *Phys Med Biol* (2015) **60**(11):4551–64. doi:10.1088/0031-9155/60/11/4551

29. Asur R, Butterworth KT, Penagaricano JA, Prise KM, Griffin RJ. High dose bystander effects in spatially fractionated radiation therapy. *Cancer Lett* (2015) 356(1):52–7. doi:10.1016/j.canlet.2013.10.032

30. Willers H, Dahm-Daphi J, Powell SN. Repair of radiation damage to DNA. *Br J Cancer* (2004) 90:1297–301. doi:10.1038/sj.bjc.6601729

31. Hiom K. Coping with DNA double strand breaks. *DNA Repair (Amst)* (2010) 9(12):1256–63. doi:10.1016/j.dnarep.2010.09.018

32. Lieber MR. The mechanism of double-strand DNA break repair by the nonhomologous DNA end-joining pathway. *Annu Rev Biochem* (2010) 79:181–211. doi:10.1146/annurev.biochem.052308.093131

33. Jeggo PA, Geuting V, Lobrich M. The role of homologous recombination in radiation-induced double-strand break repair. *Radiother Oncol* (2011) 101(1):7–12. doi:10.1016/j.radonc.2011.06.019

34. Willers H, Pfaffle HN, Zou L. Targeting homologous recombination repair in cancer. In: Kelley MR, editor. *DNA Repair in Cancer Therapy: Molecular Targets and Clinical Applications*. Waltham, MA: Academic Press (2012). p. 119–60.

35. Klein Douwel D, Boonen RA, Long DT, Szypowska AA, Raschle M, Walter JC, et al. XPF-ERCC1 acts in unhooking DNA interstrand crosslinks in cooperation with FANCD2 and FANCP/SLX4. *Mol Cell* (2014) 54(3):460–71. doi:10.1016/j.molcel.2014.03.015

36. Frankenberg-Schwager M, Gebauer A, Koppe C, Wolf H, Pralle E, Frankenberg D. Single-strand annealing, conservative homologous recombination, nonhomologous DNA end joining, and the cell cycle-dependent repair of DNA double-strand breaks induced by sparsely or densely ionizing radiation. *Radiat Res* (2009) 171(3):265–73. doi:10.1667/RR0784.1

37. Zafar F, Seidler SB, Kronenberg A, Schild D, Wiese C. Homologous recombination contributes to the repair of DNA double-strand breaks induced by high-energy iron ions. *Radiat Res* (2010) 173(1):27–39. doi:10.1667/RR1910.1

38. Yajima H, Fujisawa H, Nakajima NI, Hirakawa H, Jeggo PA, Okayasu R, et al. The complexity of DNA double strand breaks is a critical factor enhancing end-resection. *DNA Repair (Amst)* (2013) 12(11):936–46. doi:10.1016/j.dnarep.2013.08.009

39. Takahashi A, Kubo M, Ma H, Nakagawa A, Yoshida Y, Isono M, et al. Nonhomologous end-joining repair plays a more important role than homologous recombination repair in defining radiosensitivity after exposure to high-LET radiation. *Radiat Res* (2014) 182(3):338–44. doi:10.1667/RR13782.1

40. Steinstrater O, Scholz U, Friedrich T, Kramer M, Grun R, Durante M, et al. Integration of a model-independent interface for RBE predictions in a treatment planning system for active particle beam scanning. *Phys Med Biol* (2015) 60(17):6811–31. doi:10.1088/0031-9155/60/17/6811

41. Inaniwa T, Kanematsu N, Matsufuji N, Kanai T, Shirai T, Noda K, et al. Reformulation of a clinical-dose system for carbon-ion radiotherapy treatment planning at the National Institute of Radiological Sciences, Japan. *Phys Med Biol* (2015) 60(8):3271–86. doi:10.1088/0031-9155/60/8/3271

42. Paganetti H. Relative biological effectiveness (RBE) values for proton beam therapy. Variations as a function of biological endpoint, dose, and linear energy transfer. *Phys Med Biol* (2014) 59(22):R419–72. doi:10.1088/0031-9155/59/22/R419

43. Grosse N, Fontana A, Hug EB, Lomax A, Coray A, Augsburger M, et al. Deficiency in homologous recombination renders mammalian cells more sensitive to proton versus photon irradiation. *Int J Radiat Oncol Biol Phys* (2014) 88(1):175–81. doi:10.1016/j.ijrobp.2013.09.041

44. Liu Q, Ghosh P, Magpayo N, Testa M, Tang S, Gheorghiu L, et al. Lung cancer cell line screen links Fanconi anemia/BRCA pathway defects to increased relative biological effectiveness of proton radiation. *Int J Radiat Oncol Biol Phys* (2015) 91(5):1081–9. doi:10.1016/j.ijrobp.2014.12.046

45. Fontana AO, Augsburger MA, Grosse N, Guckenberger M, Lomax AJ, Sartori AA, et al. Differential DNA repair pathway choice in cancer cells after proton- and photon-irradiation. *Radiother Oncol* (2015) 116(3):374–80. doi:10.1016/j.radonc.2015.08.014

46. Guan F, Bronk L, Titt U, Lin SH, Mirkovic D, Kerr MD, et al. Spatial mapping of the biologic effectiveness of scanned particle beams: towards biologically optimized particle therapy. *Sci Rep* (2015) 5:9850. doi:10.1038/srep09850

47. Garnett MJ, Edelman EJ, Heidorn SJ, Greenman CD, Dastur A, Lau KW, et al. Systematic identification of genomic markers of drug sensitivity in cancer cells. *Nature* (2012) 483(7391):570–5. doi:10.1038/nature11005

48. Imielinski M, Berger AH, Hammerman PS, Hernandez B, Pugh TJ, Hodis E, et al. Mapping the hallmarks of lung adenocarcinoma with massively parallel sequencing. *Cell* (2012) 150(6):1107–20. doi:10.1016/j.cell.2012.08.029

49. Network CGAR. Comprehensive genomic characterization of squamous cell lung cancers. *Nature* (2012) 489(7417):519–25. doi:10.1038/nature11404

50. Wang AT, Smogorzewska A. SnapShot: Fanconi anemia and associated proteins. *Cell* (2015) 160(1–2):354–e1. doi:10.1016/j.cell.2014.12.031

51. Rostek C, Turner EL, Robbins M, Rightnar S, Xiao W, Obenaus A, et al. Involvement of homologous recombination repair after proton-induced DNA damage. *Mutagenesis* (2008) 23(2):119–29. doi:10.1093/mutage/gem055

52. Gulston M, Fulford J, Jenner T, de Lara C, O'Neill P. Clustered DNA damage induced by gamma radiation in human fibroblasts (HF19), hamster (V79-4) cells and plasmid DNA is revealed as Fpg and Nth sensitive sites. *Nucleic Acids Res* (2002) 30(15):3464–72. doi:10.1093/nar/gkf467

53. Sutherland BM, Bennett PV, Sutherland JC, Laval J. Clustered DNA damages induced by X-rays in human cells. *Radiat Res* (2002) 157:611–6. doi:10.1667/0033-7587(2002)157[0611:CDDIBX]2.0.CO;2

54. Ando K. Review of RBE data on ion beams from Chiba: influence of LET and biological system. *Dose Reporting in Ion Beam Therapy*. Vienna: International Atomic Energy Agency (2007). p. 89–98.

55. Ando K, Kase Y. Biological characteristics of carbon-ion therapy. *Int J Radiat Biol* (2009) 85(9):715–28. doi:10.1080/09553000903072470

56. Ando S, Nojima K, Ishihara H, Suzuki M, Ando M, Majima H, et al. Induction by carbon-ion irradiation of the expression of vascular endothelial growth factor in lung carcinoma cells. *Int J Radiat Biol* (2000) 76(8):1121–7. doi:10.1080/09553000050111596

57. Belli M, Bettega D, Calzolari P, Cherubini R, Cuttone G, Durante M, et al. Effectiveness of monoenergetic and spread-out Bragg peak carbon-ions for inactivation of various normal and tumour human cell lines. *J Radiat Res* (2008) 49(6):597–607. doi:10.1269/jrr.08052

58. Combs SE, Bohl J, Elsasser T, Weber KJ, Schulz-Ertner D, Debus J, et al. Radiobiological evaluation and correlation with the local effect model (LEM) of carbon ion radiation therapy and temozolomide in glioblastoma cell lines. *Int J Radiat Biol* (2009) 85(2):126–37. doi:10.1080/09553000802641151

59. Furusawa Y, Fukutsu K, Aoki M, Itsukaichi H, Eguchi-Kasai K, Ohara H, et al. Inactivation of aerobic and hypoxic cells from three different cell lines by accelerated (3)He-, (12)C- and (20)Ne-ion beams. *Radiat Res* (2000) 154(5):485–96. doi:10.1667/0033-7587(2000)154[0485:IOAAHC]2.0.CO;2

60. Ito A, Nakano H, Kusano Y, Hirayama R, Furusawa Y, Murayama C, et al. Contribution of indirect action to radiation-induced mammalian cell inactivation: dependence on photon energy and heavy-ion LET. *Radiat Res* (2006) 165(6):703–12. doi:10.1667/RR3557.1

61. Iwadate Y, Mizoe J, Osaka Y, Yamaura A, Tsujii H. High linear energy transfer carbon radiation effectively kills cultured glioma cells with either mutant or wild-type p53. *Int J Radiat Oncol Biol Phys* (2001) 50(3):803–8. doi:10.1016/S0360-3016(01)01514-0

62. Kagawa K, Murakami M, Hishikawa Y, Abe M, Akagi T, Yanou T, et al. Preclinical biological assessment of proton and carbon ion beams at Hyogo Ion Beam Medical Center. *Int J Radiat Oncol Biol Phys* (2002) 54(3):928–38. doi:10.1016/S0360-3016(02)02949-8

63. Kamlah F, Hanze J, Arenz A, Seay U, Hasan D, Juricko J, et al. Comparison of the effects of carbon ion and photon irradiation on the angiogenic response in human lung adenocarcinoma cells. *Int J Radiat Oncol Biol Phys* (2011) 80(5):1541–9. doi:10.1016/j.ijrobp.2011.03.033

64. Matsui Y, Asano T, Kenmochi T, Iwakawa M, Imai T, Ochiai T. Effects of carbon-ion beams on human pancreatic cancer cell lines that differ in genetic status. *Am J Clin Oncol* (2004) 27(1):24–8. doi:10.1097/01.coc.0000046037.75545.AD

65. Matsumoto Y, Iwakawa M, Furusawa Y, Ishikawa K, Aoki M, Imadome K, et al. Gene expression analysis in human malignant melanoma cell lines exposed to carbon ions. *Int J Radiat Biol* (2008) 84:299–314. doi:10.1080/09553000801953334

66. Matsuzaki H, Miyamoto T, Miyazawa Y, Okazumi S, Koide Y, Isono K. Biological effects of heavy ion beam on human breast cancers. *Breast Cancer* (1998) 5(3):261–8. doi:10.1007/BF02966706

67. Ofuchi T, Suzuki M, Kase Y, Ando K, Isono K, Ochiai T. Chromosome breakage and cell lethality in human hepatoma cells irradiated with X rays and carbon-ion beams. *J Radiat Res* (1999) 40(2):125–33. doi:10.1269/jrr.40.125

68. Persson LM, Edgren MR, Stenerlow B, Lind BK, Hedlof I, Jernberg AR, et al. Relative biological effectiveness of boron ions on human melanoma cells. *Int J Radiat Biol* (2002) 78(8):743–8. doi:10.1080/09553000210140091

69. Stenerlow B, Pettersson OA, Essand M, Blomquist E, Carlsson J. Irregular variations in radiation sensitivity when the linear energy transfer is increased. *Radiother Oncol* (1995) 36(2):133–42. doi:10.1016/0167-8140(95)01591-4

70. Suzuki M, Kase Y, Yamaguchi H, Kanai T, Ando K. Relative biological effectiveness for cell-killing effect on various human cell lines irradiated with heavy-ion medical accelerator in Chiba (HIMAC) carbon-ion beams. *Int J Radiat Oncol Biol Phys* (2000) 48(1):241–50. doi:10.1016/S0360-3016(00)00568-X

71. Suzuki M, Kase Y, Nakano T, Kanai T, Ando K. Residual chromatin breaks as biodosimetry for cell killing by carbon ions. *Adv Space Res* (1998) 22(12):1663–71. doi:10.1016/S0273-1177(99)00031-9

72. Suzuki M, Kase Y, Kanai T, Ando K. Correlation between cell killing and residual chromatin breaks measured by PCC in six human cell lines irradiated with different radiation types. *Int J Radiat Biol* (2000) 76(9):1189–96. doi:10.1080/09553000050134429

73. Suzuki M, Kase Y, Kanai T, Ando K. Change in radiosensitivity with fractionated-dose irradiation of carbon-ion beams in five different human cell lines. *Int J Radiat Oncol Biol Phys* (2000) 48(1):251–8. doi:10.1016/S0360-3016(00)00606-4

74. Takahashi A, Ohnishi K, Tsuji K, Matsumoto H, Aoki H, Wang X, et al. WAF1 accumulation by carbon-ion beam and alpha-particle irradiation in human glioblastoma cultured cells. *Int J Radiat Biol* (2000) 76(3):335–41. doi:10.1080/095530000138673

75. Takahashi A, Ohnishi K, Ota I, Asakawa I, Tamamoto T, Furusawa Y, et al. p53-dependent thermal enhancement of cellular sensitivity in human squamous cell carcinomas in relation to LET. *Int J Radiat Biol* (2001) 77(10):1043–51. doi:10.1080/09553000110066095

76. Takahashi A, Matsumoto H, Yuki K, Yasumoto J, Kajiwara A, Aoki M, et al. High-LET radiation enhanced apoptosis but not necrosis regardless of p53 status. *Int J Radiat Oncol Biol Phys* (2004) 60(2):591–7. doi:10.1016/j.ijrobp.2004.05.062

77. Takahashi A, Matsumoto H, Furusawa Y, Ohnishi K, Ishioka N, Ohnishi T. Apoptosis induced by high-LET radiations is not affected by cellular p53 gene status. *Int J Radiat Biol* (2005) 81:581–6. doi:10.1080/09553000500280484

78. Tsuboi K, Tsuchida Y, Nose T, Ando K. Cytotoxic effect of accelerated carbon beams on glioblastoma cell lines with p53 mutation: clonogenic survival and cell-cycle analysis. *Int J Radiat Biol* (1998) 74(1):71–9. doi:10.1080/095530098141744

79. Tsuboi K, Moritake T, Tsuchida Y, Tokuuye K, Matsumura A, Ando K. Cell cycle checkpoint and apoptosis induction in glioblastoma cells and fibroblasts irradiated with carbon beam. *J Radiat Res* (2007) 48(4):317–25. doi:10.1269/jrr.06081

80. Tsuchida Y, Tsuboi K, Ohyama H, Ohno T, Nose T, Ando K. Cell death induced by high-linear-energy transfer carbon beams in human glioblastoma cell lines. *Brain Tumor Pathol* (1998) 15(2):71–6. doi:10.1007/BF02478886

81. Yamakawa N, Takahashi A, Mori E, Imai Y, Furusawa Y, Ohnishi K, et al. High LET radiation enhances apoptosis in mutated p53 cancer cells through caspase-9 activation. *Cancer Sci* (2008) 99(7):1455–60. doi:10.1111/j.1349-7006.2008.00818.x

82. Ferrandon S, Magne N, Battiston-Montagne P, Hau-Desbat NH, Diaz O, Beuve M, et al. Cellular and molecular portrait of eleven human glioblastoma cell lines under photon and carbon ion irradiation. *Cancer Lett* (2015) 360(1):10–6. doi:10.1016/j.canlet.2015.01.025

83. Schlaich F, Brons S, Haberer T, Debus J, Combs SE, Weber KJ. Comparison of the effects of photon versus carbon ion irradiation when combined with chemotherapy in vitro. *Radiat Oncol* (2013) 8:260. doi:10.1186/1748-717X-8-260

84. Beuve M, Alphonse G, Maalouf M, Colliaux A, Battiston-Montagne P, Jalade P, et al. Radiobiologic parameters and local effect model predictions for head-and-neck squamous cell carcinomas exposed to high linear energy transfer ions. *Int J Radiat Oncol Biol Phys* (2008) 71(2):635–42. doi:10.1016/j.ijrobp.2007.10.050

85. Kato TA, Tsuda A, Uesaka M, Fujimori A, Kamada T, Tsujii H, et al. In vitro characterization of cells derived from chordoma cell line U-CH1 following

86. Takiguchi Y, Miyamoto T, Nagao K, Kuriyama T. Assessment of the homogeneous efficacy of carbon ions in the spread-out Bragg peak for human lung cancer cell lines. *Radiat Med* (2007) 25(6):272–7. doi:10.1007/s11604-007-0134-6

87. Habermehl D, Ilicic K, Dehne S, Rieken S, Orschiedt L, Brons S, et al. The relative biological effectiveness for carbon and oxygen ion beams using the raster-scanning technique in hepatocellular carcinoma cell lines. *PLoS One* (2014) 9(12):e113591. doi:10.1371/journal.pone.0113591

88. Fujisawa H, Genik PC, Kitamura H, Fujimori A, Uesaka M, Kato TA. Comparison of human chordoma cell-kill for 290 MeV/n carbon ions versus 70 MeV protons in vitro. *Radiat Oncol* (2013) 8:91. doi:10.1186/1748-717X-8-91

89. Oonishi K, Cui X, Hirakawa H, Fujimori A, Kamijo T, Yamada S, et al. Different effects of carbon ion beams and X-rays on clonogenic survival and DNA repair in human pancreatic cancer stem-like cells. *Radiother Oncol* (2012) 105(2):258–65. doi:10.1016/j.radonc.2012.08.009

90. El Shafie RA, Habermehl D, Rieken S, Mairani A, Orschiedt L, Brons S, et al. In vitro evaluation of photon and raster-scanned carbon ion radiotherapy in combination with gemcitabine in pancreatic cancer cell lines. *J Radiat Res* (2013) 54(Suppl 1):i113–9. doi:10.1093/jrr/rrt052

91. Combs SE, Zipp L, Rieken S, Habermehl D, Brons S, Winter M, et al. In vitro evaluation of photon and carbon ion radiotherapy in combination with chemotherapy in glioblastoma cells. *Radiat Oncol* (2012) 7:9. doi:10.1186/1748-717X-7-9

92. Ando K, Kase Y, Matsufuji N. Light ion radiation biology. In: Brahme A, editor. *Comprehensive Biomedical Physics*. Amsterdam: Elsevier (2014). p. 195–210.

93. Brown JM, Attardi LD. The role of apoptosis in cancer development and treatment response. *Nat Rev Cancer* (2005) 5(3):231–7. doi:10.1038/nrc1560

94. Held KD. Radiation-induced apoptosis and its relationship to loss of clonogenic survival. *Apoptosis* (1997) 2:265–82. doi:10.1023/A:1026485003280

95. Tommasino F, Durante M. Proton radiobiology. *Cancers* (2015) 7(1):353–81. doi:10.3390/cancers7010353

96. Brown JM, Wouters BG. Apoptosis, p53, and tumor cell sensitivity to anti-cancer agents. *Cancer Res* (1999) 59:1391–9.

97. Grun R, Friedrich T, Kramer M, Zink K, Durante M, Engenhart-Cabillic R, et al. Assessment of potential advantages of relevant ions for particle therapy: a model based study. *Med Phys* (2015) 42(2):1037–47. doi:10.1118/1.4905374

98. Wulf H, Kraft-Weyrather W, Miltenburger HG, Blakely EA, Tobias CA, Kraft G. Heavy-ion effects on mammalian cells: inactivation measurements with different cell lines. *Radiat Res Suppl* (1985) 8:S122–34. doi:10.2307/3576639

99. Belli M, Cera F, Cherubini R, Haque AMI, Ianzini F, Moschini G, et al. The RBE of protons for cell inactivation: the experience with V79 cells. In: Amaldi U, Larsson B, editors. *Hadrontherapy in Oncology*. Amsterdam: Elsevier Science (1994). p. 702–5.

100. Cucinotta FA, Kim MH, Chappell LJ. *Space Radiation Cancer Risk Projections and Uncertainties – 2012. NASA/TP-2013-217375* (2013). Available from: http://ston.jsc.nasa.gov/collections/TRS

101. Friedrich T, Scholz U, Elsasser T, Durante M, Scholz M. Calculation of the biological effects of ion beams based on the microscopic spatial damage distribution pattern. *Int J Radiat Biol* (2012) 88(1–2):103–7. doi:10.3109/09553002.2011.611213

102. Bassler N, Toftegaard J, Luhr A, Sorensen BS, Scifoni E, Kramer M, et al. LET-painting increases tumour control probability in hypoxic tumours. *Acta Oncol* (2014) 53(1):25–32. doi:10.3109/0284186X.2013.832835

103. Kamada T, Tsujii H, Blakely EA, Debus J, De Neve W, Durante M, et al. Carbon ion radiotherapy in Japan: an assessment of 20 years of clinical experience. *Lancet Oncol* (2015) 16(2):e93–100. doi:10.1016/S1470-2045(14)70412-7

104. Steel GG, McMillan TJ, Peacock JH. The radiobiology of human cells and tissues. In vitro radiosensitivity. The picture has changed in the 1980s. *Int J Radiat Biol* (1989) 56(5):525–37. doi:10.1080/09553008914551691

105. Steel GG, Peacock JH. Why are some human tumours more radiosensitive than others? *Radiother Oncol* (1989) 15(1):63–72. doi:10.1016/0167-8140(89)90119-9

106. Bao S, Wu Q, McLendon RE, Hao Y, Shi Q, Hjelmeland AB, et al. Glioma stem cells promote radioresistance by preferential activation of the DNA damage response. *Nature* (2006) **444**:756–60. doi:10.1038/nature05236

107. Phillips TM, McBride WH, Pajonk F. The response of CD24(-/low)/CD44+ breast cancer-initiating cells to radiation. *J Natl Cancer Inst* (2006) **98**:1777–85. doi:10.1093/jnci/djj495

108. Diehn M, Cho RW, Lobo NA, Kalisky T, Dorie MJ, Kulp AN, et al. Association of reactive oxygen species levels and radioresistance in cancer stem cells. *Nature* (2009) **458**(7239):780–3. doi:10.1038/nature07733

109. Cui X, Oonishi K, Tsujii H, Yasuda T, Matsumoto Y, Furusawa Y, et al. Effects of carbon ion beam on putative colon cancer stem cells and its comparison with X-rays. *Cancer Res* (2011) **71**(10):3676–87. doi:10.1158/0008-5472.CAN-10-2926

110. Pardal R, Clarke MF, Morrison SJ. Applying the principles of stem-cell biology to cancer. *Nat Rev Cancer* (2003) **3**:895–902. doi:10.1038/nrc1232

111. Khan IN, Al-Karim S, Bora RS, Chaudhary AG, Saini KS. Cancer stem cells: a challenging paradigm for designing targeted drug therapies. *Drug Discov Today* (2015) **20**(10):1205–16. doi:10.1016/j.drudis.2015.06.013

112. Pajonk F, Vlashi E, McBride WH. Radiation resistance of cancer stem cells: the 4 R's of radiobiology revisited. *Stem Cells* (2010) **28**:639–48. doi:10.1002/stem.318

113. Vlashi E, Kim K, Lagadec C, Donna LD, McDonald JT, Eghbali M, et al. In vivo imaging, tracking, and targeting of cancer stem cells. *J Natl Cancer Inst* (2009) **101**(5):350–9. doi:10.1093/jnci/djn509

114. Calabrese C, Poppleton H, Kocak M, Hogg TL, Fuller C, Hamner B, et al. A perivascular niche for brain tumor stem cells. *Cancer Cell* (2007) **11**(1):69–82. doi:10.1016/j.ccr.2006.11.020

115. Ishimoto T, Nagano O, Yae T, Tamada M, Motohara T, Oshima H, et al. CD44 variant regulates redox status in cancer cells by stabilizing the xCT subunit of system xc(-) and thereby promotes tumor growth. *Cancer Cell* (2011) **19**(3):387–400. doi:10.1016/j.ccr.2011.01.038

116. Yang G, Quan Y, Wang W, Fu Q, Wu J, Mei T, et al. Dynamic equilibrium between cancer stem cells and non-stem cancer cells in human SW620 and MCF-7 cancer cell populations. *Br J Cancer* (2012) **106**(9):1512–9. doi:10.1038/bjc.2012.126

117. Piao LS, Hur W, Kim TK, Hong SW, Kim SW, Choi JE, et al. CD133+ liver cancer stem cells modulate radioresistance in human hepatocellular carcinoma. *Cancer Lett* (2012) **315**(2):129–37. doi:10.1016/j.canlet.2011.10.012

118. Shimura T, Noma N, Oikawa T, Ochiai Y, Kakuda S, Kuwahara Y, et al. Activation of the AKT/cyclin D1/Cdk4 survival signaling pathway in radioresistant cancer stem cells. *Oncogenesis* (2012) **1**:e12. doi:10.1038/oncsis.2012.12

119. Xia P, Xu XY. PI3K/Akt/mTOR signaling pathway in cancer stem cells: from basic research to clinical application. *Am J Cancer Res* (2015) **5**(5):1602–9.

120. Sai S, Wakai T, Vares G, Yamada S, Kamijo T, Kamada T, et al. Combination of carbon ion beam and gemcitabine causes irreparable DNA damage and death of radioresistant pancreatic cancer stem-like cells in vitro and in vivo. *Oncotarget* (2015) **6**(8):5517–35. doi:10.18632/oncotarget.3584

121. Quan Y, Wang W, Fu Q, Mei T, Wu J, Li J, et al. Accumulation efficiency of cancer stem-like cells post γ-ray and proton irradiation. *Nucl Instr Meth Phys Res B* (2012) **286**:341–5. doi:10.1016/j.nimb.2011.11.019

122. Fu Q, Quan Y, Wang W, Mei T, Wu J, Li J, et al. Response of cancer stem-like cells and non-stem cancer cells to proton and γ-ray irradiation. *Nucl Instr Meth Phys Res B* (2012) **286**:346–50. doi:10.1016/j.nimb.2012.01.032

123. Blakely EA, Tobias CA, Yang TCH, Smith KC, Lyman JT. Inactivation of human kidney cells by high-energy monoenergetic heavy-ion beams. *Radiat Res* (1979) **80**:122–60. doi:10.2307/3575121

124. Nakagawa Y, Takahashi A, Kajihara A, Yamakawa N, Imai Y, Ota I, et al. Depression of p53-independent Akt survival signals in human oral cancer cells bearing mutated p53 gene after exposure to high-LET radiation. *Biochem Biophys Res Commun* (2012) **423**(4):654–60. doi:10.1016/j.bbrc.2012.06.004

125. Hamada N, Imaoka T, Masunaga S, Ogata T, Okayasu R, Takahashi A, et al. Recent advances in the biology of heavy-ion cancer therapy. *J Radiat Res* (2010) **51**(4):365–83. doi:10.1269/jrr.09137

126. Takahashi A, Ma H, Nakagawa A, Yoshida Y, Kanai T, Ohno T, et al. Carbon-ion beams efficiently induce cell killing in X-ray resistant human squamous

127. tongue cancer cells. *Int J Med Phys Clin Eng Radiat Oncol* (2014) **3**:133–42. doi:10.4236/ijmpcero.2014.33019

127. Bertrand G, Maalouf M, Boivin A, Battiston-Montagne P, Beuve M, Levy A, et al. Targeting head and neck cancer stem cells to overcome resistance to photon and carbon ion radiation. *Stem Cell Rev* (2014) **10**(1):114–26. doi:10.1007/s12015-013-9467-y

128. Joiner MC, Van der Kogel AJ. *Basic Clinical Radiobiology*. London: Hodder Arnold (2009).

129. Fleming IN, Manavaki R, Blower PJ, West C, Williams KJ, Harris AL, et al. Imaging tumour hypoxia with positron emission tomography. *Br J Cancer* (2015) **112**(2):238–50. doi:10.1038/bjc.2014.610

130. Vaupel P, Harrison L. Tumor hypoxia: causative factors, compensatory mechanisms, and cellular response. *Oncologist* (2004) **9**(Suppl 5):4–9. doi:10.1634/theoncologist.9-90005-4

131. Tinganelli W, Ma NY, Von Neubeck C, Maier A, Schicker C, Kraft-Weyrather W, et al. Influence of acute hypoxia and radiation quality on cell survival. *J Radiat Res* (2013) **54**(Suppl 1):i23–30. doi:10.1093/jrr/rrt065

132. Ma NY, Tinganelli W, Maier A, Durante M, Kraft-Weyrather W. Influence of chronic hypoxia and radiation quality on cell survival. *J Radiat Res* (2013) **54**(Suppl 1):i13–22. doi:10.1093/jrr/rrs135

133. Zolzer F, Streffer C. Increased radiosensitivity with chronic hypoxia in four human tumor cell lines. *Int J Radiat Oncol Biol Phys* (2002) **54**(3):910–20. doi:10.1016/S0360-3016(02)02963-2

134. Wenzl T, Wilkens JJ. Modelling of the oxygen enhancement ratio for ion beam radiation therapy. *Phys Med Biol* (2011) **56**(11):3251–68. doi:10.1088/0031-9155/56/11/006

135. Scifoni E, Tinganelli W, Weyrather WK, Durante M, Maier A, Kramer M. Including oxygen enhancement ratio in ion beam treatment planning: model implementation and experimental verification. *Phys Med Biol* (2013) **58**(11):3871–95. doi:10.1088/0031-9155/58/11/3871

136. Hirayama R, Furusawa Y, Fukawa T, Ando K. Repair kinetics of DNA-DSB induced by X-rays or carbon ions under oxic and hypoxic conditions. *J Radiat Res* (2005) **46**(3):325–32. doi:10.1269/jrr.46.325

137. Nakano T, Suzuki Y, Ohno T, Kato S, Suzuki M, Morita S, et al. Carbon beam therapy overcomes the radiation resistance of uterine cervical cancer originating from hypoxia. *Clin Cancer Res* (2006) **12**(7 Pt 1):2185–90. doi:10.1158/1078-0432.CCR-05-1907

138. Antonovic L, Lindblom E, Dasu A, Bassler N, Furusawa Y, Toma-Dasu I. Clinical oxygen enhancement ratio of tumors in carbon ion radiotherapy: the influence of local oxygenation changes. *J Radiat Res* (2014) **55**(5):902–11. doi:10.1093/jrr/rru020

139. Schlaff CD, Krauze A, Belard A, O'Connell JJ, Camphausen KA. Bringing the heavy: carbon ion therapy in the radiobiological and clinical context. *Radiat Oncol* (2014) **9**(1):88. doi:10.1186/1748-717X-9-88

140. Bentzen SM, Ritter MA. The alpha/beta ratio for prostate cancer: what is it, really? *Radiother Oncol* (2005) **76**(1):1–3. doi:10.1016/j.radonc.2005.06.009

141. Bentzen SM, Overgaard J, Thames HD, Overgaard M, Vejby Hansen P, von der Maase H, et al. Clinical radiobiology of malignant melanoma. *Radiother Oncol* (1989) **16**(3):169–82.

142. Williams MV, Denekamp J, Fowler JF. A review of alpha/beta ratios for experimental tumors: implications for clinical studies of altered fractionation. *Int J Radiat Oncol Biol Phys* (1985) **11**(1):87–96. doi:10.1016/0360-3016(85)90366-9

143. Lo SS, Fakiris AJ, Chang EL, Mayr NA, Wang JZ, Papiez L, et al. Stereotactic body radiation therapy: a novel treatment modality. *Nat Rev Clin Oncol* (2010) **7**(1):44–54. doi:10.1038/nrclinonc.2009.188

144. Kupelian PA, Thakkar VV, Khuntia D, Reddy CA, Klein EA, Mahadevan A. Hypofractionated intensity-modulated radiotherapy (70 gy at 2.5 Gy per fraction) for localized prostate cancer: long-term outcomes. *Int J Radiat Oncol Biol Phys* (2005) **63**(5):1463–8. doi:10.1016/j.ijrobp.2005.05.054

145. Schulz-Ertner D, Nikoghosyan A, Hof H, Didinger B, Combs SE, Jakel O, et al. Carbon ion radiotherapy of skull base chondrosarcomas. *Int J Radiat Oncol Biol Phys* (2007) **67**(1):171–7. doi:10.1016/j.ijrobp.2006.08.027

146. Denekamp J, Waites T, Fowler JF. Predicting realistic RBE values for clinically relevant radiotherapy schedules. *Int J Radiat Biol* (1997) **71**(6):681–94. doi:10.1080/095530097143694

147. Denekamp J, Harris SR, Morris C, Field SB. The response of a transplantable tumor to fractionated irradiation. II. Fast neutrons. *Radiat Res* (1976) **68**(1):93–103. doi:10.2307/3574537

148. Ando K, Koike S, Uzawa A, Takai N, Fukawa T, Furusawa Y, et al. Biological gain of carbon-ion radiotherapy for the early response of tumor growth delay and against early response of skin reaction in mice. *J Radiat Res* (2005) **46**(1):51–7. doi:10.1269/jrr.46.51

149. Field SB, Hornsey S. RBE values for cyclotron neutrons for effects on normal tissues and tumours as a function of dose and dose fractionation. *Eur J Cancer* (1971) **7**(2):161–9. doi:10.1016/0014-2964(71)90011-9

150. Leith JT, Woodruff KH, Lyman JT. Early effects of single doses of 375 MeV/nucleon 20Neon ions on the skin of mice and hamsters. *Radiat Res* (1976) **65**(3):440–50. doi:10.2307/3574375

151. Joiner MC. Linear energy transfer and relative biological effectiveness. 4th ed. In: Joiner MC, van der Kogel AJ, editors. *Basic Clinical Radiobiology*. London: Hodder Arnold (2009). p. 68–77.

152. Jones B. The apparent increase in the {beta}-parameter of the linear quadratic model with increased linear energy transfer during fast neutron irradiation. *Br J Radiol* (2010) **83**(989):433–6. doi:10.1259/bjr/68792966

153. Yoshida Y, Ando K, Ando K, Murata K, Yoshimoto Y, Musha A, et al. Evaluation of therapeutic gain for fractionated carbon-ion radiotherapy using the tumor growth delay and crypt survival assays. *Radiother Oncol* (2015) **117**(2):351–7. doi:10.1016/j.radonc.2015.09.027

154. Uzawa A, Ando K, Kase Y, Hirayama R, Matsumoto Y, Matsufuji N, et al. Designing a ridge filter based on a mouse foot skin reaction to spread out Bragg-peaks for carbon-ion radiotherapy. *Radiother Oncol* (2015) **115**(2):279–83. doi:10.1016/j.radonc.2015.04.007

155. Ando K, Koike S, Uzawa A, Takai N, Fukawa T, Furusawa Y, et al. Repair of skin damage during fractionated irradiation with gamma rays and low-LET carbon ions. *J Radiat Res* (2006) **47**(2):167–74. doi:10.1269/jrr.47.167

156. Karger CP, Peschke P, Sanchez-Brandelik R, Scholz M, Debus J. Radiation tolerance of the rat spinal cord after 6 and 18 fractions of photons and carbon ions: experimental results and clinical implications. *Int J Radiat Oncol Biol Phys* (2006) **66**(5):1488–97. doi:10.1016/j.ijrobp.2006.08.045

157. Ando K, Koike S, Ohira C, Chen YJ, Nojima K, Ando S, et al. Accelerated reoxygenation of a murine fibrosarcoma after carbon-ion radiation. *Int J Radiat Biol* (1999) **75**(4):505–12. doi:10.1080/095530099140438

158. Oya N, Sasai K, Shibata T, Takagi T, Shibuya K, Koike S, et al. Time course of reoxygenation in experimental murine tumors after carbon-beam and X-ray irradiation. *J Radiat Res* (2001) **42**(2):131–41. doi:10.1269/jrr.42.131

159. Kanai T, Matsufuji N, Miyamoto T, Mizoe J, Kamada T, Tsuji H, et al. Examination of GyE system for HIMAC carbon therapy. *Int J Radiat Oncol Biol Phys* (2006) **64**(2):650–6. doi:10.1016/j.ijrobp.2005.09.043

160. Kanai T, Furusawa Y, Fukutsu K, Itsukaichi H, Eguchi-Kasai K, Ohara H. Irradiation of mixed beam and design of spread-out Bragg peak for heavy-ion radiotherapy. *Radiat Res* (1997) **147**(1):78–85. doi:10.2307/3579446

161. Shibamoto Y, Otsuka S, Iwata H, Sugie C, Ogino H, Tomita N. Radiobiological evaluation of the radiation dose as used in high-precision radiotherapy: effect of prolonged delivery time and applicability of the linear-quadratic model. *J Radiat Res* (2012) **53**(1):1–9. doi:10.1269/jrr.11095

162. Song CW, Kim MS, Cho LC, Dusenbery K, Sperduto PW. Radiobiological basis of SBRT and SRS. *Int J Clin Oncol* (2014) **19**(4):570–8. doi:10.1007/s10147-014-0717-z

163. Park HJ, Griffin RJ, Hui S, Levitt SH, Song CW. Radiation-induced vascular damage in tumors: implications of vascular damage in ablative hypofractionated radiotherapy (SBRT and SRS). *Radiat Res* (2012) **177**(3):311–27. doi:10.1667/RR2773.1

164. Williams JP, Brown SL, Georges GE, Hauer-Jensen M, Hill RP, Huser AK, et al. Animal models for medical countermeasures to radiation exposure. *Radiat Res* (2010) **173**:557–78. doi:10.1667/RR1880.1

165. Brown JM, Carlson DJ, Brenner DJ. Dose escalation, not "new biology," can account for the efficacy of stereotactic body radiation therapy with non-small cell lung cancer. In reply to Rao et al. *Int J Radiat Oncol Biol Phys* (2014) **89**(3):693–4. doi:10.1016/j.ijrobp.2014.03.014

166. Brown JM, Carlson DJ, Brenner DJ. The tumor radiobiology of SRS and SBRT: are more than the 5 Rs involved? *Int J Radiat Oncol Biol Phys* (2014) **88**(2):254–62. doi:10.1016/j.ijrobp.2013.07.022

167. Fowler JF. The radiobiology of prostate cancer including new aspects of fractionated radiotherapy. *Acta Oncol* (2005) **44**(3):265–76. doi:10.1080/02841860410002824

168. Garcia-Barros M, Paris F, Cordon-Cardo C, Lyden D, Rafii S, Haimovitz-Friedman A, et al. Tumor response to radiotherapy regulated by endothelial cell apoptosis. *Science* (2003) **300**(5622):1155–9. doi:10.1126/science.1082504

169. Fuks Z, Kolesnick R. Engaging the vascular component of the tumor response. *Cancer Cell* (2005) **8**(2):89–91. doi:10.1016/j.ccr.2005.07.014

170. Lee Y, Auh SL, Wang Y, Burnette B, Meng Y, Beckett M, et al. Therapeutic effects of ablative radiation on local tumor require CD8+ T cells: changing strategies for cancer treatment. *Blood* (2009) **114**(3):589–95. doi:10.1182/blood-2009-02-206870

171. Matsumura S, Wang B, Kawashima N, Braunstein S, Badura M, Cameron TO, et al. Radiation-induced CXCL16 release by breast cancer cells attracts effector T cells. *J Immunol* (2008) **181**(5):3099–107. doi:10.4049/jimmunol.181.5.3099

172. Ogata T, Teshima T, Kagawa K, Hishikawa Y, Takahashi Y, Kawaguchi A, et al. Particle irradiation suppresses metastatic potential of cancer cells. *Cancer Res* (2005) **65**(1):113–20.

173. Tamaki T, Iwakawa M, Ohno T, Imadome K, Nakawatari M, Sakai M, et al. Application of carbon-ion beams or gamma-rays on primary tumors does not change the expression profiles of metastatic tumors in an in vivo murine model. *Int J Radiat Oncol Biol Phys* (2009) **74**(1):210–8. doi:10.1016/j.ijrobp.2008.12.078

174. Matsunaga A, Ueda Y, Yamada S, Harada Y, Shimada H, Hasegawa M, et al. Carbon-ion beam treatment induces systemic antitumor immunity against murine squamous cell carcinoma. *Cancer* (2010) **116**(15):3740–8. doi:10.1002/cncr.25134

175. Ohkubo Y, Iwakawa M, Seino K, Nakawatari M, Wada H, Kamijuku H, et al. Combining carbon ion radiotherapy and local injection of alpha-galactosyl-ceramide-pulsed dendritic cells inhibits lung metastases in an in vivo murine model. *Int J Radiat Oncol Biol Phys* (2010) **78**(5):1524–31. doi:10.1016/j.ijrobp.2010.06.048

176. Yoshimoto Y, Oike T, Okonogi N, Suzuki Y, Ando K, Sato H, et al. Carbon-ion beams induce production of an immune mediator protein, high mobility group box 1, at levels comparable with X-ray irradiation. *J Radiat Res* (2015) **56**(3):509–14. doi:10.1093/jrr/rrv007

177. Durante M, Reppingen N, Held KD. Immunologically augmented cancer treatment using modern radiotherapy. *Trends Mol Med* (2013) **19**(9):565–82. doi:10.1016/j.molmed.2013.05.007

178. Ogata T, Teshima T, Inaoka M, Minami K, Tsuchiya T, Isono M, et al. Carbon ion irradiation suppresses metastatic potential of human non-small cell lung cancer A549 cells through the phosphatidylinositol-3-kinase/Akt signaling pathway. *J Radiat Res* (2011) **52**(3):374–9. doi:10.1269/jrr.10102

179. Karger CP, Scholz M, Huber PE, Debus J, Peschke P. Photon and carbon ion irradiation of a rat prostate carcinoma: does a higher fraction number increase the metastatic rate? *Radiat Res* (2014) **181**(6):623–8. doi:10.1667/RR13611.1

5

Exposure to Carbon Ions Triggers Proinflammatory Signals and Changes in Homeostasis and Epidermal Tissue Organization to a Similar Extent as Photons

Palma Simoniello[1†], Julia Wiedemann[1,2†], Joana Zink[1], Eva Thoennes[1], Maike Stange[1], Paul G. Layer[2], Maximilian Kovacs[3], Maurizio Podda[3], Marco Durante[1,2] and Claudia Fournier[1,4*]

[1] Department of Biophysics, GSI Helmholtzzentrum für Schwerionenforschung, Darmstadt, Germany, [2] Department of Biology, Technische Universität Darmstadt, Darmstadt, Germany, [3] Department of Dermatology, Darmstadt Hospital, Darmstadt, Germany, [4] Hochschule Darmstadt, Darmstadt, Germany

*Correspondence:
Claudia Fournier
c.fournier@gsi.de

†Palma Simoniello and Julia Wiedemann have contributed equally to this work.

The increasing application of charged particles in radiotherapy requires a deeper understanding of early and late side effects occurring in skin, which is exposed in all radiation treatments. We measured cellular and molecular changes related to the early inflammatory response of human skin irradiated with carbon ions, in particular cell death induction and changes in differentiation and proliferation of epidermal cells during the first days after exposure. Model systems for human skin from healthy donors of different complexity, i.e., keratinocytes, coculture of skin cells, 3D skin equivalents, and skin explants, were used to investigate the alterations induced by carbon ions (spread-out Bragg peak, dose-averaged LET 100 keV/µm) in comparison to X-ray and UV-B exposure. After exposure to ionizing radiation, in none of the model systems, apoptosis/necrosis was observed. Carbon ions triggered inflammatory signaling and accelerated differentiation of keratinocytes to a similar extent as X-rays at the same doses. High doses of carbon ions were more effective than X-rays in reducing proliferation and inducing abnormal differentiation. In contrast, changes identified following low-dose exposure ($\leq$0.5 Gy) were induced more effectively after X-ray exposure, i.e., enhanced proliferation and change in the polarity of basal cells.

Keywords: human skin equivalent, keratinocytes, differentiation, apoptosis, inflammation, proliferation, ionizing irradiation, carbon ions

---

Abbreviations: cl, cleaved; D, dermis; fl, full length; HSE, human skin equivalent; M, marker; PC, positive control; SB, stratum basale; SC, stratum corneum; SG, stratum granulosum; SS, stratum spinosum.

INTRODUCTION

The increasing application of charged particles in radiotherapy motivates our assessment of inflammatory reactions and homeostasis of tissue exposed to carbon ions and to compare the response to X-rays. In the current study, we focus on the analysis of cell death, proliferation, differentiation, and reorganization of different layers of the epidermis.

Charged particles display particular physical characteristics, such as high mass and electrical charge, resulting in an inverted depth dose profile compared to photons with a high relative dose deposition at the end of their trajectory. This enables a volume conform treatment of deep-seated tumors (1) as well as sparing of critical organs. In addition, when using ions heavier than protons, the exposure of cells or tissue in the "Bragg Peak" region at the end of the trajectory leads to a higher local intensity of ionizing events, and thereby clusters of DNA damage (2). As a consequence, an enhanced biological efficiency compared to photons is observed (3, 4).

New treatment approaches with carbon ions make use of these advantages by increasing the dose to the tumor to enhance the tumor control probability (1, 2). However, this also implies the delivery of a higher dose to the surrounding normal tissue, including skin (5). Skin reactions associated with carbon ion therapy for deep-seated tumors are reported to be moderate and comparable to classical photon exposure (6). However, dose escalation trials in particle therapy applying a higher dose via only 1–2 entrance channels may cause skin toxicity (5). A typical case is breast cancer proton therapy, where the target (lumpectomy cavity) is shallow, and therefore skin toxicity is the limiting factor for beam arrangement and prescription doses (7, 8).

Skin is of interest because a considerable part of the side effects occurring after radiotherapy are observed in this organ due to its sensitivity (9) and its involvement in all radiation exposures (10). Radiation effects observed in the epidermis of the skin are erythema, desquamation and, for very high doses, late necrosis. In the dermis late effects occur, i.e., persisting vascular damage and fibrosis (11–13). In addition, anti-inflammatory effects induced by low-dose radiation (14) exposure can be anticipated as they are already shown for UV exposure (15, 16).

In the work presented here, we aimed to investigate the cellular and molecular changes related to the early inflammatory response of irradiated skin, in particular the occurrence of cell death and changes in differentiation and proliferation of the epidermal cells. In this context, a comparison between X-rays and carbon ions was intended. The first experiments were performed in monolayer- and cocultures of skin cells (keratinocytes, cocultured with fibroblasts); the respective results are reported in the supplement.

Based on these results obtained in cell cultures, we used a 3D human skin equivalent (HSE) and human skin explants to approach the physiological conditions in tissue and tested the following working hypotheses:

(1) Cell death of keratinocytes does not play a major role in the inflammatory response to ionizing radiation within the first days postexposure.

(2) An early release of inflammatory cytokines in irradiated skin tissue may be elicited by other typical changes (proliferation, differentiation, and tissue organization) than cell death.

(3) Taking into account previous knowledge about irradiation-induced changes in tissue, we hypothesize that activation of proliferation, differentiation, and tissue organization may be affected.

(4) Carbon ions, delivered to normal skin under therapy conditions, induce similar effects related to inflammation, proliferation, differentiation, and tissue organization compared to the same physical doses of photons.

Throughout the assessment of cell death, cytokine release, homeostasis, and tissue organization, the effects of carbon ions, using an extended Bragg Peak as a therapy-like configuration, were compared to X-rays. As the efficiency of carbon ions in inducing the respective effects has not been reported for skin cells and tissue before, we have chosen the same low and moderate doses to compare the radiation qualities and, in addition, a high X-ray dose to take into account a potential higher but not yet determined efficiency of carbon ions. A considerable number of data sets on non-ionizing UV-B exposure are available, and therefore UV-B irradiation served as a reference, and the respective results for all model systems used are reported in the supplement.

MATERIALS AND METHODS

Tissue Culture

Human full-thickness skin equivalent constructs (EpiDermFT™), referred to as HSE herein, were purchased from MatTek Corporation (Ashland, MA, USA) and cultured according to the manufacturer's protocol. The HSE consists of an epidermal layer composed of normal human epidermal keratinocytes, which is not submerged in culture medium and a dermal layer built up of fibroblasts and extracellular matrix (collagen1). All HSE constructs were equilibrated for at least 16 h before the experiments were started. During irradiation, the samples were maintained in PBS (Biochrom; Berlin, Germany) and fresh medium was added after irradiation. Media exchange was repeated on a daily basis until the experiment was terminated.

Human skin tissue explants were obtained from surgical discard (Dermatology Clinic, Darmstadt, Germany). The study was approved by the Local Ethics Committee (FF136/2014). The skin was washed in PBS, cut into small pieces (5 mm × 5 mm) and explanted in cell culture inserts (BD Falcon, Heidelberg Germany). The membrane of the inserts was in contact with medium (RPMI 1640, with 10% FCS and 2% Pen/Strep; all Biochrom, Berlin, Germany). The skin explants were cultured under standard conditions.

Irradiation

X-ray irradiation (X-RAD 320 R X, 250 kV, 16 mA) of HSE was performed with a dose rate of 1 Gy/min (0.5–10 Gy).

Carbon ion irradiation (0.5–2 Gy) was performed using a pencil beam in a spread-out Bragg peak (SOBP) with 20.0 mm width equivalent to a depth of 5 cm in water (110–145 MeV/μm;

LET 100 keV/μm), at the heavy-ion synchrotron (SIS) at GSI Helmholtzzentrum für Schwerionenforschung (Darmstadt, Germany). A subset of carbon ion irradiations has been performed with the same parameters of exposure at the heavy-ion synchrotron of the Heidelberg Ion-Beam Therapy Center HIT (Heidelberg, Germany).

For carbon ion irradiation, the HSE were positioned vertically. In order to protect the samples from drying out, a sterile gaze soaked with prewarmed PBS was put in the wells under the membrane, and the wells were closed with Parafilm during exposure, which typically took 10 min.

Histochemistry, Immunohistochemistry, Imaging, and Quantitative Analysis

For histological analyses, HSE was fixed in a 4% PFA-solution, processed for paraffin embedding, and cut into 5 μm sections using a microtome (RM2235; Leica Microsystems, Wetzlar, Germany). For hematoxylin and eosin (H&E) staining, slides were deparaffinized, rehydrated, and stained according to commonly used procedures (17).

For immunostaining, the sections were deparaffinized, rehydrated, treated with 10 mM citrate acid buffer (pH 6.0), and heated in a microwave to unmask the antigens. After rinsing in deionized water, the slides were incubated in 0.3% H_2O_2 for 30 min to block the endogenous peroxidase activity. After washing in PBS (three times), non-specific binding sites were blocked by incubating the sections with blocking solution (1.5% normal goat serum in PBS with 0.1% (v/v) Triton X-100). Finally, the slides were incubated with the primary antibody at 4°C overnight. Used antibodies and dilutions were: rabbit anti-active caspase-3 (Ab-2; Calbiochem, San Diego, CA, USA; 1:100), rabbit anti-Ki67 (SP6, ab16667; Abcam, Cambridge, UK; 1:100), and rabbit anti-E-Cadherin (EP700Y; ab40772; Abcam, Cambrigde, UK; 1:500). The detection of the binding of the primary antibody was performed with the Ultra-Sensitive ABC Peroxidase rabbit IgG staining kit (Thermo Scientific, Waltham, MA, USA) and the ImmPACT VIP-Peroxidase substrate kit (Vector, Burlingame, CA, USA) or SigmaFast-DAB-Tablets (Sigma, St. Louis, MO, USA) according to the manufacturer's protocol. The nuclei were counterstained with hematoxylin and the slides were dehydrated, cleared in xylene, and mounted. HSE, submerged entirely with medium, was used as positive control for apoptosis.

Tissue sections were imaged using an Olympus BX61 microscope with an E-330 camera (Olympus, Hamburg, Germany). For the quantitative or semiquantitative analysis, 20 pictures per sample were taken with a 40-fold magnification. Pyknotic cells in the stratum corneum (parakeratosis) and in the viable epidermis were counted by eye and the mean per field of view was calculated. Ki67-positive cells (proliferation) were also counted by eye and normalized on the total number of basal cells. The thickness of the stratum corneum and the viable epidermis were measured using the software Image J. The thickness of the stratum corneum was normalized on the thickness of the viable epidermis. For the semiquantitative analysis of the structure of the basal layer, for each picture, it was evaluated if the cells in the basal layer were palisadic, in part or completely cobblestoned; the fraction of pictures displaying the respective characteristic is given. Each analysis was performed from two independent experiments, in total for four samples ($n = 4$, $N = 2$); values are given as SEM.

Western Blot

The HSE epidermis was separated mechanically from dermis and lysed separately in RIPA buffer as previously described (18). In addition, tissue was homogenized with a pestle and with ultrasound treatment. Proteins were loaded (10 μg) and separated on 12% SDS-polyacrylamide gels, and then transferred to polyvinylidenfluoride membranes (Immobilon-P; Merck Millipore, Billerica, MA, USA). After blotting, the membranes were washed and incubated overnight at 4°C in 5% dry milk (Carl Roth GmbH, Karlsruhe, Germany) in Tris-buffered saline to reduce non-specific binding. Membranes were incubated with the primary antibodies for 2 h at room temperature.

Primary antibodies used were rabbit anti-caspase-3 (Cell Signaling, Danvers, MA, USA; 1:1000) and rabbit anti-PARP (46D11; Cell Signaling, Danvers, MA, USA; 1:1000). GAPDH (rabbit anti-GAPDH, Cell Signaling, Danvers, MA, USA; 1:1000) and α-Tubulin (mouse anti-α-Tubulin; Sigma, Steinheim, Germany; 1:4000) were used as a loading control. HaCaT cells, irradiated with 10 Gy X-rays and lysed 5 days after exposure, were used as a positive control. After washing, the membrane was incubated with a horseradish peroxidase-conjugated secondary antibody for 1 h at room temperature (anti-mouse IgG or anti-rabbit IgG HRP linked antibody; GE Healthcare, München, Germany; 1:10,000). Protein expression was visualized using enhanced chemiluminescence (Pierce ECL Plus Western; Thermo Scientific, Waltham, MA, USA) according to the manufacturer's instructions and detected on a X-ray film.

Enzyme-Linked Immunosorbent Assay

To quantify the levels of released cytokines in the medium of HSE, ELISA kits for the detection of TNF-α, IL-2, IL-6, IL-8, IL-10, TGF-β (all ELISA Ready-SET-go!; eBioscience, San Diego, CA, USA), and IL-1α (Platinum ELISA, eBioscience, San Diego, CA, USA) were used according to the manufacturer's protocol. The measured values for each sample were normalized on the controls. In the first step, we checked the cytokine release from each sample before irradiation separately, but as the values were very similar to each other, this additional normalization step according to Varnum et al. (19) was not pursued. The concentration of HMGB1 in the medium of HSE was measured using an ELISA kit (human HMGB1; Cloud-Clone-Corp., Houston, TX, USA), according to the manufacturer's instructions and normalized on the controls.

Statistical Analysis

Unless stated otherwise, the error bars represent the mean ± SEM. Statistical significance was tested using a Student's t-test. The number of independent irradiation experiments (N) and the total number of samples (n) are mentioned in the figure legends. At least two irradiation experiments and four samples were analyzed.

RESULTS

The results obtained in keratinocytes (normal human epidermal keratinocytes; NHEK), either in monolayers or cocultured with fibroblasts (normal human epidermal fibroblasts; NHDF), are presented in the supplement. The results obtained in a 3D HSE and in human skin explants are presented in the following paragraphs for X-ray and carbon irradiation, for UVB exposure in the supplement.

Induction of Apoptosis

We first assessed clonogenic cell survival after radiation exposure (Figure S1 in Supplementary Material). As expected, the dose–response curve shows a typical shoulder for X-ray, whereas the curve is linear for carbon ions, indicating a higher efficiency of carbon ions compared to X-ray in terms of cell inactivation. Please note that for cell inactivation, monoenergetic carbon ions (170 keV/μm) were used, whereas all the following experiments have been performed with SOBP carbon ions (100 keV/μm), which corresponds to the conditions used in radiotherapy.

Then, we investigated if this cell inactivation is due to the induction of cell death during 144 h after exposure to ionizing radiation (X-rays and SOBP carbon ions) in a monolayer culture of keratinocytes. In addition, we repeated this experiment in cocultures of keratinocytes and fibroblasts. The results are shown in Figures S1, S2, and S4 in Supplementary Material. In spite of clearly detectable cytogenetic damage in terms of micronuclei formation for both radiation qualities, the results did not indicate an occurrence of apoptosis (no detection of annexin V positive cells, pyknotic nuclei, apoptotic bodies, activated caspase-3, and cleaved PARP), not even at high doses, and showed only low levels of necrosis (release of HMGB, High Mobility Group Box 1 protein, an established marker for necrosis (20, 21), Figure S5 in Supplementary Material).

From these results, we hypothesized that cell death of keratinocytes does not play a major role in the inflammatory response to ionizing radiation, at least not within the first days after exposure. To test this in tissue, we moved on using a model system of higher complexity, i.e., a commercially available, three-dimensional HSE, and for selected experiments also human skin explants. We used the same physical doses of photons and carbon ions (0.5 and 2 Gy), and in addition a higher dose (10 Gy) of photon irradiation.

The occurrence of apoptosis was assessed in irradiated HSE and human skin up to 72 h after exposure. **Figure 1A** shows representative pictures of the immunodetection of active caspase-3 in HSE tissue sections, 24 h after exposure to moderate/high doses. In the positive control, apoptotic cells were identified in the basal layer by positive caspase-3 staining and condensed pyknotic nuclei. In contrast, no pyknotic nuclei or cells positive for active caspase-3 could be detected after irradiation, regardless of radiation quality and dose. This also applies for 72 h after irradiation (Figure S6A in Supplementary Material). Consistently, no cleaved caspase-3 and PARP (only assessed for X-ray exposure) were detected in lysates of irradiated HSE (western blot analysis for 24 h after exposure, **Figure 1B**, additional time points shown in Figure S6B in Supplementary Material). For X-ray exposure,

these observations were confirmed in sections of *ex vivo* irradiated human skin explants where no active caspase-3 and no pyknotic nuclei were observed (**Figure 1C**). The use of TUNEL assay turned out to be inappropriate to detect apoptotic cells because differentiating keratinocytes showed intensive staining, irrespective of radiation exposure, and can therefore not be distinguished from apoptotic cells (not shown), which is in line with independent observations (22).

In addition, signs of necrosis were not observed morphologically and release of HMGB1 was not detectable after irradiation neither in the medium of HSE nor in the medium of human skin explants (not shown).

All in all, our results indicate no major role for early apoptosis and necrosis neither for photon nor for carbon ion exposure within 72 h after irradiation. This we conclude from the absence of caspase-3-dependent apoptosis, HMGB1 release, and typical morphological alterations, observed in a 3D HSE, and confirmed in human skin explants, irradiated *ex vivo*.

Release of Cytokines Related to Inflammation

By analyzing cytokine release after irradiation of NHEK, an upregulation of proinflammatory cytokines on the level of gene and protein expression has been shown (12). In good agreement with published data, our own results have shown an enhanced release of IL-1α, IL-2, and TGF-β (Figure S7A in Supplementary Material, only assessed for X-rays). For IL-6 and IL-8, the measured cytokine concentration in the supernatant of the controls was below the detection limit. Thus, the relative radiation-induced increase could not be calculated reliably. The induction of IL-6 was induced by moderate doses of X-ray and UV-B irradiation, whereas IL-8 was only inducible by a high UV-B intensity (40 mJ/cm², not shown).

Of note, when the keratinocytes have been cocultured with normal dermal fibroblasts, a significant influence on the pattern of release, i.e. an inhibitory feedback loop between release of IL-1α and TGF-β, has been observed in the non-irradiated cells, which is in agreement with published data (Figure S7B in Supplementary Material) (23–26). Despite this modulating effect, a radiation-induced moderate increase in the release of IL-1α, and a clear increment of IL-6 and IL-8 release, has been detected 24 h after photon irradiation, whereas no significant change of TGF-β has been measured (Figure S7C in Supplementary Material, only assessed for X-ray).

Based on these findings, we assessed the cytokine release for relevant candidates after exposure to X-rays and carbon ions in the HSE. The results are summarized in **Figure 2**. As the kinetics of cytokine release turned out to be different for low versus high doses and for X-ray versus carbon ion exposure, the intended comparison of the respective impact of both radiation qualities was difficult. Furthermore, the release of TNF-α und IL-2 was very low, below the detection limit in all HSE experiments, except in positive controls of human skin, which were generated by submerging the skin explant with liquid. When these human skin explants were irradiated additionally, an increase of TNF-α could be measured (not shown).

For X-ray exposure (**Figure 2A**), we observed a trend for an enhancement of IL-1α release 24 h after 2 and 10 Gy, whereas after

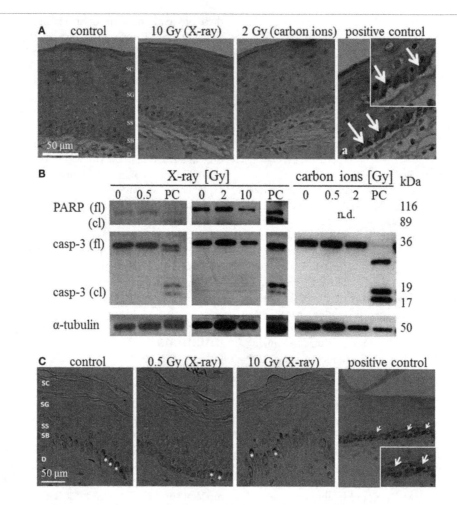

FIGURE 1 | Detection of apoptosis *in situ* and in western blot in HSE and human skin explants 24 h after irradiation with high doses of X-ray and carbon ions. **(A)** Immunodetection of active caspase-3 (brown) in HSE; cleaved caspase-3 was not detected in the epidermis after irradiation, but in the PCs (arrows in a); $N = 3$, $n = 5$. **(B)** Western blot analysis of caspase-3 and PARP in HSE; apoptosis is detected by the presence of caspase-3 and PARP cleavage fragments (17 and 19 kDa; 89 kDa) in PCs; active/cleaved caspase-3 and cleaved PARP were not detected in the epidermis of HSE after irradiation; $N = 2$, $n = 4$. **(C)** Immunodetection of cleaved caspase-3 (pink) in human skin explants; cleaved caspase-3 was not found after low or high doses of X-rays; *: melanocytes in the basal layer (brown); $N = 3$, $n = 5$.

48 h, the increment was around threefold compared to the level of controls, although not significant. For the highest X-ray dose (10 Gy), the increase was the same as for 2 Gy, and for 0.5 Gy, the release was unchanged at both time points. However, this was the only change observed after exposure to 10 Gy X-rays. The release of IL-6 after X-ray irradiation was only slightly, albeit significantly enhanced for 2 Gy at both time points (1.5-fold).

The level of the chemoattractant IL-8 protein showed a more than twofold enhancement after exposure to 0.5 Gy as early as 24 h after irradiation, and the increment for 2 Gy was significant at 24 h and also at 48 h postirradiation. As in the case of IL-6, no change in IL-8 release was observed for 10 Gy at none of the time points assessed.

Notably, for carbon ions (**Figure 2B**), after 24 h, no increment in the release of any of the measured cytokines was observed. At 48 h after exposure, there was a trend for an enhancement of IL-1α, but not for IL-6 release. The release of IL-8 was significantly increased about a factor of two.

The cytokines that are considered to have an anti-inflammatory effect at early times after irradiation, TGF-β and IL-10 (12, 27, 28), were not enhanced up to 48 h after exposure, regardless of the radiation quality. Although for IL-10, a significant enhancement was measured 48 h after carbon ion exposure (**Figure 2B**), the increment was around 1.5-fold compared to controls, raising the question about the biological significance of this modification.

Taken together, for the inflammatory cytokines IL-6 and IL-8, an enhancement within 48 h was detected after X-ray irradiation (**Figure 2A**). However, the observed changes were not strictly dose-dependent, and after carbon ion exposure (**Figure 2B**), only small changes were measured compared to the same physical doses of X-rays (0.5 and 2 Gy).

Abnormal and Accelerated Differentiation

Epidermal homeostasis is maintained by a balance between proliferating and differentiating keratinocytes. For epithelial and other tissues (29, 30), early radiation-induced changes in

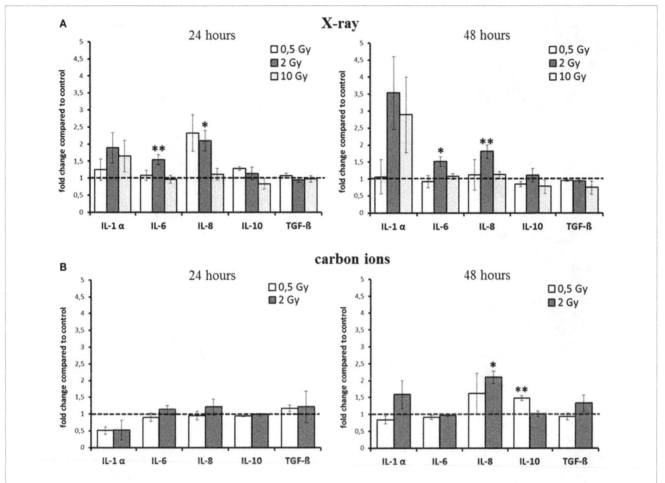

FIGURE 2 | Detection of cytokine release from HSE after irradiation with X-ray and carbon ions. **(A)** Enhancement of IL-6 and IL-8 release 24 and 48 h after exposure to moderate doses of X-rays. **(B)** No changes 24 h after carbon ion irradiation, enhanced release of IL-10 and IL-8 was detected 48 h after irradiation with carbon ions; SEM; *$p \leq 0.05$, **$p \leq 0.01$; $N = 2–3$, $n = 3–10$; IL-2 and TNF-α were not detectable.

proliferation, differentiation of keratinocytes, and reorganization of the epidermal layer are discussed to play a crucial role in early inflammation of the skin (31). Keratinocytes are organized in stratified layers. The basal layer (stratum basale) contains proliferating keratinocytes, which migrate into the upper layers (stratum spinosum and stratum granulosum) during their differentiation process by disconnecting from the basal membrane. During this process, morphology and protein expression profiles change. When keratinocytes finally reach the outer layer of the epidermis (stratum corneum), they have lost their nuclei and are terminally differentiated to cornified cells, which constitute the mechanical barrier of the skin, protecting the organisms against any type of external stress (10).

An abnormal pattern of morphology and differentiation is the occurrence of keratinocytes with pyknotic nuclei. If they are observed in the stratum corneum, which in healthy tissue consists of denucleated keratinocytes, this phenomenon is called parakeratosis and is associated with skin diseases (32, 33). These cells are also found in the viable part of the epidermis and in this case they are termed "sunburn cells", as they were first described after UV exposure (34, 35).

We assessed parakeratosis and "sunburn cells" in irradiated HSE at 24 and 72 h after exposure (**Figure 3**). In **Figure 3A**, a representative picture of parakeratosis is shown. Quantification was achieved by counting the number of pyknotic cells in the stratum corneum per field of view. As can be seen in **Figure 3B**, we observed parakeratosis at a low level in non-irradiated HSE (0.1–0.6 pyknotic nuclei in the stratum corneum per field of view) and an indication for an increase, albeit not statistically significant in HSE after carbon ion exposure. In **Figure 3C**, so-called "sunburn cells" are shown, which are not only characterized by pyknotic nuclei but also by an eosinophilic cytoplasm and the occurrence in the viable epidermis (34, 35). Quantification (**Figure 3D**) of these cells in the viable epidermis revealed a comparable increase 24 h after exposure to a moderate dose of X-ray and carbon ions (2 Gy), which was still persisting 72 h after irradiation. Notably, the increment was not observed for a low (0.5 Gy) and a high X-ray dose (10 Gy).

In some studies, sunburn cells are reported to be apoptotic, because the morphological alteration overlaps for part of the cells with positive staining for activated, cleaved caspase-3 (36). This was clearly not the case for the HSE in our study; in none of the

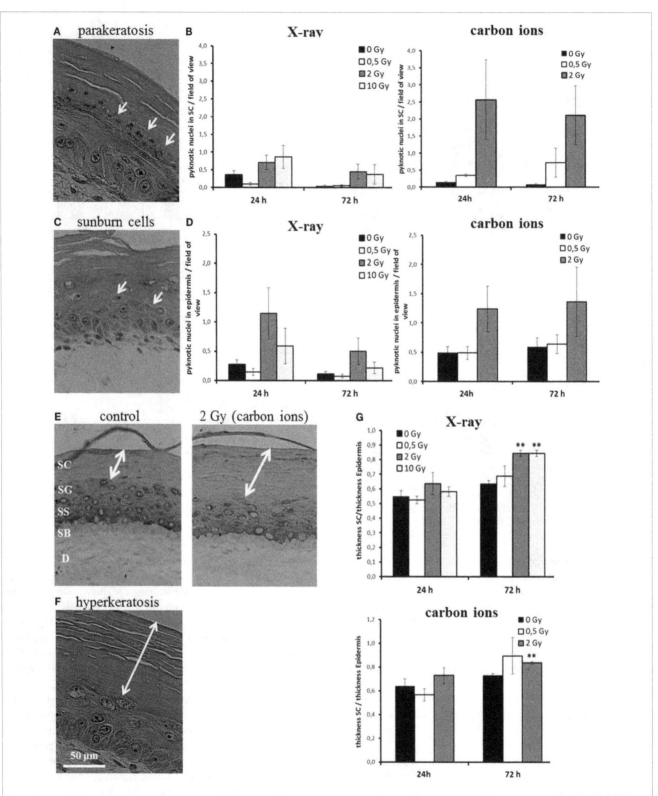

FIGURE 3 | Abnormal and accelerated differentiation in HSE after irradiation with X-ray and carbon ions. (A) Pyknotic keratinocytes are observed in the stratum corneum (parakeratosis). **(B)** Quantification of parakeratosis shows a slight increase after X-ray and a more pronounced increase after carbon ion exposure. **(C)** Morphology of typical "sunburn cells" characterized by pyknotic nuclei and an eosinophilic cytoplasm. **(D)** Quantification of "sunburn cells" shows a clear increase after 2 Gy of X-ray and carbon ions exposure. **(E)** Cytokeratin 10 expression (only in differentiating layers) in HSE 72 h after irradiation with carbon ions shows an enhanced thickness of the stratum corneum, where Cytokeratin 10 is not expressed. **(F)** Thickening of the stratum corneum (hyperkeratosis). **(G)** Quantification of hyperkeratosis shows an increase of the thickness of the stratum corneum 72 h after X-ray and carbon ion irradiation; SEM; *$p \leq 0.05$, **$p \leq 0.01$; $N = 2, n = 4$.

experimental conditions, a colocalization of sunburn cells and caspase-3 positive staining was detected (see **Figure 1**; Figure S6 in Supplementary Material).

Another physiological change reported after UV-B exposure (37) is the thickening of the stratum corneum. The stratum corneum is the epidermal layer where the differentiation is terminal and Cytokeratin 10 is not expressed (38) (example shown in **Figure 3E**). The thickening of the stratum corneum corresponds to an accelerated differentiation leading to an accumulation of cornified cells and is considered as a protective mechanism (39). In **Figure 3F**, a thickened stratum corneum (so-called "hyperkeratosis") of an irradiated HSE is depicted. For quantification, we measured the thickness of the stratum corneum and normalized this value to the thickness of the viable epidermis. As shown in **Figure 3G**, an increase of the stratum corneum was observed 72 h after exposure. The enhancement was significant for 2 and 10 Gy X-rays and 2 Gy carbon ions, whereas irradiation with a low dose (0.5 Gy) did not yield an effect.

The results show that abnormal differentiation patterns occur for moderate doses and were more pronounced for carbon ion than for X-ray exposure, whereas accelerated differentiation is significantly enhanced for X-ray exposure, also for a high dose, and for carbon ions, only a trend is observed. Both abnormal and accelerated differentiation is not detectable for low doses.

Proliferation

Enhanced proliferation due to a chronically activated state of keratinocytes has been reported for human skin, where skin biopsies have been taken from patients who had undergone radiotherapy and investigated months later (31). As we have observed accelerated differentiation for moderate and high doses, we set out to investigate a potential association with enhanced proliferation at early times after irradiation.

Proliferation activity was measured by Ki67 staining 72 h after irradiation of HSE. **Figure 4A** shows Ki67-positive cells in the basal layer. In controls, around 5% of the basal cells were positive for Ki67. Quantification of the fraction of Ki67-positive cells is depicted in **Figure 4B**, normalized on the level of non-irradiated HSE. An enhanced proliferation activity was observed after irradiation with a low X-ray dose (0.5 Gy), though not significant due to interexperimental variation. For higher X-ray doses and a low dose of carbon ions (0.5 Gy), no changes were observed, whereas following exposure to 2 Gy carbon ions a reduced fraction of proliferating cells was detected.

An increase in proliferation activity of the basal cells for 0.5 Gy and an unchanged activity for 10 Gy was confirmed in first experiments using explants of human skin (**Figure 4C**), which were *ex vivo* exposed to X-ray irradiation (24 and 48 h).

These results show an enhanced proliferation occurring only after exposure to a low dose of X-rays, but not for carbon ions, pointing to a specific effect, which is inversely correlated to increasing dose and ionizing density. According to this, at higher doses, no changes or even a reduced proliferation activity have been detected, the latter indicating an inhibition of cell cycle progression. This is consistent with the results obtained in NHEK (Figure S8 in Supplementary Material).

Changed Polarity of the Basal Cells

The polarity of the basal keratinocytes is a prerequisite for a balanced homeostasis of the epidermal layer (40). The typical palisade-like morphology of the basal cells allows for an attachment to the basal membrane and for a regular alignment, determining the polarity of the basal cells. When the basal cells are not attached to the basal membrane, the order and structure of the basal layer is disturbed, potentially leading to uncontrolled proliferation and migration (41).

After irradiation, we observed a transition from the typical palisade-like morphology to a cobblestoned morphology of the basal cells, as shown in a representative picture in **Figure 5A**. As quantification is difficult, we performed a semiquantitative scoring by determining if in the field of view all basal cells display a palisade-like morphology or if the cells have undergone a partial or a complete transition to a cobblestoned morphology. The semiquantitative evaluation in **Figure 5B** shows a shift to a cobblestoned morphology for X-ray exposure compared to controls. A transition to more areas with cobblestoned morphology was observed 24 and 72 h after irradiation, and in some fields of view, all basal cells displayed a cobblestoned morphology. Interestingly, the effect was inversely correlated with increasing dose and most pronounced after 0.5 Gy. Similar changes were found after carbon ion irradiation (**Figure 5B**) but less pronounced comparing the low dose (0.5 Gy) for both radiation qualities. In addition, we observed an alteration, which may be related to the described changes in morphology and polarity of basal keratinocytes, i.e., a delocalization of E-Cadherin from the cytoplasmic membrane to the cytoplasm (**Figure 5C**).

In summary, the transition of basal cells from a palisade-like to a cobblestoned morphology, indicating a change in polarity and disorganization of the basal layer, occurs for low and high doses, and for all radiation qualities. However, the effect is clearly more pronounced for low compared to high doses and for X-rays compared to carbon ions comparing the same physical doses.

DISCUSSION

The early and late skin response to ionizing radiation in classical photon therapy is clinically well known (31, 42) and constitutes a dose-limiting factor (43, 44). However, for reactions occurring within the first days in the epidermal layer of the skin, the cellular and molecular basis is explored much more intensive for UV exposure than for ionizing irradiation. For carbon ion exposure, the early radiation response of skin tissue has been investigated for the first time on a cellular level in our current study.

Cell Death Does Not Play a Major Role in the Early Radiation Response of Skin

The onset of an inflammatory reaction is one of the first events after irradiation of skin (45), and cell death can trigger this response (14, 46). Given the well-known enhanced efficiency for cell inactivation and higher relative biological effectiveness (RBE) of two to five of carbon ions (depending on the energy) compared to photons in mammalian cell types (47–49), a careful investigation of cell death induction in epidermal cells within the first days after exposure was conducted. As expected, clonogenic survival

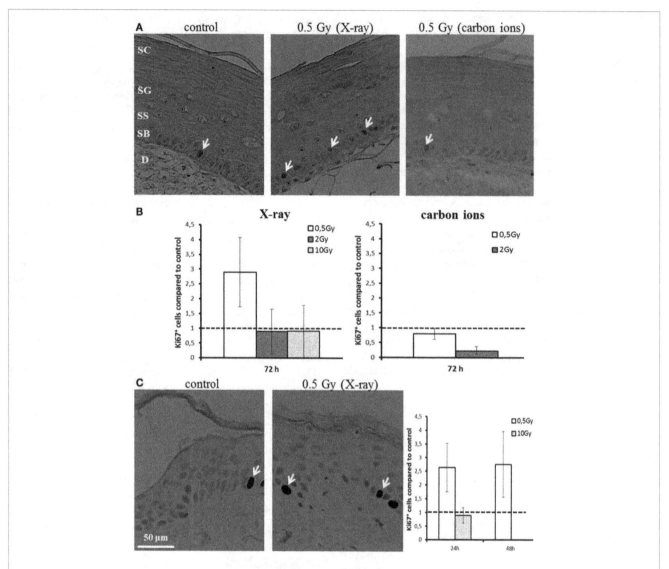

FIGURE 4 | Proliferation activity measured by Ki67 staining in HSE and human skin explants after irradiation with X-ray and carbon ions. (A)
Ki67-positive cells (arrows) in the basal layer of HSE. **(B)** Number of Ki67-positive cells in the HSE, normalized on the total number of cells in the basal layer and shown relative to the controls, shows enhanced proliferation after 0.5 Gy X-ray irradiation. **(C)** Ki67-positive cells in human skin explants (arrows); quantification shows an increase of proliferation after low dose of X-rays; $N = 2$, $n = 4$.

of NHEK was reduced after X-ray exposure and even more pronounced after high LET carbon ion irradiation (170 keV/μm, Figure S1A in Supplementary Material). However, cell death was not detectable in mono and coculture of NHEK (Figures S1 and S4 in Supplementary Material, assessed for X-rays), which is consistent with reported results, where no or only a minor early increment in apoptotic cells was observed in primary keratinocytes exposed to moderate and high doses of γ-rays (50, 51). This indicates different mechanisms of clonogenic inactivation, such as accelerated differentiation, as shown for other primary cells (49, 52).

Using the more complex skin models, HSE and human skin explants, we confirmed that caspase-3-dependent apoptosis and necrosis do not play a role within the first days after radiation exposure to both X-rays and carbon ions in the assessed dose range (**Figure 1**). A low level of apoptosis, remaining unchanged after irradiation of the same HSE as used in our experiments,

was also mentioned in an independent study (53). In biopsies of radiotherapy patients, the low basic level of apoptosis was increased only after more than 6 weeks (42), and in animal experiments, caspase-3-dependent apoptosis (22) and epidermal cell loss (54) were shown for very high doses. We conclude that apoptosis occurs only for very high doses and/or later than a few days. Early after exposure to low and moderate doses, apoptosis and necrosis do not contribute to inflammatory reactions.

Carbon Ions and X-Rays Trigger an Early Release of ProInflammatory Signals in Irradiated HSE with Similar Efficiency

For X-ray exposure, an early upregulation of inflammatory pathways on the transcriptional level in the irradiated epidermis is well established and has been investigated in skin biopsies of

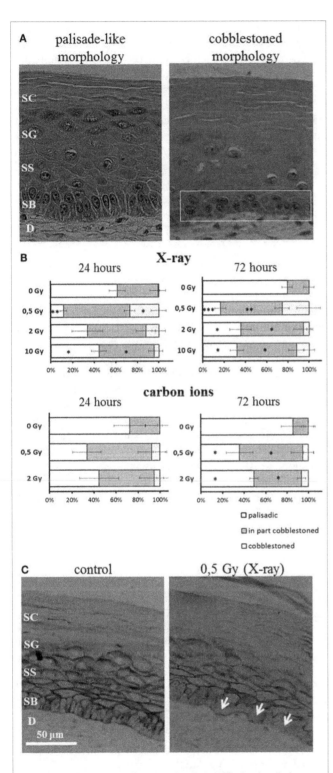

FIGURE 5 | Changed polarity of basal cells in HSE after irradiation with X-ray and carbon ions. (A) Transition of palisade-like morphology of basal cells to a cobblestoned morphology indicating a change in polarity and disorganization of the basal layer. **(B)** Quantification of palisade-like morphology and cobblestoned (partial or total) morphology shows a transition for all doses of X-ray and carbon ions; most pronounced and highly significant for 0.5 Gy. **(C)** E-Cadherin staining shows a delocalization of the protein in the cells from the basal layer (arrows) 72 h after irradiation with 0.5 Gy X-rays; SEM; $^*p \leq 0.05$, $^{**}p \leq 0.01$; $^{***}p \leq 0.001$; $N = 2$, $n = 4$.

radiotherapy patients, in HSE (12, 53, 55, 56), and in keratinocytes in animal and cell culture studies (50, 57). We could show in a HSE that both photon and carbon ion irradiation induce an early, significantly increased release of cytokines, which are known to trigger inflammation, such as IL-6 and IL-8, and a trend in increase of IL-1α. Anti-inflammatory cytokines (TGF-β and IL-10) were not elevated after exposure, except for a small enhancement of IL-10 at 48 h following carbon ion irradiation. This argues against an anti-inflammatory response at low doses elicited in the model systems investigated here. However, TGF-β mRNA was reported to be upregulated for high γ-ray doses (58), probably related to its key role in the late fibrotic response of skin.

In our study, comparing the same physical doses, the response to carbon ion irradiation compared to X-ray exposure was weak, detectable only after 48 h and significant only for IL-8 release (**Figure 2**). This indicates a similar enhancement in the release of proinflammatory cytokines after X-ray and carbon ion exposure. However, this is more a relative statement concerning the efficiency of carbon ions compared to X-rays than a result which fully represents the inflammatory response in a skin model such as a HSE, because a partially, but not fully overlapping pattern of X-ray induced cytokine release was detected in a study conducted by an independent group in the same HSE (19).

The Differentiation of Epidermal Cells After Irradiation is in Part Abnormal and Accelerated

Typical features that might contribute to the onset of an inflammatory reaction in skin are changes in proliferation and differentiation of keratinocytes, as reported for radiotherapy patients and irradiated animals (31, 59, 60). The normal differentiation and migration process implies nuclear disintegration of the keratinocytes that have reached the stratum corneum (10). When nucleated cells are found in the stratum corneum, the differentiation process is abnormal and called "parakeratosis". We observed parakeratosis after exposure to carbon ions (2 Gy), whereas only a weak induction was detected after irradiation with moderate and high X-ray doses (**Figure 3B**). In line with a change occurring at higher ionizing densities, parakeratosis was reported also for proton irradiation in an epidermis equivalent (61).

Another indicator of abnormal development is the occurrence of cells with pyknotic nuclei and eosinophilic cytoplasm, which are located in the viable epidermis. We found an increased number of those cells, albeit at a low level, after exposure to moderate doses of X-rays and, longer persisting, for carbon ions (2 Gy; **Figure 3D**). However, unlike "sunburn cells", which have been observed after UV exposure (34, 35), these cells did not show positive staining for activated caspase-3 and were not found in the basal layer. This result indicates that cells with a sunburn-like morphology detected after X-ray and carbon ion irradiation can be ascribed to abnormal differentiation and that this process is not necessarily associated with classical caspase-3-dependent apoptosis. Based on the morphological similarity, the occurrence of these cells might be a prestep for parakeratosis.

In contrast to the aberrant features (parakeratosis, "sunburn cells"), which occur to a higher extent after carbon ion exposure, we found indications for non-aberrant, but accelerated differentiation after exposure to moderate and high but not for a low X-ray dose. Quantitative analysis revealed a significant enhancement of thickness of the stratum corneum (hyperkeratosis) for X-rays and for carbon ions. Similar observations in an epidermal skin equivalent are reported for proton exposure (61) and less pronounced for higher LET ions (62). All in all, our own and published data indicate for X-ray and charged particles of the lower LET range that the induced imbalance of the differentiation process manifests as accelerated and not really aberrant as observed for higher LET radiation qualities.

The Proliferation Activity of Basal Cells is Enhanced for a Low Dose of X-Rays

Differentiation and cell proliferation are directly associated; therefore, we also studied the proliferation activity of the basal cells in the HSE, which we found to be enhanced for a low X-ray dose (**Figure 4**). Notably, in human *ex vivo* irradiated skin, we could confirm the enhanced proliferation activity of epidermal cells induced by low X-ray doses (**Figure 4C**). For higher X-ray doses and for carbon ions, the proliferation activity was unchanged or even inhibited, which is in line with results from animal photon studies (22, 54, 60, 63) and consistent with the cell cycle arrest that we observed in NHEK (**Figures 4A,B**; Figure S8 in Supplementary Material).

Our results suggest that increased proliferation is a low-dose effect, which is induced within a few days after exposure. Furthermore, the effect seems to be related to ionizing density, which is endorsed by the observation of an increased proliferation after exposure to charged particles with a relatively low LET [protons (61) and oxygen (62)], which was not detected for heavy ions with a higher LET in the HSE construct used in our study (62). These findings and our results indicate a low-dose effect, which is induced by low or moderate LET radiation, and may correspond to an early onset of tissue regeneration but does not occur at high doses and high LET, where cell cycle arrest and terminal differentiation are dominating.

Obvious Changes in the Organization of the Basal Layer Occur After Exposure to Low Doses of X-Rays

In addition to changed differentiation and proliferation, we observed a radiation-induced transition from the typical palisade-like to a cobblestoned morphology of the basal cells for X-rays and carbon ions (**Figure 5A**). This is independent of the anchorage to the basal membrane, indicating a changed polarity of the basal cells. Semiquantitative analysis revealed a more pronounced effect for low compared to higher doses and comparing the same physical doses, a more pronounced effect for X-rays than for carbon ions (see **Figure 5B**) and comparing the same physical doses, a more pronounced effect for X-rays than for carbon ions.

A changed polarity has been characterized as a cellular change concomitant to the onset of proliferation and/or to migration (64), in particular in carcinogenic development. Anchorage-independent growth of epidermal cells can be evoked by irradiation as established

in a murine epidermal cell line. Interestingly, we detected a delocalization of E-Cadherin from the cytoplasma membrane in HSE after X-ray and carbon ion exposure (**Figure 5C**). E-Cadherin is involved in cell–cell contacts of keratinocytes, and the transition to a cobblestoned morphology of the basal keratinocytes implies a dissociation of the intercellular contacts in the basal layer. The translocalization of E-Cadherin could be involved in the molecular mechanisms of radiation-induced anchorage independence, which was observed in our study. According to the results obtained so far, changed epidermal tissue organization plays a role for both X-ray and carbon ion exposure.

CONCLUSION

Our results show that ionizing irradiation has an effect on the differentiation and organization of the epidermal layers in the skin equivalent. Densely ionizing charged particle are more effective than X-rays per unit dose in the induction of several biological endpoints, including DNA damage, chromosome aberrations, mutations, and cell killing. Our results suggest that exposure to carbon ions under therapy-like conditions triggers proinflammatory signals and changes in homeostasis and epidermal tissue organization to a similar extent as photons, independent of cell death. On the other hand, heavy ions and X-rays modify epidermal tissue organization at low doses and differentiation at high doses. How these tissue-specific effects can be related to the initial DNA damage, whose quality is different after low and high LET radiation, is unclear yet. Recently, Kang et al. (65) have shown that DNA damage response activates the GATA4 pathway, thus inducing inflammatory responses and reducing proliferation. The establishment of a direct link between DNA repair and late changes in homeostasis is important to explain why some effects can be differently revealed at low/high doses or low/high LET.

ACKNOWLEDGMENTS

We want to acknowledge the dedicated help of G. Alphonse and C. Rodriguez-Lafrasse (University Lyon, France) in establishing methods for the assessment of apoptosis in cells. We would like to thank K. Petschick, C. Caliendo, A. Bentzer, and L. Madl for their excellent help with the experiments. We thank M. Scholz, T. Friedrich, W. Becher (GSI); S. Brons, K. Weber, T. Haberer (HIT); and the respective dosimetry teams from GSI and HIT for the dedicated support during the experimental runs. We acknowledge the hospital team of the dermatology clinic (Darmstadt, Germany) for providing skin tissue samples.

FUNDING

This work was supported by DFG (GRK1657), BMBF (GREWIS; 02NUK017A), PARTNER Project, HGS-hire, and Verein zur Förderung der Tumortherapie mit schweren Ionen e.V.

REFERENCES

1. Durante M, Loeffler JS. Charged particles in radiation oncology. *Nat Rev Clin Oncol* (2010) 7:37–43. doi:10.1038/nrclinonc.2009.183

2. Loeffler JS, Durante M. Charged particle therapy – optimization, challenges and future directions. *Nat Rev Clin Oncol* (2013) 10:411–24. doi:10.1038/nrclinonc.2013.79

3. Scholz M. Effects of ion radiation on cells and tissues. In: Kausch H, editor. *Radiation Effects on Polymers for Biological Use*. Berlin Heidelberg: Springer-Verlag (2003). p. 95–155. doi:10.1007/3-540-45668-6

4. Kraft G. Radiobiological effects of very heavy ions: inactivation, induction of chromosome aberrations and strand breaks. *Nucl Sci Appl* (1987) 3:1–28.

5. Yanagi T, Kamada T, Tsuji H, Imai R, Serizawa I, Tsujii H. Dose-volume histogram and dose-surface histogram analysis for skin reactions to carbon ion radiotherapy for bone and soft tissue sarcoma. *Radiother Oncol* (2010) 95:60–5. doi:10.1016/j.radonc.2009.08.041

6. Rieber JG, Kessel KA, Witt O, Behnisch W, Kulozik AE, Debus J, et al. Treatment tolerance of particle therapy in pediatric patients. *Acta Oncol* (2015) 54:1049–55. doi:10.3109/0284186X.2014.998273

7. Whaley JT, Kirk M, Cengel K, McDonough J, Bekelman J, Christodouleas JP. Protective effect of transparent film dressing on proton therapy induced skin reactions. *Radiat Oncol* (2013) 8:19. doi:10.1186/1748-717X-8-19

8. Galland-Girodet S, Pashtan I, MacDonald SM, Ancukiewicz M, Hirsch AE, Kachnic LA, et al. Long-term cosmetic outcomes and toxicities of proton beam therapy compared with photon-based 3-dimensional conformal accelerated partial-breast irradiation: a phase 1 trial. *Int J Radiat Oncol Biol Phys* (2014) 90:493–500. doi:10.1016/j.ijrobp.2014.04.008

9. Shore RE. Radiation-induced skin cancer in humans. *Med Pediatr Oncol* (2001) 36:549–54. doi:10.1002/mpo.1128

10. Kolarsick PAJ, Kolarsick MA, Goodwin C. Anatomy and physiology of the skin. *J Dermatol Nurs Assoc* (2011) 3:203–13. doi:10.1097/JDN.0b013e3182274a98

11. Peter R. The cutaneous radiation syndrome. In: MacVittie TJ, Weiss JF, Browne D, editors. *Advances in the Treatment of Radiation Injuries*. Oxford: Elsevier (1996). p. 237–41.

12. Müller K, Meineke V. Radiation-induced alterations in cytokine production by skin cells. *Exp Hematol* (2007) 35:96–104. doi:10.1016/j.exphem.2007.01.017

13. Berkey FJ. Managing the adverse effects of radiation therapy. *Am Fam Physician* (2010) 82(381–8):394.

14. Rödel F, Frey B, Manda K, Hildebrandt G, Hehlgans S, Keilholz L, et al. Immunomodulatory properties and molecular effects in inflammatory diseases of low-dose x-irradiation. *Front Oncol* (2012) 2:120. doi:10.3389/fonc.2012.00120

15. Aubin F. Mechanisms involved in ultraviolet light-induced immunosuppression. *Eur J Dermatol* (2003) 13:515–23.

16. Schwarz T. Mechanisms of UV-induced immunosuppression. *Keio J Med* (2005) 54:165–71. doi:10.2302/kjm.54.165

17. Suvarna KS, Layton C, Bancroft JD. *Bancroft's Theory and Practice of Histological Techniques*. 7th ed. Elsevier Health Sciences (2012). Available from: http://books.google.com/books?id=wPPI4NyGm3gC&pgis=1

18. Fournier C, Wiese C, Taucher-Scholz G. Accumulation of the cell cycle regulators TP53 and CDKN1A (p21) in human fibroblasts after exposure to low- and high-LET radiation. *Radiat Res* (2004) 161:675–84. doi:10.1667/RR3182

19. Varnum SM, Springer DL, Chaffee ME, Lien KA, Webb-Robertson B-JM, Waters KM, et al. The effects of low-dose irradiation on inflammatory response proteins in a 3D reconstituted human skin tissue model. *Radiat Res* (2012) 178:591–9. doi:10.1667/RR2976.1

20. Bell CW, Jiang W, Reich CF, Pisetsky DS. The extracellular release of HMGB1 during apoptotic cell death. *Am J Physiol Cell Physiol* (2006) 291:C1318–25. doi:10.1152/ajpcell.00616.2005

21. Raucci A, Palumbo R, Bianchi ME. HMGB1: a signal of necrosis. *Autoimmunity* (2007) 40:285–9. doi:10.1080/08916930701356978

22. Ahmed EA, Agay D, Schrock G, Drouet M, Meineke V, Scherthan H. Persistent DNA damage after high dose in vivo gamma exposure of minipig skin. *PLoS One* (2012) 7:e39521. doi:10.1371/journal.pone.0039521

23. Le Poole IC, Boyce ST. Keratinocytes suppress transforming growth factor-beta1 expression by fibroblasts in cultured skin substitutes. *Br J Dermatol* (1999) 140:409–16. doi:10.1046/j.1365-2133.1999.02700.x

24. Maas-Szabowski N, Stark HJ, Fusenig NE. Keratinocyte growth regulation in defined organotypic cultures through IL-1-induced keratinocyte growth factor expression in resting fibroblasts. *J Invest Dermatol* (2000) 114:1075–84. doi:10.1046/j.1523-1747.2000.00987.x

25. Matsumura T, Hayashi H, Takii T, Thorn CF, Whitehead AS, Inoue J-I, et al. TGF-beta down-regulates IL-1alpha-induced TLR2 expression in murine hepatocytes. *J Leukoc Biol* (2004) 75:1056–61. doi:10.1189/jlb.0104108

26. Lian X, Yang L, Gao Q, Yang T. IL-1alpha is a potent stimulator of keratinocyte tissue plasminogen activator expression and regulated by TGF-beta1. *Arch Dermatol Res* (2008) 300:185–93. doi:10.1007/s00403-007-0828-8

27. Martin M, Lefaix J, Delanian S. TGF-beta1 and radiation fibrosis: a master switch and a specific therapeutic target? *Int J Radiat Oncol Biol Phys* (2000) 47:277–90. doi:10.1016/S0360-3016(00)00435-1

28. King A, Balaji S, Le LD, Crombleholme TM, Keswani SG. Regenerative wound healing: the role of interleukin-10. *Adv Wound Care* (2014) 3:315–23. doi:10.1089/wound.2013.0461

29. Grivennikov SI, Greten FR, Karin M. Immunity, inflammation, and cancer. *Cell* (2010) 140:883–99. doi:10.1016/j.cell.2010.01.025

30. Barcellos-Hoff MH, Nguyen DH. Radiation carcinogenesis in context: how do irradiated tissues become tumors? *Health Phys* (2009) 97:446–57. doi:10.1097/HP.0b013e3181b08a10

31. Sivan V, Vozenin-Brotons M-C, Tricaud Y, Lefaix J-L, Cosset J-M, Dubray B, et al. Altered proliferation and differentiation of human epidermis in cases of skin fibrosis after radiotherapy. *Int J Radiat Oncol Biol Phys* (2002) 53:385–93. doi:10.1016/S0360-3016(01)02732-8

32. Lowes MA, Bowcock AM, Krueger JG. Pathogenesis and therapy of psoriasis. *Nature* (2007) 445:866–73. doi:10.1038/nature05663

33. Johnson-Huang LM, Lowes MA, Krueger JG. Putting together the psoriasis puzzle: an update on developing targeted therapies. *Dis Model Mech* (2012) 5:423–33. doi:10.1242/dmm.009092

34. Lippens S, Hoste E, Vandenabeele P, Agostinis P, Declercq W. Cell death in the skin. *Apoptosis* (2009) 14:549–69. doi:10.1007/s10495-009-0324-z

35. Van Laethem A, Claerhout S, Garmyn M, Agostinis P. The sunburn cell: regulation of death and survival of the keratinocyte. *Int J Biochem Cell Biol* (2005) 37:1547–53. doi:10.1016/j.biocel.2005.02.015

36. Qin J-Z, Chaturvedi V, Denning MF, Bacon P, Panella J, Choubey D, et al. Regulation of apoptosis by p53 in UV-irradiated human epidermis, psoriatic plaques and senescent keratinocytes. *Oncogene* (2002) 21:2991–3002. doi:10.1038/sj.onc.1205404

37. Elias PM. Stratum corneum defensive functions: an integrated view. *J Invest Dermatol* (2005) 125:183–200. doi:10.1111/j.0022-202X.2005.23668.x

38. Maverakis E, Miyamura Y, Bowen MP, Correa G, Ono Y, Goodarzi H. Light, including ultraviolet. *J Autoimmun* (2010) 34:J247–57. doi:10.1016/j.jaut.2009.11.011

39. Elias PM, Gruber R, Crumrine D, Menon G, Williams ML, Wakefield JS, et al. Formation and functions of the corneocyte lipid envelope (CLE). *Biochim Biophys Acta* (2014) 1841:314–8. doi:10.1016/j.bbalip.2013.09.011

40. Muroyama A, Lechler T. Polarity and stratification of the epidermis. *Semin Cell Dev Biol* (2012) 23:890–6. doi:10.1016/j.semcdb.2012.08.008

41. Jamal S, Schneider RJ. UV-induction of keratinocyte endothelin-1 downregulates E-cadherin in melanocytes and melanoma cells. *J Clin Invest* (2002) 110:443–52. doi:10.1172/JCI13729

42. Turesson I, Nyman J, Qvarnström F, Simonsson M, Book M, Hermansson I, et al. A low-dose hypersensitive keratinocyte loss in response to fractionated radiotherapy is associated with growth arrest and apoptosis. *Radiother Oncol* (2010) 94:90–101. doi:10.1016/j.radonc.2009.10.007

43. Hopewell JW. Mechanisms of the action of radiation on skin and underlying tissues. *Br J Radiol Suppl* (1986) 19:39–47.

44. Bentzen SM, Saunders MI, Dische S, Bond SJ. Radiotherapy-related early morbidity in head and neck cancer: quantitative clinical radiobiology as deduced from the CHART trial. *Radiother Oncol* (2001) 60:123–35. doi:10.1016/S0167-8140(01)00358-9

45. Gottlöber P, Steinert M, Weiss M, Bebeshko V, Belyi D, Nadejina N, et al. The outcome of local radiation injuries: 14 years of follow-up after the Chernobyl accident. *Radiat Res* (2001) 155:409–16. doi:10.1667/0033-7587(2001)155[0409:TOOLRI]2.0.CO;2

46. Fink SL, Cookson BT. Apoptosis, pyroptosis, and necrosis: mechanistic description of dead and dying eukaryotic cells. *Infect Immun* (2005) 73:1907–16. doi:10.1128/IAI.73.4.1907-1916.2005

47. Weyrather WK, Ritter S, Scholz M, Kraft G. RBE for carbon track-segment irradiation in cell lines of differing repair capacity. *Int J Radiat Biol* (1999) **75**:1357–64. doi:10.1080/095530099139232

48. Suzuki M, Kase Y, Yamaguchi H, Kanai T, Ando K. Relative biological effectiveness for cell-killing effect on various human cell lines irradiated with heavy-ion medical accelerator in Chiba (HIMAC) carbon-ion beams. *Int J Radiat Oncol Biol Phys* (2000) **48**:241–50. doi:10.1016/S0360-3016(00)00568-X

49. Fournier C, Scholz M, Weyrather WK, Rodemann HP, Kraft G. Changes of fibrosis-related parameters after high- and low-LET irradiation of fibroblasts. *Int J Radiat Biol* (2001) **77**:713–22. doi:10.1080/09553000110045025

50. Petit-Frere C, Capulas E, Lyon DA, Norbury CJ, Lowe JE, Clingen PH, et al. Apoptosis and cytokine release induced by ionizing or ultraviolet B radiation in primary and immortalized human keratinocytes. *Carcinogenesis* (2000) **21**:1087–95. doi:10.1093/carcin/21.6.1087

51. Rachidi W, Harfourche G, Lemaitre G, Amiot F, Vaigot P, Martin MT. Sensing radiosensitivity of human epidermal stem cells. *Radiother Oncol* (2007) **83**:267–76. doi:10.1016/j.radonc.2007.05.007

52. Fournier C, Winter M, Zahnreich S, Nasonova E, Melnikova L, Ritter S. Interrelation amongst differentiation, senescence and genetic instability in long-term cultures of fibroblasts exposed to different radiation qualities. *Radiother Oncol* (2007) **83**:277–82. doi:10.1016/j.radonc.2007.04.022

53. Von Neubeck C, Shankaran H, Karin NJ, Kauer PM, Chrisler WB, Wang X, et al. Cell type-dependent gene transcription profile in a three-dimensional human skin tissue model exposed to low doses of ionizing radiation: implications for medical exposures. *Environ Mol Mutagen* (2012) **53**:247–59. doi:10.1002/em.21682

54. Morris GM, Hopewell JW. Changes in the cell kinetics of pig epidermis after single doses of X rays. *Br J Radiol* (1988) **61**:205–11. doi:10.1259/0007-1285-61-723-205

55. Berglund SR, Rocke DM, Dai J, Schwietert CW, Santana A, Stern RL, et al. Transient genome-wide transcriptional response to low-dose ionizing radiation in vivo in humans. *Int J Radiat Oncol Biol Phys* (2008) **70**:229–34. doi:10.1016/j.ijrobp.2007.09.026

56. Goldberg Z, Rocke DM, Schwietert C, Berglund SR, Santana A, Jones A, et al. Human in vivo dose-response to controlled, low-dose low linear energy transfer ionizing radiation exposure. *Clin Cancer Res* (2006) **12**:3723–9. doi:10.1158/1078-0432.CCR-05-2625

57. Liu W, Ding I, Chen K, Olschowka J, Xu J, Hu D, et al. Interleukin 1beta (IL1B) signaling is a critical component of radiation-induced skin fibrosis. *Radiat Res* (2006) **165**:181–91. doi:10.1667/RR3478.1

58. Martin M, Lefaix JL, Pinton P, Crechet F, Daburon F. Temporal modulation of TGF-beta 1 and beta-actin gene expression in pig skin and muscular fibrosis after ionizing radiation. *Radiat Res* (1993) **134**:63–70. doi:10.2307/3578502

59. Dörr W. Modulation of repopulation processes in oral mucosa: experimental results. *Int J Radiat Biol* (2003) **79**:531–7. doi:10.1080/09553002310001600925

60. Liu K, Kasper M, Trott KR. Changes in keratinocyte differentiation during accelerated repopulation of the irradiated mouse epidermis. *Int J Radiat Biol* (1996) **69**:763–9. doi:10.1080/095530096145508

61. Mezentsev A, Amundson SA. Global gene expression responses to low- or high-dose radiation in a human three-dimensional tissue model. *Radiat Res* (2011) **175**:677–88. doi:10.1667/RR2483.1

62. Von Neubeck C, Geniza MJ, Kauer PM, Robinson RJ, Chrisler WB, Sowa MB. The effect of low dose ionizing radiation on homeostasis and functional integrity in an organotypic human skin model. *Mutat Res* (2015) **775**:10–8. doi:10.1016/j.mrfmmm.2015.03.003

63. Dörr W, Emmendörfer H, Weber-Frisch M. Tissue kinetics in mouse tongue mucosa during daily fractionated radiotherapy. *Cell Prolif* (1996) **29**:495–504. doi:10.1111/j.1365-2184.1996.tb00992.x

64. Steude J, Kulke R, Christophers E. Interleukin-1-stimulated secretion of interleukin-8 and growth-related oncogene-alpha demonstrates greatly enhanced keratinocyte growth in human raft cultured epidermis. *J Invest Dermatol* (2002) **119**:1254–60. doi:10.1046/j.1523-1747.2002.19616.x

65. Kang C, Xu Q, Martin TD, Li MZ, Demaria M, Aron L, et al. The DNA damage response induces inflammation and senescence by inhibiting autophagy of GATA4. *Science* (2015) **349**:aaa5612. doi:10.1126/science.aaa5612

6

Correlation of Particle Traversals with Clonogenic Survival Using Cell-Fluorescent Ion Track Hybrid Detector

Ivana Dokic[1,2,3]*, Martin Niklas[1,2,3], Ferdinand Zimmermann[1,2,3], Andrea Mairani[2,4], Philipp Seidel[1,2,3], Damir Krunic[5], Oliver Jäkel[2,3,6], Jürgen Debus[1,2,3], Steffen Greilich[3,6] and Amir Abdollahi[1,2,3]*

[1] German Cancer Consortium, Translational Radiation Oncology, National Center for Tumor Diseases, German Cancer Research Center, Heidelberg University Medical School, Heidelberg, Germany, [2] Heidelberg Ion Therapy Center, Heidelberg, Germany, [3] Heidelberg Institute of Radiation Oncology, National Center for Radiation Research in Oncology, Heidelberg, Germany, [4] National Center for Oncological Hadrontherapy, Pavia, Italy, [5] Light Microscopy Facility, German Cancer Research Center, Heidelberg, Germany, [6] Division of Medical Physics in Radiation Oncology, German Cancer Research Center, Heidelberg, Germany

*Correspondence:
Ivana Dokic
i.dokic@dkfz.de;
Amir Abdollahi
a.amir@dkfz.de

Development of novel approaches linking the physical characteristics of particles with biological responses are of high relevance for the field of particle therapy. In radiobiology, the clonogenic survival of cells is considered the gold standard assay for the assessment of cellular sensitivity to ionizing radiation. Toward further development of next generation biodosimeters in particle therapy, cell-fluorescent ion track hybrid detector (Cell-FIT-HD) was recently engineered by our group and successfully employed to study physical particle track information in correlation with irradiation-induced DNA damage in cell nuclei. In this work, we investigated the feasibility of Cell-FIT-HD as a tool to study the effects of clinical beams on cellular clonogenic survival. Tumor cells were grown on the fluorescent nuclear track detector as cell culture, mimicking the standard procedures for clonogenic assay. Cell-FIT-HD was used to detect the spatial distribution of particle tracks within colony-initiating cells. The physical data were associated with radiation-induced foci as surrogates for DNA double strand breaks, the hallmark of radiation-induced cell lethality. Long-term cell fate was monitored to determine the ability of cells to form colonies. We report the first successful detection of particle traversal within colony-initiating cells at subcellular resolution using Cell-FIT-HD.

Keywords: clonogenic survival, fluorescent nuclear track detector, carbon ion irradiation, 53BP1, DNA damage foci

INTRODUCTION

Radiotherapy with protons and heavier ions has become a swiftly growing field, and it is becoming an integrative part of therapy of solid tumors, due to its high success rate in treating certain tumors (1). Nevertheless, intracellular molecular events caused by interactions between the charged particles and cellular structures are not yet well understood. Development of novel approaches that will facilitate deciphering those processes is of high relevance for the field.

Recently, a cell-fluorescent ion track hybrid detector (Cell-FIT-HD) was engineered by our group. It provides information on spatial correlation between single ion traversals and the events within a cell (2, 3). Cell-FIT-HD technology is based on growing a cellular monolayer (biological compartment) on a surface of a fluorescent nuclear track detector [FNTD; physical compartment (4)]. Due to its unique design, Cell-FIT-HD enables simultaneous investigation of microscopic beam parameters and their effect on various cellular structures and biological processes, using confocal laser scanning microscope (5).

In this work, we investigated the feasibility of Cell-FIT-HD for colony formation analysis. Colony formation assay (also called clonogenic assay), developed in 1950s (6), is the most reliable and relevant method for studying the efficacy of the radiation treatment *in vitro*. It has been named "gold standard" in radiation research as it combines contribution of all types of cell death, as well as ability of surviving cells' to indefinitely proliferate and form colonies (7, 8). For particle therapy planning, clonogenic survival data are of utmost importance for studying radiobiological effectiveness (RBE) and they continue to be used as the main biological experimental outcome for testing biophysical models for predicting tumor response to irradiation (9). Colony formation and cellular clonogenic survival after irradiation are highly depend on radiation potential to induce complex, difficult to repair, DNA damage [such as DNA double-strand breaks (DSB)] (10). Commonly used molecular surrogate for detecting DNA damage and DNA DSB is p53 binding protein 1 (53BP1), which localizes at the sites of DSB and forms nuclear radiation-induced foci (RIF) (11, 12). In irradiated cells, on DNA DSB sites, 53BP1 foci colocalize with Serine 139 phosphorylated histone H2AX foci (γ-H2AX) flanking a larger area around a DSB and hence considered another sensitive marker for DNA DSB damage (13, 14).

Combination of Cell-FIT-HD technology, clonogenic assay, and RIF detection should provide a platform for simultaneous analysis of microscopic beam parameters, particle effects on RIF formation and the ability of cells to form colonies as a function of particle number, quality, and spatial distribution.

MATERIALS AND METHODS

Cell Culture

Cell lines used in this study were murine (Balb/c) renal adenocarcinoma cells (RENCA) and human alveolar adenocarcinoma cell line (A549), obtained from ATCC. RENCA were cultured in RPMI-1640 Medium (Gibco) supplemented with 10% fetal bovine serum (FBS, Gibco), non-essential amino acids (0.1 mM, Sigma), sodium pyruvate (1 mM, Sigma), and L-glutamine (2 mM, Sigma). A549 cells were cultured in Dulbecco's Modified Eagle Medium (DMEM, ATCC) supplemented with 10% heat-inactivated FBS (Millipore), 2 mM glutamine, and 1% penicillin/streptomycin (complete DMEM).

Cells Transduction and Immune Staining

A549 cells were transduced using a retroviral construct containing mCherry-53BP1-2 pLPC-Puro [Addgene plasmid # 19836; (15)]. Retrovirus production and cells transduction

with mCherry-53BP1 construct were carried out, as previously described (15). Retrovirus production was performed using Retro-X Universal Packaging System (Clontech), according to manufacturer's instructions. Transduction was conducted by the incubation of cells and viral particles in a complete medium containing 8 μg/ml Polybrene (Sigma) at 37°C, 5% CO_2. Selection of transduced cells was performed using 2 μg/ml of Puromycin (Gibco). A549 cells expressing mCherry-53BP1 were cultured in complete DMEM containing 0.4 μg/ml of Puromycin (Gibco). All cells were incubated at 37°C at 5% CO_2 atmosphere. A549 cells expressing mCherry-53BP1 construct were counterstained for γ-H2AX marker as described (16). Fixed (4% paraformaldehyde, for 10 min) and permeabilized (0.1% Triton-X for 10 min) cells were labeled using primary anti-γ-H2AX antibody (1:100, Cell Biolabs) and secondary Alexa Fluor 488-conjugated donkey anti-mouse antibody (Molecular Probes).

Colony-Forming Cell Assay and Irradiation

For preparation of colony-forming cell assay using FNTD as a substrate (Cell-FIT-HD), FNTDs were first washed in an ultrasonic bath (Bandelin Sonorex) for 15 min at room temperature (RT). FNTDs were then placed in 70% ethanol overnight at RT. FNTDs were thoroughly washed in PBS, before used for cell culture.

Standard clonogenic assay (8) was performed using RENCA cells in six-well cell culture plates (200 cells/well). After attachment, cells were irradiated with ^{12}C ion beam at Heidelberg Ion-Beam Therapy Center (HIT). Cells were positioned in the middle of a 1-cm widespread out Bragg peak (SOBP, 1 Gy) centered at approximately 3.5 cm water-equivalent depth, mimicking the clinical-like settings. Dose averaged linear energy transfer (LET) was 95 keV/μm. Non-irradiated cells were used as control. After colonies were formed, cells were fixed with 75% methanol and 25% acetic acid for 10 min at RT and stained with 0.1% crystal violet for 15 min.

Standard clonogenic assay was modified for studying the colony formation on FNTDs. Forty microliters of growth medium drop containing 50 cells were placed on the polished surface of the FNTD. The growth area was approximately 4 mm × 8 mm. For studying the ability of cells to grow on FNTD surface and form colonies, FNTDs containing cells (Cell-FIT-HD) were either irradiated as described above, or left without irradiation (control) and incubated for 7 days. After colony formation, cells were fixed and stained as in standard clonogenic assay (as above). FNTDs containing colonies were scanned (EPSON Scan). All obtained images were corrected for brightness and contrast by ImageJ (http://rsb.info.nih.gov/ij/) using the same image processing settings.

To correlate colony forming ability of a single cell and microscopic ion beam parameters, mCherry-53BP1 A549 cells were allowed to attach (100 cells/FNTD for control and 200 cells/FNTD for irradiated sample) at 37°C at 5% CO_2 for at least 8 h prior to irradiation. Cell-FIT-HD was irradiated perpendicularly with respect to the incident ^{12}C ion beam, as described above.

Approximately 30 min post-irradiation ($t = 30$ min), the entire area of the Cell-FIT-HD was imaged by widefield microscopy (see below). After the initial imaging, Cell-FIT-HD was placed in the incubator (37°C at 5% CO_2 atmosphere) for 7 days to allow colony formation on the polished surface of the FNTD. The ability of colony formation with/without irradiation after 7 days ($t = 7$ days) was assessed by additional imaging of Cell-FIT-HD by widefield microscopy.

Read-Out of Cell-FIT-HD

The read-outs of the physical compartment (FNTD) and of the biological compartment (single cells or colonies) of Cell-FIT-HD were uncoupled. 53BP1 (mCherry signal) and γ-H2AX (Alexa Fluor 488) in **Figure 2** were imaged by Zeiss LSM710, Confocor 3 confocal laser scanning microscope, as previously described (3), at 30 min post-irradiation.

Initial cell attachment and colonies were imaged by the inverted widefield microscope Cell Observer (Carl Zeiss AG). To record the initial cell attachment, an overview scan of the entire cell attachment area (polished surface of the FNTD) was performed. Image stacks of regions of interests (ROIs) containing single cells were subsequently recorded. The stacks contained 41 and 45 image planes (each separated by 2 μm) for the imaging at $t = 30$ min, and at $t = 7$ days, respectively. The entire depth of the cell layer was covered. For each imaging plane, the bright field (BF) as well as the mCherry fluorescent channel (mPlum filter set) was recorded. After recording the overview scan, single ROI was subsequently imaged to allow for visualization of 53BP1 foci formation in individual cell nuclei of the colony. ROIs were chosen to match approximately the positions of time point 0. Individual tiles of the overview scan were corrected for shading and stitched using the ZEN software. The cells were washed away from FNTDs after the last widefield microscopy read-out. ROIs in the FNTD were then imaged by the Zeiss LSM710, Confocor 3 confocal laser scanning microscope. The imaging parameters were adjusted to gain optimal read-outs for the primary particles (5). The frequency distribution of fluorescence intensity of the ion tracks was assessed as a proxy for the LET spectrum. There are two distinct peaks that can be attributed to the primary carbon ions and the lighter fragments, respectively. A threshold was set to separate between the two species. Obviously, some heavier fragments might be considered as primaries, what, however, does not affect the generality of the results of this study. For each position, a z-stack of 35 imaging planes was recorded by 633 nm HeNe laser line (17). T-PMT detection was recorded in parallel. For widefield and for confocal imaging uncoated glass bottom, culture dishes (MatTek Corp.) were used.

Registration of Biological and Physical Beam Data

Widefield (biological compartment) and confocal images (physical compartment) were registered employing point mapping to correlate cellular response to microscopic ion beam parameters spatially at time point 0. To this end, non-fluorescent Al–Al spinel cubical inclusions in the Al2O3:C, Mg crystal – both visible in the T-PMT and the BF channel – were used as point pairs. At least four point pairs were used yielding an accuracy of the projective registration smaller than 0.3 μm, i.e., on a sub-pixel scale. The same registration procedure was performed when projecting the nuclei positions at

time point 0 into the cell layer at time point 7 days post-irradiation. It was ensured that the fluorescence (mCherry) and the brightfield channels of the widefield microscopy were spatially aligned.

Ion-Hit Statistics

Due to perpendicular irradiation setup, all track spot centers at $z = -3$ μm (measuring from the FNTD surface, $z = 0$ μm) were projected onto the maximum intensity projection (MIP) of the 53BP1 mCherry signal of the cell layer. Positions of single ion traversals were assessed by using an in-house developed thresholding algorithm. To determine intranuclear ion hits, the positions of the track spot center (rounded to pixel values) were projected onto the nuclei mask of the MIP of the 53BP1 mCherry signal. Trajectory reconstruction and angle assessment confirmed the validity of perpendicular extrapolation (3, 5). In the imaging plane at approximately $z = -3$ μm each track spot was masked and the maximum intensity value assessed. The maximum intensity value was converted into count-rate and was corrected for non-linearity in APD detection (18).

RESULTS

Colony Formation on FNTD

To study the feasibility of a FNTD's surface for colony formation, murine renal adenocarcinoma cells (RENCA) were used. As shown in **Figure 1A**, the cells were able to attach and form

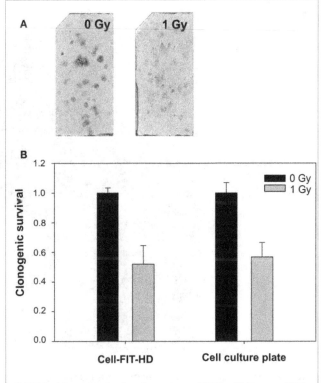

FIGURE 1 | **Example of colony formation on FNTDs. (A)** Spots on FNTD surface: crystal violet staining of cell colonies. Brightness/contrast was adjusted for better visualization. **(B)** Comparison of clonogenic survival on FNTDs and in culture flasks. Means and SDs of triplicates are shown.

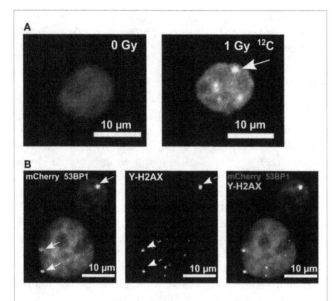

FIGURE 2 | mCherry 53BP1 and γ-H2AX signal in cell nuclei of A549 cells. (A) Pan-nuclear expression of 53BP1-mCherry fusion protein in a control sample (panel left). Irradiated (1 Gy ¹²C) nucleus showing accumulation of 53BP1-mCherry signal (53BP1 foci, arrow). **(B)** mCherry-53BP1 signal (left panel, arrows point to 53BP1 foci), γ-H2AX signal (middle panel; dashed arrows point to γ-H2AX foci) in irradiated mCherry-53BP1 cells. Colocalization of 53BP1 and γ-H2AX foci (panel right). Sum of intensities of Z-stack slices is shown. Brightness and contrast were adjusted for better visualization.

colonies on FNTD surface. The mean plating efficacy and SD on FNTD surface was $33 \pm 1.2\%$, whereas in a six-well plate it was $37 \pm 6\%$. The results for colony formation and clonogenic survival on FNTDs correspond to those obtained using the standard clonogenic assay in cell culture dishes (**Figure 1B**).

To investigate colony formation on FNTDs, on a microscopic level, as well as DNA damage foci formation, we utilized human A549 cells expressing mCherry-53BP1 fusion protein. A549 cell line was selected because of its low level of background foci (2). The stable expression of the fluorescent fusion protein, localized in cell nuclei, provided homogeneous pan-nuclear staining, which enabled microscopic imaging of cellular nuclei, as well as individual foci formation after irradiation (**Figure 2A**). 53BP1 signal in irradiated cells colocalizes with γ-H2AX signal, which confirms the fact that 53BP1 accumulates at the DNA DSB sites (**Figure 2B**).

In order to localize colony-initiating cell within a respective colony, the whole surface of Cell-FIT-HD was imaged at early ($t = 30$ min; red pseudocolor) and late ($t = 7$ days; green pseudocolor) time point, and the images were overlaid (**Figure 3**). At the seventh day post-irradiation, A549 cells formed dense colonies. This stands particularly true in case of control samples, where most of the cells were able to produce colonies (**Figure 3A**). Irradiated cells showed lower capability for clonogenic growth when compared to the control cells. They produced smaller colonies in comparison to a control sample, and many cells were not dividing (**Figure 3B**).

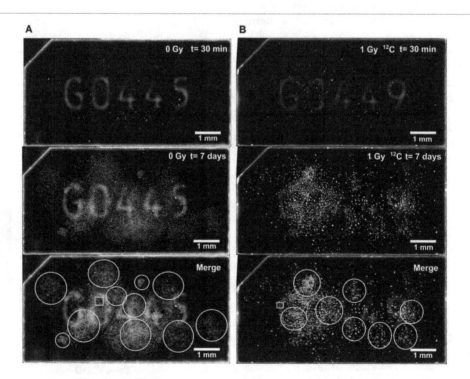

FIGURE 3 | Microscopic visualization of Cell-FIT-HD. (A) Control sample (mock irradiation) and **(B)** irradiated sample (1 Gy ¹²C-irradiation). FNTD surface was imaged at two time points: 30 min post irradiation ($t = 30$ min) and at 7 days ($t = 7$ days) post-irradiation. Early and late image orientations as well as brightness and contrast were adjusted and images were merged. Pan-nuclear mCherry-53BP1 signal was shown in red pseudocolor for $t = 30$ min, and in green pseudocolor for $t = 7$ days. White empty circles were used to mark different colonies. White empty squares indicate ROIs used for **Figure 4**. Numbers seen on FNTDs' surface are identification numbers engraved in each FNTD.

Even though cells can migrate on the surface during the colony formation time, it was assumed that the colony-initiating cell retained its position within the respective colony region. In the previous experiments, we observed that A549 cells can migrate up to 1 μm within 30 min in different directions, and these motion patterns of A549 cells would not be sufficient for a colony-initiating cell to leave the colony regions, especially in the case of larger colonies. Continuous live imaging of a colony formation was impossible due to the cytotoxicity induced by the long-term imaging settings.

Irradiation-Induced Foci and Ion Hits

To demonstrate the feasibility of a Cell-FIT-HD for analyzing ion traversals together with the irradiation-induced foci formation in a single cell, and investigate cell's fate in regards to colony formation, ROIs were selected in both control and irradiated Cell-FIT-HD. For the control sample, ROI containing three cells (at the early time point) was selected. These cells divided multiple times forming a large colony (**Figure 4A**). Initial positions of the colony-initiating cells' nuclei are marked by green closed lines (**Figure 4A**). At the seventh day post-irradiation, in case of irradiated samples, we analyzed the ROI containing cells that were

not capable of colony formation (**Figure 4B**, right panel). Even though those cells did not form colonies, additional cells were found in their close proximity. This could imply either cell migration, or a single division of a cell (**Figure 4B**, top right panel). For the same ROI, we extracted the particle beam information from a physical compartment (FNTD) of a Cell-FIT-HD to visualize ion tracks. Within selected ROI, two nuclei showed large 53BP1 foci formation. Respective ion track spots were assigned to these irradiation-induced 53BP1 foci based on the closest proximity (orange circles, **Figure 4B**, left panel). These track spots were induced by primary-like carbon ions, since the imaging parameters were adjusted to detect primarily carbon ions. However, secondary high LET fragments can be in principle also included. Fast protons of low LET were not visualized. The ion beam fluency assessed was approximately 7.0×10^6 particles/cm².

DISCUSSION

Colony formation assay is a quantitative, macroscopic assay, which represents the standard for studying cell's sensitivity to irradiation (8). It provides valuable information on the outcome

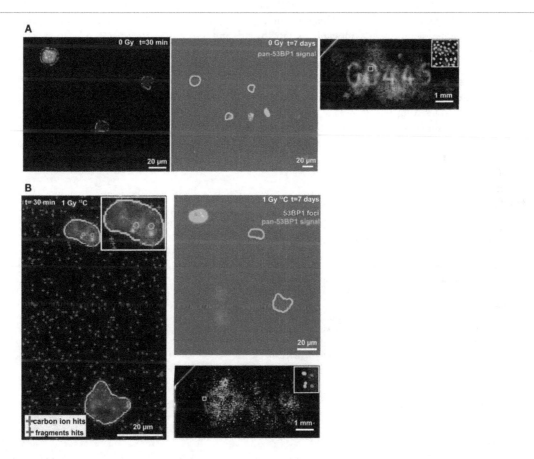

FIGURE 4 | Maximum intensity projections of 53BP1-mCherry signal and ion hits. (A) Control sample at $t = 30$ min (panel left) and $t = 7$ days (large colony formation; middle panel). Position of selected ROI on FNTD (white empty square). Insert: magnification of selected ROI (panel right). **(B)** Irradiated sample at $t = 30$ min (panel left). The cross sectional area of the nuclei at $t = 30$ min is encircled in green. The bright spots in the nuclei are 53BP1-mCherry foci most probably induced by carbon ions (highlighted by yellow circles, closest proximity). The positions of ion traversals and fragments are indicated by the red and blue crosses, respectively. Insert: magnification of the upper nucleus. Upper right panel shows the irradiated nuclei at $t = 7$ days, and no colony formation. Dense aggregation of 53BP1 signal is marked in yellow. The position of the nuclei at $t = 30$ min is labeled by green lines. The positions were registered to $t = 7$ days using the unique spinel fingerprint of spinels in the FNTD. Position of selected ROI on FNTD (white empty square). Insert: magnification of selected ROI (bottom right).

of a large cell population upon the irradiation. However, this assay does not provide an insight on a single cell fate within a population, and why certain cells within a population will stop dividing and eventually die, whereas the other ones will still be capable of clonogenic growth. It can be hypothesized that certain cells within a population accumulate lethal level of irradiation-induced damage, and lose capability to divide and form colonies, whereas the other cells remain unaffected. The unaffected cells might have higher DNA damage repair potential or may be "missed" by the irradiation particles (19, 20). The first step for addressing these questions is to develop a platform that provides direct information about spatial distribution of irradiation particles and correlates it at a single cell level with the clonogenic capacity. For that purpose, we adapted the conventional approach for colony formation assay and combined it with the usage of FNTDs (Cell-FIT-HD). This approach enables simultaneous analysis of the microscopic beam parameters together with the events in colonies, single cells, and at sub-cellular level. We were able to show that single cells can attach and grow as colonies on FNTD surface. The size of a surface area of a FNTD (4 mm × 8 mm) is not optimal for clonogenic growth, resulting in many overlapping colonies, and therefore the current design of the Cell-FIT-HD is not suitable for performing large-scale quantitative clonogenic assay. This might be restricted to certain cell types, such as the RENCA, where circumscribed colonies could be detected at an early phase of colony formation. Further studies are needed to find the optimal constraints for colony forming cell lines/primary cells in the Cell-FIT-HD setting. Nevertheless, our primary purpose was the application for analyzing single colonies, single cells, subcellular structures, and microscopic beam parameters, which was successfully demonstrated.

The current work represents a proof of principle study for correlation of particle traversal with long-term colony formation using Cell-FIT-HD. The entire workflow is established and builds a solid foundation for further improvements toward population level quantitative analysis. Further application of Cell-FIT-HD may provide necessary information for dissecting underlying mechanisms for colony formation of irradiated cells, which is important for studying time-dependent repair capability analyzing eventually correlation between fast and slow repair and the complexity of the induced damage, as well as bystander effect.

AUTHOR CONTRIBUTIONS

ID, MN, FZ, AM, PS, and DK performed experimental design, acquisition, analysis, and interpretation of the results. They participated in manuscript writing, revision, and approval of the final version for submission and publishing. ID, MN, OJ, SG, JD, and AA participated in the conception and design of the work, as well as interpretation of the data. They participated in manuscript writing, revision, and approval of the final version for submission and publishing. All authors agree to be accountable for all aspects of the work in ensuring that questions related to the accuracy or integrity of any part of the work are appropriately investigated and resolved.

FUNDING

This work was supported by German Research Council (DFG-KFO214), Deutsche Krebshilfe (Max-Eder 108876), Heidelberg School of Oncology Stipend (to MN) and intramural grants from National Center for Tumor diseases (NCT/DKFZ-DKTK, Heidelberg, Germany).

REFERENCES

1. Loeffler JS, Durante M. Charged particle therapy – optimization, challenges and future directions. *Nat Rev Clin Oncol* (2013) **10**:411–24. doi:10.1038/nrclinonc.2013.79
2. Niklas M, Abdollahi A, Akselrod MS, Debus J, Jakel O, Greilich S. Subcellular spatial correlation of particle traversal and biological response in clinical ion beams. *Int J Radiat Oncol Biol Phys* (2013) **87**:1141–7. doi:10.1016/j.ijrobp.2013.08.043
3. Niklas M, Greilich S, Melzig C, Akselrod MS, Debus J, Jakel O, et al. Engineering cell-fluorescent ion track hybrid detectors. *Radiat Oncol* (2013) **8**:141. doi:10.1186/1748-717X-8-141
4. Akselrod MS, Sykora GJ. Fluorescent nuclear track detector technology – a new way to do passive solid state dosimetry. *Radiat Meas* (2011) **46**:1671–9. doi:10.1016/j.radmeas.2011.06.018
5. Greilich S, Osinga JM, Niklas M, Lauer FM, Klimpki G, Bestvater F, et al. Fluorescent nuclear track detectors as a tool for ion-beam therapy research. *Radiat Meas* (2013) **56**:267–72. doi:10.1016/j.radmeas.2013.01.033
6. Puck TT, Marcus PI. Action of x-rays on mammalian cells. *J Exp Med* (1956) **103**:653–66. doi:10.1084/jem.103.5.653
7. Brown JM, Attardi LD. The role of apoptosis in cancer development and treatment response. *Nat Rev Cancer* (2005) **5**:231–7. doi:10.1038/nrc1560
8. Franken NA, Rodermond HM, Stap J, Haveman J, Van Bree C. Clonogenic assay of cells in vitro. *Nat Protoc* (2006) **1**:2315–9. doi:10.1038/nprot.2006.339
9. Friedrich T, Scholz U, Elsasser T, Durante M, Scholz M. Systematic analysis of RBE and related quantities using a database of cell survival experiments with ion beam irradiation. *J Radiat Res* (2013) **54**:494–514. doi:10.1093/jrr/rrs114
10. Khanna KK, Jackson SP. DNA double-strand breaks: signaling, repair and the cancer connection. *Nat Genet* (2001) **27**:247–54. doi:10.1038/85798
11. Noon AT, Goodarzi AA. 53BP1-mediated DNA double strand break repair: insert bad pun here. *DNA Repair (Amst)* (2011) **10**:1071–6. doi:10.1016/j.dnarep.2011.07.012
12. Markova E, Vasilyev S, Belyaev I. 53BP1 foci as a marker of tumor cell radiosensitivity. *Neoplasma* (2015) **62**:770–6. doi:10.4149/neo_2015_092
13. Ward IM, Minn K, Jorda KG, Chen J. Accumulation of checkpoint protein 53BP1 at DNA breaks involves its binding to phosphorylated histone H2AX. *J Biol Chem* (2003) **278**:19579–82. doi:10.1074/jbc.C300117200
14. Sharma A, Singh K, Almasan A. Histone H2AX phosphorylation: a marker for DNA damage. *Methods Mol Biol* (2012) **920**:613–26. doi:10.1007/978-1-61779-998-3_40
15. Dimitrova N, Chen YCM, Spector DL, De Lange T. 53BP1 promotes non-homologous end joining of telomeres by increasing chromatin mobility. *Nature* (2008) **456**:524–U551. doi:10.1038/nature07433
16. Dokic I, Mairani A, Brons S, Schoell B, Jauch A, Krunic D, et al. High resistance to X-rays and therapeutic carbon ions in glioblastoma cells bearing dysfunctional ATM associates with intrinsic chromosomal instability. *Int J Radiat Biol* (2015) **91**:157–65. doi:10.3109/09553002.2014.937511
17. Niklas M, Bartz JA, Akselrod MS, Abollahi A, Jokel J, Greilich S. Ion track reconstruction in 3D using alumina-based fluorescent nuclear track

detectors. *Phys Med Biol* (2013) **58**:N251–66. doi:10.1088/0031-9155/58/18/N251

18. Niklas M, Melzig C, Abdollahi A, Bartz J, Akselrod MS, Debus J, et al. Spatial correlation between traversal and cellular response in ion radiotherapy – towards single track spectroscopy. *Radiat Meas* (2013) **56**:285–9. doi:10.1016/j.radmeas.2013.01.060

19. Haynes RH, Eckardt F, Kunz BA. The DNA damage-repair hypothesis in radiation biology: comparison with classical hit theory. *Br J Cancer Suppl* (1984) **6**:81–90.

20. Schaue D, McBride WH. Counteracting tumor radioresistance by targeting DNA repair. *Mol Cancer Ther* (2005) **4**:1548–50. doi:10.1158/1535-7163.MCT-05-CO1

Translational Research to Improve the Efficacy of Carbon Ion Radiotherapy: Experience of Gunma University

7

Takahiro Oike[1], Hiro Sato[1], Shin-ei Noda[1] and Takashi Nakano[1,2]*

[1] Department of Radiation Oncology, Gunma University Graduate School of Medicine, Gunma, Japan, [2] Gunma University Heavy Ion Medical Center, Gunma, Japan

Correspondence:
Takashi Nakano
tnakano@gunma-u.ac.jp

Carbon ion radiotherapy holds great promise for cancer therapy. Clinical data show that carbon ion radiotherapy is an effective treatment for tumors that are resistant to X-ray radiotherapy. Since 1994 in Japan, the National Institute of Radiological Sciences has been heading the development of carbon ion radiotherapy using the Heavy Ion Medical Accelerator in Chiba. The Gunma University Heavy Ion Medical Center (GHMC) was established in the year 2006 as a proof-of-principle institute for carbon ion radiotherapy with a view to facilitating the worldwide spread of compact accelerator systems. Along with the management of more than 1900 cancer patients to date, GHMC engages in translational research to improve the treatment efficacy of carbon ion radiotherapy. Research aimed at guiding patient selection is of utmost importance for making the most of carbon ion radiotherapy, which is an extremely limited medical resource. Intratumoral oxygen levels, radiation-induced cellular apoptosis, the capacity to repair DNA double-strand breaks, and the mutational status of tumor protein p53 and epidermal growth factor receptor genes are all associated with X-ray sensitivity. Assays for these factors are useful in the identification of X-ray-resistant tumors for which carbon ion radiotherapy would be beneficial. Research aimed at optimizing treatments based on carbon ion radiotherapy is also important. This includes assessment of dose fractionation, normal tissue toxicity, tumor cell motility, and bystander effects. Furthermore, the efficacy of carbon ion radiotherapy will likely be enhanced by research into combined treatment with other modalities such as chemotherapy. Several clinically available chemotherapeutic drugs (carboplatin, paclitaxel, and etoposide) and drugs at the developmental stage (Wee-1 and heat shock protein 90 inhibitors) show a sensitizing effect on tumor cells treated with carbon ions. Additionally, the efficacy of carbon ion radiotherapy can be improved by combining it with cancer immunotherapy. Clinical validation of preclinical findings is necessary to further improve the treatment efficacy of carbon ion radiotherapy.

Keywords: carbon ion radiotherapy, patient selection, combination therapy, translational research, treatment planning

INTRODUCTION

Carbon ion radiotherapy holds great promise for cancer therapy. Carbon ions have two advantages over X-rays such as a sharp dose distribution and a strong cell-killing capacity (1). Clinical trials show that carbon ion radiotherapy has excellent antitumor effects (2, 3). Moreover, it is suggested that carbon ion radiotherapy is an effective treatment for tumors that are resistant to conventional X-ray radiotherapy (4–6).

The National Institute of Radiological Sciences (NIRS) initiated carbon ion radiotherapy in Japan in the year 1994 using the Heavy Ion Medical Accelerator in Chiba (HIMAC). Up until January 2016, more than 8000 patients with different types of cancer were treated at the NIRS. The excellent clinical outcomes encouraged widespread use of carbon ion radiotherapy (2). However, the high cost of constructing the accelerator system limits its practical application. New accelerator systems were designed to overcome this limitation; as a result, the cost of the accelerator systems was reduced to approximately $100,000,000 that accounts for one-third of the corresponding HIMAC parameters. Gunma University Heavy Ion Medical Center (GHMC) was launched in the year 2006 as a proof-of-principle institute for carbon ion radiotherapy based on the newly introduced compact accelerator systems. GHMC commenced operation of

the accelerator systems in 2009 and performed the first carbon ion radiotherapy for cancer in 2010. All carbon ion radiotherapy carried out at GHMC has been performed as prospective clinical trial (**Table 1**). As of January 2016, GHMC has treated more than 1900 cancer patients with carbon ion radiotherapy, without any major incidents.

Along with carbon ion radiotherapy, GHMC engages in translational research to improve the efficacy of this treatment modality with financial support from the Japan Society for the Promotion of Science through its two umbrella programs: the Twenty-First Century Centers of Excellence Program (2004–2008) and the Strategic Young Researcher Overseas Visits Program for Accelerating Brain Circulation (2013–2016). Translational research at GHMC was further accelerated by establishment of the Gunma University Initiative for Advanced Research in 2015, in which the Department of Radiation Oncology of the Massachusetts General Hospital/Harvard Medical School launched a Japanese branch to stimulate interdisciplinary collaboration in the field of heavy ion radiation biology. In addition, GHMC contributes to the education and development of global leaders in the field of heavy ion radiation therapy through the Program for Cultivating Global Leaders in Heavy Ion Therapeutics and Engineering, supported by the Japanese Ministry of Education, Culture, Sports, Science, and

TABLE 1 | Clinical trails on carbon ion radiotherapy at GHMC.

Trial ID	Patient enrollment	Cancer type	Major indication criteria	Total dose/fr.	Combined therapy
Gunma0905	2012-	Cranial base tumor	No CNS invasion	60.8 GyRBE/16 fr.	–
Gunma0901	2010–2013	H&N cancer (except Sq, melanoma, sarcoma)	N0/1M0	57.6 or 64 GyRBE/16 fr.	–
Gunma0902	2012-	H&N musculoskeletal tumor	N0/1M0	70 GyRBE/16 fr.	–
Gunma0903	2012-	H&N melanoma	N0M0	57.6 or 64 GyRBE/16 fr.	Concurrent DTIC, ACNU, and VCR
Gunma0701	2010–2015	NSCLC	Stage I, peripheral, inoperable	60 GyRBE/4 fr.	–
Gunma1201	2013–2015	NSCLC	Stage III, inoperable	40 GyRBE/10 fr. (ENI) + 20 or 24 GyRBE/6 fr. (IFI)	–
Gunma0703	2010–2013	Hepatcellular carcinoma	Tumor diameter ≤10 cm	52.8 GyRBE/4 fr.	–
Gunma1203	2013	Hepatcellular carcinoma	Tumor diameter 3–10 cm	60 GyRBE/4 fr.	–
Gunma1303	2013–2015	Hepatcellular carcinoma	Adjacent to digestive tract	60 or 64.8 GyRBE/12 fr.	–
Gunma1301	2013–2015	Pancreatic cancer	T4N0/1, inoperable	52.8 or 55.2 GyRBE/12 fr.	Concurrent gemcitabine
Gunma1501	2015-	Pancreatic cancer	T4N0/1M0	55.2 GyRBE/12 fr.	Concurrent S-1
Gunma0801	2010-	Rectal cancer	Postoperative local recurrence	73.6 GyRBE/16 fr.	–
Gunma0702	2010–2013	Prostate cancer	≤T3	57.6 GyRBE/16 fr.	± Hormone therapy
Gunma1302	2013-	Prostate cancer	≤T3	57.6 GyRBE/16 fr.	± Hormone therapy
Gunma1103	2013-	Prostate cancer	Castration resistant cancer	57.6 GyRBE/16 fr.	± Hormone therapy
Gunma1202	2013–2014	Uterine cervical cancer	Locally advanced	36 GyRBE/12 fr. (WPI) + 19.2 GyRBE/4 fr. (IFI)	Concurrent CDDP followed by ICBT
Gunma1401	2014-	Uterine cervical cancer	Locally advanced	36 GyRBE/12 fr. (WPI) + 19.2 GyRBE/4 fr. (IFI)	Concurrent CDDP followed by ICBT
Gunma0904	2010–2013	Musculoskeletal tumors	N0M0	64, 67.2, or 70.4 GyRBE/16 fr.	–
Gunma1102	2011–2013	Musculoskeletal tumors (pediatric)	Age 6–16, inoperable	60.8, 64, 67.2, or 70.4 GyRBE/16 fr.	–
Gunma1101	2011-	Lymph node metastatic tumor	1–3 nodes in 1 irradiation field	48 or 52.8 GyRBE/12 fr.	–
Gunma1304	2013-	In-field recurrent tumor	previously treated by radiotherapy	Various according to disease site	–
Gunma1204	2013-	Tumor resistant to standard Tx	known to be resistant to standard Tx	Various according to disease site	–

fr., fractions; CNS, central nervous system; H&N, head and neck; Sq, squamous cell carcinoma; NSCLC, non-small cell lung carcinoma; DTIC, dacarbazine; ACNU, nimustine; VCR, vincristine; ENI, elective nodal irradiation; IFI, involved field irradiation; WPI, whole pelvic irradiation; CDDP, cisplatin; ICBT, intracavitary brachytherapy; Tx, therapy.

Technology (2012–2018). Here, we summarize achievements in translational research on carbon ion radiotherapy performed at GHMC through these scientific endeavors.

RESEARCH TO GUIDE THE SELECTION OF PATIENTS SUITABLE FOR CARBON ION RADIOTHERAPY

The number of newly diagnosed cancer patients worldwide is ~14 million/year (7). By contrast, the maximum number of patients that can be treated by carbon ion radiotherapy worldwide is estimated to be ~2100/year (**Table 2**) (8). Thus, carbon ion radiotherapy has the capacity to treat only 0.015% of the total patient population with a newly diagnosed cancer. Moreover, even in Japan, which has the highest density of facilities for carbon ion radiotherapy in the world, carbon ion radiotherapy has the capacity to treat only 0.20% of newly diagnosed cancer cases. These facts highlight the extremely limited availability of this medical resource. Although 11 facilities for carbon ion radiotherapy are currently under construction or are planned for construction (1), the critical shortage of facilities will not be resolved in any practical way for a few decades. Therefore, selecting patients who can derive the greatest benefit from carbon ion radiotherapy is of great importance. Early clinical experience shows that carbon ion radiotherapy is an effective treatment for tumors that are resistant to conventional X-ray radiotherapy (4–6); therefore, carbon ion radiotherapy will be the most beneficial for patients with these types of tumor. From this point of view, assays that predict the X-ray sensitivity of a tumor are urgently required to facilitate appropriate selection of patients for carbon ion radiotherapy.

Histopathological typing of tumors is performed to predict treatment responses in the clinical setting of X-ray radiotherapy. Nevertheless, the response varies widely according to tumor type, and even among those with the same histological type. Thus, additional indices that support prediction of X-ray sensitivity

according to histopathological type are required. For many types of cancer, the SF2 value, i.e., the surviving fraction of X-irradiated tumor cells (irradiated *ex vivo* with a dose of 2 Gy) measured in a clonogenic survival assay, correlates with clinical outcome of X-ray radiotherapy (9). However, the SF2 value has shortcomings, i.e., primary culture of the tumor cells required for the clonogenic assay is difficult, and necessitates 2 weeks to obtain final results. Therefore, the SF2 value is not widely used in the clinic. Previously, we identified several cellular mechanisms that contribute to the resistance of cancer cells to X-rays, including intratumoral hypoxia, resistance to radiation-induced apoptosis, a high capacity for the repair of DNA double-strand breaks (DSBs), and mutations in certain oncogene and tumor suppressor genes. By focusing on these factors, we propose the following predictive assays for determining the X-ray sensitivity of cancer cells.

Intratumoral hypoxia is a major contributor to the X-ray resistance of cancer cells (10–12). Nakano et al. used a needle-type polarographic oxygen electrode to measure intratumoral oxygen partial pressure (pO₂) in patients with locally advanced uterine cervical cancer treated using X-ray radiotherapy (13) (**Figure 1**). The authors found that low pretreatment intratumoral pO₂ values correlated with poor outcomes after X-ray radiotherapy. On the other hand, carbon ion radiotherapy showed good antitumor effects in patients with locally advanced uterine cervical cancer, irrespective of pretreatment intratumoral pO₂ levels. These data indicate that assays to determine pretreatment intratumoral pO₂ values will be useful for identification of X-ray-resistant tumors profiting from carbon ion radiotherapy. Importantly, recent studies indicate that as many as 50% of tumors have hypoxic regions, which could underpin X-ray treatment failure and expand the indications for carbon ion radiotherapy (14). Cancer cell resistance to radiation-induced apoptosis is another major factor that contributes to X-ray resistance. Preclinical studies suggest that carbon ions effectively kill cancer cells that are resistant to apoptosis induced by X-ray irradiation (15, 16). Another mode

TABLE 2 | Number of cancer patients treated by carbon ion radiotherapy worldwide per year.

S. No.	Country	City	Facility	Case/year	Year
1	Japan	Chiba	NIRS	888	2013
2	Japan	Gunma	GHMC	448	2013
3	Japan	Hyogo	HIBMC	270	2013
4	Japan	Saga	HIMAT	132	2013
5	China	Lanzhou	HIRFL	27	2006–2013 in average
6	Germany	Heidelberg	HIT	274	2009–2013 in average
7	Italy	Pavia	CNAO	53	2012–2013 in average

NIRS, National Institute of Radiological Sciences; GHMC, Gunma University Heavy Ion Medical Center; HIBMC, Hyogo Ion-Beam Medical Center; HIMAT, Heavy Ion Medical Accelerator in Tosu; HIRFL, Heavy Ion Research Facility in Lanzhou; HIT, Heidelberg Ion-Beam Therapy Center; CNAO, Centro Nazionale Adroterapia Oncologica. Data on facility #1–4 are based on the website of Association for Nuclear Technology in Medicine (written in Japanese): http://www.antm.or.jp/05_treatment/01.html. Data on facility #5–7 are based on Ref. (8).

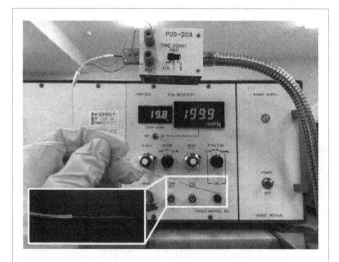

FIGURE 1 | Tools for intratumoral pO₂ measurement. A needle-type polarographic oxygen electrode is used by direct insertion into a tumor.

of clonogenic cell death, called mitotic catastrophe and necrosis, is involved in efficient killing of apoptosis-resistant cancer cells by carbon ions (15, 16). Apoptosis following irradiation is readily assessed by morphological observation of nuclei stained with 4′,6-diamidino-2-phenylindole dihydrochloride (DAPI) (**Figure 2**). Amornwichet et al. demonstrated that apoptosis in HCT116 colon cancer cells peaked at 72 h post-X-ray irradiation, as assessed by DAPI staining (16). This is consistent with the observation that radiation-induced apoptosis in solid tumors mainly corresponds to the so-called late apoptosis, which occurs a few days post-irradiation (17). Furthermore, the DAPI-based assay is easier and faster to perform than the clonogenic survival assay used to calculate the SF2 value. Therefore, DAPI staining of *ex vivo*-irradiated tumor specimens at 72 h post-irradiation is useful for identifying tumors that are resistant to X-ray-induced apoptosis and would therefore benefit from carbon ion radiotherapy.

Double-strand breaks are major cytotoxic lesions that cause cancer cell death after exposure to ionizing radiation (17). Preclinical studies indicate that the high capacity of cancer cells for DSB repair contributes to X-ray resistance (18, 19). Meanwhile, the cell-killing actions of carbon ions are less affected by intrinsic DSB repair capacity (18, 19). Most likely, complex carbon ion-induced DSBs are more difficult to repair than X-ray-induced DSBs; these persistent unrepaired DSBs then lead to mitotic catastrophe (16). These data indicate that tumors with a high capacity for DSB repair are suitable for carbon ion radiotherapy. DSB repair capacity can be evaluated by immuno-fluorescence staining for Ser139-phosphorylated histone H2AX (γH2AX) or p53-binding protein 1 (53BP1) because DSBs are detected as foci of γH2AX or 53BP1 (**Figure 3**) (20–22). The number of foci at 30 min post-irradiation can be used as an index for radiation-induced DSBs. On the other hand, the number of foci in irradiated cells decreases by more than 90% within 24 h post-irradiation, indicating that a major proportion of radiation-induced DSBs is repaired by that time point (20). Thus, the ratio of the foci number at 24 h post-irradiation to that at 30 min post-irradiation can be used as an index for DSB repair capacity.

Importantly, the high DSB repair capacity (as indicated by low number of foci at 24 h post-irradiation) is associated with a high rate of clonogenic survival (19). Hence, assay of γH2AX or 53BP1 foci in *ex vivo*-irradiated tumor specimens can be performed to identify tumors with a high capacity for DSB repair and suitable for carbon ion radiotherapy.

Cancer cells harbor modifications in a number of molecular pathways that affect intrinsic radiosensitivity. Mutations in oncogenes and tumor suppressor genes are common, and these mutations result in alterations in signaling pathways. We previously showed that inactivating mutations in the gene encoding tumor suppressor protein 53 (*TP53*) confer X-ray resistance on cancer cells (15, 16, 23). We also showed that epidermal growth factor receptor gene (*EGFR*) mutation-negative non-small cell lung cancer (NSCLC) cells are more resistant to X-rays than *EGFR* mutation-positive NSCLC cells (19). These findings were validated by clinical studies (24–27). Interestingly, investigations using isogenic cancer cell lines demonstrated that carbon ions can kill cancer cells irrespective of the mutational status of *TP53* and *EGFR* (15, 16, 19, 23). Taken together, these data indicate that the mutational status of *TP53/EGFR* is useful for selecting patients who are suited for carbon ion radiotherapy. Nevertheless, a recent genome-wide analysis revealed the presence of hundreds of gene mutations in a single tumor (28). Because the overall radiosensitivity of a tumor should be the result of this highly complex genetic context, the mutational

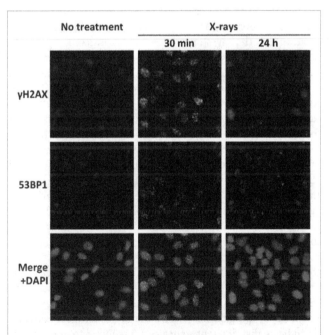

FIGURE 3 | **Radiation-induced DSBs visualized by immunofluorescence staining of γH2AX and 53BP1**. Cultured A549 lung cancer cells were immunostained for γH2AX and 53BP1 at 30 min or 24 h post-irradiation using X-rays at a dose of 1 Gy. DSBs are identified as foci of γH2AX and 53BP1. Merged images show high consistency between γH2AX foci and 53BP1 foci. A markedly smaller number of γH2AX and 53BP1 foci at 24 h compared with 30 min indicate the high capacity of the X-ray-resistant cell line for DSB repair.

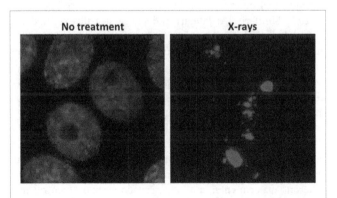

FIGURE 2 | **Radiation-induced apoptosis, as assessed by DAPI staining**. Cultured Ma-24 lung cancer cells were stained with DAPI at 72 h after irradiation using X-rays at a dose of 4 Gy. Apoptotic cells are identified by the appearance of apoptotic bodies, characterized by condensed and fragmented nuclei, under a fluorescence microscope.

status of only a small subset of well-known cancer-related genes (e.g., *TP53* and *EGFR*) may not be the best predictor of radiosensitivity. Thus, studies aimed at elucidating detailed gene mutation profiles to facilitate better prediction of tumor radiosensitivity are warranted.

RESEARCH AIMED AT OPTIMIZING CARBON ION RADIOTHERAPY

Optimization of carbon ion radiotherapy can be addressed using two approaches such as radiation physics and radiation biology. Both physics and biology play intertwining roles in treatment planning; therefore, advances in one field benefit the other. For example, increased irradiation accuracy results in less normal tissue toxicity. By contrast, accurate information about the biological characteristics of tumors and normal tissues aids optimal treatment planning. Biological factors that affect the treatment procedure, including biological responses to dose fractionation, normal tissue toxicity, tumor cell motility, and the bystander effect, are discussed below.

In X-ray radiotherapy, the rationale for dose fractionation is provided by the re-oxygenation and cell cycle redistribution of tumor cells, as well as a higher capacity for the repair of sublethal damage in normal tissues versus tumors (17). The cell-killing effect of carbon ions versus X-rays is less dependent on these factors (13, 17); therefore, the responses of tumors and normal tissues to carbon ions may be different from those to X-rays, even when the same dose fractionation schedule is utilized. To address this issue, Ando et al. used a mouse model to explore the effects of carbon ion dose fractionation on tumor and normal tissues (29). The investigators treated fibrosarcoma xenografts and host mouse skin with γ rays or carbon ion beams with three different linear energy transfer (LET) values (20, 42, and 77 keV/µm) and with different fractionation schedules (i.e., one to seven fractions). Interestingly, the relative biological effectiveness (RBE) values for tumor growth delay were higher than those for early skin reaction when 42- and 77-keV/µm carbon ion beams, but not γ rays or 20-keV/µm carbon ion beams, were employed in intermediate fractionation schedules (i.e., two to six fractions). The therapeutic gain (calculated as the ratio of the RBE value for tumor growth delay to that for early skin reaction) was maximized for the 42 keV/µm beams delivered in four fractions. Yoshida et al. examined the impact of carbon ion dose fractionation on the small intestine by assessing crypt survival in the mouse model employed above (30). In contrast to the results for early skin reaction, no therapeutic gain was observed for the intermediate fractionation schedules. This might be because intestinal crypt cells have a low capacity to repair sublethal damage induced by carbon ions. These two studies indicate that different strategies are required to optimize the dose fractionation schedules used for carbon ion radiotherapy in the skin versus the small intestine. With respect to the skin, the therapeutic window for carbon ion irradiation can be expanded by employing an intermediate hypofractionation strategy. Therefore, the actual fractionation schedule that corresponds to "intermediate" hypofractionation in the mouse model should be further explored in the clinic. On the other hand, the therapeutic

window for carbon ions and X-rays in the small intestine may be comparable, and the benefit of dose fractionation may be lower for carbon ions than for X-rays. This indicates that, in abdominal irradiation to treat tumors such as uterine cervical cancer, the maximum tolerable carbon ion dose can be delivered in a smaller number of fractions, resulting in a shorter treatment period. In addition, hypofractionated carbon ion radiotherapy that results in the shorter treatment period compared with X-ray radiotherapy utilizing conventional 2 Gy/day fractionation can contribute to reduce tumor repopulation effect. Assessment of the effect of carbon ion dose fractionation in different tumors and normal tissues in the same mouse model should be further investigated, together with concomitant evaluation of factors that can affect the results of fractionated irradiation (i.e., oxygen levels, cell cycle profiles, and DSB repair capacity).

Carbon ion radiotherapy shows a steep dose fall-off; therefore, the treatment plans are more susceptible to target motion than the plan for three-dimensional conformal radiotherapy (3D-CRT) with X-rays. A larger target volume setting increases the robustness of the dose delivered to the tumor; however, it also increases toxicity to adjacent normal tissues. Therefore, it is necessary to determine the sensitivity of normal tissues to obtain the optimal target volume setting. The nervous system is critically at risk of radiotherapy toxicity, because it is a serial organ with low redundancy and low capacity for regeneration. The sensitivity of the central nervous system to carbon ions has been examined in multiple experimental models. Isono et al. evaluated the sensitivity of human neural stem cells to carbon ions and found that the RBE value, as assessed by cell proliferation, was 2.0 (31). Yoshida et al. examined the effects of carbon ion irradiation in normal rat brain (32). The authors used an organotypic slice culture of cerebellum excised from 10-day-old rats and assessed morphological changes and cellular apoptosis, defined as disorganization of the external granule cell layer and positive staining for TdT-mediated dUTP-biotin nick-end labeling (TUNEL), respectively. They found that the RBE value for rat cerebellum was 1.4–1.5. Kaminuma et al. also explored carbon ion-provoked apoptosis in the rat brain by performing a TUNEL assay in a primary culture of fetal hippocampal neurons (33). The RBE value was strikingly high at 10.2. Similarly, Al-Jahdari and colleagues investigated the sensitivity of the peripheral nervous system to carbon ions by employing dorsal root ganglia and sympathetic ganglion chains prepared from the chick embryo at days 8 and 16, representing the immature and mature peripheral nervous system (34). Growth cone collapse was assessed as an index of malfunction in the neuronal network, yielding an RBE value of 3.1–3.2 in day 8 neurons and 1.5–2.1 in day 16 neurons. Meanwhile, the RBE value assessed by TUNEL staining was 2.5–2.9 in day 8 neurons and 1.4–1.8 in day 16 neurons. Although it is difficult to draw a firm conclusion from the above studies employing different experimental models, nervous systems (central and peripheral) and endpoints, the data collectively indicate that the RBE value of the adult nervous system is ~1.4–2.1 when morphological changes and cellular apoptosis are utilized as endpoints. Given the fact that the RBE value for carbon ions in cancer cells is generally ~2–3, these findings suggest that carbon ion radiotherapy has a wider therapeutic window than X-rays when used to treat tumors adjacent to the components of the central and peripheral nervous systems. Notably, these data also indicate that immature neurons are more sensitive to carbon ion irradiation than mature neurons. Thus, careful attention should be paid to neural toxicity when carbon ion radiotherapy is used to treat pediatric tumors.

The lung is another critical organ at risk in radiotherapy. Radiation-induced lung injury can be lethal in some patients and is a major dose-limiting factor for thoracic irradiation (35). Okano et al. used a crystal violet staining assay to examine the effect of carbon ions on the proliferation of immortalized human small airway epithelial cells (iSAECs) and normal human lung fibroblasts (36). The resultant RBE value was 3.2 for iSAECs and 2.2 for normal lung fibroblasts. On the other hand, ionizing radiation can indirectly damage normal lung tissue by triggering inflammatory reactions. Upregulation of intercellular adhesion molecule-1 (ICAM-1) expression on the surface of pulmonary endothelial cells participates in this inflammation-related process by increasing macrophage infiltration into the lung (37, 38). Kiyohara et al. compared ICAM-1 expression on the surface of human umbilical vein endothelial cells after irradiation with carbon ions and X-rays. The data showed that post-irradiation ICAM-1 expression levels were 2.56- and 2.47-fold higher after carbon ion irradiation than after X-ray irradiation at 1 and 2 Gy, respectively (39). These data signify that the estimated RBE values in normal lung tissue and lung cancer cells are comparable (~2–3) (19).

Several studies demonstrate that X-ray irradiation increases the motility of cancer cells (40, 41). The migration of irradiated cancer cells may influence the setting of target volumes, i.e., the margin from the gross tumor volume (GTV) to the clinical target volume (CTV). Murata et al. used a wound healing assay and F-actin staining to examine the effect of carbon ions on the motility of A549 lung cancer cells (42). Carbon ion irradiation promoted the healing of scratch wounds in cell monolayers and increased the formation of F-actin protrusions, both indicators of increased cancer cell motility. Interestingly, the RBE value based on cell motility was consistent with that based on cell survival (i.e., ~4 versus 3.9). This finding provides important insight into treatment planning, i.e., the GTV–CTV margin can be set in a comparable manner for X-rays and carbon ions.

The bystander effect is a phenomenon whereby non-irradiated cells adjacent to irradiated cells are killed (43). Previous research shows that the bystander effect is universal among most types of normal cells and tumor cells (43). However, the significance of the bystander effect among different types of cells after carbon ion irradiation is not fully understood. Harada et al. investigated the bystander effect in carbon ion-irradiated A549 cells by using carbon ion microbeams (diameter = 20 μm) to irradiate only 0.0001–0.002% of the cells in a culture plate (44). The entire cell population was then subjected to a clonogenic survival assay, resulting in an 8–14% reduction in cell survival. Thus, the bystander effect plays a highly significant role in carbon ion-induced killing of A549 lung cancer cells. By contrast, Wakatsuki et al. found that the bystander effect played no role in the killing

of a HTB-94 chondrosarcoma cell line (45). These data highlight the fact that different cell types show different susceptibilities to the bystander effect induced by carbon ion irradiation by up to ~10%. Further research into the carbon ion radiotherapy-induced bystander effects in different tumor cells and normal cells is necessary to optimize treatment planning.

RESEARCH INTO COMBINATION THERAPY TO ENHANCE THE EFFICACY OF CARBON ION RADIOTHERAPY

Theoretically, a sufficiently high dose of ionizing radiation can sterilize any type of tumor (46). However, clinically applicable doses are delivered within a range that is tolerable by normal tissues (47). Dose escalation trials are underway to identify the maximum tolerable dose for carbon ion radiotherapy according to disease site (2). To date, clinical experience indicates that carbon ion radiotherapy can be delivered to many disease sites at higher biologically equivalent doses than 3D-CRT using X-rays. Carbon ion radiotherapy can also achieve nearly 100% tumor control probability in tumors that are uncontrollable by other radiation therapy modalities using X-rays and protons, such as spinal chordomas (1). Nonetheless, local recurrence occurs within the GTV, indicating the presence of a subset of carbon ion-resistant tumors.

To eradicate carbon ion-resistant tumors, it is important to establish an optimal form of combination treatment that increases the efficacy of carbon ion radiotherapy. To this end, several clinically available chemotherapeutic drugs have been tested in a preclinical setting. Kubo et al. examined the ability of carboplatin and paclitaxel to sensitize H460 lung cancer cells to carbon ion beams (48). Both sensitized cancer cells to carbon ion irradiation, with sensitizing ratios of 1.21 and 1.22, respectively (NB, a sensitizing ratio of >1 indicates that the radiation and the drug have a synergistic effect). These sensitizing ratios were comparable with those of X-rays. Similarly, Takahashi et al. demonstrated that etoposide sensitized X-ray-resistant rat yolk sac tumor cells to carbon ions, reporting a sensitizing ratio of ~1.2 (23). Carboplatin, paclitaxel, and etoposide are all currently used in combination with X-rays for clinical tumor treatment; carboplatin and paclitaxel are used to treat NSCLC, uterine cervical cancer, and esophageal cancer, and etoposide is used to treat small cell lung cancer. The combination of these drugs with carbon ions should likewise be tested in the clinic.

Several drugs currently under development have been tested for their ability to sensitize cells to carbon ion irradiation. Ma and colleagues examined the sensitizing effects of the Wee-1 inhibitor, MK-1775, using H1299 lung cancer cells (49). Wee-1 is a nuclear kinase protein involved in activating the G2 cell cycle checkpoint. Pretreatment for lung cancer cells with MK-1775 abrogated the induction of G2/M arrest after carbon ion irradiation, leading to an increase in mitotic catastrophe-mediated cell death. The sensitizing ratio of MK-1775 was 1.21 at 200 nM, a concentration at which MK-1775 alone reduces the surviving cell fraction by 50%. Musha et al. evaluated the sensitizing effect of the heat shock protein 90 (Hsp90) inhibitor, 17-AAG, in LMF4 oral squamous cell carcinoma cells (50). Hsp90 forms a chaperone complex with client proteins, thereby stabilizing them. Because various Hsp90 client proteins [e.g., Akt, ErbB2, and hypoxia-inducible factor-1α (HIF-1α)] are associated with malignant cancer phenotypes, Hsp90 is regarded as a potent molecular target (51–53). 17-AAG sensitized tumor cells to carbon ions with a sensitizing ratio of 1.14 at 100 nM, a concentration at which 17-AAG alone reduces the surviving cell fraction by 30–40%, although the underlying mechanism is unclear. These data indicate that Wee-1 or Hsp90 inhibition is a viable strategy for sensitization of carbon ions, but the sensitizing effect requires further testing in animal models. As a monomodality treatment for cancer, MK-1775 is currently under investigation in phase I and phase II clinical trials (54). Meanwhile, a phase II clinical trial for 17-AAG was terminated due to the lack of adequate tumor response and the presence of normal tissue toxicity (55). Nevertheless, a number of next-generation Hsp90 inhibitors are now being tested in multiple clinical trials (55).

Cancer immunotherapy has recently provoked a great deal of interest. Novel molecular targeting therapies (including those targeting programed cell death 1, programed cell death-ligand 1, and cytotoxic T-lymphocyte-associated protein 4) all demonstrate marked antitumor effects (56–58). Evidence suggests that the antitumor immune response plays an important role in the antitumor efficacy of X-ray radiotherapy. Nakano et al. showed that pretreatment levels of intratumoral infiltration by Langerhans cells and T cells, the key players in antitumor immune responses, correlates with a favorable outcome in patients with uterine cervical cancer treated using X-ray radiotherapy (59). They also showed that concomitant use of X-rays and intratumoral injection of sizofiran, an immune-response modifying drug, increases intratumoral infiltration of Langerhans cells and T-cells in patients with uterine cervical cancer (60). Recently, Suzuki et al. demonstrated that an antigen-specific T cell response is activated in esophageal cancer patients receiving combined X-ray radiotherapy and chemotherapy (61). These data suggest that the efficacy of X-ray radiotherapy can be improved upon combination with assorted cancer immunotherapies.

To investigate whether the antitumor immune response contributes to the antitumor efficacy of carbon ion radiotherapy, Yoshimoto et al. examined the impact of carbon ion irradiation on the release of high-mobility group box 1 protein (HMGB1) after irradiation in various cancer cell lines (62). HMGB1 is released from tumor cells damaged by radiotherapy and/or chemotherapy. Elevated serum HMGB1 levels are associated with activation of the antigen-specific T cell responses after chemoradiotherapy (61). The investigators found that HMGB1 levels in conditioned culture media were significantly higher after carbon ion irradiation. The RBE values based on HMGB1 release were similar to those based on clonogenic survival. These data suggest that the antitumor immune response contributes to an antitumor effect not only in X-ray radiotherapy but also in carbon ion radiotherapy. Additional preclinical research investigating the effects of combinations of carbon ion radiotherapy and cancer immunotherapy is currently underway.

PERSPECTIVES

Carbon ion radiotherapy is a promising therapy for cancer. Appropriate patient selection based on individual tumor radiosensitivity is key to making the most of this medical resource with extremely limited availability. Recent advances in molecular biology research emphasize the need for functional predictive assays using tumor biopsy specimens for the practice of precision medicine (63). The utility of predictive assays for determining intratumoral oxygen levels, radiation-induced cellular apoptosis, DSB repair capacity, and gene mutational status should be tested in the clinic. Of note, recent studies demonstrate that a combination of distinct tumor features can work synergistically to predict prognosis in a subset of tumors, indicating the benefit of combined usage of these predictive assays (64). In addition, progress in the field of metabolomics indicates that non-invasive predictive assays based on biofluids, such as blood or urine, will be established in the near future (65, 66).

Researchers have accumulated extensive data concerning radiobiological properties of cancers and normal tissues. However, translation of biological data to the clinic remains far from satisfactory. This may be partially due the huge diversity in experimental systems used in radiation biology studies, making it difficult to draw solid conclusions for clinical applications. A meta-analytic approach to integrate the existing data is suggested. Moreover, specification of carbon ion beams including LET values employed in the studies must be carefully considered during the data translation process. Most in vitro studies used mono-energetic high-LET (i.e., ~100 keV/μm) carbon ion beams. However, several facilities, including NIRS and GHMC, now utilize spread-out Bragg peak (SOBP) carbon ion beams, which comprise a mixture of different LET beams, in the clinic. The biological effect of SOBP carbon ion beams likely differs from that of mono-energetic high-LET beams. Studies during the early era of carbon ion radiobiology provide plenty of data on the biological effect of SOBP carbon ion beams. Nevertheless, these data are difficult to interpret in the context of modern molecular biology and in a clinical setting because the biological effects were analyzed using biophysics models to deconvolute the mixed LET spectrum. Therefore, future studies should investigate the effects of SOBP carbon ion beams using current molecular biological techniques, particularly with respect to tumor hypoxia, radiation-induced apoptosis, and DSB repair.

Emerging molecular biology techniques are expected to contribute to further advancement of translational research in carbon ion radiobiology. First, next-generation sequencing technologies will almost certainly identify specific genomic and epigenomic profiles that affect radiosensitivity (28, 67) and can be combined with existing data concerning expression profiles related to radiosensitivity (68, 69). Second, advanced high-resolution microscopy techniques will clarify the molecular processes that occur following carbon ion irradiation. For example, Britton et al. visualized recruitment of a single Ku molecule at DSB sites, which is essential for the repair of DSBs induced by ionizing irradiation (70). Thus, advanced high-resolution microscopy will promote our understanding of the repair kinetics of complex DSBs induced by carbon ions. Third, emerging imaging technologies will enable detailed visualization of intratumoral oxygen levels and metabolomic states (71). We anticipate that integration and translation of data in radiation biology will greatly improve the efficacy of carbon ion radiotherapy.

AUTHOR CONTRIBUTIONS

TO, HS and S-eN summarized data and drafted the manuscript. TN supervised the manuscript. All authors read and approved the final manuscript.

ACKNOWLEDGMENTS

We sincerely thank Dr. Atsushi Shibata and Dr. Atsuko Niimi (Gunma University) for their generous support in obtaining the data used in the figures. We thank Ms. Yuka Kimura and Ms. Yuka Hirota (Gunma University) for technical assistance.

FUNDING

This work was supported by Grants-in-Aid from the Ministry of Education, Culture, Sports, Science, and Technology of Japan for programs for Leading Graduate Schools, Cultivating Global Leaders in Heavy Ion Therapeutics and Engineering, and for Strategic Young Researcher Overseas Visits Program for Accelerating Brain Circulation. This work was also supported by Grants-in-Aid from the Japan Society for the Promotion of Science for Scientific Research (B) KAKENHI (24390288) and for the Twenty-First Century Centers of Excellence Program (K05).

REFERENCES

1. Loeffler JS, Durante M. Charged particle therapy-optimization, challenges and future directions. *Nat Rev Clin Oncol* (2013) 10:411–24. doi:10.1038/nrclinonc.2013.79

2. Kamada T, Tsujii H, Blakely EA, Debus J, De Neve W, Durante M, et al. Carbon ion radiotherapy in Japan: an assessment of 20 years of clinical experience. *Lancet Oncol* (2015) 16:e93–100. doi:10.1016/S1470-2045(14)70412-7

3. Combs SE, Debus J. Treatment with heavy charged particles: systematic review of clinical data and current clinical (comparative) trials. *Acta Oncol* (2013) 52:1272–86. doi:10.3109/0284186X.2013.818254

4. Shinoto M, Yamada S, Yasuda S, Imada H, Shioyama Y, Honda H, et al. Phase 1 trial of preoperative, short-course carbon-ion radiotherapy for patients with resectable pancreatic cancer. *Cancer* (2013) 119:45–51. doi:10.1002/cncr.27723

5. Jingu K, Tsujii H, Mizoe JE, Hasegawa A, Bessho H, Takagi R, et al. Carbon ion radiation therapy improves the prognosis of unresectable adult bone and soft-tissue sarcoma of the head and neck. *Int J Radiat Oncol Biol Phys* (2012) 82:2125–31. doi:10.1016/j.ijrobp.2010.08.043

6. Mizoe JE, Hasegawa A, Jingu K, Takagi R, Bessyo H, Morikawa T, et al. Results of carbon ion radiotherapy for head and neck cancer. *Radiother Oncol* (2012) 103:32–7. doi:10.1016/j.radonc.2011.12.013

7. Website: Cancer Research UK (2016). Available from: http://www.cancerresearchuk.org/health-professional/cancer-statistics/worldwide-cancer

8. Jermann M. Particle therapy statistics in 2013. *Int J Part Ther* (2014) 1:40–3. doi:10.14338/IJPT.14-editorial-2.1

9. Torres-Roca JF. A molecular assay of tumor radiosensitivity: a roadmap towards biology-based personalized radiation therapy. *Per Med* (2012) 9:547–57. doi:10.2217/pme.12.55

10. Kallman RF. The phenomenon of reoxygenation and its implications for fractionated radiotherapy. *Radiology* (1972) 105:135–42. doi:10.1148/105.1.135

11. Gatenby RA, Kessler HB, Rosenblum JS, Coia LR, Moldofsky PJ, Hartz WH, et al. Oxygen distribution in squamous cell carcinoma metastases and its relationship to outcome of radiation therapy. *Int J Radiat Oncol Biol Phys* (1988) 14:831–8. doi:10.1016/0360-3016(88)90002-8

12. Nordsmark M, Overgaard M, Overgaard J. Pretreatment oxygenation predicts radiation response in advanced squamous cell carcinoma of the head and neck. *Radiother Oncol* (1996) 41:31–9. doi:10.1016/S0167-8140(96)91811-3

13. Nakano T, Suzuki Y, Ohno T, Kato S, Suzuki M, Morita S, et al. Carbon beam therapy overcomes the radiation resistance of uterine cervical cancer originating from hypoxia. *Clin Cancer Res* (2006) 12:2185–90. doi:10.1158/1078-0432.CCR-05-1907

14. Hill RP, Bristow RG, Fyles A, Koritzinsky M, Milosevic M, Wouters BG. Hypoxia and predicting radiation response. *Semin Radiat Oncol* (2015) 25:260–72. doi:10.1016/j.semradonc.2015.05.004

15. Takahashi A, Matsumoto H, Yuki K, Yasumoto J, Kajiwara A, Aoki M, et al. High-LET radiation enhanced apoptosis but not necrosis regardless of p53 status. *Int J Radiat Oncol Biol Phys* (2004) 60:591–7. doi:10.1016/j.ijrobp.2004.05.062

16. Amornwichet N, Oike T, Shibata A, Ogiwara H, Tsuchiya N, Yamauchi M, et al. Carbon-ion beam irradiation kills X-ray-resistant p53-null cancer cells by inducing mitotic catastrophe. *PLoS One* (2014) 9:e115121. doi:10.1371/journal.pone.0115121

17. Joiner MC, van der Kogel A. *Basic Clinical Radiobiology.* Florida: CRC Press (2009).

18. Takahashi A, Kubo M, Ma H, Nakagawa A, Yoshida Y, Isono M, et al. Nonhomologous end-joining repair plays a more important role than homologous recombination repair in defining radiosensitivity after exposure to high-LET radiation. *Radiat Res* (2014) 182:338–44. doi:10.1667/RR13782.1

19. Amornwichet N, Oike T, Shibata A, Nirodi CS, Ogiwara H, Makino H, et al. The EGFR mutation status affects the relative biological effectiveness of carbon-ion beams in non-small cell lung carcinoma cells. *Sci Rep* (2015) 5:11305. doi:10.1038/srep11305

20. Löbrich M, Shibata A, Beucher A, Fisher A, Ensminger M, Goodarzi AA, et al. gammaH2AX foci analysis for monitoring DNA double-strand break repair: strengths, limitations and optimization. *Cell Cycle* (2010) 9:662–9. doi:10.1158/0008-5472.CAN-03-3207

21. Stiff T, O'Driscoll M, Rief N, Iwabuchi K, Löbrich M, Jeggo PA. ATM and DNA-PK function redundantly to phosphorylate H2AX after exposure to ionizing radiation. *Cancer Res* (2004) 64:2390–6. doi:10.1158/0008-5472.CAN-03-3207

22. Markova E, Vasilyev S, Belyaev I. 53BP1 foci as a marker of tumor cell radiosensitivity. *Neoplasma* (2015) 62:770–6. doi:10.4149/neo_2015_092

23. Takahashi T, Fukawa T, Hirayama R, Yoshida Y, Musha A, Furusawa Y, et al. In vitro interaction of high-LET heavy-ion irradiation and chemotherapeutic agents in two cell lines with different radiosensitivities and different p53 status. *Anticancer Res* (2010) 30:1961–7.

24. Ishikawa H, Mitsuhashi N, Sakurai H, Maebayashi K, Niibe H. The effects of p53 status and human papillomavirus infection on the clinical outcome of patients with stage IIIB cervical carcinoma treated with radiation therapy alone. *Cancer* (2001) 91:80–9. doi:10.1002/1097-0142(20010101)91:1<80:AID-CNCR11>3.0.CO;2-E

25. Huerta S, Hrom J, Gao X, Saha D, Anthony T, Reinhart H, et al. Tissue microarray constructs to predict a response to chemoradiation in rectal cancer. *Dig Liver Dis* (2010) 42:679–84. doi:10.1016/j.dld.2010.02.003

26. Nakano T, Oka K, Taniguchi N. Manganese superoxide dismutase expression correlates with p53 status and local recurrence of cervical carcinoma treated with radiation therapy. *Cancer Res* (1996) 56:2771–5.

27. Yagishita S, Horinouchi H, Katsui Taniyama T, Nakamichi S, Kitazono S, Mizugaki H, et al. Epidermal growth factor receptor mutation is associated with longer local control after definitive chemoradiotherapy in patients with

stage III nonsquamous non-small-cell lung cancer. *Int J Radiat Oncol Biol Phys* (2015) 91:140–8. doi:10.1016/j.ijrobp.2014.08.344

28. Alexandrov LB, Nik-Zainal S, Wedge DC, Aparicio SA, Behjati S, Biankin AV, et al. Signatures of mutational processes in human cancer. *Nature* (2013) 500:415–21. doi:10.1038/nature12477

29. Ando K, Koike S, Uzawa A, Takai N, Fukawa T, Furusawa Y, et al. Biological gain of carbon-ion radiotherapy for the early response of tumor growth delay and against early response of skin reaction in mice. *J Radiat Res* (2005) 46:51–7. doi:10.1269/jrr.46.51

30. Yoshida Y, Ando K, Ando K, Murata K, Yoshimoto Y, Musha A, et al. Evaluation of therapeutic gain for fractionated carbon-ion radiotherapy using the tumor growth delay and crypt survival assays. *Radiother Oncol* (2015) 117:351–7. doi:10.1016/j.radonc.2015.09.027

31. Isono M, Yoshida Y, Takahashi A, Oike T, Shibata A, Kubota Y, et al. Carbon-ion beams effectively induce growth inhibition and apoptosis in human neural stem cells compared with glioblastoma A172 cells. *J Radiat Res* (2015) 56:856–61. doi:10.1093/jrr/rrv033

32. Yoshida Y, Suzuki Y, Al-Jahdari WS, Hamada N, Funayama T, Shirai K, et al. Evaluation of the relative biological effectiveness of carbon ion beams in the cerebellum using the rat organotypic slice culture system. *J Radiat Res* (2012) 53:87–92. doi:10.1269/jrr.11139A

33. Kaminuma T, Suzuki Y, Shirai K, Mizui T, Noda SE, Yoshida Y, et al. Effectiveness of carbon-ion beams for apoptosis induction in rat primary immature hippocampal neurons. *J Radiat Res* (2010) 51:627–31. doi:10.1269/jrr.10050

34. Al-Jahdari WS, Suzuki Y, Yoshida Y, Hamada N, Shirai K, Noda SE, et al. The radiobiological effectiveness of carbon-ion beams on growing neurons. *Int J Radiat Biol* (2009) 85:700–9. doi:10.1080/09553000903020032

35. Yamashita H, Nakagawa K, Nakamura N, Koyanagi H, Tago M, Igaki H, et al. Exceptionally high incidence of symptomatic grade 2-5 radiation pneumonitis after stereotactic radiation therapy for lung tumors. *Radiat Oncol* (2007) 2:21. doi:10.1186/1748-717X-2-21

36. Okano N, Oike T, Saitoh J, Shirai K, Kiyono T, Enari M, et al. In vitro determination of the relative biological effectiveness of carbon ion beam irradiation in cells derived from human normal lung tissues. *Int J Radiat Oncol Biol Phys* (2014) 90:S787. doi:10.1016/j.ijrobp.2014.05.2275

37. Quarmby S, Kumar P, Kumar S. Radiation-induced normal tissue injury: role of adhesion molecules in leukocyte-endothelial cell interactions. *Int J Cancer* (1999) 82:385–95. doi:10.1002/(SICI)1097-0215(19990730)82:3<385:AID-IJC12>3.0.CO;2-5

38. Mollà M, Gironella M, Miquel R, Tovar V, Engel P, Biete A, et al. Relative roles of ICAM-1 and VCAM-1 in the pathogenesis of experimental radiation-induced intestinal inflammation. *Int J Radiat Oncol Biol Phys* (2003) 57:264–73. doi:10.1016/S0360-3016(03)00523-6

39. Kiyohara H, Ishizaki Y, Suzuki Y, Katoh H, Hamada N, Ohno T, et al. Radiation-induced ICAM-1 expression via TGF-β1 pathway on human umbilical vein endothelial cells; comparison between X-ray and carbon-ion beam irradiation. *J Radiat Res* (2011) 52:287–92. doi:10.1269/jrr.10061

40. Fujita M, Otsuka Y, Yamada S, Iwakawa M, Imai T. X-ray irradiation and Rho-kinase inhibitor additively induce invasiveness of the cells of the pancreatic cancer line, MIAPaCa-2, which exhibits mesenchymal and amoeboid motility. *Cancer Sci* (2011) 102:792–8. doi:10.1111/j.1349-7006.2011.01852.x

41. Zhai GG, Malhotra R, Delaney M, Latham D, Nestler U, Zhang M, et al. Radiation enhances the invasive potential of primary glioblastoma cells via activation of the Rho signaling pathway. *J Neurooncol* (2006) 76:227–37. doi:10.1007/s11060-005-6499-4

42. Murata K, Noda SE, Oike T, Takahashi A, Yoshida Y, Suzuki Y, et al. Increase in cell motility by carbon ion irradiation via the Rho signaling pathway and its inhibition by the ROCK inhibitor Y-27632 in lung adenocarcinoma A549 cells. *J Radiat Res* (2014) 55:658–64. doi:10.1093/jrr/rru002

43. Prise KM, O'Sullivan JM. Radiation-induced bystander signalling in cancer therapy. *Nat Rev Cancer* (2009) 9:351–60. doi:10.1038/nrc2603

44. Harada K, Nonaka T, Hamada N, Sakurai H, Hasegawa M, Funayama T, et al. Heavy-ion-induced bystander killing of human lung cancer cells: role of gap junctional intercellular communication. *Cancer Sci* (2009) 100:684–8. doi:10.1111/j.1349-7006.2009.01093.x

45. Wakatsuki M, Magpayo N, Kawamura H, Held KD. Differential bystander signaling between radioresistant chondrosarcoma cells and fibroblasts after

x-ray, proton, iron ion and carbon ion exposures. *Int J Radiat Oncol Biol Phys* (2012) 84:e103–8. doi:10.1016/j.ijrobp.2012.02.052

46. Thariat J, Hannoun-Levi JM, Sun Myint A, Vuong T, Gérard JP. Past, present, and future of radiotherapy for the benefit of patients. *Nat Rev Clin Oncol* (2013) 10:52–60. doi:10.1038/nrclinonc.2012.203

47. Nakano T, Suzuki M, Abe A, Suzuki Y, Morita S, Mizoe J, et al. The phase I&II clinical study of carbon ion therapy for cancer of the uterine cervix. *Cancer J Sci Am* (1999) 5:362–9.

48. Kubo N, Noda SE, Takahashi A, Yoshida Y, Oike T, Murata K, et al. Radiosensitizing effect of carboplatin and paclitaxel to carbon-ion beam irradiation in the non-small-cell lung cancer cell line H460. *J Radiat Res* (2015) 56:229–38. doi:10.1093/jrr/rru085

49. Ma H, Takahashi A, Sejimo Y, Adachi A, Kubo N, Isono M, et al. Targeting of carbon ion-induced G(2) checkpoint activation in lung cancer cells using Wee-1 inhibitor MK-1775. *Radiat Res* (2015) 184:660–9. doi:10.1667/RR14171.1

50. Musha A, Yoshida Y, Takahashi T, Ando K, Funayama T, Kobayashi Y, et al. Synergistic effect of heat shock protein 90 inhibitor, 17-allylamino-17-demethoxygeldanamycin and X-rays, but not carbon-ion beams, on lethality in human oral squamous cell carcinoma cells. *J Radiat Res* (2012) 53:545–50. doi:10.1093/jrr/rrs012

51. Schulte TW, Blagosklonny MV, Ingui C, Neckers L. Disruption of the Raf-1-Hsp90 molecular complex results in destabilization of Raf-1 and loss of Raf-1-Ras association. *J Biol Chem* (1995) 270:24585–8. doi:10.1074/jbc.270.41.24585

52. Sato S, Fujita N, Tsuruo T. Modulation of Akt kinase activity by binding to Hsp90. *Proc Natl Acad Sci U S A* (2000) 97:10832–7. doi:10.1073/pnas.170276797

53. Peng X, Guo X, Borkan SC, Bharti A, Kuramochi Y, Calderwood S, et al. Heat shock protein 90 stabilization of ErbB2 expression is disrupted by ATP depletion in myocytes. *J Biol Chem* (2005) 280:13148–52. doi:10.1074/jbc.M410838200

54. De Witt Hamer PC, Mir SE, Noske D, Van Noorden CJ, Wurdinger T. WEE1 kinase targeting combined with DNA-damaging cancer therapy catalyzes mitotic catastrophe. *Clin Cancer Res* (2011) 17:4200–7. doi:10.1158/1078-0432.CCR-10-2537

55. Tatokoro M, Koga F, Yoshida S, Kihara K. Heat shock protein 90 targeting therapy: state of the art and future perspective. *EXCLI J* (2015) 14:48–58. doi:10.17179/excli2015-586

56. Robert C, Long GV, Brady B, Dutriaux C, Maio M, Mortier L, et al. Nivolumab in previously untreated melanoma without BRAF mutation. *N Engl J Med* (2015) 372:320–30. doi:10.1056/NEJMoa1412082

57. Powles T, Eder JP, Fine GD, Braiteh FS, Loriot Y, Cruz C, et al. MPDL3280A (anti-PD-L1) treatment leads to clinical activity in metastatic bladder cancer. *Nature* (2014) 515:558–62. doi:10.1038/nature13904

58. Hodi FS, O'Day SJ, McDermott DF, Weber RW, Sosman JA, Haanen JB, et al. Improved survival with ipilimumab in patients with metastatic melanoma. *N Engl J Med* (2010) 363:711–23. doi:10.1056/NEJMoa1003466

59. Nakano T, Oka K, Takahashi K, Morita S, Arai T. Roles of Langerhans cells and T-lymphocytes infiltrating cancer tissues in patients treated by radiation therapy for cervical cancer. *Cancer* (1992) 70:2839–44. doi:10.1002/1097-0142(19921215)70:12<2839:AID-CNCR2820701220>3.0.CO;2-7

60. Nakano T, Oka K, Hanba K, Morita S. Intratumoral administration of sizofiran activates Langerhans cell and T-cell infiltration in cervical cancer. *Clin Immunol Immunopathol* (1996) 79:79–86. doi:10.1006/clin.1996.0053

61. Suzuki Y, Mimura K, Yoshimoto Y, Watanabe M, Ohkubo Y, Izawa S, et al. Immunogenic tumor cell death induced by chemoradiotherapy in patients with esophageal squamous cell carcinoma. *Cancer Res* (2012) 72:3967–76. doi:10.1158/0008-5472.CAN-12-0851

62. Yoshimoto Y, Oike T, Okonogi N, Suzuki Y, Ando K, Sato H, et al. Carbon-ion beams induce production of an immune mediator protein, high mobility group box 1, at levels comparable with X-ray irradiation. *J Radiat Res* (2015) 56:509–14. doi:10.1093/jrr/rrv007

63. Friedman AA, Letai A, Fisher DE, Flaherty KT. Precision medicine for cancer with next-generation functional diagnostics. *Nat Rev Cancer* (2015) 15:747–56. doi:10.1038/nrc4015

64. Okayama H, Schetter AJ, Ishigame T, Robles AI, Kohno T, Yokota J, et al. The expression of four genes as a prognostic classifier for stage I lung

adenocarcinoma in 12 independent cohorts. *Cancer Epidemiol Biomarkers Prev* (2014) 23:2884–94. doi:10.1158/1055-9965.EPI-14-0182

65. Wikoff WR, Hanash S, DeFelice B, Miyamoto S, Barnett M, Zhao Y, et al. Diacetylspermine is a novel prediagnostic serum biomarker for non-small-cell lung cancer and has additive performance with pro-surfactant protein B. *J Clin Oncol* (2015) 33:3880–6. doi:10.1200/JCO.2015.61.7779

66. Mathé EA, Patterson AD, Haznadar M, Manna SK, Krausz KW, Bowman, et al. Noninvasive urinary metabolomic profiling identifies diagnostic and prognostic markers in lung cancer. *Cancer Res* (2014) 74:3259–70. doi:10.1158/0008-5472.CAN-14-0109

67. Roadmap Epigenomics Consortium, Kundaje A, Meuleman W, Ernst J, Bilenky M, Yen A, et al. Integrative analysis of 111 reference human epigenomes. *Nature* (2015) 518:317–30. doi:10.1038/nature14248

68. Tamaki T, Iwakawa M, Ohno T, Imadome K, Nakawatari M, Sakai M, et al. Application of carbon-ion beams or gamma-rays on primary tumors does not change the expression profiles of metastatic tumors in an in vivo murine model. *Int J Radiat Oncol Biol Phys* (2009) 74:210–8. doi:10.1016/j.ijrobp.2008.12.078

69. Nakano T, Oka K. Differential values of Ki-67 index and mitotic index of proliferating cell population: an assessment of cell cycle and prognosis in radiation therapy for cervical cancer. *Cancer* (1993) 72:2401–8.

doi:10.1002/1097-0142(19931015)72:8<2401:AID-CNCR2820720818>3.0.CO;2-D

70. Britton S, Coates J, Jackson SP. A new method for high-resolution imaging of Ku foci to decipher mechanisms of DNA double-strand break repair. *J Cell Biol* (2013) 202:579–95. doi:10.1083/jcb.201303073

71. Matsuo M, Matsumoto S, Mitchell JB, Krishna MC, Camphausen K. Magnetic resonance imaging of the tumor microenvironment in radiotherapy: perfusion, hypoxia, and metabolism. *Semin Radiat Oncol* (2014) 24:210–7. doi:10.1016/j.semradonc.2014.02.002

8

Efficient Rejoining of DNA Double-Strand Breaks Despite Increased Cell-Killing Effectiveness Following Spread-Out Bragg Peak Carbon-Ion Irradiation

Nicole B. Averbeck[1]*, Jana Topsch[1†], Michael Scholz[1], Wilma Kraft-Weyrather[1], Marco Durante[1,2] and Gisela Taucher-Scholz[1,2]

[1] Department of Biophysics, GSI Helmholtzzentrum für Schwerionenforschung GmbH, Darmstadt, Germany, [2] Technische Universität Darmstadt, Darmstadt, Germany

*Correspondence:
Nicole B. Averbeck
n.averbeck@gsi.de

Radiotherapy of solid tumors with charged particles holds several advantages in comparison to photon therapy; among them conformal dose distribution in the tumor, improved sparing of tumor-surrounding healthy tissue, and an increased relative biological effectiveness (RBE) in the tumor target volume in the case of ions heavier than protons. A crucial factor of the biological effects is DNA damage, of which DNA double-strand breaks (DSBs) are the most deleterious. The reparability of these lesions determines the cell survival after irradiation and thus the RBE. Interestingly, using phosphorylated H2AX as a DSB marker, our data in human fibroblasts revealed that after therapy-relevant spread-out Bragg peak irradiation with carbon ions DSBs are very efficiently rejoined, despite an increased RBE for cell survival. This suggests that misrepair plays an important role in the increased RBE of heavy-ion radiation. Possible sources of erroneous repair will be discussed.

Keywords: heavy ions, carbon-ion radiotherapy, DSB complexity, DSB repair, error-prone DNA repair, RBE

INTRODUCTION

Radiotherapy is an indispensable tool for treating solid tumors (1). Advances in conventional radiation therapy with photons and especially new approaches using charged particles have led to an improved physical delivery of dose in radiation therapy (2–4). Irradiation with accelerated ions heavier than protons, namely carbon ions, has additional advantage as it is characterized by an increased relative biological effectiveness (RBE) in the targeted tumor volume (4). This allows the irradiation of deep-seated tumors, minimizing at the same time the dose to normal tissue or in organs at risk (2). Accelerated ions of a linear energy transfer (LET) of >10 keV/µm are considered high-LET radiation. Due to their characteristic energy deposition within a confined volume, they cause DNA damage of greater complexity (5–7). A special feature of this densely ionizing radiation is the induction of clustered lesions – two or more DNA lesions within one or two helix turns (8) – comprising double-strand breaks (DSBs) in close proximity that are more difficult to repair (9, 10). An additional level of complexity arises due to the localized microscopic energy deposition occurring along the particle track when traversing nuclear chromatin. At different size scales, from the nucleosome to chromatin fiber loops, the induction of spatially correlated DSBs within chromatin subunits can increase the severity of the induced lesions (11, 12), resulting in a decreased probability of DSB repair (13). Damage clustering at different levels is thus a crucial factor for the enhanced biological effects of radiotherapeutical heavy-ion irradiation and was shown earlier (14, 15).

Several studies have analyzed the repair capacity of heavy ion radiation-induced DSBs with different kinds of methods (13, 16–20). All studies revealed that with increasing LET repair slows down and the number of DSBs remaining unrepaired increases. Furthermore, chromosome studies applying premature chromosome condensation (PCC) on cells exposed to radiation of different LET agree with these data; with increasing LET, the fraction of excess PCC fragments increases and correspondingly the unrejoined breaks (21–25). In addition, high-LET radiation is also more effective in inducing mutations and chromosome aberrations, especially of the complex type, i.e., involving at least two or more chromosomes, which indicates misrepair of DSBs (26–30). Likely sources for misrepair are the close proximity of the breaks, which could facilitate the ligation of wrong break ends and the choice of the DSB-repair pathway (7, 31). The latter is supported by our findings that repair of carbon ion-induced DSBs is dependent on resection (32), a process that clearly influences the repair pathway choice (33). Thus, the increased RBE of high-LET radiation is presumably based on an increased number of unrejoined and misrepaired DSBs.

In carbon-ion radiotherapy the target volume is typically irradiated with ions from opposing fields. Beams with different ion energies are superimposed, resulting in a spread-out Bragg peak (SOBP) with the desired homogeneous distribution of dose (4). Consequently, the cells within the SOBP are exposed to a wide spectrum of carbon ions with different individual energies and LET. Due to this mixed radiation field, DNA damage of different complexity is expected to occur, from rather simple lesions induced by high-energy ions to very complex damage induced by low-energy ions. The DNA damage of different quality will likely influence the efficiency of cell killing and thus the RBE.

Earlier survival studies have shown that the RBE depends on the capacity to repair the induced DNA damage (14, 15). These and most of the above mentioned research, which revealed an increased number of unrejoined DSBs in repair studies and misrepaired DSBs in cytogenetic analyses, was performed using mainly monoenergetic ions or hamster cells (13, 16–20, 26–29). Aimed at a better understanding of the relationship between DSB repair and the RBE of therapeutic carbon-ion irradiation, we examined the effect of radiation quality on the survival of human fibroblasts and DSB repair.

RESULTS

Within this study, we used normal human fibroblasts to first examine the systematics of survival depending on the changing radiation quality along the penetration path of carbon ions. Furthermore, we compared the repair of DSBs after exposure to the different radiation qualities in the carbon-ion entrance channel (EC) and SOBP, where the target tumor volume would

be seated. The confluent fibroblast cells analyzed in this study preclude the interference of cell cycle changes and are thus especially suitable for reliable repair measurements using phosphorylated H2AX (γH2AX) as a marker for DSBs (34).

Cell Survival in Dependence of the Penetration Depth of Carbon Ions

To study cell survival along the carbon-ion EC and SOBP, we applied an experimental setup that allows irradiating cells at different positions within a polyacrylic tank previously described (35) (**Figure 1A**). Following the one-field irradiation with a 4-cm SOBP of carbon ions in a water-equivalent depth of 6–10 cm, the survival data obtained for confluent, human fibroblasts show the expected depth profile with higher survival levels in the EC and a decline of cell survival in the target SOBP region, yielding a region with clearly reduced cell survival compared to the EC (**Figure 1C**). The increase of the RBE with penetration depth – represented by the ratio of the two depth-dose curves in **Figure 1B** – becomes obvious from the fact that despite the reduction of absorbed dose toward the distal end of the SOBP the biological effect still increases, i.e., the survival drops within the SOBP. The RBE reaches a value of 2.3 at the distal edge, whereas in the EC, it is approximately 1.1.

These data have been also used to validate the local effect model (LEM) that has been developed for biological optimization in treatment planning (35). Very good agreement is found between the model prediction and the experimental data both in the EC and in the target region.

Repair Kinetics of DSBs Induced in the Carbon-Ion EC and SOBP

Aimed at mimicking a therapy-like configuration, we studied the DSB-repair capacity of confluent (G0/G1-phase) human fibroblasts upon a two-field SOBP carbon-ion irradiation. The irradiation from two opposing sides, typical for patient treatment, has the advantage of compensating for the variations in LET and RBE gradients observed in **Figure 1**. The applied physical dose within the SOBP was 2 Gy according to a typical therapeutic fraction; the corresponding EC dose was 0.6 Gy. We adapted the previously described experimental setup (**Figure 1A**) placing cells grown on coverslips (to allow DSB microscopy analysis; see below) at positions equivalent to those in the EC and the SOBP (**Figure 2A**). The irradiation geometry was verified by the measured clonogenic cell survival. The experimental data showing clearly lower survival in the SOBP compared to the EC (**Figure 2B**, circles) agree very well with the calculated survival from the LEM (**Figure 2B**, line). In this case, it has been taken into account that cells growing on glass typically show a higher sensitivity as compared to cells grown on plastic material (36). Subsequently, this setup was used to measure the repair of DSBs induced in the EC and SOBP. We first directly compared the repair of DSBs induced by 0.6 Gy carbon ions in the EC with that after the same dose of X-rays (**Figure 3A**) using immunofluorescence microscopy to detect the DSB marker γH2AX (34). This method had proven most appropriate at the dose applied here and represents a suitable DSB-repair assay in G0/G1-phase cells

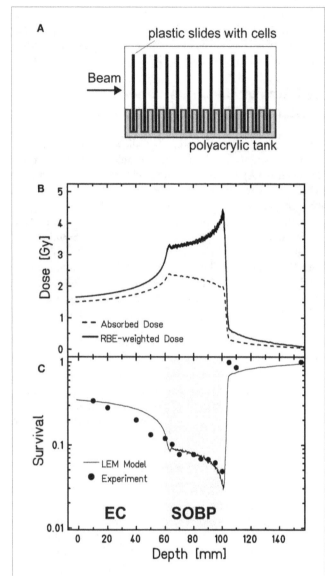

FIGURE 1 | Survival of human fibroblasts upon a one-field carbon-ion irradiation along the beam penetration path. **(A)** Experimental setup for a one-field irradiation. Confluent, human fibroblasts (AG1522D) grown on slides were placed perpendicular to the beam direction in a medium filled tank at different positions from the beam entrance side, as described earlier (35). The irradiation at the heavy-ion synchrotron (SIS), GSI Darmstadt, was done with a 4-cm SOBP in a water-equivalent depth of 6–10 cm (LET: 45 keV/μm at the proximal edge, 150 keV/μm at the distal edge). **(B)** Depth-dose distribution of the absorbed dose (dashed line) and the RBE-weighted dose (LEM calculated; solid line) of the carbon ions. **(C)** Measured (circles; $n = 1$) and calculated (line; LEM) clonogenic cell survival of human fibroblasts along the beam axes.

SOBP, a significant fraction of γH2AX foci is still remaining 24 h post exposure (**Figure 3A**). These results emphasize the impact of radiation quality on DSB repair and show that repair of clustered DSBs is impaired, which is in line with earlier findings (18–20, 37). It should be noted, however, that despite irradiation with the beam almost parallel to the cell monolayer enabling improved foci counting along the ion tracks, γH2AX foci induced by these densely ionizing ions may not represent individual DSBs (38–41).

We next applied the two-field carbon-ion irradiation to measure the repair of DSBs induced in the center of an SOBP at a dose of 2 Gy. In order to avoid inconsistencies in foci counting due to overlapping foci at the higher dose and LET (41, 44, 45), flow cytometry was used to quantify the global γH2AX signal. This method is suggested to give an enhanced resolution in measuring DSB damage induced by high-LET high-energy ion irradiation compared to γH2AX-foci counting (20, 46). The γH2AX signal was measured up to 65 h post exposure and the DSB-repair data for irradiation in the SOBP are compared with the corresponding γH2AX values obtained after exposure of the cells to the same dose (2 Gy) of ions in the EC (**Figure 3B**). As expected, DSBs induced within the EC are mostly repaired within 12 h, similar to the result obtained by the γH2AX-foci assay upon irradiation with 0.6 Gy. Interestingly, also the cells placed in the SOBP region repaired the carbon ion-induced DSBs very efficiently to the same extent as in the EC. Although the decay of the γH2AX signal appeared to be slightly slower up to 24 h post SOBP irradiation, it declined similar to the EC almost to control values within 48 h.

DISCUSSION

Here, we aimed at clarifying the relationship between DSB repair and RBE of therapeutic carbon-ion irradiation. We confirmed that the repair capacity represents an important factor in this relationship, and our data further suggest that the quality of the repair also affects the RBE.

Efficiency of Cell Killing and DSB Rejoining along the Penetration Path of Carbon Ions

The survival data of the G0/G1-phase human fibroblasts and the calculated RBE in the EC and the SOBP demonstrate that the RBE is highest in the SOBP. This is in accordance with data obtained with hamster cells in a similar setup (35). Interestingly, the smallest survival and highest RBE are observed within the SOBP where the ion energy is smallest, at the very distal edge. Our repair data on ion irradiation of this quality, i.e., high LET, low-energy carbon ions (9.9 keV/u on target) in **Figure 3A**, show impaired repair of DSBs. Thus, the decreased survival at the distal edge of a one-field SOBP irradiation corresponds well with the decreased repair capacity we observed for low-energy ions and as it was seen earlier (16, 19). The notion that the decreased DSB-repair capacity is responsible for the decreased survival upon low-energy carbon-ion irradiation is further supported by earlier data on survival of confluent, human fibroblasts upon fractionated and non-fractionated irradiation with low-energy carbon ions (11 MeV/u, 153.5 keV/μm); fractionating the dose with

(34). The repair of DSBs for both types of irradiation was similar and mostly completed within 12 h, as determined by γH2AX-foci loss. This agrees well with earlier findings on DSB rejoining along the irradiation axis of therapy-relevant carbon ions or X-rays (16). By contrast, following irradiation with a comparable dose (0.8 Gy) of high LET (168 keV/μm), low-energy (9.9 MeV/u on target) carbon ions, which correspond to stopping ions in the

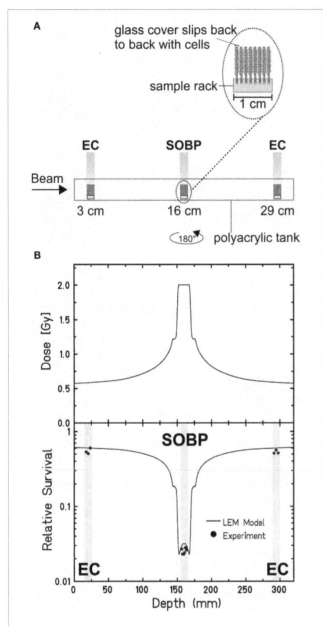

FIGURE 2 | Verification of the experimental setup to mimic therapy-like carbon-ion irradiation. (A) Experimental setup for a two-field irradiation. Confluent, human fibroblasts (AG1522D) were exposed at different positions from the beam entrance side within a medium filled tank. At the SIS, GSI Darmstadt, the two-field configuration typical for patient irradiation was simulated by irradiating the tank from both sides with a horizontal turn of 180°. The irradiation was done with an SOBP of 2.4 cm at a water-equivalent depth of 16 cm. The dose in the SOBP was 2 Gy (dose-averaged LET: 70–85 keV/μm). Samples in the EC region were irradiated with a corresponding dose of 0.6 Gy (dose-averaged LET: 13 keV/μm). **(B)** Top: distribution of the absorbed dose upon two-sided therapy-like irradiation. Bottom: corresponding calculated (line; LEM) and measured (circles; $n = 1$) cell survival. The gray boxes indicate the position of the samples during irradiation.

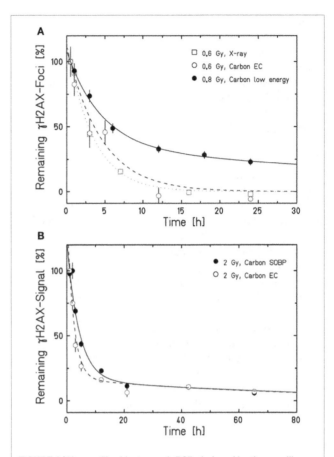

FIGURE 3 | Human fibroblasts repair DSBs induced by therapy-like carbon-ion irradiation. DSB-repair kinetics of confluent (G0/G1-phase) human AG1522 fibroblasts was measured after exposure to different radiation qualities. The average γH2AX-foci number **(A)** or γH2AX signal **(B)** of mock irradiated cells was subtracted from all data measured after irradiation. The curves are a guide to the eye obtained by exponential fits after normalization to the initial or extrapolated γH2AX values at 30 min **(A)** or 1 h **(B)** post irradiation. Data points represent the average of 2–4 experiments ± SEM [exception: low-energy carbon-ion irradiation in **(A)**; $n = 1$ ± SEM foci number/nucleus, at least 100 cells were analyzed]. **(A)** Kinetics after irradiation with 0.6 Gy X-rays, 0.6 Gy carbon ions in the EC (for irradiation conditions see **Figure 2A**), or 0.8 Gy low-energy carbon ions almost parallel to the cell monolayer (9.9 MeV/u on target; 168 keV/μm). DSBs were revealed by a γH2AX-foci analysis after γH2AX immunostaining performed as described in Meyer et al. (42). **(B)** Comparison of the DSB-repair capacity in human fibroblasts after 2 Gy carbon-ion irradiation in the EC or SOBP (for irradiation conditions see **Figure 2A**). The global immunofluorescent γH2AX signal was analyzed by flow cytometry according to Tommasino et al. (43).

The survival data and repair kinetics of cells irradiated within the EC (**Figures 2** and **3**) show that the cells can cope well with this irradiation. DSB rejoining is complete and its kinetics comparable to the rejoining kinetics of X-ray-induced DSBs (**Figure 3A**). This suggests that the repair is successful and hence ensures survival. This conclusion is supported by earlier work with the same cell system. This work revealed an RBE_{10} of 1.2 ± 0.3 for high-energy carbon ions (266 keV/u; 13.7 keV/μm) (14), which are in the range of carbon ions within the EC in the here presented experiment. In addition, Wang et al. showed clearly increased survival for both radiation qualities upon fractionated irradiation, which

a 24 h interval between fractions did not improve the survival indicating that the capacity to repair the induced DNA damage is very low (14).

further corroborates that DNA damage in the EC can be effectively repaired (14).

Our data in **Figure 2** revealed that the survival within the SOBP is smallest, yet DSBs induced within this region are repaired only slightly slower than DSBs induced within the EC (**Figure 3B**). This result is most likely based on the mixed energy and LET of the ions within this region. The fraction of low-energy ions is small, and this is mirrored in the repair capacity. Similar results were obtained with one-field SOBP–carbon-ion irradiation (50 keV/μm dose-averaged LET) of non-synchronized hamster cells (47). Nonetheless, although the DSBs induced in the SOBP are repaired the RBE of therapy-relevant carbon-ion irradiation is increased [see above and Ref. (48)]. This leads to the assumption that misrepair plays a non-negligible role in the increased RBE. The proximity of the DSBs within clusters may enhance the probability of misrejoining. In addition, the pathway choice has an important impact on the accuracy of the DNA repair, and hence, will be discussed in greater detail. **Figure 4** summarizes known and proposed repair activities at complex, ion-induced DSBs.

Repair Pathways of Complex DSBs

The observation that DSBs induced in G0/G1-phase human fibroblasts within the SOBP are repaired slightly slower than DSBs induced within the EC (**Figure 3B**) suggests that DNA-repair pathways involving different types of end processing might be used. This is supported by earlier findings showing that with increasing LET an increasing number of resected DSBs is found.

This occurs independent of the cell cycle phase (32, 49, 50) and is important for DSB repair (32). Notably, DSB repair involving resected ends represents a potential source of erroneous repair (33). The observed resection is dependent on MRE11, CtIP, and EXO1 (32, 49, 50). In addition, break-end processing by Artemis may take also place as this nuclease was shown to be important for the survival upon ion irradiation (9, 51) and was suggested to be involved in the repair of α particle-induced DSBs (52).

Which pathways repair DSBs induced by therapy-relevant carbon ions is still under investigation. Based on data on X-ray and carbon-ion irradiated human G2-phase cells, it was proposed that classical non-homologous end joining (c-NHEJ) will make an initial attempt to repair the DSBs (37, 53). This hypothesis is supported by data on proliferating hamster cells irradiated with SOBP–carbon ions, which show that c-NHEJ is vital to repair the induced DSBs (47). The choice of this pathway is supported by the findings that the repair of high-LET iron-ion (150 keV/μm) and α-particle (130 ± 10 keV/μm)-induced DSBs require DNA-PKcs, an important component of c-NHEJ (54). In addition, recruitment of GFP-tagged Ku80, a further important component of c-NHEJ, to DSBs induced by single gold ions was observed in living murine cells (55). If due to DNA fragmentation generated by ion irradiation the Ku complex cannot form fast enough (56), c-NHEJ may fail to proceed quickly. Then, resection of ion-induced DSBs by MRE11, CtIP, and EXO1 and break-end processing by Artemis may occur (32, 49, 50, 57). It is conceivable that Artemis in its function as endonuclease trims the resected

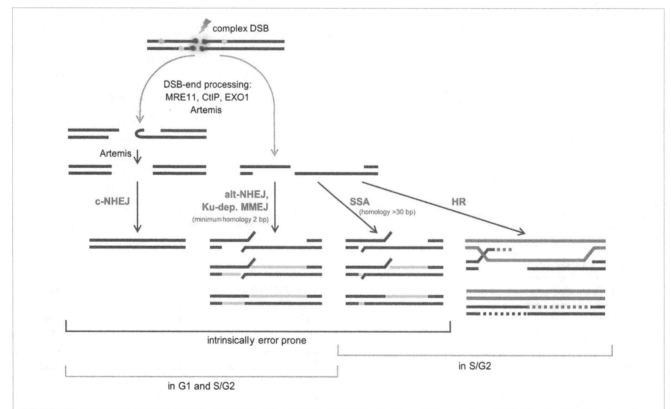

FIGURE 4 | Scheme of the repair of complex, carbon ion-induced DSBs. DSBs that cannot be rapidly repaired by c-NHEJ will undergo break-end resection by MRE11, CtIP, EXO1, and break-end processing by Artemis. Blue arrow: resected DSBs can be repaired by alt-NHEJ, a potentially Ku-dependent MMEJ, SSA, or HR. The latter two pathways operate in S- and G2-phase only. Green arrow: Artemis may make resected DSB ends available for c-NHEJ.

DSB ends – either by opening hairpins that form from single-stranded stretches or by trimming off single-stranded areas (58, 59) – to make the break ends available for the c-NHEJ repair machinery (45, 52). DSBs with single-stranded overhangs will be channeled into homology-mediated repair. In G2-phase cells, this might be single strand annealing (SSA), but it mainly represents homologous recombination (HR) as was shown upon irradiation with carbon or iron ions (37, 47, 60). The fate of resected DSBs in G1-phase cells is mainly unknown. They are not repaired by HR (32, 60). c-NHEJ factors are discussed to be involved in a repair option involving a Ku-dependent microhomology-mediated end joining (MMEJ) pathway in G1-phase cells (45, 61). However, c-NHEJ itself is considered to be unable to repair DSB break ends with long single-stranded overhangs (33). Ku- and LIG4-independent alternative (alt)-NHEJ represents a further repair choice for G1-phase DSBs with long single-stranded overhangs (62, 63), since it frequently involves CtIP- and MRE11-dependent break resection and microhomologies for ligation (64–69). Although it was described to operate only if Ku is absent (70, 71), it was proposed to operate in repair proficient cells if c-NHEJ fails locally (7). The choice of microhomology-mediated pathways is supported by the fact that ion-induced, rejoined DSBs are often characterized by deletions and flanking microhomologies (72). It should be noted that besides HR all repair pathways using processed break ends are inherently erroneous.

An increased use of error-prone repair and the close proximity of the breaks, which could facilitate the ligation of wrong break ends, represent likely reasons for the increased mutation and chromosome-aberration rate seen in cells treated with high-LET radiation (72). Considering our here presented data, we propose that misrepair and thus mutations and aberrations play a non-negligible role in the increased RBE for cell killing of therapy-relevant carbon radiation.

MATERIALS AND METHODS

Cells, Cell Culture, and Survival Assay
Normal human foreskin fibroblasts AG1522 (Coriell Cell Repository, Camden, NJ, USA; passage 11–15) were cultured in EMEM with EBSS salts, 15% FCS, 2 mM L-glutamine, and 1% penicillin/streptomycin at 37°C, 5% CO_2. To obtain confluent cultures enriched in G1 cells, 10^4 cells/cm^2 were seeded and used for experiments 10 days later. For the survival assays, the clonogenic survival was determined, as described earlier (14). For the survival data in **Figure 1**, cells were cultivated on polystyrene slides (35). For the repair kinetics and the associated survival data, cells were cultivated on glass cover slips (ø 30 mm or 24 mm × 24 mm).

Irradiation
Cells were irradiated with X-rays (250 keV, 16 mA; X-ray tube IV320-13, Seifert, Germany) or carbon ions at the GSI Helmholtz Center for Heavy Ion Research (Darmstadt, Germany). Irradiations with low-energy carbon ions were performed at the UNILAC beam line (11.4 MeV/u primary energy, 9.9 MeV/u on target, LET 168 keV/µm) and with high-energy carbon ions at the heavy-ion synchrotron (SIS) using active energy variation and raster scanning (48). Since the selection of ions available is limited

some data are from single experiments only. For the survival data in **Figure 1**, cells were irradiated in a medium filled polyacrylic tank (35) (**Figure 1A**). The one-field carbon-ion irradiation was done with a 4-cm SOBP in a water-equivalent depth of 6–10 cm (LET: 45 keV/µm at the proximal edge, 150 keV/µm at the distal edge). For the repair kinetics and corresponding survival data, cells were exposed at different positions within a medium filled polyacrylic tank (**Figure 2A**). Cells seeded on glass cover slips were positioned approximately 3, 16, and 29 cm from the beam entrance side. To simulate the two-field configuration typical for patient irradiation, the tank was first irradiated from one side and after turning it horizontally by 180°, it was irradiated from the other side with the same dose distribution. An SOBP with a width of 2.4 cm at a water-equivalent depth of 16 cm was applied. The dose in the SOBP was 2 Gy and the dose-averaged LET values were about 70 and 85 keV/µm in the center and at the edges of the SOBP, respectively. Samples for SOBP irradiation were placed in the middle of the SOPB to minimize the influence of variations in positioning. Samples in the EC region were irradiated at a depth of a few millimeter, corresponding to a dose-averaged LET of 13 keV/µm and a dose of 0.6 Gy.

Model Calculations
Model calculations were performed using the LEM, as described by Elsässer et al. (35). The model allows predicting the effects of ion radiation based on the localized, microscopic energy deposition pattern of particle tracks in combination with the knowledge of the photon dose–response curve for the endpoint under consideration. The corresponding parameters of the photon cell survival curve were $\alpha = 0.54$ Gy^{-1}, $\beta = 0.062$ Gy^{-2}, and $D_t = 13.5$ Gy, where D_t characterizes the transition from a curvilinear shape at low and intermediate doses to a linear shape at high doses [for details see, e.g., Ref. (73)]. The dose–response of AG1522D cells on glass cover slips was estimated by scaling the dose values by a factor of 1.3 according to the information given in Furre et al. (36).

Immunostaining
For the γH2AX-foci analyses, DSBs were visualized by γH2AX immunostaining performed, as described in Meyer et al. (42). The global immunofluorescent γH2AX signal was analyzed by flow cytometry according to Tommasino et al. (43).

AUTHOR CONTRIBUTIONS
GTS designed research; WKW and JT performed research; NBA, WKW, MS, and JT analyzed data; and NBA, MD, MS, and GTS wrote the paper. All authors approved the work for publication.

ACKNOWLEDGMENTS

We thank M. Herrlitz and B. Meyer for irradiation and γH2AX-foci counting using X-rays and monoenergetic carbon ions, respectively, and Y. Schweinfurth for carbon-ion irradiation in the EC and γH2AX-foci analysis with Image-Pro Plus (Media Cybernetics, USA) as well as for the survival data in **Figure 2**. This project was partially funded by the German Federal Ministry of Education and Research (grant number 02NUK001A).

REFERENCES

1. Loeffler JS, Durante M. Charged particle therapy – optimization, challenges and future directions. *Nat Rev Clin Oncol* (2013) **10**(7):411–24. doi:10.1038/nrclinonc.2013.79

2. Durante M, Loeffler JS. Charged particles in radiation oncology. *Nat Rev Clin Oncol* (2010) **7**(1):37–43. doi:10.1038/nrclinonc.2009.183

3. Schulz-Ertner D, Tsujii H. Particle radiation therapy using proton and heavier ion beams. *J Clin Oncol* (2007) **25**(8):953–64. doi:10.1200/JCO.2006.09.7816

4. Schardt D, Elsässer T, Schulz-Ertner D. Heavy-ion tumor therapy: physical and radiobiological benefits. *Rev Mod Phys* (2010) **82**(1):383–425. doi:10.1103/RevModPhys.82.383

5. Kramer M, Kraft G. Track structure and DNA damage. *Adv Space Res* (1994) **14**(10):151–9. doi:10.1016/0273-1177(94)90465-0

6. Nikjoo H, O'Neill P, Wilson WE, Goodhead DT. Computational approach for determining the spectrum of DNA damage induced by ionizing radiation. *Radiat Res* (2001) **156**(5 Pt 2):577–83. doi:10.1667/0033-7587(2001)156[0577:CAFDTS]2.0.CO;2

7. Schipler Λ, Iliakis G. DNA double-strand-break complexity levels and their possible contributions to the probability for error-prone processing and repair pathway choice. *Nucleic Acids Res* (2013) **41**(16):7589–605. doi:10.1093/nar/gkt556

8. Sage E, Harrison L. Clustered DNA lesion repair in eukaryotes: relevance to mutagenesis and cell survival. *Mutat Res* (2011) **711**(1–2):123–33. doi:10.1016/j.mrfmmm.2010.12.010

9. Asaithamby A, Chen DJ. Mechanism of cluster DNA damage repair in response to high-atomic number and energy particles radiation. *Mutat Res* (2011) **711**(1–2):87–99. doi:10.1016/j.mrfmmm.2010.11.002

10. Lorat Y, Brunner CU, Schanz S, Jakob B, Taucher-Scholz G, Rube CE. Nanoscale analysis of clustered DNA damage after high-LET irradiation by quantitative electron microscopy – the heavy burden to repair. *DNA Repair (Amst)* (2015) **28**:93–106. doi:10.1016/j.dnarep.2015.01.007

11. Rydberg B. Radiation-induced DNA damage and chromatin structure. *Acta Oncol* (2001) **40**(6):682–5. doi:10.1080/02841860152619070

12. Friedrich T, Scholz U, Elsasser T, Durante M, Scholz M. Calculation of the biological effects of ion beams based on the microscopic spatial damage distribution pattern. *Int J Radiat Biol* (2012) **88**(1–2):103–7. doi:10.3109/09553002.2011.611213

13. Tommasino F, Friedrich T, Scholz U, Taucher-Scholz G, Durante M, Scholz M. A DNA double-strand break kinetic rejoining model based on the local effect model. *Radiat Res* (2013) **180**(5):524–38. doi:10.1667/RR13389.1

14. Wang J, Li R, Guo C, Fournier C, K-Weyrather W. The influence of fractionation on cell survival and premature differentiation after carbon ion irradiation. *J Radiat Res* (2008) **49**(4):391–8. doi:10.1269/jrr.08012

15. Weyrather WK, Ritter S, Scholz M, Kraft G. RBE for carbon track-segment irradiation in cell lines of differing repair capacity. *Int J Radiat Biol* (1999) **75**(11):1357–64. doi:10.1080/095530099139232

16. Heilmann J, Taucher-Scholz G, Haberer T, Scholz M, Kraft G. Measurement of intracellular DNA double-strand break induction and rejoining along the track of carbon and neon particle beams in water. *Int J Radiat Oncol Biol Phys* (1996) **34**(3):599–608. doi:10.1016/0360-3016(95)02112-4

17. Hoglund H, Stenerlow B. Induction and rejoining of DNA double-strand breaks in normal human skin fibroblasts after exposure to radiation of different linear energy transfer: possible roles of track structure and chromatin organization. *Radiat Res* (2001) **155**(6):818–25. doi:10.1667/0033-7587(2001)155[0818:IARODD]2.0.CO;2

18. Asaithamby A, Uematsu N, Chatterjee A, Story MD, Burma S, Chen DJ. Repair of HZE-particle-induced DNA double-strand breaks in normal human fibroblasts. *Radiat Res* (2008) **169**(4):437–46. doi:10.1667/RR1165.1

19. Schmid TE, Dollinger G, Beisker W, Hable V, Greubel C, Auer S, et al. Differences in the kinetics of gamma-H2AX fluorescence decay after exposure to low and high LET radiation. *Int J Radiat Biol* (2010) **86**(8):682–91. doi:10.3109/09553001003734543

20. Whalen MK, Gurai SK, Zahed-Kargaran H, Pluth JM. Specific ATM-mediated phosphorylation dependent on radiation quality. *Radiat Res* (2008) **170**(3):353–64. doi:10.1667/RR1354.1

21. Wu H, Furusawa Y, George K, Kawata T, Cucinotta FA. Analysis of unrejoined chromosomal breakage in human fibroblast cells exposed to low- and

high-LET radiation. *J Radiat Res* (2002) **43**(Suppl):S181–5. doi:10.1269/jrr.43.S181

22. Kawata T, Durante M, George K, Furusawa Y, Gotoh E, Takai N, et al. Kinetics of chromatid break repair in G2-human fibroblasts exposed to low- and high-LET radiations. *Phys Med* (2001) **17**(Suppl 1):226–8.

23. Kawata T, Durante M, Furusawa Y, George K, Ito H, Wu H, et al. Rejoining of isochromatid breaks induced by heavy ions in G2-phase normal human fibroblasts. *Radiat Res* (2001) **156**(5 Pt 2):598–602. doi:10.1667/0033-7587(2001)156[0598:ROIBIB]2.0.CO;2

24. Nasonova E, Ritter S. Cytogenetic effects of densely ionising radiation in human lymphocytes: impact of cell cycle delays. *Cytogenet Genome Res* (2004) **104**(1–4):216–20. doi:10.1159/000077492

25. Deperas-Standylo J, Lee R, Nasonova E, Ritter S, Gudowska-Nowak E. Production and distribution of aberrations in resting or cycling human lymphocytes following Fe-ion or Cr-ion irradiation: emphasis on single track effects. *Adv Space Res* (2012) **50**(5):584–97. doi:10.1016/j.asr.2012.05.007

26. Kawata T, Ito H, George K, Wu H, Cucinotta FA. Chromosome aberrations induced by high-LET radiations. *Biol Sci Space* (2004) **18**(4):216–23. doi:10.2187/bss.18.216

27. Durante M, Bedford JS, Chen DJ, Conrad S, Cornforth MN, Natarajan AT, et al. From DNA damage to chromosome aberrations: joining the break. *Mutat Res* (2013) **756**(1–2):5–13. doi:10.1016/j.mrgentox.2013.05.014

28. Hill MA. Fishing for radiation quality: chromosome aberrations and the role of radiation track structure. *Radiat Prot Dosimetry* (2015) **166**(1–4):295–301. doi:10.1093/rpd/ncv151

29. Yatagai F. Mutations induced by heavy charged particles. *Biol Sci Space* (2004) **18**(4):224–34. doi:10.2187/bss.18.224

30. Blakely EA, Kronenberg A. Heavy-ion radiobiology: new approaches to delineate mechanisms underlying enhanced biological effectiveness. *Radiat Res* (1998) **150**(5 Suppl):S126–45. doi:10.2307/3579815

31. Mladenov E, Iliakis G. Induction and repair of DNA double strand breaks: the increasing spectrum of non-homologous end joining pathways. *Mutat Res* (2011) **711**(1–2):61–72. doi:10.1016/j.mrfmmm.2011.02.005

32. Averbeck NB, Ringel O, Herrlitz M, Jakob B, Durante M, Taucher-Scholz G. DNA end resection is needed for the repair of complex lesions in G1-phase human cells. *Cell Cycle* (2014) **13**(16):2509–16. doi:10.4161/15384101.2015.941743

33. Grabarz A, Barascu A, Guirouilh-Barbat J, Lopez BS. Initiation of DNA double strand break repair: signaling and single-stranded resection dictate the choice between homologous recombination, non-homologous end-joining and alternative end-joining. *Am J Cancer Res* (2012) **2**(3):249–68.

34. Lobrich M, Shibata A, Beucher A, Fisher A, Ensminger M, Goodarzi AA, et al. gammaH2AX foci analysis for monitoring DNA double-strand break repair: strengths, limitations and optimization. *Cell Cycle* (2010) **9**(4):662–9. doi:10.4161/cc.9.4.10764

35. Elsässer T, Weyrather WK, Friedrich T, Durante M, Iancu G, Kramer M, et al. Quantification of the relative biological effectiveness for ion beam radiotherapy: direct experimental comparison of proton and carbon ion beams and a novel approach for treatment planning. *Int J Radiat Oncol Biol Phys* (2010) **78**(4):1177–83. doi:10.1016/j.ijrobp.2010.05.014

36. Furre T, Bergstrand ES, Pedersen E, Koritzinsky M, Olsen DR, Hole EO, et al. Measurement of dose rate at the interface of cell culture medium and glass dishes by means of ESR dosimetry using thin films of alanine. *Radiat Res* (1999) **152**(1):76–82. doi:10.2307/3580052

37. Shibata A, Conrad S, Birraux J, Geuting V, Barton O, Ismail A, et al. Factors determining DNA double-strand break repair pathway choice in G2 phase. *EMBO J* (2011) **30**(6):1079–92. doi:10.1038/emboj.2011.27

38. Antonelli F, Campa A, Esposito G, Giardullo P, Belli M, Dini V, et al. Induction and repair of DNA DSB as revealed by H2AX phosphorylation foci in human fibroblasts exposed to low- and high-LET radiation: relationship with early and delayed reproductive cell death. *Radiat Res* (2015) **183**(4):417–31. doi:10.1667/RR13855.1

39. Desai N, Davis E, O'Neill P, Durante M, Cucinotta FA, Wu H. Immunofluorescence detection of clustered gamma-H2AX foci induced by HZE-particle radiation. *Radiat Res* (2005) **164**(4 Pt 2):518–22. doi:10.1667/RR3431.1

40. Jakob B, Scholz M, Taucher-Scholz G. Biological imaging of heavy charged-particle tracks. *Radiat Res* (2003) **159**(5):676–84. doi:10.1667/0033-7587(2003)159[0676:BIOHCT]2.0.CO;2

41. Jakob B, Splinter J, Taucher-Scholz G. Positional stability of damaged chromatin domains along radiation tracks in mammalian cells. *Radiat Res* (2009) **171**(4):405–18. doi:10.1667/RR1520.1

42. Meyer B, Voss KO, Tobias F, Jakob B, Durante M, Taucher-Scholz G. Clustered DNA damage induces pan-nuclear H2AX phosphorylation mediated by ATM and DNA-PK. *Nucleic Acids Res* (2013) **41**(12):6109–18. doi:10.1093/nar/gkt304

43. Tommasino F, Friedrich T, Jakob B, Meyer B, Durante M, Scholz M. Induction and processing of the radiation-induced gamma-H2AX signal and its link to the underlying pattern of DSB: a combined experimental and modelling study. *PLoS One* (2015) **10**(6):e0129416. doi:10.1371/journal.pone.0129416

44. Costes SV, Chiolo I, Pluth JM, Barcellos-Hoff MH, Jakob B. Spatiotemporal characterization of ionizing radiation induced DNA damage foci and their relation to chromatin organization. *Mutat Res* (2010) **704**(1–3):78–87. doi:10.1016/j.mrrev.2009.12.006

45. Goodarzi AA, Jeggo PA. The repair and signaling responses to DNA double-strand breaks. *Adv Genet* (2013) **82**:1–45. doi:10.1016/B978-0-12-407676-1.00001-9

46. Sridharan DM, Chappell LJ, Whalen MK, Cucinotta FA, Pluth JM. Defining the biological effectiveness of components of high-LET track structure. *Radiat Res* (2015) **184**(1):105–19. doi:10.1667/RR13684.1

47. Gerelchuluun A, Manabe E, Ishikawa T, Sun L, Itoh K, Sakae T, et al. The major DNA repair pathway after both proton and carbon-ion radiation is NHEJ, but the HR pathway is more relevant in carbon ions. *Radiat Res* (2015) **183**(3):345–56. doi:10.1667/RR13904.1

48. Weyrather WK, Debus J. Particle beams for cancer therapy. *Clin Oncol* (2003) **15**(1):S23–8. doi:10.1053/clon.2002.0185

49. Barton O, Naumann SC, Diemer-Biehs R, Kunzel J, Steinlage M, Conrad S, et al. Polo-like kinase 3 regulates CtIP during DNA double-strand break repair in G1. *J Cell Biol* (2014) **206**(7):877–94. doi:10.1083/jcb.201401146

50. Yajima H, Fujisawa H, Nakajima NI, Hirakawa H, Jeggo PA, Okayasu R, et al. The complexity of DNA double strand breaks is a critical factor enhancing end-resection. *DNA Repair (Amst)* (2013) **12**(11):936–46. doi:10.1016/j.dnarep.2013.08.009

51. Sridharan DM, Whalen MK, Almendrala D, Cucinotta FA, Kawahara M, Yannone SM, et al. Increased Artemis levels confer radioresistance to both high and low LET radiation exposures. *Radiat Oncol* (2012) **7**:96. doi:10.1186/1748-717X-7-96

52. Riballo E, Kuhne M, Rief N, Doherty A, Smith GC, Recio MJ, et al. A pathway of double-strand break rejoining dependent upon ATM, Artemis, and proteins locating to gamma-H2AX foci. *Mol Cell* (2004) **16**(5):715–24. doi:10.1016/j.molcel.2004.10.029

53. Jeggo PA, Geuting V, Lobrich M. The role of homologous recombination in radiation-induced double-strand break repair. *Radiother Oncol* (2011) **101**(1):7–12. doi:10.1016/j.radonc.2011.06.019

54. Anderson JA, Harper JV, Cucinotta FA, O'Neill P. Participation of DNA-PKcs in DSB repair after exposure to high- and low-LET radiation. *Radiat Res* (2010) **174**(2):195–205. doi:10.1667/RR2071.1

55. Merk B, Voss KO, Müller I, Fischer BE, Jakob B, Taucher-Scholz G, et al. Photobleaching setup for the biological end-station of the darmstadt heavy-ion microprobe. *Nucl Instrum Methods Phys Res B* (2013) **306**(0):81–4. doi:10.1016/j.nimb.2012.11.043

56. Wang H, Wang X, Zhang P, Wang Y. The Ku-dependent non-homologous end-joining but not other repair pathway is inhibited by high linear energy transfer ionizing radiation. *DNA Repair (Amst)* (2008) **7**(5):725–33. doi:10.1016/j.dnarep.2008.01.010

57. Moscariello M, Wieloch R, Kurosawa A, Li F, Adachi N, Mladenov E, et al. Role for Artemis nuclease in the repair of radiation-induced DNA double strand breaks by alternative end joining. *DNA Repair (Amst)* (2015) **31**:29–40. doi:10.1016/j.dnarep.2015.04.004

58. Gu J, Li S, Zhang X, Wang LC, Niewolik D, Schwarz K, et al. DNA-PKcs regulates a single-stranded DNA endonuclease activity of Artemis. *DNA Repair (Amst)* (2010) **9**(4):429–37. doi:10.1016/j.dnarep.2010.01.001

59. Ma Y, Pannicke U, Schwarz K, Lieber MR. hairpin opening and overhang processing by an Artemis/DNA-dependent protein kinase complex in nonhomologous end joining and V(D)J recombination. *Cell* (2002) **108**(6):781–94. doi:10.1016/S0092-8674(02)00671-2

60. Zafar F, Seidler SB, Kronenberg A, Schild D, Wiese C. Homologous recombination contributes to the repair of DNA double-strand breaks induced by high-energy iron ions. *Radiat Res* (2010) **173**(1):27–39. doi:10.1667/RR1910.1

61. Katsura Y, Sasaki S, Sato M, Yamaoka K, Suzukawa K, Nagasawa T, et al. Involvement of Ku80 in microhomology-mediated end joining for DNA double-strand breaks in vivo. *DNA Repair (Amst)* (2007) **6**(5):639–48. doi:10.1016/j.dnarep.2006.12.002

62. Iliakis G. Backup pathways of NHEJ in cells of higher eukaryotes: cell cycle dependence. *Radiother Oncol* (2009) **92**(3):310–5. doi:10.1016/j.radonc.2009.06.024

63. Mansour WY, Rhein T, Dahm-Daphi J. The alternative end-joining pathway for repair of DNA double-strand breaks requires PARP1 but is not dependent upon microhomologies. *Nucleic Acids Res* (2010) **38**(18):6065–77. doi:10.1093/nar/gkq387

64. Rahal EA, Henricksen LA, Li Y, Williams RS, Tainer JA, Dixon K. ATM regulates Mre11-dependent DNA end-degradation and microhomology-mediated end joining. *Cell Cycle* (2010) **9**(14):2866–77. doi:10.4161/cc.9.14.12363

65. Rass E, Grabarz A, Plo I, Gautier J, Bertrand P, Lopez BS. Role of Mre11 in chromosomal nonhomologous end joining in mammalian cells. *Nat Struct Mol Biol* (2009) **16**(8):819–24. doi:10.1038/nsmb.1641

66. Xie A, Kwok A, Scully R. Role of mammalian Mre11 in classical and alternative nonhomologous end joining. *Nat Struct Mol Biol* (2009) **16**(8):814–8. doi:10.1038/nsmb.1640

67. Bennardo N, Cheng A, Huang N, Stark JM. Alternative-NHEJ is a mechanistically distinct pathway of mammalian chromosome break repair. *PLoS Genet* (2008) **4**(6):e1000110. doi:10.1371/journal.pgen.1000110

68. Zhang Y, Jasin M. An essential role for CtIP in chromosomal translocation formation through an alternative end-joining pathway. *Nat Struct Mol Biol* (2011) **18**(1):80–4. doi:10.1038/nsmb.1940

69. Truong LN, Li Y, Shi LZ, Hwang PY, He J, Wang H, et al. Microhomology-mediated end joining and homologous recombination share the initial end resection step to repair DNA double-strand breaks in mammalian cells. *Proc Natl Acad Sci U S A* (2013) **110**(19):7720–5. doi:10.1073/pnas.1213431110

70. Fattah F, Lee EH, Weisensel N, Wang Y, Lichter N, Hendrickson EA. Ku regulates the non-homologous end joining pathway choice of DNA double-strand break repair in human somatic cells. *PLoS Genet* (2010) **6**(2):e1000855. doi:10.1371/journal.pgen.1000855

71. Wang M, Wu W, Rosidi B, Zhang L, Wang H, Iliakis G. PARP-1 and Ku compete for repair of DNA double strand breaks by distinct NHEJ pathways. *Nucleic Acids Res* (2006) **34**(21):6170–82. doi:10.1093/nar/gkl840

72. Singleton BK, Griffin CS, Thacker J. Clustered DNA damage leads to complex genetic changes in irradiated human cells. *Cancer Res* (2002) **62**(21):6263–9.

73. Elsasser T, Scholz M. Cluster effects within the local effect model. *Radiat Res* (2007) **167**(3):319–29. doi:10.1667/RR0467.1

9

DNA Damage Response Proteins and Oxygen Modulate Prostaglandin E$_2$ Growth Factor Release in Response to Low and High LET Ionizing Radiation

Christopher P. Allen[1], Walter Tinganelli[2,3], Neelam Sharma[1], Jingyi Nie[1], Cory Sicard[1], Francesco Natale[2], Maurice King III[1], Steven B. Keysar[4], Antonio Jimeno[4], Yoshiya Furusawa[3,5], Ryuichi Okayasu[6], Akira Fujimori[6], Marco Durante[2] and Jac A. Nickoloff[1]*

[1] Department of Environmental and Radiological Health Sciences, Colorado State University, Fort Collins, CO, USA, [2] GSI Helmholtzzentrum für Schwerionenforschung GmbH, Darmstadt, Germany, [3] Research Development and Support Center, National Institute of Radiological Sciences, Chiba, Japan, [4] Division of Medical Oncology, University of Colorado School of Medicine, Aurora, CO, USA, [5] Research Center for Radiation Protection, National Institute of Radiological Sciences, Chiba, Japan, [6] Research Center for Charged Particle Therapy, National Institute of Radiological Sciences, Chiba, Japan

*Correspondence:
Jac A. Nickoloff
j.nickoloff@colostate.edu

Common cancer therapies employ chemicals or radiation that damage DNA. Cancer and normal cells respond to DNA damage by activating complex networks of DNA damage sensor, signal transducer, and effector proteins that arrest cell cycle progression, and repair damaged DNA. If damage is severe enough, the DNA damage response (DDR) triggers programed cell death by apoptosis or other pathways. Caspase 3 is a protease that is activated upon damage and triggers apoptosis, and production of prostaglandin E$_2$ (PGE$_2$), a potent growth factor that can enhance growth of surviving cancer cells leading to accelerated tumor repopulation. Thus, dying tumor cells can promote growth of surviving tumor cells, a pathway aptly named Phoenix Rising. In the present study, we surveyed Phoenix Rising responses in a variety of normal and established cancer cell lines, and in cancer cell lines freshly derived from patients. We demonstrate that IR induces a Phoenix Rising response in many, but not all cell lines, and that PGE$_2$ production generally correlates with enhanced growth of cells that survive irradiation, and of unirradiated cells co-cultured with irradiated cells. We show that PGE$_2$ production is stimulated by low and high LET ionizing radiation, and can be enhanced or suppressed by inhibitors of key DDR proteins. PGE$_2$ is produced downstream of caspase 3 and the cyclooxygenases COX1 and COX2, and we show that the pan COX1–2 inhibitor indomethacin blocks IR-induced PGE$_2$ production in the presence or absence of DDR inhibitors. COX1–2 require oxygen for catalytic activity, and we further show that PGE$_2$ production is markedly suppressed in cells cultured under low (1%) oxygen concentration. Thus, Phoenix Rising is most likely to cause repopulation of tumors with relatively high oxygen, but not in hypoxic tumors. This survey lays a foundation for future studies to further define tumor responses to radiation and inhibitors of the DDR and Phoenix Rising to enhance the efficacy of radiotherapy with the ultimate goal of precision medicine informed by deep understanding of specific tumor responses to radiation and adjunct chemotherapy targeting key factors in the DDR and Phoenix Rising pathways.

Keywords: radiotherapy, DNA damage response, growth factor, apoptosis, caspase

INTRODUCTION

The majority of cancer patients receive radiotherapy (RT), and virtually all cancer treatments employ chemical or physical genotoxins that directly damage DNA, or inhibit DNA metabolism (such as topoisomerase inhibitors). DNA damage activates DNA damage response (DDR) pathways, but the specific DDR pathways activated, the degree of activation, and cell fate depend on many factors, including the amount and type of damage, as well as the genetic and environmental state of the cell (cell type, cell cycle phase, normal vs. tumor, hypoxic vs. normoxic, etc). Low and high LET IR yield different dose distributions in tissue and induce different types of damage, and may, thus, differentially activate DDR pathways. Solid tumors are genetically heterogeneous, which contributes to therapeutic resistance (1), and it is difficult to achieve 100% elimination of tumor cells while minimizing normal tissue toxicity. Rare surviving tumor cells, thus, pose a risk of tumor repopulation. A long recognized problem is that following RT, tumors may be rapidly repopulated, a phenomenon termed "accelerated tumor repopulation." The Li lab identified a paracrine growth factor signaling pathway that contributes to accelerated repopulation called "Phoenix Rising" (2–4). This pathway is initiated when lethally irradiated tumor cells activate caspase 3/7 (a key step in caspase-dependent apoptosis), leading to production of prostaglandin E^2 (PGE^2), a potent growth factor (**Figure 1A**). Thus, dying cells trigger growth of neighboring viable cells, a process akin to wound healing. PGE$_2$ produced via Phoenix Rising stimulates cell growth in culture and tumor repopulation in mice (2). Given the high radiation doses required to kill high fractions of tumor cells, the rare surviving cells are likely to experience significant DNA damage, and rapid proliferation of such cells is expected to enhance mutagenesis and may drive tumor progression toward a more aggressive metastatic state. There is accumulating evidence that PGE$_2$/Phoenix Rising is clinically relevant. Patients with head and neck squamous cell carcinoma or breast cancers that express caspase 3 show reduced survival (2), PGE$_2$ promotes renal carcinoma cell invasion that may contribute to metastasis (5), and recent studies indicate that blocking PGE$_2$ production with cyclooxygenase inhibitors improves outcomes in bladder and breast cancer patients treated with chemotherapy or RT (6, 7).

The DDR comprises complex networks of DNA repair and DNA damage signaling (checkpoint) pathways that control cell fate in response to DNA damage; a simplified view of DDR responses to ionizing radiation is shown in **Figure 1B**. The most fundamental cell fate decision is survival vs. death. Central to the DDR are protein kinases, including upstream PI3-like kinases ATM, ATR, and DNA-PKcs, that converge on downstream checkpoint kinases Chk1 and Chk2 (8). When cells experience limited damage, these factors promote cell survival and suppress cancer by effecting cell cycle arrest, stimulating repair, and promoting genome stability. Above a certain DNA damage threshold, these pathways promote senescence or programed cell death by apoptosis, necrosis, or autophagy (9, 10). Thus, DDR pathways are not "on or off" but show graded responses depending on the level of damage, and DDR thresholds are known to be genetically regulated (11, 12), and may vary for each checkpoint (13). There is substantial crosstalk among checkpoint and DNA repair pathways (14–22), and a major goal in the field is to identify synthetic (genetic) lethal interactions to exploit in cancer therapy (23).

There is considerable interest in targeting DDR proteins to augment therapeutic responses to chemotherapy and/or RT (24–26), for example, by sensitizing tumor cells to DNA damage. A common goal in cancer therapy is to kill tumor cells by inducing apoptosis. However, increasing caspase 3-dependent apoptosis may be a double-edged sword, leading initially to increased tumor killing, but accompanied by increased PGE$_2$ secretion and subsequent growth stimulation of rare surviving tumor cells. The present study was designed to determine whether modulating the DDR (by chemical inhibition of DNA-PKcs, ATM, or Chk1) influences Phoenix Rising in a variety of normal or tumor cells following exposure to low and high LET IR. Phoenix Rising can be blocked at many steps along the pathway from caspase-3 cleavage, to PGE$_2$ production/receptor binding (2, 27), and we tested whether chemical inhibition of COX1 and COX2 (COX1–2) blocked PGE$_2$ production. Certain tumors are hypoxic, and because oxygen is a necessary co-factor for COX1–2 activity, we also tested whether PGE$_2$ production differed under normoxic vs. hypoxic conditions. We show that PGE$_2$ production, and proliferation of co-cultured unirradiated cells vary widely among cell lines. In some cell lines, we observed enhanced PGE$_2$ production with inhibition of DNA-PKcs, suppression by inhibition of ATM, and both COX1–2 inhibition and hypoxia robustly suppressed PGE$_2$ production. In general, PGE$_2$ production did not affect short-term growth of irradiated cells (up to 48 h post IR), but PGE$_2$ levels correlated with growth of co-cultured, unirradiated cells in longer-term growth assays. Interestingly, both oxygen concentration and LET alter PGE$_2$ production. Together, these findings suggest that RT of certain tumor types may be enhanced by specific combinations of DDR and/or COX1–2 inhibitors that enhance tumor cell killing and mitigate accelerated tumor repopulation.

MATERIALS AND METHODS

Cell Culture and Chemical Inhibitors

Human cell lines HeLa, HT1080, HCT116, MCF7, BJ1hTERT, and HFL3, and mouse melanoma D17 cells, were cultured in Dulbecco's minimal essential medium (DMEM, Gibco) with 10% fetal bovine serum (Sigma or Atlas Biologicals), 100 IU/mL penicillin, 100 µg/mL streptomycin, 2.5 µg/mL amphotericin B (antibiotic/antimycotic, LifeTechnologies), 1 mM sodium pyruvate (Gibco) and incubated at 37°C with 5% CO$_2$ in air. For the hypoxia experiments, HeLa cells were maintained in a hypoxic incubator in the same media and growth conditions except that the oxygen concentration was limited to 1%. Primary head and neck tumor [patient-derived xenograft (PDX)] cell lines CUHN013, CUHN036 (28), CUHN065, and CUHN067 were cultured in Rhesus Monkey Kidney, *Mucaca mulatta* (RM$_K$)

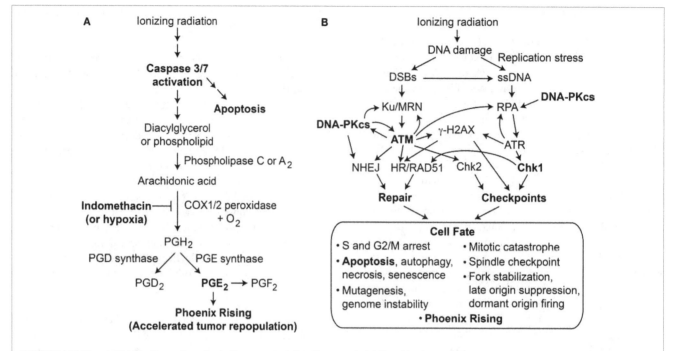

FIGURE 1 | (A) Phoenix Rising pathway of accelerated tumor repopulation. The cascade is initiated by cleavage and activation of caspase 3, which also promotes programed cell death by apoptosis. Activated caspase 3 cleaves and activates phospholipase 2 that hydrolyzes fatty acid phospholipid bonds, releasing arachidonic acid and lysophospholipids. Arachidonic acid is converted to PGH_2 by COX1 and COX2 peroxidases in the presence of oxygen; this step can be blocked by COX1–COX2 inhibitor indomethacin or hypoxia. Prostaglandin synthases generate the family of prostanoids, including PGD_2, PGE_2, and PGF_2. PGE_2 (and possibly other PGs) excreted from dying cells promote growth of surviving cells, accelerating tumor repopulation. **(B)** The DDR regulates cell fate after radiation damage. Proteins involved in DNA repair and damage checkpoint pathways crosstalk with programed cell death pathways to determine a variety of short- and long-term cell fates. Phoenix Rising and the DDR are linked through apoptosis and possibly other processes.

primary cell line media consisting of DMEM:F12 (3:1) with 10% FBS, insulin (5 µg/mL), hEGF (10 ng/mL), hydrocortisone (0.4 µg/mL), transferrin (5 µg/mL), penicillin (200 units/mL), and streptomycin (200 µg/mL).

Inhibitors of ATM (KU55933), Chk1 (UCN-01) DNA-PKcs (NU7026), and COX1–2 [indomethacin (Indo)] were purchased from Tocris Bioscience or Sigma and stored in powdered form at −20 or 4°C (NU7026). All compounds were freshly solubilized in DMSO to 100× working concentrations immediately prior to addition to cell cultures. Master mixes containing 1× final concentration of inhibitors in fresh media were prepared and added to wells pre- and post-irradiation. Final inhibitor concentrations were: 10 µM for ATMi, DNA-PKi, and COX1–2i, and 100 nM for Chk1i.

Human-Derived Head and Neck Squamous Cell Carcinoma Cell Lines

Head and neck squamous cell carcinoma patients were consented at the University of Colorado Hospital in accordance with the protocol approved by the Colorado Multiple Institutional Review Board (COMIRB #: 08-0552). CUHN013, CUHN065, and CUHN067 cell lines were derived directly from fresh patient post-surgical tumor tissue. Due to minimal tissue procured, the CUHN036 cell line required expansion and was, therefore, derived from PDX tumors. Tumor tissue was processed into ~2 mm × 2 mm × 2 mm pieces using a scalpel and forceps and

two to three pieces were placed in wells of cell culture grade six-well dishes without media. Uncovered plates were placed in the back of a cell culture hood and tumor pieces were allowed to dry/adhere to the plate for 15 min, then 2 mL of RM_K media was added to each well. Fresh media was added to tumor slices twice per week.

Outgrowing cells were characterized by flow cytometry (Cyan-ADP, Beckman Coulter) to confirm the presence of epithelial cancer cells (anti-CD44-APC, anti-EPCAM-FITC, anti-EGFR-PE) within the cancer-associated fibroblast cells (anti-mouse H2kd-PerCP–Cy5.5 for PDX tissue). Once cell populations had expanded sufficiently (~10^7 cells), cells were sorted (MoFlo-XDP, Beckman Coulter) twice in succession using the above combination of cell surface markers to eliminate contaminating fibroblasts. To confirm the origin of resulting cell lines, we conducted short tandem repeat (STR) analysis comparing sorted cells to the originating patient tissue. Finally, tumors generated in immune-compromised nude mice from these human-derived cell lines recapitulated the morphology and histology of the original patient or PDX tumors.

PGE_2 Detection by ELISA

Cells (10,000–20,000) were seeded into individual wells of 96-well microtiter dishes and incubated overnight using two to three replicate wells per treatment group. The dishes were irradiated with 10 Gy γ-rays (CSU, ^{137}Cs source), or 3 or 10 Gy X-rays

(NIRS) low LET IR. The cells were treated with either DDR or COX-1/COX-2 inhibitors 12–16 h prior to IR and the inhibitors were present in the media during and after IR. PGE_2 concentrations in growth media were measured at 0, 24, and 48 h after IR using a PGE_2 Parameter ELISA kit (R & D Systems) according to the manufacturer's directions. PGE_2 standard concentration curves (Figure S1 in Supplementary Material) were derived from dilutions of pure PGE_2 (R & D Systems) and fit to asymmetric 5-parameter logistic non-linear regressions using Prism software (Graphpad).

Cell Proliferation Assay

Cell proliferation was measured using sulforhodamine B (SRB) assays (29) performed on cells adhering to PGE_2 assay plates, since PGE_2 assays required only the growth media, and SRB assays required only adherent cells. Optical densities were measured at 560 nm wavelength in a 96-well microtiter plate reader and baseline readings for controls (empty wells and media only wells) were subtracted to yield final O.D. values. The resultant data were processed using Excel and Prism software.

PGE₂ Detection by Liquid Chromatography-Tandem Mass Spectrometry

BJ1hTERT or HT1080 cells (300,000) were seeded into T-25 flasks, incubated overnight and pretreated with DDR inhibitors as above. Supernatants from non-irradiated samples and samples irradiated with 3 Gy high LET (70 keV/μm) carbon ion IR were collected 48 h post irradiation and stabilized by the addition of 0.1% (v/v) butylated hydroxytoluene. The samples were immediately frozen, stored, and shipped to the CSU Center for Environmental Medicine Analytical Laboratory for liquid chromatography-tandem mass spectrometry (LC-MS/MS) analysis using methods developed to detect PGD_2, PGE_2, and PGF_2 (manuscript in preparation).

PGE₂ Detection After Low or High LET IR Under Normoxic or Hypoxic Conditions

HeLa cells were maintained in either normoxic (ambient) or 1% oxygen concentrations for 72 h after irradiation with low LET X-ray, either of two moderately high LET carbon ion beams (290 MeV/nucleon monoenergetic beam at 30 keV/μm, or 290 MeV/nucleon monoenergetic beam at 70 keV/μm), or a higher LET silicon ion beam (135 or 490 MeV/nucleon monoenergetic beam at 300 keV/μm). PGE_2 in the supernatant media was detected by ELISA. Normoxic and hypoxic cells that did not receive IR served as controls. Pretreatment with 10 μM COX-1/COX-2 inhibitor (Indo) was the same as described above.

Functional Assay for IR-Induced, PGE₂-Stimulated Growth of Co-cultured, Unirradiated Cells

Twenty-four hours prior to IR, 30,000 (no IR) or 100,000 (to be irradiated) HeLa cells were seeded into wells of six-well plates and incubated at 37°C in 5% CO_2 air. Additionally, 1,000 or 1,500

HeLa cells were seeded into ThinCert transwell inserts with 1 μm pores (Greiner), placed into 10 cm dishes and incubated at 37°C in 5% CO_2 in air. Once cells had attached, transwells were transferred into their corresponding wells. Control wells were prepared with equal numbers of cells in the transwells but no cells below. Twelve hours prior to IR, cells were treated with DDR inhibitors and/or Indo as above. Six-centimeter spread out Bragg Peak (SOBP) beams of moderately high LET carbon ions (290 MeV/nucleon, dose average LET of 50 keV/μm at the center of the SOBP) were generated at the Heavy Ion Medical Accelerator (HIMAC) facility of the National Institute of Radiological Sciences (NIRS), Chiba, Japan. The transwells for the irradiated plates were transferred to six-well holding plates immediately preceding irradiation and the media in the remaining wells was aspirated. Vertically oriented plates containing the cells were irradiated with 4 Gy carbon ion IR. Following irradiation, fresh media containing DDR inhibitor was added to the wells and the transwells, and the transwells were returned to their previous position. For the no IR controls, the media (in wells and transwells) was aspirated and fresh media containing DDR inhibitor was added and dishes were incubated for 3–6 days. On day 3 or day 6 post-irradiation, PGE_2 concentrations in transwell media was analyzed by ELISA. On day 7, sufficient media was added to transwells to allow cell growth for two more days, and on day 9 post-irradiation, transwell cells were trypsinized, and resuspended in 500–1000 μL of PBS and counted using a Coulter Counter or Scepter cell counting device (EMD Millipore).

Analysis of Apoptosis by Caspase 3/7 Cleavage and Annexin V Assays

Duplicate dishes were prepared for apoptosis assays as follows. Twenty-four hours prior to IR, 60,000 (no IR control) or 250,000 (to be irradiated), HeLa cells were seeded into wells of six-well plates and incubated at 37°C in 5% CO_2 in air. Twelve hours prior to IR, cells were treated with DDR and/or COX-1/COX-2 inhibitors and irradiated in parallel as described in the previous section. Following irradiation cells were incubated for 72 h and subsequently assayed by flow cytometry for two apoptosis endpoints. Caspase 3/7 cleavage/activation was monitored by cleavage of a DEVD peptide substrate conjugated to Alexafluor 488 (Cell Event 3/7 Caspase Green Reagent, Life Technologies) as follows. Cells from non-irradiated and irradiated treatment groups were trypsinized, harvested, and combined with supernatants from each well (containing potential apoptotic cells), centrifuged at 1200 rpm for 5 min, and the media was removed by aspiration. Cells were suspended in 500 μL of fresh media containing 1 μL Cell Event reagent (4 μM final concentration) and incubated at 37°C in 5% CO_2 in air for 15 min, then 500 uL of PBS was added to each sample and cells were analyzed on a BD FACSCaliber flow cytometer using 488 nm excitation and collecting fluorescent emissions with a 530/30 filter set. Gates were set using unstained and no treatment/no IR cells as negative control populations. Data represent the percent caspase-positive cells among 10,000 cells analyzed per sample. Data were acquired with CellQuest (Becton Dickinson) software, and analyzed using FloJo (Version 7.6.5, Tree Star Inc.) and Prism (Version 5.04, GraphPad) software.

Annexin V (AV) is a Ca^{2+}-dependent phospholipid binding protein that binds with high affinity to phosphatidyl serine residues that have translocated to the outer leaflet of the plasma membrane as a result of upstream apoptotic signaling, representing an early marker of apoptosis. Propidium iodide (PI) is a cell impermeant DNA binding dye that will penetrate into cells with compromised (leaky) membranes indicative of cellular necrosis, representing late-stage apoptosis. It is possible to discriminate the early (AV only), middle (AV and PI double positive), and late (PI-positive only) stages of cell death by co-staining with AV and PI. Approximately 5×10^5 cells (and supernatants containing potential apoptotic cells) were harvested from wells processed as above to generate cell pellets which were washed once in cold PBS, harvested by centrifugation, and suspended in 500 μL annexin binding buffer (10 mM HEPES, 140 mM NaCl, 2.5 mM $CaCl_2$, pH 7.4) yielding cell concentrations of approximately 1×10^6 cells/mL. Three microliters of Annexin V, Alexa Fluor 488® conjugate (Life Technologies) and 150 μL of annexin binding buffer were aliquoted to flow cytometry tubes, and 150 μL of cell suspensions were added, samples were mixed, incubated at room temperature for 15 min, and an additional 300 μL of annexin binding buffer was added, samples were mixed, stored on ice, and analyzed on a BD FACSCaliber flow cytometer using 488 nm excitation and collecting fluorescent emissions for FL1 and FL2 parameters using 530/30 and 585/42 filter sets, respectively. Compensation was established using the single-stained samples for the +IR treatment group and quadrant gating was established to identify AV^-/PI^- (apoptosis negative), AV^+/PI^- (early apoptotic), AV^+/PI^+ (middle apoptotic), and AV^-/PI^+ (late apoptotic/necrotic) populations. Data represent the percentage of cells in each quadrant from 5,000–10,000 cells collected per sample, using data acquisition and analysis software as above.

Clonogenic Cell Survival Assay

T25 flasks were seeded to ~20% confluence with cell lines to be tested, and incubated overnight. Cells were pretreated with DDR inhibitors at least 12 h prior to exposure to low or high LET IR. Cells were irradiated at ~50% confluence and allowed to recover for 30 min before they were trypsinized, harvested, suspended in fresh media, and counted using a Coulter Counter. Appropriate numbers of cells to yield ~100 colonies per 6 cm dish were suspended in fresh medium and distributed to three replicate dishes per treatment group. Forty-eight hours post irradiation, the media was aspirated and replaced with fresh media without drug. The cells were incubated for 8–11 days to allow colonies to develop. The dishes were stained with 0.5% (w/v) crystal violet in 70% methanol solution and the colonies were counted. Survival fractions were calculated and plotted using Excel and Prism software. We derived p-values for statistical analysis by using student's t-tests.

RESULTS

PGE$_2$ Production and Cell Viability After IR Vary Among Cell Types and Are Regulated by the DDR

The goals of this study were to determine whether DDR inhibitors and/or oxygen alter PGE$_2$ production and cell growth of irradiated cells in response to low and high LET ionizing radiation. We initially surveyed PGE$_2$ production in five cancer cell lines (HT1080 fibrosarcoma, HCT116 colorectal carcinoma, MCF7 breast adenocarcinoma, HeLa cervical adenocarcinoma, and B16 mouse melanoma) and two normal cell lines (BJ1hTERT, hTERT-immortalized human foreskin fibroblasts, and HFL3 spontaneously immortalized human fetal lung cells) following exposure to low LET γ-rays or X-rays. In the absence of DDR inhibitors, PGE$_2$ levels increased several fold 24 or 48 h after 10 Gy γ-rays with most cell lines, with statistically significant differences in MCF7 and BJ1hTERT, and trending toward significance in HT1080 ($p = 0.06$); HCT116 showed an approximately eightfold increase at 48 h, but significance could not be calculated because only a single determination was made at this time point (**Figure 2A**). In parallel with the PGE$_2$ assays, we measured cell survival/proliferation by SRB assay and found significant increases in cell number 48 h after IR in HT1080 and BJ1hTERT, but not HCT116 nor MCF7 (**Figure 2A**). PGE$_2$ effects on growth were previously observed at later times after IR (>5 days) (2) so the absence of a consistent early growth effect is not surprising. These PGE$_2$ effects were observed at IR doses of 3–10 Gy, higher than the 2 Gy doses typically used in fractionated photon RT, but well within the range of doses used in hypofractionated stereotactic body RT. PGE$_2$ production is likely proportional to levels of caspase activation (and apoptosis), but more studies are required to determine whether PGE$_2$ production follows a standard dose–response or displays threshold effects. These data demonstrate that basal and IR-induced PGE$_2$ levels, and early effects on survival/proliferation, vary among cell types.

DNA damage response inhibitors affected IR-induced PGE$_2$ production that again varied among cell types. In control experiments, we confirmed that inhibitors of DNA-PK, ATM, and Chk1 reduced clonogenic survival (Figure S2 in Supplementary Material and data not shown). DNA-PKi slightly increased PGE$_2$ production in HT1080 cells 48 h after IR, but the difference was not significant, and DNA-PKi had no effect on PGE$_2$ production in HCT116, MCF7, or BJ1hTERT cells (**Figure 2A**). ATMi suppressed PGE$_2$ levels in HT1080 cells 48 h post IR by ~1.5-fold, but ATMi did not affect PGE$_2$ in other cell types. Chk1i significantly enhanced PGE$_2$ production in HCT116, but other cell types showed no Chk1i effects. At 48 h after IR, ATMi dramatically decreased cell number (by ~20-fold) of both HT1080 and BJ1hTERT cells, whereas HCT116 and MCF7 cells were not affected. Because the SRB assay provides an estimate of survival/proliferation based on the amount of protein in attached cells (29), the sharp decrease in the number of attached HT1080 and BJ1hTERT cells with ATMi reflects massive cell death/detachment in response to the combined IR + ATMi treatment. Note that in both HT1080 and BJ1hTERT cells ATMi sharply reduced PGE$_2$, but only HT1080 showed reduced cell numbers, suggesting that PGE$_2$ is reduced by distinct mechanisms in these cell lines, with death and detachment preceding PGE$_2$ production in HT1080, but not BJ1hTERT.

Prostaglandin E$_2$ production depends on COX1–2 (**Figure 1A**) that can be inhibited with Indo. We next measured PGE$_2$ and cell survival/proliferation with HeLa, B16, BJ1hTERT, and HFL3 cells 48 h after 3 or 10 Gy doses of X-rays in presence or absence of Indo

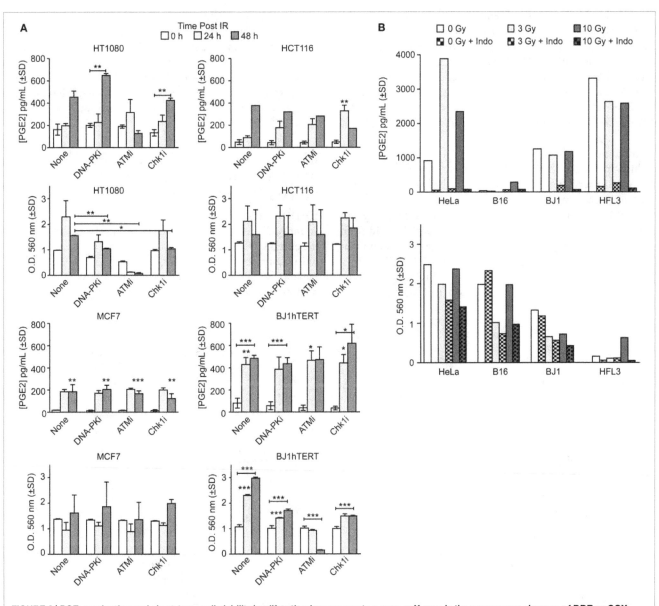

FIGURE 2 | PGE₂ production and short-term cell viability/proliferation in response to γ-rays or X-rays in the presence or absence of DDR or COX inhibitors. PGE₂ and cell growth were measured by ELISA and SRB assay in response to **(A)** 10 Gy γ-rays or **(B)** 3 or 10 Gy X-rays in the presence or absence of indomethacin (Indo). Data are averages ±SD for two to four replicates per treatment group **(A)** or single determinations **(B)**. In this and all subsequent figures, statistical significance was determined by t-tests, * indicates $p < 0.05$, **$p < 0.01$, ***$p < 0.001$.

(**Figure 2B**). With HeLa cells, PGE₂ levels increased approximately fourfold with an X-ray dose of 3 Gy, and approximately twofold with 10 Gy. B16 cells produced very little PGE₂ without IR or with a 3 Gy X-ray dose, but PGE₂ increased eightfold at 10 Gy. HFL3 and BJ1hTERT cells had high basal levels of PGE₂ that did not change substantially in response to X-rays. Uniformly, Indo dramatically suppressed PGE₂ levels (>20-fold), including basal and X-ray induced levels in both cancer and normal cells (**Figure 2B**). These data concur with numerous studies showing that inflammatory prostaglandin production can be mitigated by COX1–2 inhibitors (30). The variable basal levels of PGE₂ among cell lines may reflect differential expression or activation of PGE₂ pathway proteins, including caspase 3, which may be activated

when rapidly growing cells reach confluence and deplete growth media. There was a general trend toward decreased cell growth with increased IR dose. HeLa cells showed both stronger PGE₂ induction with X-rays, and greater radioresistance than the other cell lines. Note that HFL3 cells showed poor viability/proliferation after IR, and high basal PGE₂ levels, yet PGE₂ was not induced with IR in these cells. These features may be specific to HFL3 cells or perhaps reflect general properties of fetal cells.

To determine if low and high LET IR produce similar PGE₂ responses, absolute PGE₂ levels in media from HT1080 and BJ1hTERT cultures were determined by LC-MS/MS in response to 3 Gy high LET (70 keV/μm) carbon ions (**Figure 3**). This alternate PGE₂ assay helped us validate and expand on findings from the ELISA assay. In the absence of DDR inhibitors, HT1080 cells showed robust PGE$_2$ induction with carbon ions, similar to the effect of low LET IR, and BJ1hTERT cells were unresponsive to both low and high LET IR (**Figures 2** and **3**). These results indicate that PGE$_2$ production is stimulated by both low and high LET IR in a cell-type-dependent manner. The variation in absolute basal levels of PGE$_2$ in BJ1hTERT cells measured by LC-MS/MS and ELISA may reflect different sensitivities of ELISA and LC-MS/MS assays.

Inhibition of DNA-PK and ATM decreased carbon ion-induction of PGE$_2$ in HT1080 cells. The decrease in PGE$_2$ with DNA-PKi after high LET contrasts with that seen with γ-rays. This difference in DNA-PKi effects with low and high LET IR could reflect DNA-PK's dual role in damage signaling and DSB repair by NHEJ (**Figure 1B**), in particular, the shift from NHEJ-dominant repair of low LET IR damage to HR-dominant repair of high LET damage (31–33). By contrast, Chk1 inhibition markedly increased PGE$_2$ in BJ1hTERT cells, with or without IR. The Chk1i effect in the absence of IR suggests that

the cytotoxicity of Chk1i alone is sufficient to trigger Phoenix Rising. This Chk1i effect may reflect aberrant signaling to the p53-directed apoptotic cascade culminating in PGE$_2$ production, since p53 is stabilized by Chk1 phosphorylation of several sites after DNA damage (34). Together the results indicate that PGE$_2$ production following low or high LET IR can be enhanced or suppressed by inhibition of different pathways in the DDR network.

IR-Induced PGE$_2$ Stimulates Proliferation of Co-Cultured, Unirradiated Cells that can be Modulated by DDR and COX1–2 Inhibitors

A transwell multiple-endpoint assay system was used to examine the effects of low and high LET IR on co-cultured irradiated and unirradiated cells (**Figure 4A**). The pore size of the transwell membranes allows free diffusion of small molecules, but cell migration is blocked. This system allows simultaneous analysis of

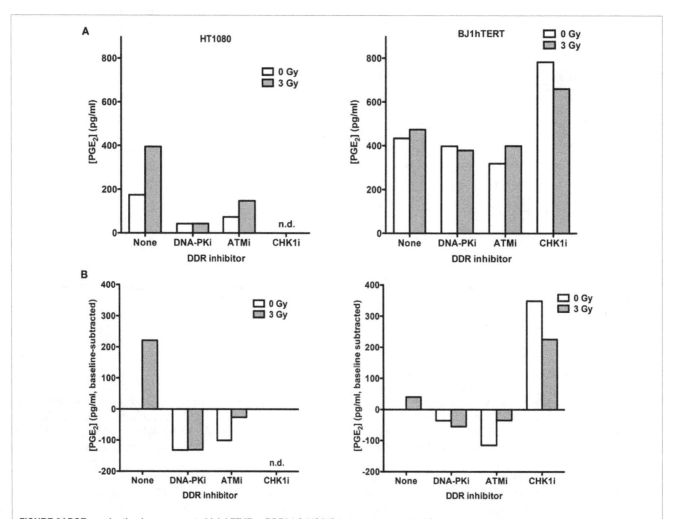

FIGURE 3 | PGE$_2$ production in response to high LET IR ± DDRi. LC-MS/MS was used to quantify PGE$_2$ levels in supernatants from HT1080 and BJ1hTERT cultures after irradiation with 3 Gy carbon ions (70 keV/μm). **(A)** Absolute PGE$_2$ levels. **(B)** PGE$_2$ levels were derived by subtracting the baseline values (no IR, no drug); n.d., not determined.

PGE$_2$ production, apoptosis, and cell growth as a key functional endpoint. We assessed the effects of radiation quality, DDR and COX1–2 inhibitors, and oxygen concentration on these endpoints. We chose HeLa cells for these studies because the cell line survey showed that HeLa cells have low basal PGE$_2$ levels, and relatively robust PGE$_2$ production after IR that is blocked by cyclooxygenase inhibition. A preliminary test of cell proliferation of unirradiated co-cultured cells 7 days after "feeder" cells received 10 Gy γ-rays showed a 2.7-fold increase in growth compared to control with mock-irradiated feeder cells, and that COX1–2i suppressed this growth (**Figure 4B**). This result is similar to a prior report in which luciferase-expressing cancer cell growth was enhanced two- to fivefold when in direct contact with irradiated feeder cells (2). The transwell system eliminates any influence of cell-to-cell contact, measuring only the growth effects of diffusible factors through the transwell membrane.

To investigate whether high LET IR would elicit similar growth effects on co-cultured unirradiated cells, we used the transwell system to monitor PGE$_2$ production and cell growth in response to 70 keV/μm carbon ions. We also tested whether DDR inhibitors and/or the COX1–2 inhibitor Indo would modulate growth stimulation. PGE$_2$ production and growth of unirradiated HeLa cells was measured 6 days after IR. PGE$_2$ levels increased >20-fold in response to IR in the absence of inhibitors (**Figure 5A**), similar to the increase seen with X-rays (**Figure 2B**). Both DNA-PKi and ATMi significantly decreased IR-induced PGE$_2$ levels (approximately fourfold), and these were further reduced by approximately twofold by Indo (**Figure 5A**), although the latter differences were not statistically significant. Growth of unirradiated co-cultured

HeLa cells was also monitored 6 days after IR. At this time point, moderate effects on growth were observed in the absence of DDR inhibitors, DNA-PKi increased growth but ATMi had no effect (**Figure 5B**). The increased growth with DNA-PKi does not appear to correlate with the lower PGE$_2$ level, but we note that PGE$_2$ levels were approximately twofold higher with DNA-PKi than untreated cells 3 days after IR (data not shown); the growth stimulation seen 6 days after IR may reflect this early burst of PGE$_2$, and the higher PGE$_2$ levels without DNA-PKi 6 days after IR would enhance growth at later times. The increased growth with DNA-PKi relative to untreated cells was dependent on feeder cells; no growth stimulation occurred without feeder cells (**Figure 5C**). As expected, blocking PGE$_2$ production with Indo (**Figure 5A**) also blocked growth stimulation (**Figures 5A,B**). As noted above, inhibiting DNA-PKcs or ATM radiosensitized cells (Figure S2 in Supplementary Material); thus, the differences in PGE$_2$ and growth effects with DNA-PKi and ATMi cannot be traced to differential degrees of cell killing, suggesting that inhibition of different DDR pathways can differentially affect Phoenix Rising and death pathway choice.

The transwell assay system is versatile in that in addition to PGE$_2$ and growth, simultaneous measures of apoptotic stages can be determined with the same cultures, including early apoptosis (caspase cleavage, detected with a cell-permeable caspase 3/7 DEVD peptide conjugated to a quenched fluorophore, which becomes fluorescent upon peptide cleavage), mid-apoptosis (Annexin V staining), and late apoptosis (revealed as gross membrane changes with propidium iodide staining). These endpoints were measured 3 and 6 days after high LET IR by flow

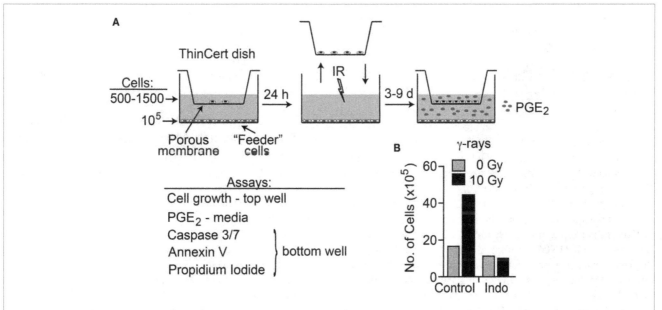

FIGURE 4 | (A) Transwell multiple-endpoint assay system. Cells were seeded into the top (500–1,500 cells) and bottom (feeder, 100,000 cells) sections of the transwell system and incubated for 24 h. The top section was transferred to a separate dish while the bottom section was irradiated, and then replaced. PGE$_2$ was measured in the media 3 and 6 days after IR; growth of unirradiated cells was determined 7–9 days after IR. Apoptotic endpoints (caspase 3/7 activation, Annexin V, and membrane changes by propidium iodide staining) were measured at 3, 6, or 9 days post IR in irradiated feeder cells. When used, DDR or cyclooxygenase inhibitors were present during the entire experiment. **(B)** HeLa cells assayed for growth stimulation using the transwell assay system after irradiation with 10 Gy low LET γ-rays. Indomethacin (Indo) inhibits COX1–2 and suppresses PGE$_2$ production.

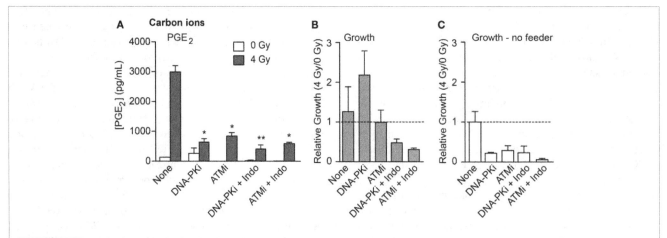

FIGURE 5 | PGE₂ production and stimulated proliferation of unirradiated HeLa cells in response to high LET carbon ions. (A) ELISA measurements from media in transwells containing HeLa cells 6 days after 0 or 4 Gy carbon ion irradiation. (B) Relative growth of unirradiated cells in transwells with or without DDR inhibitors or indomethacin, 6 days after irradiation of feeder cells. (C) As in (B) but without feeder cells. Data are averages (±SEM) for two determinations per condition.

cytometry (**Figure 6**). Minimal caspase activation was detected in unirradiated controls, and ~30% of cells activated caspase 3 and 6 days after IR. DDRi and Indo moderately suppressed caspase activation at both time points. Caspase is activated upstream of arachidonic acid that is processed by the Indo target, COX1–2, in the Phoenix Rising pathway (**Figure 1A**). This raises the possibility of a caspase–COX1–2 feedback loop, although the present experiments cannot rule out off target effects of Indo. Strikingly, ATMi appeared to completely block progression to later apoptotic stages; to a lesser extent DNA-PKi and Indo also suppressed progression to later apoptotic stages. Since ATMi is a strong radiosensitizer, the lack of progression to late apoptosis indicates that cells are shunted to one or more alternative death or senescence pathways.

Robust Phoenix Rising Responses in Cell Lines Derived From Fresh Tumor Tissue

Cell lines freshly derived from patient tumor tissue have emerged as important models for cancer cell biology studies (28, 35–37). We chose HNSCC-derived cell lines because head and neck cancers are treated with low and high LET RT. Low passage tumor cell lines were tested within 3 months of culture expansion. Two cell lines, CUHN036 and CUHN065, senesced or grew too slowly to study. Two others, CUHN013 and CUHN067, were reproductively robust and viable throughout the course of the experiments. CUHN013 is from a moderately focally keratinizing submental mass tumor. CUHN067 is from a base of tongue tumor that displayed extensive perineural invasion. Radiosensitivity was evaluated by clonogenic survival after X-rays or a clinical, 6 cm SOBP, high LET (~50 keV/μm) carbon ion beam. CUHN013 was more radiosensitive than CUHN067 to both X-rays and carbon ions, and both cell lines showed typical carbon ion RBEs of ~2–3 (Figure S3B in Supplementary Material).

Doses of 4 Gy SOBP carbon ions significantly increased caspase 3/7 activation compared to mock-irradiated controls, and DDRi and Indo had little effect on this endpoint (**Figure 7A**).

These results demonstrated that the initiating event of Phoenix Rising was functioning in these clinically relevant models. As with HeLa, in transwell experiments the CUHN cell lines showed moderate to strong growth stimulation of unirradiated cells that was dependent on irradiated feeder cells (**Figures 7B–E**). Neither CUHN cell line showed significant alterations in growth with DDRi or Indo. These early (caspase activation), late (growth stimulation, suppressible with Indo) Phoenix Rising markers indicate that Phoenix Rising is functioning in CUHN067. By contrast, CUHN013 displayed the early caspase marker and modest, but statistically significant ($p < 0.01$) growth stimulation, but Indo failed to suppress this growth, suggesting a late-stage defect. The distinct phenotypes of the two CUHN cell lines, in radiosensitivity and growth responses with or without inhibition of DNA-PK or COX1–2, highlight the challenges associated with targeting DDR and Phoenix Rising pathways for precision medicine.

Oxygen Concentration and LET Attenuate PGE₂ Production After Exposure to Carbon or Silicon Ion Beams

COX1 and COX2 require sufficient oxygen to function efficiently. A number of tumor types are naturally hypoxic and/or have hypoxic regions. We tested the hypothesis that hypoxic cells will produce less PGE₂ after IR than normoxic cells due to impaired COX1–2 function (**Figure 1A**). HeLa cells were incubated under normal conditions (5% CO_2 in air, ~20% oxygen), or hypoxic conditions (1% oxygen) for 72 h after IR and PGE₂ production was determined by ELISA. Normoxic and hypoxic cultures that did not receive IR served as controls. As above, 10 Gy X-irradiation increased PGE₂ production by ~20-fold under normoxic conditions, but this was significantly reduced (to less than fivefold) under hypoxic conditions (**Figure 8**). Oxygen concentration had no effect on PGE₂ levels without IR. We next tested the effects of oxygen on particle radiation at three LET values, 30 keV/μm carbon ion, 70 keV/μm carbon ion, and 300 keV/μm silicon ions.

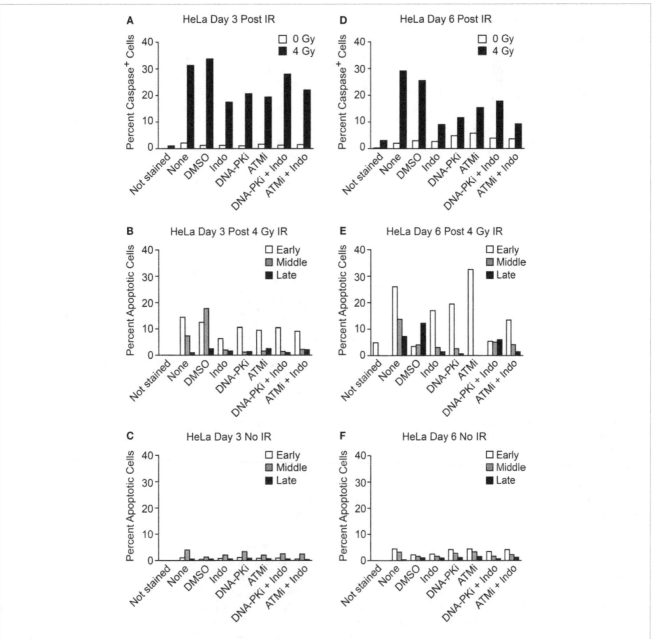

FIGURE 6 | Flow cytometric analysis of apoptotic phenotypes of feeder cells (from Figure 5) irradiated with high LET carbon ion IR. Duplicate plates were irradiated in parallel for assays 3 days post IR. Feeder cells co-cultured with transwell inserts were assayed 6 days post IR. Each sample was split at the time of harvest for two assay endpoints. Caspase cleavage and activation was assayed in live cells **(A)** 3 or **(D)** 6 days post IR using a fluorescent caspase 3/7 peptide fragment. Annexin V/propidium iodide co-staining of fixed cells discriminates between early, mid, or late apoptotic stages and was assayed **(B)** 3 or **(E)** 6 days post IR. No IR controls for the annexin V/PI assay **(C)** 3 or **(F)** 6 days post IR; ~10,000 cells were interrogated per determination. Unstained cells served as negative controls.

In all cases, hypoxia markedly reduced PGE_2 production, and with 30 or 70 keV/μm carbon ions, treatment with Indo further reduced PGE_2 production, in both normoxic and hypoxic treatment groups (**Figure 8**). Interestingly, 70 keV/μm carbon ions consistently caused approximately two- to threefold greater induction of PGE_2 than 30 keV/μm carbon ions under normoxic or hypoxic conditions, and in the presence or absence of Indo. While this suggests an LET dependence for PGE_2 production,

this is questionable given that PGE_2 induction was greatest with low LET X-rays, and that the highest LET radiation (300 keV/μm silicon ions) induced PGE_2 no more than 70 keV/μm carbon ions; this parallels earlier findings that RBE peaks at 150–200 keV/μm. Further studies are required to determine whether LET dependence follows a complex pattern (e.g., plateaus above a certain LET), and whether there are signaling differences with photons vs. particle radiation that account for the high level of PGE_2

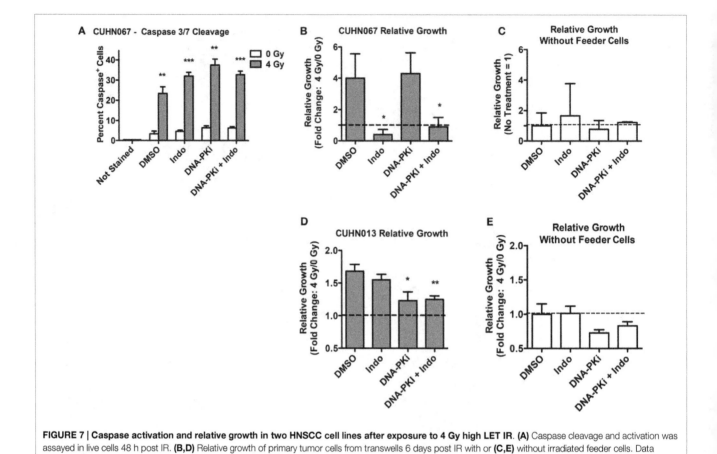

FIGURE 7 | Caspase activation and relative growth in two HNSCC cell lines after exposure to 4 Gy high LET IR. (A) Caspase cleavage and activation was assayed in live cells 48 h post IR. **(B,D)** Relative growth of primary tumor cells from transwells 6 days post IR with or **(C,E)** without irradiated feeder cells. Data represent the averages and SDs for three replicate measurements per determination.

induction with X-rays. Our results clearly indicate that, regardless of radiation quality, PGE_2 production is very sensitive to oxygen concentration. Thus, hypoxic tumor regions are unlikely to contribute to tumor repopulation via Phoenix Rising.

DISCUSSION

The Phoenix Rising pathway correlates with tumor repopulation *in vitro* and *in vivo* (27, 38, 39). The present study revealed several important features of IR-induced PGE_2 responses of normal and cancer cells. IR-induced, caspase 3-dependent, PGE_2 production (whether associated with apoptosis or other death pathways), is a common response of irradiated tumor cells, and some normal cells. PGE_2 levels generally enhanced growth of neighboring viable cells. Such growth, if unchecked, could spawn cells with high mutation rates, through replication of damaged genomes, as well as by an alternative mechanism activated in cells with moderately active caspase 3, that induces genome instability and carcinogenesis (40). Such small- and large-scale genetic change can drive rapid evolution of tumors, converting a local problem into lethal metastases.

Here, we focused on PGE_2 production, cell viability, and proliferation of irradiated and unirradiated cells in response to signaling factor(s) from co-cultured irradiated, apoptotic "feeder" cells; the modulation of these responses by DDR and COX1–2 inhibition

and by varying oxygen concentration; and the effects of radiation quality. Interconnected DDR and growth pathways coordinate responses radiation and chemotherapy-induced DNA injury and conspire with programed cell death pathways to determine cell fate (**Figure 1B**). In this study, we found that PGE_2 production and growth responses varied among cancer and normal cell lines, including cell lines freshly derived from patient tumors.

Although DDR inhibition enhanced radiosensitivity (Figure S2 in Supplementary Material), this did not correlate with a single pattern (increase or decrease) in PGE_2 production. Inherent radiosensitivity, and DDRi effects on radiosensitivity, varies widely among different cell types (4, 41) as observed here (Figures S2 and S3 in Supplementary Material). In general, the effects of radiation on the various endpoints (caspase activation, PGE_2 production, growth) were consistent across all radiation types tested. This suggests that targeting PGE_2-driven accelerated tumor repopulation may be an effective adjunct to both photon and particle radiotherapies. A fairly common response of ATMi and DNA-PKi was suppression of PGE2 production. A plausible explanation for this effect stems from the observations that ATM and DNA-PK activate the NFκB transcription factor in response to IR and other genotoxins (42–45), and COX-2, the upstream regulator of PGE2, is one of many NFκB targets (46). Because of the extensive crosstalk between DDR and growth factor networks, considerably more effort is required to define the multitude of

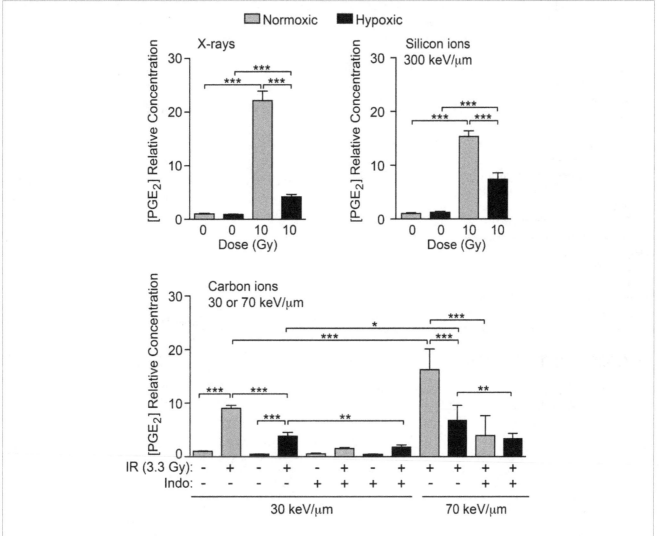

FIGURE 8 | IR-induced PGE2 production is suppressed by hypoxia. PGE$_2$ levels were determined by ELISA 3 days after X-ray, silicon ion, or carbon ion radiation at indicated LET and doses. Cells were incubated under normoxic, or hypoxic (1% O2) conditions. Data represent the averages and SDs for nine replicate measurements per determination.

tumor type responses to genetic and chemotherapeutic manipulation of DDR/growth regulatory factors. Phenotypic patterns emerging from such studies will guide mechanistic understanding of these various pathways, and may lead to rapid, inexpensive screening tools that will inform RT practice.

One facet that is consistent throughout our study and several others (2, 27, 47) is caspase activation and PGE$_2$ production. This is important because caspase status in tumors correlates with patient survival: patients with caspase 3-positive tumors do not survive as long as those with caspase 3-negaitve tumors (2, 48, 49). In addition, a recent study showed that low doses of radiation cause partial caspase 3 activation that leads to genome instability *in vitro* and *in vivo* through the generation of persistent DNA strand breaks (40). Another recent study demonstrated that caspase 3 defects created by shRNA, dominant negative gene expression, or gene deletion suppressed tumor growth *in vitro* and *in vivo* (47). Together, these findings

implicate caspase 3 as a promising target to improve chemotherapy or RT outcomes.

COX1 and COX2 are also promising targets to enhance cancer therapy. The present study and others (2, 40, 47, 50) demonstrate that PGE$_2$ production and stimulated growth can be effectively suppressed by Indo and other COX1 and COX2 inhibitors. Nonsteroidal anti-inflammatory compounds (NSAIDS) effectively target cyclooxygenase enzymes and are generally safe. Our study focused on Indo, a pan-COX1–2 inhibitor; other well-characterized examples are Naproxen and Ibuprofen, which are widely used and well tolerated. Selective COX2 inhibitors, such as Celecoxib, have been marketed but many have been withdrawn due to increased risk of myocardial infarction; it is possible that such risk is minimal for short-term courses during cancer therapy. A body of literature is beginning to emerge that describes tests of cyclooxygenase inhibitors in combination with RT or chemotherapy. In one study, Celecoxib delivered between rounds of gemcitabine and cisplatin substantially suppressed bladder urothelial carcinoma xenograft regrowth, and enhanced the chemotherapeutic response in xenografts from a chemoresistant patient (7). An earlier study of LNCaP-COX2 mouse xenografts showed that topical application of the NSAID Diclofenac significantly reduced tumor growth in combination with 3 Gy IR (51).

Finally, we demonstrate that PGE_2 production in response to IR is highly sensitive to oxygen concentration, including low and high LET radiation. Hypoxic regions of tumors are typically resistant to low LET IR. By contrast, high LET IR has a minimal oxygen enhancement ratio and, therefore, has greater efficacy than photons against these hypoxic regions (52). PGE_2-stimulated tumor repopulation may not be a critical issue to consider during treatment planning for hypoxic regions of tumors. We stand at a new frontier on the path toward personalized precision medicine. As basic scientists and clinicians look to improve the efficacy and safety of cancer treatment in the future, it will be important to develop techniques for rapid, accurate detection of Phoenix Rising biomarkers to personalize patient care. Preventing accelerated tumor repopulation during RT and chemotherapy will improve local control and reduce the likelihood that early stage cancer will progress to more dangerous invasive and metastatic stages.

AUTHOR CONTRIBUTIONS

CA, WT, NS, YF, RO, AF, MD, and JN conceived and designed experiments; CA, WT, NS, CS, FN, MK, and AF conducted experiments; CA, WT, NS, FN, MK, AF, MD, and JN participated in data analysis; CA, WT, SK, AJ, and JN wrote the manuscript; all authors participated in critical revision.

ACKNOWLEDGMENTS

We thank Greg Dooley of Colorado State University Center for Environmental Medicine Analytical Toxicology Laboratory, for assay development and technical assistance with the LC-MS/MS analysis, and the Japan National Institute of Radiological Sciences for generous provision of heavy ion beam time.

FUNDING

This work was supported by funding from the Japan National Institute of Radiological Sciences International Open Laboratory, NIH grant R01 GM084020 to JN and CA; R01 CA149456 to AJ; JSPS KAKENHI grants #24249067 and #23390301 and National Cancer Center Research and Development Funds (H23-A-43) to RO; and Research Projects with Heavy Ions at NIRS-HIMAC (18B468, 21B468, 12J468) to YF.

REFERENCES

1. Calderwood SK. Tumor heterogeneity, clonal evolution, and therapy resistance: an opportunity for multitargeting therapy. *Discov Med* (2013) **15**(82):188–94.
2. Huang Q, Li F, Liu X, Li W, Shi W, Liu F-F, et al. Caspase-mediated paracrine signaling from dying cells potently stimulate tumor cell repopulation during cancer radiotherapy. *Nat Med* (2011) **17**:860–6. doi:10.1038/nm.2385
3. Ng WL, Huang Q, Liu X, Zimmerman M, Li F, Li CY. Molecular mechanisms involved in tumor repopulation after radiotherapy. *Transl Cancer Res* (2013) **2**(5):442–8. doi:10.3978/j.issn.2218-676X.2013.10.03
4. Zimmerman MA, Huang Q, Li F, Liu X, Li CY. Cell death-stimulated cell proliferation: a tissue regeneration mechanism usurped by tumors during radiotherapy. *Semin Radiat Oncol* (2013) **23**(4):288–95. doi:10.1016/j.semradonc.2013.05.003
5. Li Z, Zhang Y, Kim WJ, Daaka Y. PGE2 promotes renal carcinoma cell invasion through activated RalA. *Oncogene* (2013) **32**(11):1408–15. doi:10.1038/onc.2012.161
6. Generali D, Buffa FM, Deb S, Cummings M, Reid LE, Taylor M, et al. COX-2 expression is predictive for early relapse and aromatase inhibitor resistance in patients with ductal carcinoma in situ of the breast, and is a target for treatment. *Br J Cancer* (2014) **111**(1):46–54. doi:10.1038/bjc.2014.236
7. Kurtova AV, Xiao J, Mo Q, Pazhanisamy S, Krasnow R, Lerner SP, et al. Blocking PGE2-induced tumour repopulation abrogates bladder cancer chemoresistance. *Nature* (2015) **517**(7533):209–13. doi:10.1038/nature14034
8. Stracker TH, Usui T, Petrini JH. Taking the time to make important decisions: the checkpoint effector kinases Chk1 and Chk2 and the DNA damage response. *DNA Repair* (2009) **8**(9):1047–54. doi:10.1016/j.dnarep.2009.04.012
9. Ciccia A, Elledge SJ. The DNA damage response: making it safe to play with knives. *Mol Cell* (2010) **40**(2):179–204. doi:10.1016/j.molcel.2010.09.019
10. Reinhardt HC, Yaffe MB. Kinases that control the cell cycle in response to DNA damage: Chk1, Chk2, and MK2. *Curr Opin Cell Biol* (2009) **21**(2):245–55. doi:10.1016/j.ceb.2009.01.018
11. Putnam CD, Jaehnig EJ, Kolodner RD. Perspectives on the DNA damage and replication checkpoint responses in *Saccharomyces cerevisiae*. *DNA Repair* (2009) **8**(9):974–82. doi:10.1016/j.dnarep.2009.04.021
12. Peng A, Lewellyn AL, Schiemann WP, Maller JL. Repo-man controls a protein phosphatase 1-dependent threshold for DNA damage checkpoint activation. *Curr Biol* (2010) **20**(5):387–96. doi:10.1016/j.cub.2010.01.020
13. Fernet M, Megnin-Chanet F, Hall J, Favaudon V. Control of the G2/M checkpoints after exposure to low doses of ionising radiation: implications for hyper-radiosensitivity. *DNA Repair* (2010) **9**(1):48–57. doi:10.1016/j.dnarep.2009.10.006
14. Allen C, Ashley AK, Hromas R, Nickoloff JA. More forks on the road to replication stress recovery. *J Mol Cell Biol* (2011) **3**:4–12. doi:10.1093/jmcb/mjq049
15. Kastan MB, Lim DS, Kim ST, Yang D. ATM – a key determinant of multiple cellular responses to irradiation. *Acta Oncol* (2001) **40**(6):686–8. doi:10.1080/02841860152619089
16. Kitagawa R, Bakkenist CJ, McKinnon PJ, Kastan MB. Phosphorylation of SMC1 is a critical downstream event in the ATM-NBS1-BRCA1 pathway. *Genes Dev* (2004) **18**(12):1423–38. doi:10.1101/gad.1200304
17. Baskaran R, Wood LD, Whitaker LL, Canman CE, Morgan SE, Xu Y, et al. Ataxia telangiectasia mutant protein activates c-Abl tyrosine kinase in response to ionizing radiation. *Nature* (1997) **387**(6632):516–9. doi:10.1038/387516a0
18. Burma S, Chen BP, Murphy M, Kurimasa A, Chen DJ. ATM phosphorylates histone H2AX in response to DNA double-strand breaks. *J Biol Chem* (2001) **276**(45):42462–7. doi:10.1074/jbc.C100466200
19. Chen BP, Uematsu N, Kobayashi J, Lerenthal Y, Krempler A, Yajima H, et al. Ataxia telangiectasia mutated (ATM) is essential for DNA-PKcs phosphorylations at the Thr-2609 cluster upon DNA double strand break. *J Biol Chem* (2007) **282**(9):6582–7. doi:10.1074/jbc.M611605200
20. Shrivastav M, Miller CA, De Haro LP, Durant ST, Chen BP, Chen DJ, et al. DNA-PKcs and ATM co-regulate DNA double-strand break repair. *DNA Repair* (2009) **8**(8):920–9. doi:10.1016/j.dnarep.2009.05.006
21. Yajima H, Lee K-J, Chen BPC. ATR-dependent DNA-PKcs phosphorylation in response to UV-induced replication stress. *Mol Cell Biol* (2006) **26**:7520–8.

22. Matsuoka S, Ballif BA, Smogorzewska A, McDonald ER III, Hurov KE, Luo J, et al. ATM and ATR substrate analysis reveals extensive protein networks responsive to DNA damage. *Science* (2007) **316**(5828):1160–6. doi:10.1126/science.1140321

23. Shaheen M, Allen C, Nickoloff JA, Hromas R. Synthetic lethality: exploiting the addiction of cancer to DNA repair. *Blood* (2011) **117**:6074–82. doi:10.1182/blood-2011-01-313734

24. Kelley MR, Logsdon D, Fishel ML. Targeting DNA repair pathways for cancer treatment: what's new? *Future Oncol* (2014) **10**(7):1215–37. doi:10.2217/fon.14.60

25. Hosoya N, Miyagawa K. Targeting DNA damage response in cancer therapy. *Cancer Sci* (2014) **105**(4):370–88. doi:10.1111/cas.12366

26. Basu B, Yap TA, Molife LR, de Bono JS. Targeting the DNA damage response in oncology: past, present and future perspectives. *Curr Opin Oncol* (2012) **24**(3):316–24. doi:10.1097/CCO.0b013e32835280c6

27. Li F, Huang Q, Chen J, Peng Y, Roop DR, Bedford JS, et al. Apoptotic cells activate the "phoenix rising" pathway to promote wound healing and tissue regeneration. *Sci Signal* (2010) **3**(110):ra13. doi:10.1126/scisignal.2000634

28. Keysar SB, Astling DP, Andersona RT, Vogler BW, Bowles DW, Morton JJ, et al. A patient tumor transplant model of squamous cell cancer identifies PI3K inhibitors as candidate therapeutics in defined molecular bins. *Mol Oncol* (2013) **7**(4):776–90. doi:10.1016/j.molonc.2013.03.004

29. Skehan P, Storeng R, Scudiero D, Monks A, McMahon J, Vistica D, et al. New colorimetric cytotoxicity assay for anticancer-drug screening. *J Natl Cancer Inst* (1990) **82**(13):1107–12. doi:10.1093/jnci/82.13.1107

30. Hawkey CJ. COX-1 and COX-2 inhibitors. *Best Pract Res Clin Gastroenterol* (2001) **15**(5):801–20. doi:10.1053/bega.2001.0236

31. Okayasu R, Okada M, Okabe A, Noguchi M, Takakura K, Takahashi S. Repair of DNA damage induced by accelerated heavy ions in mammalian cells proficient and deficient in the non-homologous end-joining pathway. *Radiat Res* (2006) **165**(1):59–67. doi:10.1667/RR3489.1

32. Hirakawa H, Fujisawa H, Masaoka A, Noguchi M, Hirayama R, Takahashi M, et al. The combination of Hsp90 inhibitor 17AAG and heavy-ion irradiation provides effective tumor control in human lung cancer cells. *Cancer Med* (2015) **4**:426–36. doi:10.1002/cam4.377

33. Wang H, Wang Y. Heavier ions with a different linear energy transfer spectrum kill more cells due to similar interference with the Ku-dependent DNA repair pathway. *Radiat Res* (2014) **182**(4):458–61. doi:10.1667/RR13857.1

34. Shieh SY, Ahn J, Tamai K, Taya Y, Prives C. The human homologs of checkpoint kinases Chk1 and Cds1 (Chk2) phosphorylate p53 at multiple DNA damage-inducible sites. *Genes Dev* (2000) **14**(3):289–300. doi:10.1101/gad.14.3.289

35. Anderson RT, Keysar SB, Bowles DW, Glogowska MJ, Astling DP, Morton JJ, et al. The dual pathway inhibitor rigosertib is effective in direct patient tumor xenografts of head and neck squamous cell carcinomas. *Mol Cancer Ther* (2013) **12**(10):1994–2005. doi:10.1158/1535-7163.MCT-13-0206

36. Jimeno A, Weiss GJ, Miller WH, Gettinger S, Eigl BJC, Chang ALS, et al. Phase I study of the hedgehog pathway inhibitor IPI-926 in adult patients with solid tumors. *Clin Cancer Res* (2013) **19**(10):2766–74. doi:10.1158/1078-0432.CCR-12-3654

37. Keysar SB, Le PN, Anderson RT, Morton JJ, Bowles DW, Paylor JJ, et al. Hedgehog signaling alters reliance on EGF receptor signaling and mediates anti-EGFR therapeutic resistance in head and neck cancer. *Cancer Res* (2013) **73**(11):3381–92. doi:10.1158/0008-5472.CAN-12-4047

38. Connell PP, Weichselbaum RR. A downside to apoptosis in cancer therapy? *Nat Med* (2011) **17**(7):780–2. doi:10.1038/nm0711-780

39. Labi V, Erlacher M. How cell death shapes cancer. *Cell Death Dis* (2015) **6**(3):e1675. doi:10.1038/cddis.2015.20

40. Liu X, He Y, Li F, Huang Q, Kato TA, Hall RP, et al. Caspase-3 promotes genetic instability and carcinogenesis. *Mol Cell* (2015) **58**(2):284–96. doi:10.1016/j.molcel.2015.03.003

41. Rich T, Allen RL, Wyllie AH. Defying death after DNA damage. *Nature* (2000) **407**(6805):777–83. doi:10.1038/35037717

42. McCool KW, Miyamoto S. DNA damage-dependent NF-kappaB activation: NEMO turns nuclear signaling inside out. *Immunol Rev* (2012) **246**(1):311–26. doi:10.1111/j.1600-065X.2012.01101.x

43. Dent P, Yacoub A, Contessa J, Caron R, Amorino G, Valerie K, et al. Stress and radiation-induced activation of multiple intracellular signaling pathways. *Radiat Res* (2003) **159**(3):283–300. doi:10.1667/0033-7587(2003)159[0283:SARIAO]2.0.CO;2

44. Basu S, Rosenberg KR, Youmell M, Price BD. The DNA-dependent protein kinase participates in the activation of NFkB following DNA damage. *Biochem Biophys Res Commun* (1998) **247**:79–83. doi:10.1006/bbrc.1998.8741

45. Sabatel H, Pirlot C, Piette J, Habraken Y. Importance of PIKKs in NF-kappaB activation by genotoxic stress. *Biochem Pharmacol* (2011) **82**(10):1371–83. doi:10.1016/j.bcp.2011.07.105

46. Tsatsanis C, Androulidaki A, Venihaki M, Margioris AN. Signalling networks regulating cyclooxygenase-2. *Int J Biochem Cell Biol* (2006) **38**(10):1654–61. doi:10.1016/j.biocel.2006.03.021

47. Donato AL, Huang Q, Liu X, Li F, Zimmerman MA, Li CY. Caspase 3 promotes surviving melanoma tumor cell growth after cytotoxic therapy. *J Invest Dermatol* (2014) **134**(6):1686–92. doi:10.1038/jid.2014.18

48. Zhang Z, Wang M, Zhou L, Feng X, Cheng J, Yu Y, et al. Increased HMGB1 and cleaved caspase-3 stimulate the proliferation of tumor cells and are correlated with the poor prognosis in colorectal cancer. *J Exp Clin Cancer Res* (2015) **34**:51. doi:10.1186/s13046-015-0166-1

49. Hu Q, Peng J, Liu W, He X, Cui L, Chen X, et al. Elevated cleaved caspase-3 is associated with shortened overall survival in several cancer types. *Int J Clin Exp Pathol* (2014) **7**(8):5057–70.

50. Yang J, Yue JB, Liu J, Sun XD, Hu XD, Sun JJ, et al. Effect of celecoxib on inhibiting tumor repopulation during radiotherapy in human FaDu squamous cell carcinoma. *Contemp Oncol (Pozn)* (2014) **18**(4):260–7. doi:10.5114/wo.2014.43932

51. Inoue T, Anai S, Onishi S, Miyake M, Tanaka N, Hirayama A, et al. Inhibition of COX-2 expression by topical diclofenac enhanced radiation sensitivity via enhancement of TRAIL in human prostate adenocarcinoma xenograft model. *BMC Urol* (2013) **13**:1. doi:10.1186/1471-2490-13-1

52. Allen CP, Borak TB, Tsujii H, Nickoloff JA. Heavy charged particle radiobiology: using enhanced biological effectiveness and improved beam focusing to advance cancer therapy. *Mutat Res* (2011) **711**:150–7. doi:10.1016/j.mrfmmm.2011.02.012

10

Ionizing Particle Radiation as a Modulator of Endogenous Bone Marrow Cell Reprogramming: Implications for Hematological Cancers

Sujatha Muralidharan[1], Sharath P. Sasi[2], Maria A. Zuriaga[1], Karen K. Hirschi[3], Christopher D. Porada[4], Matthew A. Coleman[5,6], Kenneth X. Walsh[1], Xinhua Yan[2,7] and David A. Goukassian[1,2,7]*

[1]Whitaker Cardiovascular Institute, Boston University School of Medicine, Boston, MA, USA, [2]Cardiovascular Research Center, GeneSys Research Institute, Boston, MA, USA, [3]Yale Cardiovascular Research Center, Yale School of Medicine, New Haven, CT, USA, [4]Wake Forest Institute for Regenerative Medicine, Wake Forest School of Medicine, Winston-Salem, NC, USA, [5]Radiation Oncology, School of Medicine, University of California Davis, Sacramento, CA, USA, [6]Lawrence Livermore National Laboratory, Livermore, CA, USA, [7]Tufts University School of Medicine, Boston, MA, USA

*Correspondence:
David A. Goukassian
david.goukassian@tufts.edu;
dgoukass@bu.edu

Exposure of individuals to ionizing radiation (IR), as in the case of astronauts exploring space or radiotherapy cancer patients, increases their risk of developing secondary cancers and other health-related problems. Bone marrow (BM), the site in the body where hematopoietic stem cell (HSC) self-renewal and differentiation to mature blood cells occurs, is extremely sensitive to low-dose IR, including irradiation by high-charge and high-energy particles. Low-dose IR induces DNA damage and persistent oxidative stress in the BM hematopoietic cells. Inefficient DNA repair processes in HSC and early hematopoietic progenitors can lead to an accumulation of mutations whereas long-lasting oxidative stress can impair hematopoiesis itself, thereby causing long-term damage to hematopoietic cells in the BM niche. We report here that low-dose ^{1}H- and ^{56}Fe-IR significantly decreased the hematopoietic early and late multipotent progenitor (E- and L-MPP, respectively) cell numbers in mouse BM over a period of up to 10 months after exposure. Both ^{1}H- and ^{56}Fe-IR increased the expression of pluripotent stem cell markers Sox2, Nanog, and Oct4 in L-MPPs and 10 months post-IR exposure. We postulate that low doses of ^{1}H- and ^{56}Fe-IR may induce endogenous cellular reprogramming of BM hematopoietic progenitor cells to assume a more primitive pluripotent phenotype and that IR-induced oxidative DNA damage may lead to mutations in these BM progenitors. This could then be propagated to successive cell lineages. Persistent impairment of BM progenitor cell populations can disrupt hematopoietic homeostasis and lead to hematologic disorders, and these findings warrant further mechanistic studies into the effects of low-dose IR on the functional capacity of BM-derived hematopoietic cells including their self-renewal and pluripotency.

Keywords: HSC, progenitors, radiation, endogenous reprogramming, hematological cancer

INTRODUCTION

Exposure to ionizing radiation (IR), specifically high-energy protons (^{1}H) and ions with high charge and high energy (HZE particles), is one of the major risks during spaceflight beyond low Earth orbit (LEO) (1, 2). For example, astronauts on future Mars missions are expected to encounter ~0.6 Sv of IR during 180 days transit to Mars (3). In this case, it is estimated that each cell in an astronaut's body will be traversed by a low-dose ^{1}H every 3–4 days, helium nuclei every few weeks, and HZE particles, such as iron (^{56}Fe), every few months. The radiation encountered by astronauts in LEO in proximity of the van Allen belt is mostly from ^{1}H particles from solar winds, trapped in the earth's magnetic field (4). This type of low linear energy transfer (LET) radiation, including γ rays and X-rays, deposit relatively little energy as they pass through matter. However, venturing beyond the van Allen belt and into deep space, astronauts will encounter a significant amount of galactic cosmic radiation which contains not only high-energy ^{1}H and alpha particles but also high-LET radiation from HZE particles, such as ^{56}Fe and ^{28}Si (4). These high-LET HZE ions have a greater propensity for ionization and they deposit large amounts of energy along their tracks; and thus have greater potential for causing damage to tissues. These types of low- and high-LET radiation are also encountered on earth. For example, low energy ^{1}H and HZE carbon ion IR are being used in cancer radiotherapy regimens for patients suffering from breast cancer, esophageal cancer, adenocarcinoma, and hepatocellular carcinoma (5–10). To date, the biological effects of low-dose ^{1}H and HZE ion IR have not been fully investigated.

Radiation dose is an important factor for consideration in the biological effects of low- and high-LET radiation. Although epidemiological studies based on atomic bomb survivors and cancer radiotherapy patients have provided insight into the biological effects of moderate to high doses of IR (11, 12), the effects of low-dose IR over long periods of time remain to be elucidated. A single high dose of radiation may induce significant tissue and cell damage; however, the biological effects of low-dose IR may be more relevant in disease processes, owing to IR-induced aberrations at the genetic or epigenetic levels. This "reprogramming" can be propagated in surviving cells and can have long term implications in the health of the IR exposed individual.

This article focuses on the biological relevance of low-dose low-LET ^{1}H and high-LET HZE ^{56}Fe radiation. Charged ^{1}H particles are the most abundant radiation found in deep space and HZE particles (1% of galactic cosmic rays) contribute to more than 40% of the equivalent dose exposure for the astronauts (4, 13, 14). Notably, low-energy ^{1}H particles are also being used as a source of radiation for the treatment of cancers owing to their favorable radiation dose distribution in cancerous tissue (15, 16). Therefore, studying the biological consequences of these types of radiation is of significance for understanding the consequences of both space missions and cancer therapy regimens.

EFFECTS OF IONIZING RADIATION ON THE BONE MARROW

Radiation-Induced DNA Damage and Oxidative Stress in BM Cells

Ionizing radiation promotes the induction and accumulation of mutations as a result of DNA damage and inefficient DNA repair. IR deposits energy along specific "tracks" which lead to clustering of DNA lesions (17). The extent of clustering depends on the ionization density and type of radiation, with more clustered damage often observed after exposure to heavy-ion radiation, such as ^{56}Fe particles. Such clustered DNA damage caused by high-LET radiation can lead to double strand breaks (DSBs) in DNA and mutations in the absence of proper DNA repair processes (18). Such DSBs can be repaired by non-homologous end-joining (NHEJ) or homologous recombination (HR). The NHEJ pathway seems to play a significant role in DNA repair after exposure to either ^{1}H or heavy-ion radiation while HR appears to be more important after heavy-ion radiation (19). Error-prone DNA repair during NHEJ, due to lack of a suitable template, can be a source of mutations post-IR. It should be noted that cells within the bone marrow (BM) often exhibit low levels of expression of many DNA repair proteins, suggesting they may have an inherent inability to repair DNA damage induced by radiation, and therefore are at increased risk of mutations (20). In support of this contention are studies showing that BM cells from mice exposed to 0.5–3 Gy, 1 GeV/n radiation with ^{56}Fe particles showed significantly increased chromosomal damage using multi-color FISH techniques (21, 22). ^{1}H-IR of 1 Gy, 100 MeV also induced significant DNA damage in mouse BM cells, as assessed by phospho-H2AX foci and multicolor FISH analysis (23, 24).

Exposure of cells to IR can also increase oxidative stress in cells by inducing reactive oxygen or nitrogen species (ROS or RNS), which are the result of interactions between IR and water with other biomolecules in the cell (25). ^{1}H-IR of 1 Gy, 150 MeV caused increased oxidative stress as determined by ROS levels and concomitant increases in expression of Nox4 in BM cells (24). ROS and RNS thus generated can interact with DNA and cause more DNA lesions, in addition to those induced by direct DNA damage caused in the radiation tracks. Chronic exposure to oxidative stress can lead to accumulation of such DNA lesions and promote mutagenesis (26). Therefore, the DNA damage and oxidative stress induced in BM by IR, specifically ^{1}H- and ^{56}Fe-IR, could lead to accumulation of DNA lesions and result in mutations in the hematopoietic stem and progenitor cells.

Hematopoiesis in Adult Bone Marrow

The BM niche is the predominant site of hematopoiesis and the differentiation of blood cells. This unique microenvironmental niche is also extremely sensitive to low-dose IR exposure (27–29). Disruption of hematopoietic homeostasis can result in hematologic disorders and impact the function of vital organs; for example, abnormalities in hematopoietic cells in the BM can be propagated to the successive blood lineages and result in leukemia. Therefore, it is important to understand the effects of exposure to ^{1}H- and ^{56}Fe-IR on BM.

Unlike the ablative effect of gamma radiation (γ-IR) on the BM, both short- and long-term effects of particle radiation on this site of hematopoiesis are less understood. Hematopoietic stem cells (HSCs) comprise <0.1% of the BM of adults, yet they produce all of the circulating blood cells that are responsible for constant maintenance and immune protection of the body (28). This exquisitely regulated process known as hematopoiesis occurs in the BM of adults and is responsible for both the maintenance of the primitive HSC and for inducing maturation of these cells to specific blood lineages as the need arises for those particular cell types. Discrete functions performed by the hematopoietic niche may require different growth factors and diverse interactions with different cells types within the site. These various interactions between HSCs and BM stromal cells ensure appropriate cell output to the circulation that change with specific stimuli and demands. Definitive hematopoiesis in the adult BM begins with the differentiation of self-renewing HSCs to hematopoietic multipotent progenitor cells (HPCs or MPPs) (28, 30). These progenitor cells can give rise to the different blood lineages but lack self-renewal capacity. The MPPs develop into committed common lymphoid (CLP) and myeloid (CMP) progenitor cells. The CLP population differentiates into the lymphocyte (NK, B, and T cells) lineages while the CMP gives rise to megakaryocytes, erythrocytes, monocytes, and granulocytes (neutrophils, basophils, and eosinophils). These mature blood cells then exit the BM and enter circulation where they perform important functions. Erythrocytes (red blood cells) are important for oxygen transport, megakaryocytes for blood clotting, and white blood cells (WBCs; namely lymphocytes, monocytes, and granulocytes), function in adaptive and innate immune defenses. Therefore, the process of hematopoiesis in the BM controls the development of all these blood lineages and is responsible for maintaining hematologic homeostasis.

Effects of ^{1}H Radiation on Circulating Blood Cells and Hematopoietic Precursors

Many studies have examined the effects of radiation on circulating blood cells. Irradiation of mice with up to 2 Gy of ^{1}H caused significant changes to the peripheral immune cell populations, with different populations exhibiting different sensitivities (31–33). Within the lymphocyte populations, B cells were found to be most sensitive to radiation, followed by T cells and then NK cells which were the most resistant (31). Decreases in WBC populations were dependent on ^{1}H-IR dose, but not on dose rate, energy, or fractionation (32, 33). The effects of simulated solar particle events, which are comprised of ^{1}H (up to 155 MeV), with a heterogeneous ^{1}H dose distribution, also revealed significant reduction (60–90% compared to baseline) in frequencies of circulating WBCs, lymphocytes, neutrophils, monocytes, and eosinophils in both murine and porcine models (34, 35). Murine splenic immune cell populations were impaired at 4 months post-IR with 2 Gy ^{1}H, indicating a long-term radiation effect on the precursor hematopoietic populations (36). This was confirmed in recent studies demonstrating that total body irradiation of mice with 1 Gy, 150 MeV of ^{1}H caused significant reduction in HSC (Lin$^-$c-kit$^+$Sca-1$^+$) numbers and pluripotency, even at time

points as late as 22 weeks after radiation (24). These changes were attributed to the increased levels of oxidative stress in the HSCs, causing increased HSC cell cycling and reduced self-renewal capacity, and resulting in long-term HSC injury. Although ^{1}H-IR is a low-LET radiation, its effects on DNA are more damaging than X-rays, indicating the greater capacity to induce changes at the molecular level (37).

Effects of HZE ^{56}Fe Particle Radiation on Circulating Blood Cells and Hematopoietic Precursors

Exposure to HZE particles, such as ^{56}Fe, can have even more detrimental effects on BM hematopoietic precursors and mature blood cells. Rats exposed to 1–4 Gy (5 GeV/nucleon) of ^{56}Fe-IR had significantly lower counts of circulating leukocytes and monocytes compared to non-irradiated rats for as long as 9 months post-IR (38). Mice irradiated with 6–8 Gy (1 GeV/nucleon) of ^{56}Fe particles also showed significantly lower WBC counts 7 days post-IR and lower recovery at 4 weeks post-IR compared to γ-IR mice (39). Examination of the BM revealed extensive cell death, cell cycle arrest and significant selective reduction of myeloid precursor cells in mice exposed to 2–4 Gy of ^{56}Fe-IR. Cell cycle arrest of BM cells at the G_1 phase up to 66 h post-IR was also found in another study with mice irradiated with 1 Gy (1 GeV/nucleon) of ^{56}Fe ions (40). Cell cycle arrest corresponded to an increase in cells with ^{56}Fe radiation-induced chromosomal aberrations (41). At the molecular level, exposure to 600 MeV, 0.4 Gy ^{56}Fe radiation induced DNA hypermethylation in HPCs up to 22 weeks post-IR, suggesting epigenetic reprogramming (42).

Therefore, we *hypothesize* that particle radiation, such as ^{1}H and ^{56}Fe, which induce profound changes in BM hematopoietic cells, including at the molecular level, may play a significant role in the development of hematological cancers, and thus merits further studies.

EXPOSURE TO ^{1}H AND ^{56}FE RADIATION HAS LONG-TERM EFFECTS ON BONE MARROW HEMATOPOIETIC MULTIPOTENT PROGENITOR POPULATIONS

^{1}H and ^{56}Fe Radiation Induced Significant Decrease in Bone Marrow Multipotent Progenitor Cell Numbers

To extend our knowledge of the effects of particle radiation on BM hematopoietic populations, whole-body radiation was performed on mice with 0.5 Gy (1 GeV) ^{1}H and 0.15 Gy (1 GeV/n) ^{56}Fe particles. Fluorescence-activated cell sorting (FACS) was then used to isolate early and late multipotent progenitors (E- and L-MPPs) from BM cells over a time course of 40 weeks post-IR. E-MPPs were defined as Lin$^-$/c-kit$^+$/Sca1$^+$/CD34$^+$/AC133$^+$ and L-MPPs were Lin-/c-kit$^+$/Sca1$^+$/CD34$^+$/AC133$^-$ (43, 44). Compared to control mice, ^{1}H-IR caused an initial transient spike in E-MPP and L-MPP cell numbers followed by significant downregulation of these populations at 8 weeks post-IR (**Figures 1A,B; Table 1**).

In contrast, ⁵⁶Fe-IR caused significant loss of E-MPPs and L-MPPs immediately after IR, which was maintained up to 8 weeks post-IR (**Figures 1A,B; Table 1**). By 40 weeks, the E-MPP and L-MPP populations had recovered and were comparable to control levels for both ¹H and ⁵⁶Fe radiation (**Figures 1A,B**). These findings are consistent with the study that showed γ-IR, even at the low dose of 0.4 Gy, was observed to rapidly induce apoptosis in human embryonic stem (ES) cells (45).

¹H and ⁵⁶Fe Radiation Significantly Upregulated Expression of Pluripotency Markers in Bone Marrow L-MPPs

Human ES cells that survived γ-IR exposure exhibited features of pluripotency at 3 weeks post-IR exposure (45). To decipher the molecular events in our radiation study, the expression of pluripotency markers *Sox2*, *Nanog*, and *Oct4* was examined in

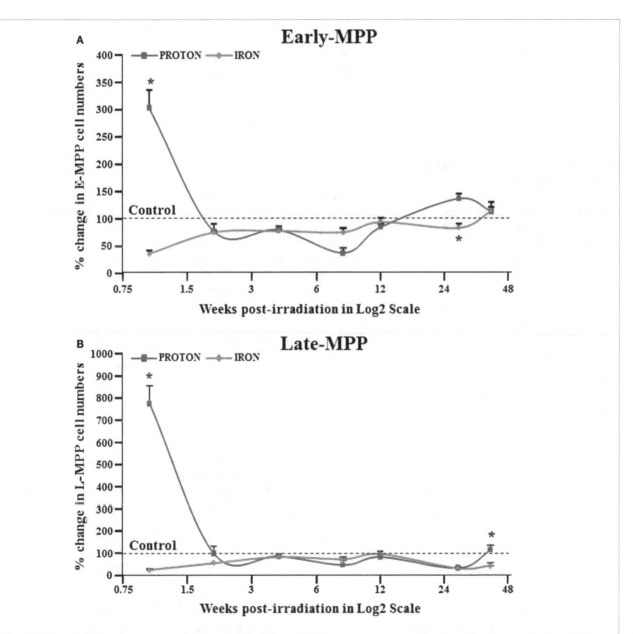

FIGURE 1 | E-MPP and L-MPP cell numbers are downregulated by ⁵⁶Fe- and ¹H-IR but recover to control levels by 40 weeks post-IR. Effect of full-body single dose of proton (¹H) at 0.5 Gy, 1 GeV and iron (⁵⁶Fe) at 0.15 Gy, 1 GeV/nucleon of ionizing radiation (IR) on survival of multipotent progenitor cell populations was examined. The survival of **(A)** E-MPPs and **(B)** L-MPPs in the BM after particle IR in C57BL/6NT mice were determined at 1, 2, 4, 8, 12, 28, and 40 weeks post-IR. Total BM-derived mononuclear cells were triple-stained with FITC-labeled RAM34 antibody (that consists of CD34, c-kit, and Sca1 antibodies), PE-Cy7-AC133, and PE-hematopoietic lineage cocktail (CD3e, Ly-6G/Ly-6C, CD11b, CD45R/B220, TER-119), then sorted by FASC for **(A)** E-MPPs (CD34⁺/c-kit⁺/Sca-1⁺/AC133⁺/Lin⁻) and **(B)** L-MPPs (CD34⁺/c-kit⁺/Sca-1⁺/AC133⁻/Lin⁻). Percentage changes in cell numbers were calculated relative to control sham irradiated mice, which was set to 100% for each time point. Solid lines represent mean ± SEM (*n* = 6/group) for ¹H-IR (solid blue lines) and ⁵⁶Fe-IR (solid red lines). "*" represents statistically significant differences compared to control with *p* < 0.05.

TABLE 1 | ^{56}Fe- and ^{1}H-IR resulted in decreased E-MPP and L-MPP cell numbers.

IR type	Weeks						
	1	2	4	8	12	28	40
(A) E-MPP							
^{1}H%	665↑*	3↓	13↓	52↓	17↓	66↓	15↑
^{56}Fe%	74↓	44↓	16↓	26↓	3↓	69↓	55↓**
(B) L-MPP							
^{1}H%	203↑*	23↓	21↓	63↓	16↓	36↑***	13↑
^{56}Fe%	65↓	25↓	23↓	25↓	6↓	17↓	15↑

Representation of % change difference in cell number for (A) E-MPPs (CD34+/c-kit+/Sca-1+/AC133+/Lin−) and (B) L-MPPs (CD34+/c-kit+/Sca-1+/AC133−/Lin−) from full-body ^{1}H-IR and ^{56}Fe-IR mice when compared to respective control cell numbers at each time point set at 100%. The arrows show the direction up or down for the population change.

*p < 0.001.
**p < 0.01.
***p < 0.03.

the L-MPPs for a period of 40 weeks following irradiation with ^{1}H or ^{56}Fe particles. The qRT-PCR analysis revealed a significant increase in expression of these markers at 8 and 40 weeks after both ^{1}H and ^{56}Fe irradiation (**Figures 2A–C**). Of note, it has been shown that ES cells exposed to 3 Gy high-LET carbon ion radiation also maintain their pluripotent state and express Oct3/4 and Sox2; data which agree with our current observations (46). Based on these observations, one could hypothesize that the increase in expression of the pluripotency markers in L-MPPs at 8 weeks post-radiation with ^{1}H or ^{56}Fe in our study could be the result of preferential expansion of radio-resistant cells. Indeed, this contention is supported by cancer biology studies that have shown a correlation between expression of Oct4 and Sox2 protein and increased resistance of cancer cells to radiotherapy (47, 48). However, the reduced cell numbers we observed at the 8-week time point post-IR (**Figure 1B**; **Table 1**) argues against this explanation. An alternative hypothesis to explain our observations is that ^{1}H- or ^{56}Fe-IR-induced genetic "reprogramming" of the existing L-MPPs. Consistent with this notion, γ-IR was reported to induce reprogramming of cancer stem cells that express the pluripotency genes Oct4, Sox2, Nanog, and Klf4 in a Notch-dependent manner for up to 5 days post-IR (47, 49). Furthermore, forced expression of Nanog, Oct4, Sox2, and Lin28 were sufficient to reprogram human somatic cells into pluripotent stem cells (50). Constitutive overexpression of Nanog alone is sufficient to promote proliferation of human ES cells while maintaining pluripotency and Oct4 expression (51, 52). Collectively, our data and previously published data strongly suggest that low doses of ^{1}H- or ^{56}Fe-IR may induce reprogramming of the L-MPPs to a state of pluripotency while promoting proliferation to replenish the progenitor populations.

Analysis of L-MPPs After Exposure to ^{1}H and ^{56}Fe Radiation Revealed Distinct Long-Term Genetic Programming

A significant increase in expression of these genes was also observed at 40 weeks post-irradiation with ^{1}H and ^{56}Fe particles

(**Figures 2A–C**). In order to examine this more closely, a multitude of hematopoiesis-related genes were analyzed in the L-MPPs at the 40-week time point, employing a PCR array for a pilot study (**Table 2**). Overall, ^{1}H- and ^{56}Fe-IR induced distinct genetic programs in the L-MPPs, with observable similarities and differences. We found that exposure of L-MPPs to either ^{56}Fe- or ^{1}H-IR markedly downregulated the expression of several genes that play key functions in the process of hematopoiesis, including CD164 (sialomucin), which increases adhesion of CD34 + cells to BM stroma and downregulates HPC proliferation (53, 54), and Fut10, which can fucosylate selectins for recruitment of progenitors to BM stroma (55, 56) (**Table 2**). It is possible that downregulation of adhesion molecules could be involved in mobilization of progenitor cells and increase their proliferation. Transcription factors that play an important role in hematopoiesis, such as Cbfb and Ash2l, were downregulated to a greater extent in L-MPPs exposed to ^{56}Fe-IR compared to ^{1}H-IR indicating a larger insult by ^{56}Fe radiation on BM cells (**Table 2**) (57, 58). This conclusion is also supported by the observed decrease in expression of immune receptors TLR3 and TLR4, and the co-receptor CD14 in ^{56}Fe-IR L-MPPs, indicating compromised immune responses and immune cell mobilization (**Table 2**) (59, 60). However, ^{1}H-IR L-MPPs showed an increase in expression of these genes, signifying activation of a different epigenetic program. Increased TLR3, TLR4, and CD14 expression on hematopoietic progenitor cells has been correlated with skewing toward myeloid cell differentiation as observed in aging (61, 62). It is possible that the ^{1}H- and ^{56}Fe-IR may promote the differentiation of these progenitors into the myeloid and lymphoid lineages, respectively. ^{1}H-IR exposed L-MPPs showed increased expression of Notch1 and its downstream target, Rbpj. In contrast, L-MPP cells from mice exposed to ^{56}Fe-IR showed a discernable decrease in expression of these genes (**Table 2**). Since activation of Notch1 was shown to promote myeloid differentiation via Rbpj (63), these data may be indicative of myeloid and lymphoid skewing in MPPs induced by ^{1}H- and ^{56}Fe-IR, respectively. On the other hand, expression of other Notch signaling molecules (Notch4, Jag1, and Jag2) were increased in L-MPPs exposed to ^{1}H- and ^{56}Fe-IR (**Table 2**). Interestingly, increased Notch signaling could potentially promote endogenous reprogramming of the cells, as indicated by reports of increased differentiation of cancer stem cells in response to Notch inhibition (64, 65). Therefore, these preliminary gene expression data also supports the possibility of radiation-induced reprogramming of BM progenitors to maintain pluripotency.

Other studies illustrating radiation-induced endogenous reprogramming have been largely conducted in cancer models. For example, inhibition of Notch signaling partially prevented radiation-induced reprogramming of differentiated breast cancer cells (isolated from patients) into cancer stem cells, thereby preventing their re-acquisition of expression of pluripotency genes Oct4, Nanog, and Klf4 (47). High doses of γ-IR was also shown to re-program hepatocellular cancer cell lines to acquire stemness phenotype (49). At the molecular level, radiation can induce epigenetic reprogramming in terms of DNA methylation which can also have important implications in BM progenitor populations (66). Mouse mesenchymal stem cells exposed to non-IR promoted an adipose phenotype (67). Collectively, these observations lend

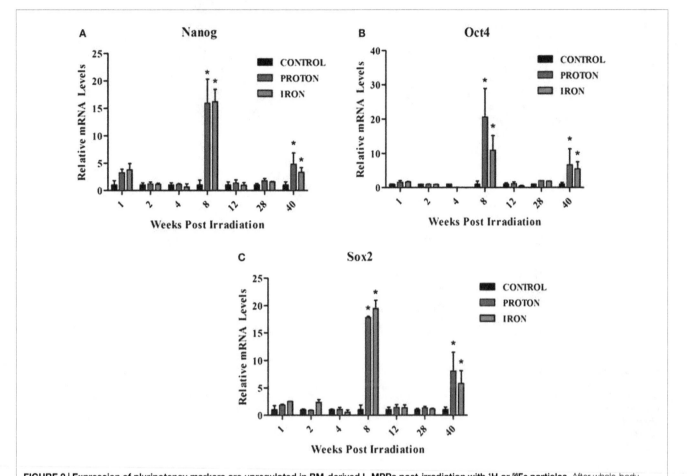

FIGURE 2 | Expression of pluripotency markers are upregulated in BM-derived L-MPPs post-irradiation with ¹H or ⁵⁶Fe particles. After whole-body irradiation with 0.5 Gy, 1 GeV ¹H and 0.15 Gy, 1 GeV/n ⁵⁶Fe particles, mononuclear cells from bone marrow of C57BL/6NT mice were sorted into L-MPPs (CD34⁺/c-kit⁺/Sca-1⁺/AC133⁻/Lin⁻) by FACS at multiple time points over 40 weeks post-IR. Levels of **(A)** *Nanog*, **(B)** *Oct4*, and **(C)** *Sox2* were analyzed using Taqman probes by qRT-PCR. Relative mRNA levels were calculated with respect to control sham irradiated animals. Bars represent mean ± SEM (*n* = 6/group) for control (solid black bars), ¹H-IR (solid blue bars), and ⁵⁶Fe-IR (solid red bars). "*" represents statistically significant differences compared to control with *p* < 0.05.

TABLE 2 | Exposure to ¹H or ⁵⁶Fe particles caused notable changes in hematopoietic genes in L-MPPs at 40 weeks post-radiation.

Group	Gene	Relative mRNA levels in ¹H-IR L-MPPs	Relative mRNA levels in ⁵⁶Fe-IR L-MPPs
Transcription factors	Cbfb	0.75↓	0.30↓
	Ash2l	0.98↓	0.45↓
Adhesion molecules	CD164	0.484↓	0.28↓
	FutIO	0.22↓	0.06↓
Immune receptors	TLR4	2.91↑	0.73↓
	TLR3	12.81↑	0.63↓
	CD14	1.32↑	0.03↓
Notch signaling	Notch1	1.83↑	0.60↓
	Notch4	5.24↑	2.29↑
	JagI	7.22↑	2.72↑
	Jag2	2.152↑	1.75↑
	Rbpj	1.622↑	0.32↓

After whole-body irradiation with 0.5 Gy, 1 GeV ¹H and 0.15 Gy, 1 GeV/n ⁵⁶Fe particles, mononuclear cells from bone marrow of C57BL/6NT mice were sorted into L-MPPs (CD34⁺/c-kit⁺/Sca-1⁺/AC133⁻/Lin⁻) by FACS at 40 weeks post-IR. These experiments were repeated at least twice. Expression of multiple hematopoietic gene transcripts was analyzed using a RT² PCR array. Fold changes were calculated with respect to control sham irradiated animals. The arrows show the direction up or down for the fold change.

further credibility to our postulation of radiation-induced reprogramming of BM cells, at the molecular level.

IMPLICATIONS OF RADIATION-INDUCED CHANGES IN BONE MARROW HEMATOPOIETIC PROGENITOR CELLS

In our studies into the effects of low-dose low-LET ¹H and high-LET ⁵⁶Fe-IR on BM hematopoietic progenitor populations, the most striking results were the significant loss of cell numbers and the changes in pluripotent markers in the surviving cells. The long-lasting decrease in the E-MPP and L-MPP populations in the irradiated mice over the course of 40 weeks suggests disrupted hematopoietic homeostasis. Such perturbation of hematopoiesis has the potential to lead to hematological disorders including blood cancers. With regard to the observed genetic changes induced by IR in the surviving L-MPP cell fractions at the 8- and 40-week time point, and supported by the literature reviewed herein, we posit that low-dose IR, especially particle radiation, can induce mutations in the hematopoietic progenitor pools in

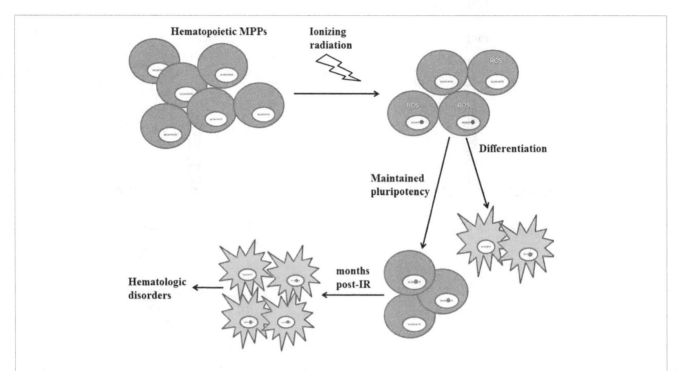

FIGURE 3 | Proposed model on the effects of low-LET ¹H and high-LET ⁵⁶Fe radiation on hematopoietic progenitor cells in the bone marrow niche. There is a significant decrease in MPP population numbers upon exposure to particle radiation. The majority of surviving cells experience DNA damage (depicted in blue) and oxidative stress (depicted by ROS), which could result in DNA mutations (depicted in red). While some MPPs continue to differentiate into blood cells, the remaining cells are "reprogrammed" to maintain pluripotency. As a result, even months post-IR, these "reprogrammed" MPPs [containing IR-induced mutations (depicted in red)] persist and give rise to differentiated blood cells, thereby propagating mutations to subsequent lineages, which may cause hematologic disorders, such as cancer. Blue cells represent multipotent progenitor cells and green cells represent differentiated blood cells.

the BM while concomitantly reprogramming them to a more primitive pluripotent state. While such reprogramming may be beneficial to replenish the progenitor cell pools within the radiation-depleted BM compartments, it may also have severe repercussions on the functions of the subsequent blood cell lineages (**Figure 3**). One can readily envision the radiation-induced reprogramming of BM progenitor cells, which may also contain radiation-induced mutations, will affect the phenotypes of multiple lymphoid and myeloid cell populations, thereby propagating the mutations to differentiated blood lineages. In particular, the propagation of mutations in oncogenes could promote risk for hematological cancers. It should be noted that high doses of IR are more likely to induce cell apoptosis, which may produce short-term effects, but low-dose radiation can cause significant long-term consequences by inducing mutations that will persist and differentiate into blood cells with altered function. Therefore, exposure to low-dose ⁵⁶Fe or ¹H particle radiation, as experienced by astronauts in spaceflight or cancer patients that undergo radiation therapy (specifically, the protracted full-body doses), can cause long-term effects in BM cells, thereby increasing their risks of developing (secondary) blood cancers.

AUTHOR CONTRIBUTIONS

SM – performed PCR, data analysis, wrote, and edited the manuscript; SS – performed and supervised all experimental studies, analyzed data, and edited the manuscript; MZ – performed PCR and data analysis; KH – reviewed and edited the manuscript; CP – reviewed and edited the manuscript; MC – reviewed and edited the manuscript; KW – reviewed and edited the manuscript; XY – reviewed and edited the manuscript; and DG – conceived the study, designed research, analyzed data, and wrote and edited the manuscript.

ACKNOWLEDGMENTS

We would like to thank members of Flow Cytometry Core at TUFTS University, School of Medicine – Allen Parmelee and Stephen Kwok. We would also like to thank members of NASA Space Radiation Laboratory (NSRL) and Biological Environmental and Climate Sciences Department at Brookhaven National Laboratory – Drs. Adam Rusek and Peter Guida and their teams for the help and support of our research studies.

FUNDING

This work was supported by the National Aeronautic and Space Administration (NASA) under Grant No. NNX11AD22G and American Heart Association (AHA) under Grant No. 14GRNT18860032 to DAG and NASA Grant No. NNX13AB67G to CDP.

REFERENCES

1. Czupalla M, Horneck G, Blome HJ. The conceptual design of a hybrid life support system based on the evaluation and comparison of terrestrial testbeds. *Adv Space Res* (2005) **35**:1609–20. doi:10.1016/j.asr.2005.06.010

2. Reitz G. Characteristic of the radiation field in low Earth orbit and in deep space. *Z Med Phys* (2008) **18**:233–43. doi:10.1016/j.zemedi.2008.06.015

3. Kerr RA. Planetary exploration. Radiation will make astronauts' trip to Mars even riskier. *Science* (2013) **340**:1031. doi:10.1126/science.340.6136.1031

4. Chancellor JC, Scott GB, Sutton JP. Space radiation: the number one risk to astronaut health beyond low earth orbit. *Life (Basel)* (2014) **4**:491–510. doi:10.3390/life4030491

5. Lomax AJ, Cella L, Weber D, Kurtz JM, Miralbell R. Potential role of intensity-modulated photons and protons in the treatment of the breast and regional nodes. *Int J Radiat Oncol Biol Phys* (2003) **55**:785–92. doi:10.1016/S0360-3016(02)04210-4

6. Sugahara S, Tokuuye K, Okumura T, Nakahara A, Saida Y, Kagei K, et al. Clinical results of proton beam therapy for cancer of the esophagus. *Int J Radiat Oncol Biol Phys* (2005) **61**:76–84. doi:10.1016/j.ijrobp.2004.04.003

7. Widesott L, Amichetti M, Schwarz M. Proton therapy in lung cancer: clinical outcomes and technical issues. A systematic review. *Radiother Oncol* (2008) **86**:154–64. doi:10.1016/j.radonc.2008.01.003

8. Newhauser WD, Fontenot JD, Mahajan A, Kornguth D, Stovall M, Zheng Y, et al. The risk of developing a second cancer after receiving craniospinal proton irradiation. *Phys Med Biol* (2009) **54**:2277–91. doi:10.1088/0031-9155/54/8/002

9. Hamada N, Imaoka T, Masunaga S, Ogata T, Okayasu R, Takahashi A, et al. Recent advances in the biology of heavy-ion cancer therapy. *J Radiat Res* (2010) **51**:365–83. doi:10.1269/jrr.09137

10. Okada T, Kamada T, Tsuji H, Mizoe JE, Baba M, Kato S, et al. Carbon ion radiotherapy: clinical experiences at National Institute of Radiological Science (NIRS). *J Radiat Res* (2010) **51**:355–64. doi:10.1269/jrr.10016

11. Hayashi T, Kusunoki Y, Hakoda M, Morishita Y, Kubo Y, Maki M, et al. Radiation dose-dependent increases in inflammatory response markers in A-bomb survivors. *Int J Radiat Biol* (2003) **79**:129–36. doi:10.1080/0955300021000038662

12. Darby SC, Mcgale P, Taylor CW, Peto R. Long-term mortality from heart disease and lung cancer after radiotherapy for early breast cancer: prospective cohort study of about 300,000 women in US SEER cancer registries. *Lancet Oncol* (2005) **6**:557–65. doi:10.1016/S1470-2045(05)70251-5

13. Simpson J. Elemental and isotopic composition of the galactic cosmic rays. *Annu Rev Nucl Part Sci* (1983) **33**:323–82. doi:10.1146/annurev.ns.33.120183.001543

14. Mewaldt RA. Galactic cosmic ray composition and energy spectra. *Adv Space Res* (1994) **14**:737–47. doi:10.1016/0273-1177(94)90536-3

15. Raju MR. Proton radiobiology, radiosurgery and radiotherapy. *Int J Radiat Biol* (1995) **67**:237–59. doi:10.1080/09553009514550301

16. Loeffler JS, Smith AR, Suit HD. The potential role of proton beams in radiation oncology. *Semin Oncol* (1997) **24**:686–95.

17. Burdak-Rothkamm S, Prise KM. New molecular targets in radiotherapy: DNA damage signalling and repair in targeted and non-targeted cells. *Eur J Pharmacol* (2009) **625**:151–5. doi:10.1016/j.ejphar.2009.09.068

18. Tokuyama Y, Furusawa Y, Ide H, Yasui A, Terato H. Role of isolated and clustered DNA damage and the post-irradiating repair process in the effects of heavy ion beam irradiation. *J Radiat Res* (2015) **56**:446–55. doi:10.1093/jrr/rru122

19. Gerelchuluun A, Manabe E, Ishikawa T, Sun L, Itoh K, Sakae T, et al. The major DNA repair pathway after both proton and carbon-ion radiation is NHEJ, but the HR pathway is more relevant in carbon ions. *Radiat Res* (2015) **183**:345–56. doi:10.1667/RR13904.1

20. So EY, Ouchi T. Decreased DNA repair activity in bone marrow due to low expression of DNA damage repair proteins. *Cancer Biol Ther* (2014) **15**:906–10. doi:10.4161/cbt.28883

21. Brooks A, Bao S, Rithidech K, Couch LA, Braby LA. Relative effectiveness of HZE iron-56 particles for the induction of cytogenetic damage in vivo. *Radiat Res* (2001) **155**:353–9. doi:10.1667/0033-7587(2001)155[0353:REOHIP]2.0.CO;2

22. Rithidech KN, Honikel L, Whorton EB. mFISH analysis of chromosomal damage in bone marrow cells collected from CBA/CaJ mice following whole body exposure to heavy ions (56Fe ions). *Radiat Environ Biophys* (2007) **46**:137–45. doi:10.1007/s00411-006-0092-x

23. Rithidech KN, Honikel LM, Reungpatthanaphong P, Tungjai M, Golightly M, Whorton EB. Effects of 100MeV protons delivered at 0.5 or 1cGy/min on the in vivo induction of early and delayed chromosomal damage. *Mutat Res* (2013) **756**:127–40. doi:10.1016/j.mrgentox.2013.06.001

24. Chang J, Feng W, Wang Y, Luo Y, Allen AR, Koturbash I, et al. Whole-body proton irradiation causes long-term damage to hematopoietic stem cells in mice. *Radiat Res* (2015) **183**:240–8. doi:10.1667/RR13887.1

25. Kryston TB, Georgiev AB, Pissis P, Georgakilas AG. Role of oxidative stress and DNA damage in human carcinogenesis. *Mutat Res* (2011) **711**:193–201. doi:10.1016/j.mrfmmm.2010.12.016

26. Cooke MS, Evans MD, Dizdaroglu M, Lunec J. Oxidative DNA damage: mechanisms, mutation, and disease. *FASEB J* (2003) **17**:1195–214. doi:10.1096/fj.02-0752rev

27. Rossi DJ, Bryder D, Seita J, Nussenzweig A, Hoeijmakers J, Weissman IL. Deficiencies in DNA damage repair limit the function of haematopoietic stem cells with age. *Nature* (2007) **447**:725–9. doi:10.1038/nature05862

28. Orkin SH, Zon LI. Hematopoiesis: an evolving paradigm for stem cell biology. *Cell* (2008) **132**:631–44. doi:10.1016/j.cell.2008.01.025

29. Mandal PK, Blanpain C, Rossi DJ. DNA damage response in adult stem cells: pathways and consequences. *Nat Rev Mol Cell Biol* (2011) **12**:198–202. doi:10.1038/nrm3060

30. Kondo M. Lymphoid and myeloid lineage commitment in multipotent hematopoietic progenitors. *Immunol Rev* (2010) **238**:37–46. doi:10.1111/j.1600-065X.2010.00963.x

31. Kajioka EH, Andres ML, Li J, Mao XW, Moyers MF, Nelson GA, et al. Acute effects of whole-body proton irradiation on the immune system of the mouse. *Radiat Res* (2000) **153**:587–94. doi:10.1667/0033-7587(2000)153[0587:AEOWBP]2.0.CO;2

32. Ware JH, Sanzari J, Avery S, Sayers C, Krigsfeld G, Nuth M, et al. Effects of proton radiation dose, dose rate and dose fractionation on hematopoietic cells in mice. *Radiat Res* (2010) **174**:325–30. doi:10.1667/RR1979.1

33. Maks CJ, Wan XS, Ware JH, Romero-Weaver AL, Sanzari JK, Wilson JM, et al. Analysis of white blood cell counts in mice after gamma- or proton-radiation exposure. *Radiat Res* (2011) **176**:170–6. doi:10.1667/RR2413.1

34. Sanzari JK, Cengel KA, Wan XS, Rusek A, Kennedy AR. Acute hematological effects in mice exposed to the expected doses, dose-rates, and energies of solar particle event-like proton radiation. *Life Sci Space Res (Amst)* (2014) **2**:86–91. doi:10.1016/j.lssr.2014.01.003

35. Sanzari JK, Wan SX, Diffenderfer ES, Cengel KA, Kennedy AR. Relative biological effectiveness of simulated solar particle event proton radiation to induce acute hematological change in the porcine model. *J Radiat Res* (2014) **55**:228–44. doi:10.1093/jrr/rrt108

36. Gridley DS, Pecaut MJ. Whole-body irradiation and long-term modification of bone marrow-derived cell populations by low- and high-LET radiation. *In vivo* (2006) **20**:781–9.

37. Hada M, Sutherland BM. Spectrum of complex DNA damages depends on the incident radiation. *Radiat Res* (2006) **165**:223–30. doi:10.1667/RR3498.1

38. Gridley DS, Obenaus A, Bateman TA, Pecaut MJ. Long-term changes in rat hematopoietic and other physiological systems after high-energy iron ion irradiation. *Int J Radiat Biol* (2008) **84**:549–59. doi:10.1080/09553000802203614

39. Datta K, Suman S, Trani D, Doiron K, Rotolo JA, Kallakury BV, et al. Accelerated hematopoietic toxicity by high energy (56)Fe radiation. *Int J Radiat Biol* (2012) **88**:213–22. doi:10.3109/09553002.2012.639434

40. Rithidech KN, Golightly M, Whorton E. Analysis of cell cycle in mouse bone marrow cells following acute in vivo exposure to 56Fe ions. *J Radiat Res* (2008) **49**:437–43. doi:10.1269/jrr.07109

41. Ritter S, Nasonova E, Furusawa Y, Ando K. Relationship between aberration yield and mitotic delay in human lymphocytes exposed to 200 MeV/u Fe-ions or X-rays. *J Radiat Res* (2002) **43**(Suppl):S175–9. doi:10.1269/jrr.43.S175

42. Miousse IR, Shao L, Chang J, Feng W, Wang Y, Allen AR, et al. Exposure to low-dose (56)Fe-ion radiation induces long-term epigenetic alterations in mouse bone marrow hematopoietic progenitor and stem cells. *Radiat Res* (2014) **182**:92–101. doi:10.1667/RR13580.1

43. Guo Y, Lubbert M, Engelhardt M. CD34- hematopoietic stem cells: current concepts and controversies. *Stem Cells* (2003) **21**:15–20. doi:10.1634/stemcells.21-1-15

44. Arndt K, Grinenko T, Mende N, Reichert D, Portz M, Ripich T, et al. CD133 is a modifier of hematopoietic progenitor frequencies but is dispensable for the maintenance of mouse hematopoietic stem cells. *Proc Natl Acad Sci U S A* (2013) **110**:5582–7. doi:10.1073/pnas.1215438110

45. Wilson KD, Sun N, Huang M, Zhang WY, Lee AS, Li Z, et al. Effects of ionizing radiation on self-renewal and pluripotency of human embryonic stem cells. *Cancer Res* (2010) **70**:5539–48. doi:10.1158/0008-5472.CAN-09-4238

46. Luft S, Pignalosa D, Nasonova E, Arrizabalaga O, Helm A, Durante M, et al. Fate of D3 mouse embryonic stem cells exposed to X-rays or carbon ions. *Mutat Res Genet Toxicol Environ Mutagen* (2014) **760**:56–63. doi:10.1016/j.mrgentox.2013.12.004

47. Lagadec C, Vlashi E, Della Donna L, Dekmezian C, Pajonk F. Radiation-induced reprogramming of breast cancer cells. *Stem Cells* (2012) **30**:833–44. doi:10.1002/stem.1058

48. Shen L, Huang X, Xie X, Su J, Yuan J, Chen X. High expression of SOX2 and OCT4 indicates radiation resistance and an independent negative prognosis in cervical squamous cell carcinoma. *J Histochem Cytochem* (2014) **62**:499–509. doi:10.1369/0022155414532654

49. Ghisolfi L, Keates AC, Hu X, Lee DK, Li CJ. Ionizing radiation induces stemness in cancer cells. *PLoS One* (2012) **7**:e43628. doi:10.1371/journal.pone.0043628

50. Yu J, Vodyanik MA, Smuga-Otto K, Antosiewicz-Bourget J, Frane JL, Tian S, et al. Induced pluripotent stem cell lines derived from human somatic cells. *Science* (2007) **318**:1917–20. doi:10.1126/science.1151526

51. Chambers I, Colby D, Robertson M, Nichols J, Lee S, Tweedie S, et al. Functional expression cloning of Nanog, a pluripotency sustaining factor in embryonic stem cells. *Cell* (2003) **113**:643–55. doi:10.1016/S0092-8674(03)00392-1

52. Zhang X, Neganova I, Przyborski S, Yang C, Cooke M, Atkinson SP, et al. A role for NANOG in G1 to S transition in human embryonic stem cells through direct binding of CDK6 and CDC25A. *J Cell Biol* (2009) **184**:67–82. doi:10.1083/jcb.200801009

53. Zannettino AC, Buhring HJ, Niutta S, Watt SM, Benton MA, Simmons PJ. The sialomucin CD164 (MGC-24v) is an adhesive glycoprotein expressed by human hematopoietic progenitors and bone marrow stromal cells that serves as a potent negative regulator of hematopoiesis. *Blood* (1998) **92**:2613–28.

54. Doyonnas R, Yi-Hsin Chan J, Butler LH, Rappold I, Lee-Prudhoe JE, Zannettino AC, et al. CD164 monoclonal antibodies that block hemopoietic progenitor cell adhesion and proliferation interact with the first mucin domain of the CD164 receptor. *J Immunol* (2000) **165**:840–51. doi:10.4049/jimmunol.165.2.840

55. Xia L, Mcdaniel JM, Yago T, Doeden A, Mcever RP. Surface fucosylation of human cord blood cells augments binding to P-selectin and E-selectin and enhances engraftment in bone marrow. *Blood* (2004) **104**:3091–6. doi:10.1182/blood-2004-02-0650

56. Wan X, Sato H, Miyaji H, Mcdaniel JM, Wang Y, Kaneko E, et al. Fucosyltransferase VII improves the function of selectin ligands on cord blood hematopoietic stem cells. *Glycobiology* (2013) **23**:1184–91. doi:10.1093/glycob/cwt055

57. Speck NA, Stacy T, Wang Q, North T, Gu TL, Miller J, et al. Core-binding factor: a central player in hematopoiesis and leukemia. *Cancer Res* (1999) **59**:1789s–93s.

58. Wang J, Zhou Y, Yin B, Du G, Huang X, Li G, et al. ASH2L: alternative splicing and downregulation during induced megakaryocytic differentiation of multi-potential leukemia cell lines. *J Mol Med (Berl)* (2001) **79**:399–405. doi:10.1007/s001090100222

59. Wieland CW, Van Lieshout MH, Hoogendijk AJ, Van Der Poll T. Host defence during *Klebsiella* pneumonia relies on haematopoietic-expressed Toll-like receptors 4 and 2. *Eur Respir J* (2011) **37**:848–57. doi:10.1183/09031936.00076510

60. Burberry A, Zeng MY, Ding L, Wicks I, Inohara N, Morrison SJ, et al. Infection mobilizes hematopoietic stem cells through cooperative NOD-like receptor and Toll-like receptor signaling. *Cell Host Microbe* (2014) **15**:779–91. doi:10.1016/j.chom.2014.05.004

61. Nagai Y, Garrett KP, Ohta S, Bahrun U, Kouro T, Akira S, et al. Toll-like receptors on hematopoietic progenitor cells stimulate innate immune system replenishment. *Immunity* (2006) **24**:801–12. doi:10.1016/j.immuni.2006.04.008

62. Granick JL, Simon SI, Borjesson DL. Hematopoietic stem and progenitor cells as effectors in innate immunity. *Bone Marrow Res* (2012) **2012**:165107. doi:10.1155/2012/165107

63. Schroeder T, Just U. Notch signalling via RBP-J promotes myeloid differentiation. *EMBO J* (2000) **19**:2558–68. doi:10.1093/emboj/19.11.2558

64. Fan X, Khaki L, Zhu TS, Soules ME, Talsma CE, Gul N, et al. NOTCH pathway blockade depletes CD133-positive glioblastoma cells and inhibits growth of tumor neurospheres and xenografts. *Stem Cells* (2010) **28**:5–16. doi:10.1002/stem.254

65. Sikandar SS, Pate KT, Anderson S, Dizon D, Edwards RA, Waterman ML, et al. NOTCH signaling is required for formation and self-renewal of tumor-initiating cells and for repression of secretory cell differentiation in colon cancer. *Cancer Res* (2010) **70**:1469–78. doi:10.1158/0008-5472.CAN-09-2557

66. Zielske SP. Epigenetic DNA methylation in radiation biology: on the field or on the sidelines? *J Cell Biochem* (2015) **116**:212–7. doi:10.1002/jcb.24959

67. Bock J, Fukuyo Y, Kang S, Phipps ML, Alexandrov LB, Rasmussen KO, et al. Mammalian stem cells reprogramming in response to terahertz radiation. *PLoS One* (2010) **5**:e15806. doi:10.1371/journal.pone.0015806

11

The Influence of C-Ions and X-Rays on Human Umbilical Vein Endothelial Cells

Alexander Helm[1]*, Ryonfa Lee[1†], Marco Durante[1,2] and Sylvia Ritter[1]

[1] Department of Biophysics, GSI Helmholtz Centre for Heavy Ion Research, Darmstadt, Germany, [2] Department of Condensed Matter Physics, Technical University of Darmstadt, Darmstadt, Germany

*Correspondence:
Alexander Helm
a.helm@gsi.de

Damage to the endothelium of blood vessels, which may occur during radiotherapy, is discussed as a potential precursor to the development of cardiovascular disease. We thus chose human umbilical vein endothelial cells as a model system to examine the effect of low- and high-linear energy transfer (LET) radiation. Cells were exposed to 250 kV X-rays or carbon ions (C-ions) with the energies of either 9.8 MeV/u (LET = 170 keV/μm) or 91 MeV/u (LET = 28 keV/μm). Subculture of cells was performed regularly up to 46 days (~22 population doublings) post-irradiation. Immediately after exposure, cells were seeded for the colony forming assay. Additionally, at regular intervals, mitochondrial membrane potential (MMP) (JC-1 staining) and cellular senescence (senescence-associated β-galactosidase staining) were assessed. Cytogenetic damage was investigated by the micronucleus assay and the high-resolution multiplex fluorescence *in situ* hybridization (mFISH) technique. Analysis of radiation-induced damage shortly after exposure showed that C-ions are more effective than X-rays with respect to cell inactivation or the induction of cytogenetic damage (micronucleus assay) as observed in other cell systems. For 9.8 and 91 MeV/u C-ions, relative biological effectiveness values of 2.4 and 1.5 were obtained for cell inactivation. At the subsequent time points, the number of micronucleated cells decreased to the control level. Analysis of chromosomal damage by mFISH technique revealed aberrations frequently involving chromosome 13 irrespective of dose or radiation quality. Disruption of the MMP was seen only a few days after exposure to X-rays or C-ions. Cellular senescence was not altered by radiation at any time point investigated. Altogether, our data indicate that shortly after exposure C-ions were more effective in damaging endothelial cells than X-rays. However, late damage to endothelial cells was not found for the applied conditions and endpoints.

Keywords: cardiovascular disease, endothelial cells, high-LET radiation, carbon ions, carbon ion therapy, chromosome 13, micronucleus formation, senescence-associated β-galactosidase

---

Abbreviations: CPD, cumulative population doublings; HUVEC, human umbilical vein endothelial cells; JC-1, 5,5′,6,6′-tetrachloro-1,1′,3,3′-tetraethylbenzimidazolyl-carbocyanine iodide; LET, linear energy transfer; mFISH, multiplex fluorescence *in situ* hybridization; MMP, mitochondrial membrane potential; RBE, relative biological effectiveness; SA-β-gal, senescence-associated β-galactosidase.

INTRODUCTION

An increased risk of cardiovascular disease (CVD), i.e., any disease involving the heart or blood vessels, such as ischemic heart disease, myocardial infarction, or hypertension, is a known consequence of radiotherapy for the treatment of certain types of cancer, such as breast cancer or Hodgkin lymphoma, where the heart is typically part of the radiation field and thus may be exposed to relatively high doses of ionizing radiation (IR) (1, 2). Although modern radiotherapy techniques aim to spare organs at risk such as the heart, coronary arteries may still be affected and thus a risk for cardiovascular damage remains (3, 4). Furthermore, there is growing evidence of an increased risk of CVD at low and moderate doses of IR stemming mainly from atomic bomb survivors and occupationally exposed groups, typically developing with a long latency (5–7). Generally, radiation-induced cell killing of endothelial cells and a subsequent induction of a pro-inflammatory response are considered as the mechanism triggering arteriosclerosis and ischemic heart disease (6, 8, 9). The mechanisms by which low and moderate doses of IR provoke CVD are still poorly understood. However, direct damage to endothelial cells followed by an inflammatory response seems to play also a role at low doses (6, 10).

Radiation-induced damage to the endothelium may simply be a consequence of cell loss due to cell killing, as discussed by Little et al. (6). Yet, also radiation-induced genomic instability, oxidative stress disrupting mitochondrial function, and accelerated cellular senescence have been implicated in the pathogenesis of arteriosclerosis (8, 11–14). So far, most data are available on the effects of low-linear energy transfer (LET) radiation, while only few data on the impact of high-LET radiation exist, yet suggesting a higher risk (10). With an increasing use of high-LET particles such as carbon ions (C-ions) in cancer therapy or radiosurgery (15–17), an assessment of their possible cardiovascular effects is important.

To gain a deeper insight into the effects of high-LET radiation on endothelial cells, we chose human umbilical vein endothelial cells (HUVEC) as a model system. HUVEC have been already used to study the radiation response to both low- and high-LET radiation investigating, e.g., cell survival, apoptosis, gene expression, or angiogenesis [e.g., Ref. (18–20)]. We exposed cells to C-ions with two different energies relevant for cancer therapy, i.e., 9.8 and 91 MeV/u corresponding to LET values of 170 and 28 keV/μm. For comparison, X-ray experiments were performed. The focus was set on doses ≤1.5 Gy. We investigated clonogenic cell survival, apoptosis, and cytogenetic damage expressed as micronuclei formation or chromosomal aberrations, premature senescence, and the integrity of the mitochondrial membrane potential (MMP). Measurements were performed up to 46 days post-irradiation.

MATERIALS AND METHODS

Cell Culture

Human umbilical vein endothelial cells were purchased from PromoCell (Heidelberg, Germany) and cultured according to the manufacturer's protocol in medium optimized for the cultivation of primary endothelial cells from large blood vessels. Briefly, cells were maintained in basal Endothelial Cell Growth Medium supplemented with Endothelial Cell Growth Kit components. The final supplement concentrations in the medium were 2% fetal calf serum, 0.1 ng/ml epidermal growth factor, 1 μg/ml hydrocortisone, 1 ng/ml basic fibroblast growth factor, and 0.4% endothelial cell growth supplement. Cells were passaged every 4–5 days upon reaching ~80% confluency. For cell detachment, a mixture of 0.05% trypsin and 0.02% EDTA was used and neutralized with trypsin neutralizing solution containing 0.05% trypsin inhibitor in 0.1% BSA and plated at a density of 6.6×10^3 cells/cm² unless otherwise stated. Medium was changed for every 2–3 days, and the cumulative population doubling (CPD) was determined. All cell culture products were purchased from PromoCell.

Irradiation

Sub-confluent cultures with a CPD level of about 6 (culture age: about 11 days) were exposed to X-rays or C-ions with an initial energy of either 11.4 or 100 MeV/u at GSI Helmholtz Centre for Heavy Ion Research (Darmstadt, Germany). For the exposure to X-rays or high energy C-ions, cells were seeded into 25 cm² culture flasks, whereas for the exposure to low energy C-ions, cells were plated into 35 mm Petri dishes.

X-ray irradiation was performed at a Seifert (Germany) X-ray machine operated at 250 kV and 16 mA with a 1 mm Al + 1 mm Cu filtering. The dose rate was about 1.5 Gy/min. Exposure to 11.4 MeV/u C-ions was done at the linear accelerator UNILAC, as described in detail elsewhere (21, 22). At sample position, the energy was 9.8 MeV/u corresponding to an LET of 170 keV/μm. Irradiation with 100 MeV/u C-ions was performed at the heavy ion synchrotron SIS with the raster scanning technique (23). The resulting energy on target was 91 MeV/u with an LET of 28 keV/μm. For C-ions, the irradiation time was in the range of 0.5–2 min depending on dose and accelerator conditions. All exposures were done at room temperature, and control samples were sham irradiated.

For longer follow-up studies (up to 46 days post-irradiation corresponding to 22 population doublings), we limited the analyses to doses at an isosurvival level of about 50 and 20%, respectively. Cell survival of 50% was expected for 0.75 Gy X-rays, 0.35 Gy 91 MeV/u C-ions, and 0.25 Gy 9.8 MeV/u C-ions, while a survival rate of 20% was estimated for 1.5, 0.75, and 0.5 Gy, respectively. Further details on particle fluences and the number of particle traversals per nucleus are given in Table S1 in Supplementary Material.

Clonogenic Cell Survival

Cell survival was measured using the standard colony forming assay (24). In brief, directly after exposure cells were trypsinized, counted, and plated in triplicate into 25 or 75 cm² tissue culture flasks. The number of cells seeded was estimated to result in a statistically significant formation of at least 100 colonies. After 12 days of incubation, cells were fixed and stained. Cell clusters consisting of at least 50 cells were counted as a colony.

Micronuclei

To assess the cytogenetic damage 24 h after radiation exposure, the micronucleus assay was applied as described in Fenech (25) with minor modifications. Briefly, cells were incubated for 4 h following irradiation and subsequently treated with 0.75 µg/ml cytochalasin-B for 20 h. Cells were then washed in PBS, fixed in 8% formaldehyde for 5 min, and stained with DAPI (0.2 µg/ml) for 15 min at room temperature. At least 1000 cells were scored, and the number of binucleated cells containing micronuclei was determined. For follow-up studies, i.e., >24 h, cells were regularly subcultured and at selected time points the spontaneously occurring frequency of cells carrying micronuclei was analyzed by scoring 1000 cells per dose and time point.

Apoptosis

For analysis at the early time point, cells were fixed in 8% formaldehyde and stained with DAPI as described for the micronuclei samples. Additionally, cells were subcultured and at consecutive time points 5×10^4 cells were seeded in 35 mm tissue culture dishes and incubated for 2 more days until fixation and staining. At least 1000 cells were scored per dose and time point. Apoptotic cells were identified under a fluorescence microscope (400× magnification) by the typical morphological changes of the cell nucleus, such as chromatin condensation or fragmentation (26, 27).

Senescence-Associated β-Galactosidase

Analysis of cellular senescence-associated β-galactosidase activity (SA-β-gal) was performed using the Senescence Cell Staining kit (Sigma-Aldrich, Germany) according to the manufacturer's protocol. At several time points after radiation exposure (2 up to 44 days), cells were seeded at a density of 5×10^4 in 35 mm tissue culture dishes. Two days later, cells were fixed and staining. At least 2000 cells were scored by light microscopy (400× magnification), and the fraction of cells exhibiting a blue stain, i.e., SA-β-gal activity, was determined.

Mitochondrial Membrane Potential

To assess the influence of radiation exposure on the MMP (also referred to as $\Delta\Psi_M$), the cationic, lipophilic dye 5,5′,6,6′-tetra chloro-1,1′,3,3′-tetraethylbenzimidazolyl-carbocyanine iodide (JC-1) was applied. The dye shifts its fluorescence signal from 525 nm (green) to 595 nm (red) due to a dimerization in the presence of protons thus indicating a functional MMP. For MMP analyses, samples were collected 12, 24, and 48 h after exposure. Measurements at later time points were performed using ~80% confluent cultures. Analysis of the MMP was performed as described previously (28) with modifications. Briefly, cells were harvested and incubated for 10 min in medium containing JC-1 (5 µg/ml) at 37°C. Thereafter, cells were washed twice with PBS analyzed by flow cytometry using a Pas III Particle Analysing System and the software FloMax (both from Partec, Germany). The fraction of predominantly red cells, i.e., cells mainly containing mitochondria with an intact MMP, was determined in at least 1×10^4 cells of each sample. As a positive control, cells were treated with 2 mM 2,4-dinitrophenol 10 min before JC-1 staining, resulting in ~5% of cells with a red fluorescent signal.

Chromosome Analysis

Chromosome aberrations were analyzed in control cultures at CPD 13 ± 2 and in the progeny of irradiated cells at CPD 22 ± 2. For cytogenetic analyses, cells were seeded into 75 cm² flasks and cultured for 2 days. Then, colcemid (0.1 µg/ml) was added for 3 h to accumulate metaphase cells. Chromosome spreads were prepared according to the standard procedures, e.g., cells were trypsinized, treated with hypotonic solution, fixed, and dropped on wet slides. Slides were stained using multiplex fluorescence in situ hybridization (mFISH). For mFISH analysis, slides were hybridized with the 24XCyte mFISH probe kit from MetaSystems (Altlussheim, Germany) following the instructions of the manufacturer. Chromosome spreads were examined using an Olympus BX61 microscope (Olympus, Tokyo, Japan) equipped with six filter sets specific for the applied fluorochromes. Images of the metaphases were captured (100× objective) with a charged coupled device camera, and karyotyping was performed using the ISIS/mFISH software. Both, structural and numerical aberrations were recorded in at least 100 metaphases per dose and time point. Structural aberrations were classified following the mPAINT system, as described in detail elsewhere (29). In the present study, breaks and simple exchanges were detected. Breaks were referred to as terminal deletions, when the centric and acentric part of the same chromosome were present within the cell. Terminal deletions involved either both chromatids at the same location (chromosome-type breaks, csb) or only one chromatid (chromatid-type break, ctb). Additionally, lone truncated chromosomes (T) were found, i.e., the acentric part of chromosome was not visible. Simple exchanges include translocations (complete, incomplete, and one-way forma) and dicentrics.

Statistics

When applicable, data were expressed as the mean value ± SEM or SD as indicated. For data stemming from one experiment only, Poisson statistics were applied to calculate the error bars as indicated, and statistical analysis was performed using a Fisher's exact test as indicated. Survival data have been normalized by evaluating the plating efficiency not considering control data (0 Gy) only, but rather by performing a fit of the form $(\alpha \times d + o)$ to the experimental data, where o is an offset term, which reflects the plating efficiency, determined from all data points. This procedure is more precise, as all measured data are subject to the same plating efficiency and consequently all data points can be exploited to derive this quantity. Deviations for 0 Gy to full survival arises, as also control measurements are affected by uncertainty. Based on the α-values derived from the linear fitting, a Student's t-test was used for statistical analysis. Curve fitting of the micronuclei formation 24 h after exposure was performed according to

$$Y = p_1 D \times e^{-p_2 D} \qquad (1)$$

where Y is the yield of micronuclei, D the dose, and p_1 and p_2 fitting parameters. Statistical analysis was performed based on the parameters derived from the fitting using a Student's *t*-test. Generally, differences were considered significant if the *p*-value ≤0.01.

RESULTS

Radiation Affects Clonogenic Cell Survival and Micronuclei Formation in a Dose- and LET-Dependent Manner 24 h after Exposure

To examine the putative radiation effect directly after exposure, a clonogenic cell survival assay was performed (**Figure 1**). For the three radiation types investigated cell survival decreased with dose and showed a clear LET dependence, i.e., 9.8 MeV/u C-ions with LET = 170 keV/μm were most effective, followed by 91 MeV/u C-ions with LET = 28 keV/μm and X-rays with 2 keV/μm. As all survival curves are linear, the relative biological effectiveness (RBE) does not depend on survival level, resulting in values of 2.4 and 1.5 for 9.8 and 91 MeV/u C-ions, respectively. Next, we measured cytogenetic damage in cells undergoing first division after exposure (24 h after exposure, cytochalasin-B treatment). The analysis showed an LET-dependent formation of micronuclei in binucleated cells (**Figure 2**). Within the limited dose range examined a saturation in the yield of cells carrying micronuclei was observed for >0.5 Gy 9.8 MeV/u C-ions (**Figure 2**) and >2 Gy X-rays. Thus, the damage induced by IR in first division cells clearly depends on the radiation quality and dose. Apoptosis was assessed 48 h after radiation exposure by investigation of morphological criteria of the cell nuclei. A slightly yet insignificantly increased fraction of apoptotic cells was observed in the irradiated samples independent of dose or radiation quality (**Figure 3**).

Radiation-Induced Damage Is Transient Rather Than Persistent in Cells Cultured up to 46 Days Following Exposure

For investigation of putative late effects of IR, we cultured both exposed cells and sham-irradiated cells up to 46 days corresponding to 22 population doublings post-irradiation (Figure S1 in Supplementary Material). Generally, radiation exposure did not severely alter the population growth compared to the control. Only in one case, i.e., after exposure to 1.5 Gy X-rays, a slightly lower CPD was found toward the end of the culture time.

Next, we determined the amount of cells harboring micronuclei after an extended culture time (**Figure 4**). To allow for a better comparison, we plotted the mean value (±SD) of all controls over time instead of single data points. As shown in **Figure 4**, in all irradiated samples, the fraction of HUVEC containing micronuclei was significantly increased 2 days after exposure. For C-ions, the increase was dose dependent. Generally, at the following time points, only small differences between irradiated and sham-irradiated control cultures were found. Yet, exposure to the high doses (0.5 and 0.75 Gy) low and high energy C-ions resulted in an increased fraction of cells containing micronuclei when comparing to the respective controls (not displayed) 21 and 20 days post-irradiation, respectively. These increases are above the range of the mean value of pooled controls from all experiments and its upper SD, as indicated in the graph (**Figure 4**). Subsequent investigation time points did not reveal significant dose effects compared to the controls. Thus, analysis of the formation of micronuclei provided no evidence for a radiation-induced chromosomal damage in the progeny of irradiated cells.

Furthermore, we investigated radiation-induced apoptosis in the descendants of irradiated cells. The morphological analysis of

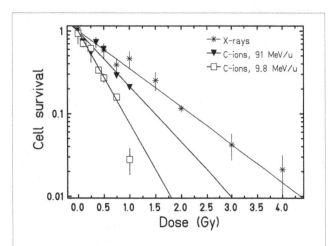

FIGURE 1 | Clonogenic cell survival of HUVEC. Cells were plated immediately after exposure to X-rays or C-ions. Data points represent the mean X ± SD from replicates stemming from one (C-ions) or three (X-rays) experiments. Curves were fitted by a linear function. Based on the α-values, clonogenic cell survival was found significantly (*p* < 0.01, Student's *t*-test) different for the three radiation types.

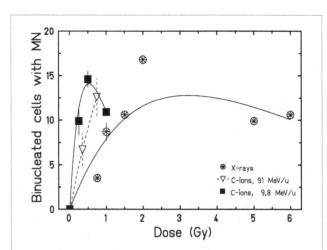

FIGURE 2 | Micronuclei formation 24 h after exposure. Following irradiation, cells were incubated with cytochalasin-B, and the amount of binucleated cells containing micronuclei was determined. Data points represent the mean X ± SEM (for data points with *n* = 2) or error was calculated according to Poisson statistics for data points stemming from one experiment. Curves for X-rays and 9.8 MeV/u C-ions were fitted as described. For 91 MeV/u C-ions, lines are drawn to guide the eye. Statistical analysis using a Student's *t*-test revealed significant differences for 9.8 MeV/u C-ions when compared to X-rays (*p* < 0.01).

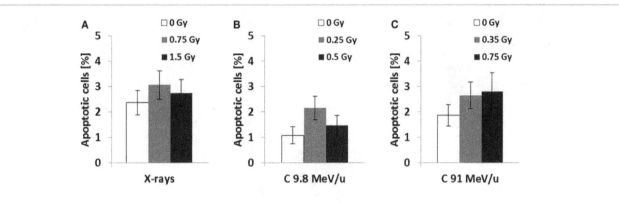

FIGURE 3 | Apoptosis 48 h after exposure. Cells were fixed 48 h following radiation exposure to X-rays **(A)**, 9.8 MeV/u C-ions **(B)**, and 91 MeV/u C-ions **(C)**. The fraction of apoptotic cells was determined according to morphological criteria of the nucleus. Error was calculated according to Poisson statistics. Fisher's exact test revealed no significant differences between all samples ($n = 1$, $p > 0.01$).

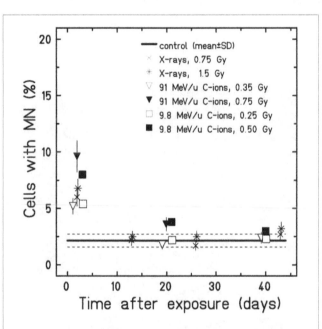

FIGURE 4 | Micronuclei formation in cells after extended culture time. Cells were fixed at several time points after exposure (w/o cytochalasin-B), and all cells harboring micronuclei were scored. The error was calculated according to Poisson statistics, and a Fisher's exact test was performed ($n = 1$). Only 2 days after exposure, micronuclei formation was found significantly higher compared to the control (mean ± SD). Note that for better visualization, the samples 2 days after exposure to the different radiation types were plotted separated from each other despite stemming from the same time point.

the cell nuclei showed no differences in the fraction of apoptotic cells in irradiated samples compared to the respective controls (data not shown).

Additionally, the putative damage on the MMP was studied by applying the proton-sensitive dye JC-1. In control cultures ($n = 4$), the proportion of cells with an intact MMP (mainly red-fluorescing cells) amounted to $79 \pm 8.4\%$ (mean ± SD) over the whole time interval investigated (data not shown). After exposure to X-rays or C-ions, we found a slight decrease in cells with an intact MMP between 3 and 8 days post-irradiation, partly falling

below the value of the lower SD (i.e., about 71%) down to 61% (for 1.5 Gy X-rays and 0.35 Gy C-ions 91 MeV/u, data not shown). To elucidate whether higher doses are required to profoundly impair mitochondrial function in HUVEC cultures within this period of time, we exposed cells to 1.5, 4, and 10 Gy X-rays and analyzed the MMP daily until 10 days after exposure (Figure S2 in Supplementary Material). We found that 2 days after exposure for all three doses applied, the amount of cells exhibiting mainly red fluorescence was lower compared to the respective control and the lower SD of all controls. Three days after irradiation with 1.5 Gy X-rays, the fraction of cells containing mitochondria with mostly intact MMP rose and reached the control level by day 5. For cells exposed to 4 Gy X-rays, recovery started at day 6 and the control value was reached by day 7, whereas the exposure to 10 Gy resulted in a persistently decreased level of cells with an intact MMP over the period investigated. Hence, the dose dependence was expressed rather in the recovery time than in the fraction of cells with intact MMP.

Furthermore, the expression of SA-β-gal was investigated in the progeny of irradiated and non-irradiated HUVEC to assess whether the radiation exposure induced premature senescence. Generally, the fraction of SA-β-gal positive cells raised with an increasing CPD. The proportion was comparable in irradiated samples and the respective controls. Only in one sample, i.e., 6 days after exposure to 0.5 Gy C-ions 9.8 MeV/u, an increased fraction of SA-β-gal positive cells was found and thus may be considered false positive (Figure S3 in Supplementary Material). Altogether, these data indicate that within the dose range investigated neither X-ray nor C-ion exposure induces a premature cellular senescence of HUVEC cultures.

Analysis of Chromosomal Aberrations by the mFISH Technique Revealed Specific Alterations in the Progeny of Non-Irradiated and Irradiated HUVEC Cultures

To verify the observation that the progeny of non-irradiated and irradiated cells do not express an elevated level of cytogenetic

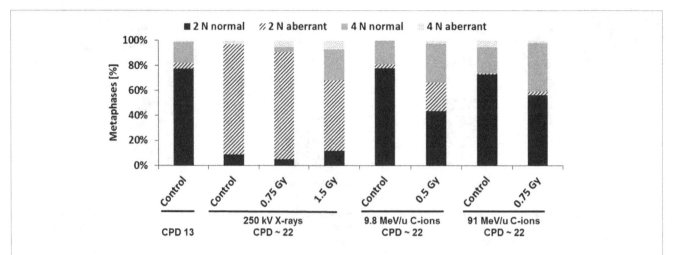

FIGURE 5 | Analysis of structural chromosome aberrations in HUVEC cultures (non-irradiated and irradiated) by means of the mFISH technique. The fractions of normal and aberrant diploid/hypodiploid cells (referred to as ~2N) and tetraploid/hypotetraploid cells (referred to as ~4N) are given (n = 1). The terms hypodiploidy or tetradiploidy indicate the loss of one or two chromosomes. Cells were analyzed in controls at a CPD level of 13 ± 2 and about 9 population doublings after exposure (CPD ~22).

damage (**Figure 4**), we measured chromosome aberrations in all cultures about 9 doublings post-irradiation corresponding to a CPD level of ~22. Additionally, the baseline level of aberrations was determined (CPD level ~13). The analyses were performed by means of the high-resolution mFISH technique. As shown in **Figure 5**, in non-irradiated HUVEC cultures at CPD ~13 most cells had a normal (2N) karyotype, occasionally the loss of one chromosome was observed. Overall, about 80% of the cells were diploid or hypodiploid. Notably, also tetraploid cells (4N) and a few cells with a hypotetraploid karyotype were registered (in total 20% of the population). Structural aberrations (mainly breaks and translocations) were detected in ~5% of cells analyzed. With increasing CPD, only small changes occurred in two control cultures (C-ion studies), but chromosome 13 appeared to be non-randomly involved. Either it was truncated or one copy was lost. In one control culture (X-ray study), the proportion of cells with a ~2N karyotype was much higher at CPD ~22, i.e., amounted to 97%. Notably, also the number of cells with structural aberrations was highly elevated, i.e., 88/97 ~2N cells and 3/3 ~4N cells were aberrant. In all affected cells, the same aberration, a large truncation of the q-arm of chromosome 13, was observed indicating a clonal origin.

Chromosome analysis in cells at CPD ~22 (**Figure 5**) consistently showed that the fraction of ~4N cells was generally higher in the progeny of irradiated cells than in the respective controls culture. Structural aberrations were found in all cultures and were generally translocations (sporadic or clonal) or truncated chromosomes. As observed in the control cultures chromosome 13 was non-randomly involved in aberrations. Likewise, the loss of one or two chromosomes was registered. Again, chromosome 13 was over-represented (**Figure 6**). A summary of the data is shown in Table S2 in Supplementary Material.

Altogether, these data show that in HUVEC chromosome 13 is inherently unstable. Frequently, cells with a lost or truncated chromosome were observed. Based on the number of

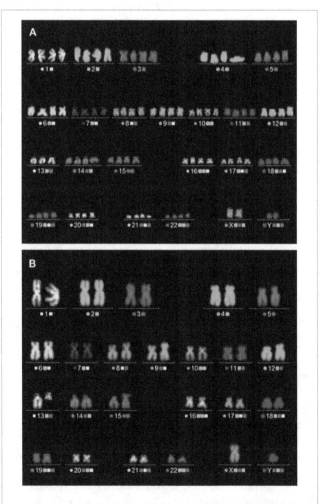

FIGURE 6 | Typical aberrations detected in HUVEC by means of the mFISH technique. (A) Hypotetraploid cell, one copy of chromosome 13 is lost. **(B)** Diploid cell, one chromosome is truncated (here: non-irradiated cells, CPD ~22).

cells affected (i.e., the clone sizes), the loss or the deletion of a large part of the q-arm of chromosome 13 results in a survival advantage. As these changes are clonal they remain undetected by micronucleus analysis.

DISCUSSION

Epidemiological data demonstrate an increased risk of CVD when the heart and its adjacent blood vessels are exposed to relatively high doses of low-LET radiation as a consequence of radiotherapy, e.g., breast cancer or Hodgkin lymphoma (1, 2, 30). An increased risk of CVD at low or moderate doses of IR is indicated by epidemiological data stemming mainly from atomic bomb survivors or occupationally exposed groups (7, 31). However, the mechanisms leading to CVD after exposure to IR remain to be elucidated. The available data point at damage to the endothelial cells as the initial event in pathogenesis (31). Hence, we chose HUVEC as a model system. This system bears two advantages. First, the umbilical cord provides a cost-effective source of endothelial cells. Second, in several studies, the effect of low LET on HUVEC has already been examined [e.g., Ref. (32, 33)]. Since data on high-LET C-ions are scarce but of great interest owing to the increased use of C-ions in modern radiotherapy (15–17), we analyzed the response of HUVEC after exposure to C-ions with energies relevant for radiotherapy (see Table S1 in Supplementary Material).

Radiation Induces a Dose- and LET-Dependent Damage in HUVEC 24 h Following Exposure

In HUVEC, radiation-induced damage in terms of clonogenic survival was found to depend on both dose and LET (**Figure 1**). For 91 MeV/u C-ions, an RBE value of 1.5 was obtained, whereas 9.8 MeV/u C-ions resulted in an RBE of 2.4. This is in line with the data reported for other cell lines [e.g., Ref. (34, 35)]. Cell survival of HUVEC after exposure to low-LET radiation was already measured by others (36, 37), but the radiosensitivity of cells used in the present study was much higher. For example, in the present study, a surviving fraction of 10% was reached after exposure to 2 Gy X-rays (**Figure 1**), whereas 4 and 5 Gy were needed for the same effect in the studies of Manti et al. and Hei et al., respectively. Furthermore, the survival data published by both authors show a shoulder, typically observed after exposure to low-LET photons. By contrast, our X-ray data display no shoulder. Lack of a shoulder points to a higher radiosensitivity and might be caused, for example, by a reduced DNA repair capacity as reported for Ku80-deficient cell lines [e.g., Ref. (34)]. Since HUVEC originate from apparently healthy donors, it is unlikely that the observed difference in the shape of the survival curves is attributable to compromised DNA repair. Yet, one possible explanation is a difference in the cell culture condition. In the present study, a specialized medium for primary endothelial cells was used with 2% serum, while Hei et al. cultured HUVEC in medium with 20% serum. Manti et al. studied also the response of HUVEC after exposure to C-ions with different LET values (13 and 100 keV/µm) and reported a clear dose and LET dependence as found in our study,

too. For C-ions with a high LET (100 keV/µm), Manti et al. did not find a shoulder either.

As observed for cell survival, C-ions were more effective than X-rays with respect to the formation of micronuclei in binucleated cells (**Figure 2**). Analogously, 9.8 MeV/u C-ions were more effective than 91 MeV/u C-ions due to the higher LET. The fraction generally increased with dose, however, after X-ray irradiation, a saturation was found for doses >2 Gy (data not shown). The available data indicate that for 9.8 MeV/u C-ions, the saturation occurred at a much lower dose (>0.5 Gy). Yet, for firm conclusions, measurements have to be performed over a wider range of doses. A dose-dependent increase in the rate of micronuclei in various rat, bovine, or human endothelial cell cultures (38, 39), and a saturation effect for doses around 2 Gy X-rays (38) has been reported by others and is in line with our findings (**Figure 2**). Since we screened for micronuclei in binucleated cells, the saturation may be correlated with a hampered cell division capacity for higher doses. Furthermore, cytochalasin-B is cytotoxic, thus an increased rate of apoptosis may compete with the formation of binucleated cells, additionally leading to an underestimation of the damage induced by IR.

In contrast to the damage induced as reduced clonogenic survival or micronuclei formation, apoptosis was found to be only slightly higher after exposure, independent from dose or applied radiation quality (**Figure 3**). A small increase in the fraction of apoptotic cells for HUVEC after exposure to low doses of X-rays is in line with literature (20).

Taken together, radiation does induce damage up to 24 h following exposure that depends both on dose and the LET value. Such damage to endothelial cells may be considered the initial event in the pathogenesis of CVD (31). However, CVD has a long latency period. Therefore, we investigated whether genetic damage persists in cultures and whether other cellular processes implicated in the pathogenesis of CVD were affected up to 46 days after exposure corresponding to 22 population doublings.

Radiation-Induced Damage Does Not Persist

Genomic instability, disrupted mitochondrial function, and accelerated replicative cellular senescence are implicated in pathogenesis of arteriosclerosis (8, 11–14). To address this topic, we assessed micronuclei formation, occurrence of chromosomal aberrations, apoptosis, and changes in the MMP as well as the expression of SA-β-gal in HUVEC cultured up to 22 population doublings after exposure (Figure S1 in Supplementary Material). For follow-up investigations, we focused on low doses up to 0.75 and 1.5 Gy for C-ions and X-rays, respectively, comparable to each other by isosurvival levels.

A dose-dependent effect on the number of cells with micronuclei was still visible at 48 h following exposure (**Figure 4**). At the later time points, the fraction of cells with micronuclei was similar in irradiated and control cultures indicating that the genomic stability of the cells was not affected by IR. Genomic instability expressed as micronuclei formation is a known consequence of exposure to IR (40). Yet, to the best of our knowledge, no other data sets for endothelial cells cultured for a prolonged time post-irradiation are available for comparison.

Premature senescence is considered as a key cellular stress response resulting, e.g., from DNA damage (41–43). Likewise, data indicate that premature senescence may contribute to the pathogenesis of arteriosclerosis (44, 45). Along this line, we examined the activation of SA-β-gal, a marker of cellular senescence (46) in the progeny of irradiated HUVEC.

Generally, no radiation-induced alterations were found over the time course investigated when compared to controls (Figure S3 in Supplementary Material). Only in one sample (0.5 Gy of 9.8 MeV/u C-ions), an elevated number of SA-β-gal positive cells was found 6 days after exposure that did not persist. Published data for endothelial cells are in contrast to our results. For example, Grossi et al. (47) registered a higher number of SA-β-gal expressing HUVEC several passages after exposure to 1.75 Gy X-rays or 0.5 Gy C-ions (13 keV/μm), i.e., doses comparable to the one in the current study. An increased number of endothelial cells, including HUVEC expressing SA-β-gal, was also observed after exposure to higher doses (2–10 Gy) of X-rays (48–50). Reasons for this different response are still unknown. Yet, studies over an extended culture time consistently showed an increase in the number of SA-β-gal positive endothelial cells with cell age (47, 51, 52). Our data support this finding.

There is evidence that radiation-induced oxidative stress and hampered mitochondrial function (53) play a role in endothelial dysfunction and CVDs (31, 54, 55). For example, in heart tissue, an impairment of mitochondrial proteins related to oxidative phosphorylation (e.g., complex I and III) was demonstrated following exposure to ≤2 Gy X-rays (56). Therefore, we examined the MMP, a key parameter of mitochondrial function. The dye JC-1, whose red fluorescence is directly correlated with the integrity of the MMP (57), was applied (data not shown). We found a slight decrease in the amount of cells containing mainly mitochondria with an intact MMP shortly after exposure (i.e., up to 8 days) independent of the radiation type and dose. Yet, by applying higher doses of X-rays (1.5, 4, and 10 Gy), we recorded an impairment of mitochondrial function in HUVEC that increased with dose (Figure S2 in Supplementary Material). Likewise, a decrease of the MMP following staining with JC-1 or other fluorescent dyes after high doses of X-rays (≤10 Gy) was reported for other cell lines (58–60).

A stress-triggered decrease of the MMP may be related to the onset of apoptosis via cytochrome c release and subsequent signaling pathways (61). In this context, our findings collectively provide no evidence for a delayed radiation-induced apoptosis in HUVEC.

Interestingly, the number of structural and numerical chromosomal aberrations increased with culture time in the progeny of unirradiated and irradiated cells. Consistently, chromosome 13 was involved. While, to the best of our knowledge, truncation of chromosome 13 in HUVEC has not yet been described, its loss has already been reported by others (51, 62, 63) and was accompanied by a growth advantage, i.e., leading to clonal expansion. Our data show that not only the complete deletion of chromosome 13 but also a deletion of a large part of the q-arm of chromosome 13 confers a growth advantage to the affected cells. Noteworthy, the q-arm of chromosome 13 harbors the Rb gene, encoding for the Rb protein, a well-known tumor suppressor and regulator of the cell cycle (64) that may account for an enhanced replication. As the number of cells with cytogenetic changes increased with time in irradiated cultures and the respective controls in a similar way, it is reasonable to assume that these cytogenetic changes are a feature of aging HUVEC that is barely affected by IR within the dose range examined (0.5–1.5 Gy). Moreover, our data revealed considerable inter-experimental differences in the number and types of aberrations in HUVEC cultures at CPD level 22 (see **Figure 4**; Table S2 in Supplementary Material). Pronounced inter-experimental differences in the aberration yield were also reported for other cell types, e.g., human foreskin fibroblasts and skin fibroblasts, subcultured up to CPD level 50 (41). Reasons underlying this phenomenon remain to be elucidated.

Taken together, our data point to a radiosensitivity for HUVEC directly after exposure to radiation, i.e., mainly by cell killing and even low or moderate doses as used in this study result in a reduced cellular survival. This is important if endothelial cell damage is taken into account as the initial step in the pathogenesis of arteriosclerosis (31). It was hypothesized that endothelial cell damage may trigger pro-inflammatory signals, which finally results in the enhanced formation of arteriosclerotic lesions [e.g., Ref. (6, 31)]. Yet, the link between radiation-induced damage and pro-inflammatory signaling remains poorly understood and requires further investigation. Since we found C-ions LET dependently more effective (RBE of 1.5 and 2.4 for 91 and 9.8 MeV/u C-ions, respectively) than X-rays, our results demonstrate the need of further studies in order to better estimate a putative risk of high-LET radiation.

AUTHOR CONTRIBUTIONS

AH, RL, MD, and SR have substantially contributed to the conception and design of the work, as well as the acquisition, analysis, and interpretation of the data.

ACKNOWLEDGMENTS

The authors acknowledge P. Hessel and D. Szypkowski for skillful assistance as well as M. Scholz, T. Friedrich, W. Becher, and G. Lenz for planning and realizing the particle exposure of cells.

REFERENCES

1. Darby SC, Ewertz M, McGale P, Bennet AM, Blom-Goldman U, Brønnum D, et al. Risk of ischemic heart disease in women after radiotherapy for breast cancer. *N Engl J Med* (2013) **368**:987–98. doi:10.1056/NEJMoa1209825

2. Aleman BMP, Moser EC, Nuver J, Suter TM, Maraldo MV, Specht L, et al. Cardiovascular disease after cancer therapy. *EJC Suppl* (2014) **12**:18–28. doi:10.1016/j.ejcsup.2014.03.002

3. Hodgson DC. Late effects in the era of modern therapy for Hodgkin lymphoma. *Hematology Am Soc Hematol Educ Program* (2011) **2011**:323–9. doi:10.1182/asheducation-2011.1.323

4. Lemanski C, Thariat J, Ampil FL, Bose S, Vock J, Davis R, et al. Image-guided radiotherapy for cardiac sparing in patients with left-sided breast cancer. *Front Oncol* (2014) **4**:257. doi:10.3389/fonc.2014.00257

5. Howe GR, Zablotska LB, Fix JJ, Egel J, Buchanan J. Analysis of the mortality experience amongst U. S. Nuclear Power Industry Workers after chronic low-dose exposure to ionizing radiation. *Radiat Res* (2004) **162**:517–26. doi:10.1667/RR3258

6. Little MP, Tawn EJ, Tzoulaki I, Wakeford R, Hildebrandt G, Paris F, et al. Review and meta-analysis of epidemiological associations between low/moderate doses of ionizing radiation and circulatory disease risks, and their possible mechanisms. *Radiat Environ Biophys* (2009) **49**:139–53. doi:10.1007/s00411-009-0250-z

7. Little MP. A review of non-cancer effects, especially circulatory and ocular diseases. *Radiat Environ Biophys* (2013) **52**:435–49. doi:10.1007/s00411-013-0484-7.A

8. Schultz-Hector S, Trott K-R. Radiation-induced cardiovascular diseases: is the epidemiologic evidence compatible with the radiobiologic data? *Int J Radiat Oncol Biol Phys* (2007) **67**:10–8. doi:10.1016/j.ijrobp.2006.08.071

9. Rader DJ, Daugherty A. Translating molecular discoveries into new therapies for atherosclerosis. *Nature* (2008) **451**:904–13. doi:10.1038/nature06796

10. Hoel DG. Ionizing radiation and cardiovascular disease. *Ann N Y Acad Sci* (2006) **1076**:309–17. doi:10.1196/annals.1371.001

11. Andreassi MG, Botto N. DNA damage as a new emerging risk factor in atherosclerosis. *Trends Cardiovasc Med* (2003) **13**:270–5. doi:10.1016/S1050-1738(03)00109-9

12. Di Lisa F, Kaludercic N, Carpi A, Menab R, Giorgio M. Mitochondria and vascular pathology. *Pharmacol Rep* (2009) **61**:123–30. doi:10.1016/S1734-1140(09)70014-3

13. Finsterer J. Is atherosclerosis a mitochondrial disorder? *Vasa* (2007) **36**:229–40. doi:10.1024/0301-1526.36.4.229

14. Ito TK, Yokoyama M, Yoshida Y, Nojima A, Kassai H, Oishi K, et al. A crucial role for CDC42 in senescence-associated inflammation and atherosclerosis. *PLoS One* (2014) **9**:e102186. doi:10.1371/journal.pone.0102186

15. Bert C, Engenhart-Cabillic R, Durante M. Particle therapy for noncancer diseases. *Med Phys* (2012) **39**:1716–27. doi:10.1118/1.3691903

16. Tsujii H, Kamada T. A review of update clinical results of carbon ion radiotherapy. *Jpn J Clin Oncol* (2012) **42**:670–85. doi:10.1093/jjco/hys104

17. Loeffler JS, Durante M. Charged particle therapy – optimization, challenges and future directions. *Nat Rev Clin Oncol* (2013) **10**:411–24. doi:10.1038/nrclinonc.2013.79

18. Takahashi Y, Teshima T, Kawaguchi N, Hamada Y, Mori S, Madachi A, et al. Heavy ion irradiation inhibits in vitro angiogenesis even at sublethal dose. *Cancer Res* (2003) **63**:4253–7.

19. Lanza V, Pretazzoli V, Olivieri G, Pascarella G, Panconesi A, Negri R. Transcriptional response of human umbilical vein endothelial cells to low doses of ionizing radiation. *J Radiat Res* (2005) **46**:265–76. doi:10.1269/jrr.46.265

20. Rombouts C, Aerts A, Beck M, De Vos WH, Van Oostveldt P, Benotmane MA, et al. Differential response to acute low dose radiation in primary and immortalized endothelial cells. *Int J Radiat Biol* (2013) **89**:841–50. doi:10.3109/09553002.2013.806831

21. Kraft G, Daues HW, Fischer B, Kopf U, Leibold S, Quis D, et al. Irradiation chamber and sample changes for biological samples. *Nucl Instrum Methods* (1980) **168**:175–9. doi:10.1016/0029-554X(80)91249-5

22. Kraft-Weyrather W, Kraft G, Ritter S, Scholz M, Stanton J. The preparation of biological targets for heavy-ion experiments up to 20 MeV/u. *Nucl Instrum Methods Phys Res A* (1989) **282**:22–7. doi:10.1016/0168-9002(89)90104-6

23. Haberer T, Becher W, Schardt D, Kraft G. Magnetic scanning system for heavy ion therapy. *Nucl Instrum Methods Phys Res A* (1993) **330**:296–305. doi:10.1016/0168-9002(93)91335-K

24. Franken NAP, Rodermond HM, Stap J, Haveman J, van Bree C. Clonogenic assay of cells in vitro. *Nat Protoc* (2006) **1**:2315–9. doi:10.1038/nprot.2006.339

25. Fenech M. The in vitro micronucleus technique. *Mutat Res* (2000) **455**:81–95. doi:10.1016/S0027-5107(00)00065-8

26. Meijer AE, Kronqvist U-SE, Lewensohn R, Harms-Ringdahl M. RBE for the induction of apoptosis in human peripheral lymphocytes exposed in vitro to high-LET radiation generated by accelerated nitrogen ions. *Int J Radiat Biol* (1998) **73**:169–77. doi:10.1080/095530098142554

27. Johnson VL, Ko SCW, Holmstrom TH, Eriksson JE, Chow SC. Effector caspases are dispensable for the early nuclear morphological changes during chemical-induced apoptosis. *J Cell Sci* (2000) **113**:2941–53.

28. Cosarizza A, Baccarani-Contri M, Kalashnikova G, Franceschi C. A new method for the cytofluorimetric analysis of mitochondrial membrane potential using the J-aggregate forming lipophilic cation 5,5',6,6'-tetra-chloro-1,1',3,3'-tetraethylbenzimidazolcarbocyanine iodide (JC-1). *Biochem Biophys Res Commun* (1993) **197**:40–5. doi:10.1006/bbrc.1993.2438

29. Cornforth M. Analyzing radiation-induced complex chromosome rearrangements by combinatorial painting. *Radiat Prot Dosimetry* (2001) **155**:643–59.

30. Hooning MJ, Botma A, Aleman BMP, Baaijens MHA, Bartelink H, Klijn JGM, et al. Long-term risk of cardiovascular disease in 10-year survivors of breast cancer. *J Natl Cancer Inst* (2007) **99**:365–75. doi:10.1093/jnci/djk064

31. Hendry JH, Akahoshi M, Wang LS, Lipshultz SE, Stewart FA, Trott KR. Radiation-induced cardiovascular injury. *Radiat Environ Biophys* (2008) **47**:189–93. doi:10.1007/s00411-007-0155-7

32. Chen Y-H, Pan S-L, Wang J-C, Kuo S-H, Cheng JC-H, Teng C-M. Radiation-induced VEGF-C expression and endothelial cell proliferation in lung cancer. *Strahlenther Onkol* (2014) **190**:1154–62. doi:10.1007/s00066-014-0708-z

33. Ebrahimian T, Le Gallic C, Stefani J, Dublineau I, Yentrapalli R, Harms-Ringdahl S, et al. Chronic gamma-irradiation induces a dose-rate-dependent pro-inflammatory response and associated loss of function in human umbilical vein endothelial cells. *Radiat Res* (2015) **183**:447–54. doi:10.1667/RR13732.1

34. Weyrather WK, Ritter S, Scholz M, Kraft G. RBE for carbon track-segment irradiation in cell lines of differing repair capacity. *Int J Radiat Biol* (1999) **75**:1357–64. doi:10.1080/095530099139232

35. Habermehl D, Ilicic K, Dehne S, Rieken S, Orschiedt L, Brons S, et al. The relative biological effectiveness for carbon and oxygen ion beams using the raster-scanning technique in hepatocellular carcinoma cell lines. *PLoS One* (2014) **9**:e113591. doi:10.1371/journal.pone.0113591

36. Hei TK, Marchese MJ, Hall EJ. Radiosensitivity and sublethal damage repair in human umbilical cord vein endothelial cells. *Int J Radiat Oncol Biol Phys* (1987) **13**:879–84. doi:10.1016/0360-3016(87)90103-9

37. Manti L, Durante M, Elsaesser T, Gialanella G, Pugliese M, Ritter S, et al. Premature senescence in human endothelial cells exposed to carbon ions. *GSI Sci Rep* (2007) **1**:350.

38. Raicu M, Vral A, Thierens H, De Ridder L. Radiation damage to endothelial cells in vitro, as judged by the micronucleus assay. *Mutagenesis* (1993) **8**:335–9. doi:10.1093/mutage/8.4.335

39. Laurent C, Voisin P, Pouget J-P. DNA damage in cultured skin microvascular endothelial cells exposed to gamma rays and treated by the combination pentoxifylline and alpha-tocopherol. *Int J Radiat Biol* (2006) **82**:309–21. doi:10.1080/09553000600733150

40. Morgan WF. Is there a common mechanism underlying genomic instability, bystander effects and other nontargeted effects of exposure to ionizing radiation? *Oncogene* (2003) **22**:7094–9. doi:10.1038/sj.onc.1206992

41. Zahnreich S, Melnikova L, Winter M, Nasonova E, Durante M, Ritter S, et al. Radiation-induced premature senescence is associated with specific cytogenetic changes. *Mutat Res* (2010) **701**:60–6. doi:10.1016/j.mrgentox.2010.03.010

42. Vavrova J, Rezacova M. The importance of senescence in ionizing radiation-induced tumour suppression. *Folia Biol (Praha)* (2011) **57**:41–6.

43. Shah DJ, Sachs RK, Wilson DJ. Radiation-induced cancer: a modern view. *Br J Radiol* (2012) **85**:1166–73. doi:10.1259/bjr/25026140

44. Yentrapalli R, Azimzadeh O, Sriharshan A, Malinowsky K, Merl J, Wojcik A, et al. The PI3K/Akt/mTOR pathway is implicated in the premature senescence of primary human endothelial cells exposed to chronic radiation. *PLoS One* (2013) **8**:e70024. doi:10.1371/journal.pone.0070024

45. Favero G, Paganelli C, Buffoli B, Rodella LF, Rezzani R. Endothelium and its alterations in cardiovascular diseases?: life style intervention. *Biomed Res Int* (2014) **2014**:801896. doi:10.1155/2014/801896

46. Dimri GP, Leet X, Basile G, Acosta M, Scorrt G, Roskelley C, et al. A biomarker that identifies senescent human cells in culture and in aging skin in vivo. *Proc Natl Acad Sci U S A* (1995) **92**:9363–7. doi:10.1073/pnas.92.20.9363

47. Grossi G, Bettega D, Calzolari P, Durante M, Elsässer T, Gialanella G, et al. Late cellular effects of 12 C ions. *Nuovo Cim* (2008) **31**:39–47. doi:10.1393/ncc/i2008-10278-4

48. Oh C, Bump EA, Kim J-S, Janigro D, Mayberg MR. Induction of a senescence-like phenotype in bovine aortic endothelial cells by ionizing radiation. *Radiat Res* (2001) **156**:232–40. doi:10.1667/0033-7587(2001)156[0232:IOASLP]2.0.CO;2

49. Igarashi K, Sakimoto I, Kataoka K, Ohta K, Miura M. Radiation-induced senescence-like phenotype in proliferating and plateau-phase vascular endothelial cells. *Exp Cell Res* (2007) **313**:3326–36. doi:10.1016/j.yexcr.2007.06.001

50. Kim KS, Kim JE, Choi KJ, Bae S, Kim DH. Characterization of DNA damage-induced cellular senescence by ionizing radiation in endothelial cells. *Int J Radiat Biol* (2014) **90**:71–80. doi:10.3109/09553002.2014.859763

51. Zhang L, Aviv H, Gardner JP, Okuda K, Patel S, Kimura M, et al. Loss of chromosome 13 in cultured human vascular endothelial cells. *Exp Cell Res* (2000) **260**:357–64. doi:10.1006/excr.2000.4997

52. Wagner M, Hampel B, Bernhard D, Hala M, Zwerschke W, Jansen-Dürr P. Replicative senescence of human endothelial cells in vitro involves G1 arrest, polyploidization and senescence-associated apoptosis. *Exp Gerontol* (2001) **36**:1327–47. doi:10.1016/S0531-5565(01)00105-X

53. Kim JH, Jenrow KA, Brown SL. Mechanisms of radiation-induced normal tissue toxicity and implications for future clinical trials. *Radiat Oncol J* (2014) **32**:103–15. doi:10.3857/roj.2014.32.3.103

54. Davidson SM, Duchen MR. Endothelial mitochondria: contributing to vascular function and disease. *Circ Res* (2007) **100**:1128–41. doi:10.1161/01.RES.0000261970.18328.1d

55. Donato AJ, Eskurza I, Silver AE, Levy AS, Pierce GL, Gates PE, et al. Direct evidence of endothelial oxidative stress with aging in humans: relation to impaired endothelium-dependent dilation and upregulation of nuclear factor-kappaB. *Circ Res* (2007) **100**:1659–66. doi:10.1161/01.RES.0000269183.13937.e8

56. Barjaktarovic Z, Schmaltz D, Shyla A, Azimzadeh O, Schulz S, Haagen J, et al. Radiation-induced signaling results in mitochondrial impairment in mouse heart at 4 weeks after exposure to X-rays. *PLoS One* (2011) **6**:e27811. doi:10.1371/journal.pone.0027811

57. Smiley ST, Reers M, Mottola-Hartshorn C, Lin M, Chen A, Smith TW, et al. Intracellular heterogeneity in mitochondrial membrane potentials revealed by a J-aggregate-forming lipophilic cation JC-1. *Proc Natl Acad Sci U S A* (1991) **88**:3671–5. doi:10.1073/pnas.88.9.3671

58. Lyng FM, Seymour CB, Mothersill C. Production of a signal by irradiated cells which leads to a response in unirradiated cells characteristic of initiation of apoptosis. *Br J Cancer* (2000) **83**:1223–30. doi:10.1054/bjoc.2000.1433

59. Wang W, Yang S, Su Y, Xiao Z, Wang C, Li X, et al. Enhanced antitumor effect of combined triptolide and ionizing radiation. *Clin Cancer Res* (2007) **13**:4891–9. doi:10.1158/1078-0432.CCR-07-0416

60. Nair S, Nair RRK, Srinivas P, Srinivas G, Pillai MR. Radiosensitizing effects of plumbagin in cervical cancer cells is through modulation of apoptotic pathway. *Mol Carcinog* (2008) **47**:22–33. doi:10.1002/mc

61. Samraj AK, Sohn D, Schulze-Osthoff K, Schmitz I. Loss of caspase-9 reveals its essential role for caspase-2 activation and mitochondrial membrane depolarization. *Mol Biol Cell* (2007) **18**:84–93. doi:10.1091/mbc.E06

62. Kimura M, Cao X, Patel S, Aviv A. Survival advantage of cultured human vascular endothelial cells that lost chromosome 13. *Chromosoma* (2004) **112**:317–22. doi:10.1007/s00412-004-0276-6

63. Anno K, Hayashi A, Takahashi T, Mitsui Y, Ide T, Tahara H. Telomerase activation induces elongation of the telomeric single-stranded overhang, but does not prevent chromosome aberrations in human vascular endothelial cells. *Biochem Biophys Res Commun* (2007) **353**:926–32. doi:10.1016/j.bbrc.2006.12.112

64. Giacinti C, Giordano A. RB and cell cycle progression. *Oncogene* (2006) **25**:5220–7. doi:10.1038/sj.onc.1209615

12

HZE Radiation Non-Targeted Effects on the Microenvironment that Mediate Mammary Carcinogenesis

Mary Helen Barcellos-Hoff[1] and Jian-Hua Mao[2]*

[1] Department of Radiation Oncology, University of California San Francisco, San Francisco, CA, USA, [2] Lawrence Berkeley National Laboratory, Berkeley, CA, USA

Correspondence:
Mary Helen Barcellos-Hoff
mary.barcellos-hoff@ucsf.edu

Clear mechanistic understanding of the biological processes elicited by radiation that increase cancer risk can be used to inform prediction of health consequences of medical uses, such as radiotherapy, or occupational exposures, such as those of astronauts during deep space travel. Here, we review the current concepts of carcinogenesis as a multicellular process during which transformed cells escape normal tissue controls, including the immune system, and establish a tumor microenvironment. We discuss the contribution of two broad classes of radiation effects that may increase cancer: radiation targeted effects that occur as a result of direct energy deposition, e.g., DNA damage, and non-targeted effects (NTE) that result from changes in cell signaling, e.g., genomic instability. It is unknown whether the potentially greater carcinogenic effect of high Z and energy (HZE) particle radiation is a function of the relative contribution or extent of NTE or due to unique NTE. We addressed this problem using a radiation/genetic mammary chimera mouse model of breast cancer. Our experiments suggest that NTE promote more aggressive cancers, as evidenced by increased growth rate, transcriptomic signatures, and metastasis, and that HZE particle NTE are more effective than reference γ-radiation. Emerging evidence suggest that HZE irradiation dampens antitumor immunity. These studies raise concern that HZE radiation exposure not only increases the likelihood of developing cancer but also could promote progression to more aggressive cancer with a greater risk of mortality.

Keywords: cosmic radiation, cancer risk models, ionizing radiation exposure, carcinogenesis process

Epidemiological data on radiation therapy, occupational exposures, and accidental or terrorist radiological events have established the carcinogenic potential of sparsely ionizing radiation that includes γ-rays and X-rays. Less is known about the carcinogenic potential of densely ionizing radiation from accelerated particles recently implemented in the clinic and that are of a concern for space flight. The galactic cosmic radiation environment consists of high atomic number (Z) and energy (HZE) charged particles that are characterized by high linear energy transfer (LET) along the particle track, i.e., densely ionizing, in contrast to most terrestrial low LET radiations that are sparsely ionizing. The unique pattern of energy deposition incurred by HZE particle traversal is of often the primary focus in evaluating the biological effects of the galactic cosmic radiation on astronauts (1, 2). During a 3-year flight in extra-magnetospheric space, 3% of the cells of the human body would be traversed on

---

Abbreviations: HZE, high Z and energy; LET, linear energy transfer; NTE, non-targeted effects; RBE, relative biological effect; RTE, radiation targeted effects; TGFβ, transforming growth factor β.

average by one Fe ion (3). Cancer risk from exposure to the deep space radiation environment could constrain mission parameters for astronauts. The cancer incidence following radiotherapy is low but significant late tissue effect and, though the favorable dose distribution that reduces dose to normal tissue is thought to provide protection, that of HZE particle radiotherapy is yet unknown.

High Z and energy particle radiation is of particular concern for cancer because the limited experimental data to date indicate that the relative biological effect (RBE) for densely ionizing HZE particles is several-to-many fold greater than sparsely ionizing radiation. HZE particles have a high RBE for many biological end points (4); however, some HZE biological effects are not observed following sparsely ionizing radiation (5) and some radiation effects, such as genomic instability, do not show classic dose dependence (6). As a consequence, measurements of individual biological events and their dose dependence do not describe how an organism will respond to radiation damage. HZE particles traversing a cell nucleus cause difficult to repair clustered DNA damage that is classified as a radiation targeted effects (RTE), i.e., due to the deposition of energy in the cell. Radiation exposure also elicits complex changes in signaling and phenotype, which are called non-targeted effects (NTE) because they are often observed in the neighbors or daughters of irradiated cells.

Radiation is classified as a complete carcinogen in the etiology of human tumors, including breast cancer, lung cancer, lymphoma, liver carcinoma, sarcoma, and glioma (7). Radiation-induced DNA damage elicits a rapid and efficient repair network, but the occasional misrepair of these lesions results in mutations, translocations, deletions, and amplifications, which are also hallmarks of cancer cells. Many risk models use the frequency of these RTE as the basis for estimating cancer risk. Such models assume that the probability of cancer is proportional to DNA damage and, hence, exposure, which is consistent with epidemiological association of cancer risk and polymorphisms in certain genes in the DNA repair pathway (8).

The risk paradigm broadly based on RTE, that is direct DNA damage, has been challenged by at least two classes of NTE: first, the demonstration that descendants of irradiated cells exhibit non-clonal damage (i.e., radiation-induced genomic instability) or altered phenotype; second, the designation of so-called "bystander" radiation effects, in which non-irradiated cells respond to signaling by irradiated cells (6). NTE can be functionally defined by particular experimental strategies (e.g., bystander experiments and media transfer) and occur by various mechanisms that involve gap junctions, soluble factors, and phenotypic transition that differ between cell types and between *in vitro* and *in vivo* models.

The crucial question is to determine under what conditions and to what extent NTE contribute to human health risks. Recent experimental studies of radiation carcinogenesis following low- and high LET radiation exposures are concerned with how complex organismal responses to radiation interact across levels of organization and time scales to impede or promote malignant processes (9). Mechanistic understanding of cancer has become much more detailed over the last two decades. There is growing recognition that cancer as a disease results from a systemic failure, in which many cells other than those with oncogenic genomes determine the frequency of clinical cancer (10). The challenge to predicting health effects in irradiated humans is to understand how complex radiation responses culminate in pathology.

CARCINOGENESIS IN CONTEXT

The understanding of cancer as a result of systemic failure, in which many cells other than those with oncogenic mutations/alterations determine the frequency and characteristics of clinical cancer, underscores tissue dysfunction, in which cancer cells are highly intertwined with the microenvironment (11, 12). Both tissue and organismal biology are subverted during malignant progression (13). More than a quarter of a century ago, studies by Mintz and Pierce demonstrated that malignancy could be suppressed by contact with normal tissues (14, 15). Many have even argued that disruption of the cell interactions and tissue architecture can be the primary drivers of carcinogenesis (16–20). Recent experiments with engineered models have focused on identifying the type and means by which normal cells mediate the development of cancer (21–24), but it is clear that host cells, e.g., stromal cells and bone marrow-derived cells (BMDC), sculpt carcinogenesis in a complex process that can either eliminate or accelerate malignancy.

Recent studies demonstrate that host biology is altered even before cancer is evident. A systems biology approach by Hanash and colleagues characterized the plasma proteome response in the inducible HER2/neu mouse model of breast cancer during tumor induction, progression, and regression. Mass spectrometry data derived from approximately 1.6 million spectra identified protein networks associated with tumor development. Some networks were derived from the tumor microenvironment and some from tumor cell secreted or shed proteins. The observed alterations developed prior to cancer detection, increased progressively with tumor growth, and reverted toward baseline with tumor regression. Importantly, these findings were mirrored with findings resulting from in-depth profiling of circulating proteins using prediagnostic plasma samples from women who participated in the Women's Health Initiative study and who subsequently developed breast cancer (25–27).

Although the prevailing radiation health paradigm focuses on radiation-induced DNA damage leading to mutations, numerous studies over the last 50 years have provided evidence that radiation carcinogenesis is more complex than generally appreciated [reviewed in Ref. (28)]. Terzaghi-Howe demonstrated that the expression of dysplasia *in vivo* and neoplastic transformation in culture of irradiated tracheal epithelial cells is inversely correlated to the number of cells seeded (29–32) and identified TGFβ as a key mediator (33). Our lab used a *Trp53* mutant mammary cell line to show that irradiating only the host increased the development of frank tumors fivefold (34). Saran and colleagues showed that partial body irradiation at a young age promotes *Ptch* mutant medulloblastoma (35).

Many studies using oncogenic mouse models indicate that the stroma is highly involved in early malignancy (36), which supports the idea of reciprocal evolution of the malignant cell and the tumor microenvironment (10). Although it is clear that stroma composition and signaling is altered in human breast cancer (37), less is known about how and when stroma contributes to carcinogenesis and how carcinogens, such as radiation, might alter these processes. We postulate that the tumor microenvironment is built through rate-limiting steps of construction, expansion, and maturation that parallel initiation, promotion, and progression during multistage carcinogenesis (10). Construction of a "pre-cancer niche" is the necessary first step to generate a tumor microenvironment that is essential for initiated cells to survive and evolve into clinically evident cancers (**Figure 1**). The evolution of the tumor microenvironment *via* stromal cells and BMDC during subsequent niche expansion during promotion is mediated by cytokines secreted by either the initiated epithelial cells or those host cells recruited to the niche. Maturation of the tumor microenvironment, as evidenced by angiogenesis escape from immune suppression and generation of a stroma permissive for growth and often invasion, occurs during progression. Importantly, signaling is not just local but can also be mediated by cells, cytokines, and exosomes transported

by the vasculature between the nascent cancer and distant sites include the bone marrow, which may reciprocate by expansion of cells, such as immature myeloid cells (IMC) that support tumor growth. Indeed, the pre-metastatic niche, first described by Lyden and colleagues, pre-dates and facilitates metastatic disease (38).

This model postulates that cancer survival and proliferation is as much a function of the successful niche construction as it is of specific cancer cell mutations. Indeed selective pressure for neoplastic mutations may be imposed by the composition of the niche, as well as by immune editing (39). Consequently, cancer represents an emergent property that requires a comprehensive analysis of the cell–cell interactions in the entire niche. Moreover, in contrast to initiation, which is a stochastic process by nature, niche construction represents a robust target for native immunosuppression and a potent target for cancer prevention. If microenvironments induced by radiation can promote neoplastic progression in unirradiated epithelial cells, events outside of the (targeted) box may significantly increase cancer risk. Understanding such non-targeted mechanisms readily lead

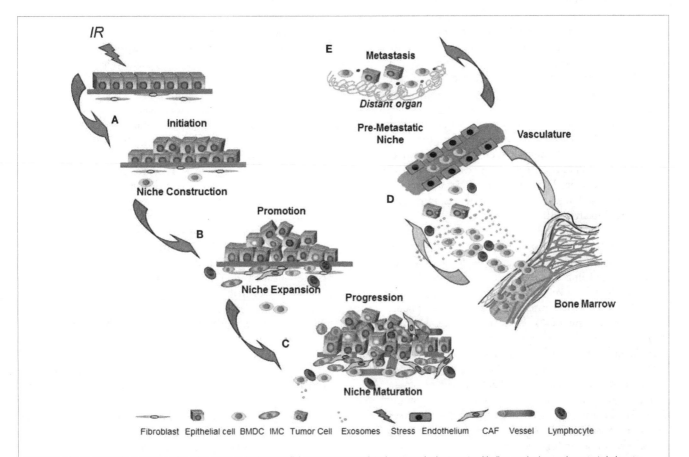

FIGURE 1 | The dynamic cancer niche. The cartoon depicts parallel processes postulated to occur in the target epithelium and microenvironment during multistage epithelial carcinogenesis. **(A)** Misrepaired DNA damage caused by radiation can malignantly *initiate* epithelial cells. Radiation effects on cell signaling and phenotype may promote concomitant niche *construction* by local or systemically recruited cells that improve initiated cell survival. **(B)** Within the epithelium, *promotion* is considered to be acquisition of additional genetic aberrations or epigenetic traits that enable malignancy. In parallel, niche *expansion*, due to signals produced by either the initiated epithelium or by the niche cells that support them, conscripts stromal cells and bone marrow-derived cells (BMDC). **(C)** *Maturation* of the tumor microenvironment that enables angiogenesis, immune suppression, and invasion is necessary for tumor *progression*. **(D)** Systemic influences, including signaling to and from *vasculature* and *bone marrow*, contribute throughout multistage carcinogenesis *via* participation of BMDC, lymphocytes, and immature myeloid cells (IMC) and their secreted cytokines and exosomes. **(E)** Some cancers are able to initiate new microenvironments, the *pre-metastatic niche*, in distant organs that facilitate *metastasis*.

to potential mechanisms for clinical interventions for health risks in future populations.

MODELING RADIATION CARCINOGENESIS

Most models of cancer risk and mitigation are focused on "targets," i.e., the cells that will undergo neoplastic transformation or the genetic alterations that initiate and promote this event. This is classically modeled in which carcinogenesis is thought to occur in four interdependent stages. The first stage is *initiation* and is typically caused by chemical, physical, or biological agents, which irreversibly and heritably alter the cell genome resulting in an enhanced growth potential. This potential is only realized, however, if the cell later undergoes *promotion*, the second stage of carcinogenesis. *Promotion* is often thought to be the rate-limiting step in carcinogenesis since it has been shown that initiation alone is not sufficient to induce cancer (40). In order to account for the observed power of age dependence in radiation-induced carcinomas, a multistage theory of carcinogenesis was introduced very early (41, 42). However, this model suggested five to seven rate-limiting stages, in contradiction with biological data. Some approaches addressed this contradiction by introducing the two-stage clonal expansion model, where a cell leads to a tumor by two separate mutations and clonal expansion (43–45). Integration of specific genetic mutations in tumor suppressor genes was originally introduced by Knudson (46). The current paradigm of carcinogenic risk remains heavily focused on predicting mutations of the genome leading to silencing of tumor suppressor genes or activation of oncogenes. However, such models neglect the influence of intercellular and extracellular interactions in the tumor growth and predict a final tumor that is unrealistic in that its cells are clonally identical.

Systems radiation biology seeks to integrate information about changes across time and scale that are determined by experimentation and to interrogate this to identify the critical events. By modeling the irradiated tissue/organ/organism as a system rather than a collection of non-interacting or minimally interacting cells, cancer can result as an emergent phenomenon of a perturbed system (47). A biological model in which radiation risk is the sum of dynamic and interacting processes could provide the impetus to reassess assumptions about radiation health effects in a healthy population and spur new approaches to prevent detrimental processes that lead to pathology.

Our studies have addressed this problem by separating RTE from NTE by using the mammary gland as a model system. The mouse mammary gland provides an experimentally malleable framework for separating the contribution of NTE on the host from the target epithelium. Mammary gland develops during the postnatal period such that the epithelium can be surgically removed and replaced, creating a tissue chimera. Transplanted syngeneic epithelium can have a specific germ line manipulation, such as a transgene or knockout, or can have received a specific type of exposure, such as radiation. We transplant *unirradiated Trp53 null* mouse mammary tissue into *irradiated* syngeneic wild-type hosts to study whether radiation NTE acting *via* the host affects the process of epithelial carcinogenesis. The *p53 null* mammary model originally described by Medina and colleagues has important features in common with human breast cancer (48). Although about a quarter of human breast cancers have p53 mutations, the utility of this model is that *Trp53 null* mouse mammary tissue develops normally until about 8 months of age, when both ductal carcinoma *in situ* and aneuploidy are evident, thus reproducing the long latency and early instability observed in most human breast cancers. Importantly, the *p53 null* tissue gives rise to histologically heterogeneous tumors that can be estrogen receptor negative or positive and genomically diverse, as are human breast cancers. Thus, the model of an oncogenically primed epithelium lacking p53 condenses the time necessary for spontaneous mutagenic events to accumulate.

The radiation-genetic chimera is used to determine whether and how radiation NTE contribute to mammary carcinogenesis (49). These data from provide strong support that NTE do contribute to radiation carcinogenesis and offer new insight into radiation quality effects that promote aggressive tumors, particularly upon exposure in middle age. Our studies summarized here have identified NTE-mediated mechanisms that include stem cell regulation, inflammation, and immune suppression that are important in determining the rate at which cancers develop and the type of cancer depends on radiation quality and genetic background.

The radiation chimera shows that NTE act *via* the microenvironment to accelerate tumorigenesis and affect critical characteristics (49). A notable observation was that the frequency of ER-negative tumors significantly doubled in irradiated hosts, which was replicated with HZE particle irradiation (50). Importantly, early radiation exposure increased ER-negative tumors in women treated with radiation for childhood cancer fourfold compared to a consecutive series of breast cancers not preceded by radiation (51). A new study by Horst and colleagues confirmed that radiation-preceded breast cancer in survivors of childhood cancer is significantly more likely to the aggressive, the so-called triple negative (negative for ER, progesterone receptor, and amplification of HER2) breast cancer (52). Interestingly, there is little evidence that the frequency of contralateral ER-negative breast cancer is increased in women treated with radiation for breast cancer (53), suggesting a physiological basis for the shift to ER-negative tumors, which are clinically less responsive and more likely to metastasize soon after detection.

To further explore how tumors arising in irradiated hosts are distinct from those that occur in non-irradiated hosts, we profiled total RNA from mammary cancers that arose in non-irradiated mice and irradiated mice (49). Permutation analysis was used to identify 156 genes that segregated tumors from irradiated or non-irradiated hosts. Significant enrichment of genes-involving leukocyte chemo-attraction and binding, monocyte maturation, and proliferation of tumor cell lines underscores the parallels between tumors forming in irradiated host and expression programs activated shortly after radiation exposure, even though the exposure occurred months before and the tumors arose from *unirradiated* epithelium.

We then used this strategy to generate a list of 323 genes and an irradiated host metaprofile (54). Bioinformatics analysis of the human orthologs of the host irradiation metaprofile was used to conduct unsupervised hierarchical clustering of radiation-associated human cancer (54). The irradiated host metaprofile segregated sporadic cancers from radiation-preceded sarcomas (55) and radiation-preceded papillary thyroid carcinomas (56). These analyses support our hypothesis that the microenvironment mediates the development of radiation-preceded human cancers.

Four gene networks representing two cell types, stem cells and macrophages, and two processes, motility and autophagy, were identified in the irradiated host tumor signature. Tissue-specific stem cells or early progenitor cells are considered to be the critical cellular target in carcinogenesis (57–63), based, in part, on the idea that stem cell transformation can lead to unlimited progeny. A mammary stem cell (MaSC) signature, defined by Visvader and colleagues (64), is enriched in the mammary gland up to 1 month after mice are exposed to 10-cGy γ-radiation. We showed this signature is functional as indicated by a doubling of mammary repopulation capacity as well as the pool of cells defined by cell surface markers as associated with mammary repopulation (49). Additional experiments in conjunction with computational modeling led us to conclude that radiation elicits a durable but transient stem cell expansion in a TGFβ and Notch-dependent fashion in juveniles, but not adults (50). In model systems, we found that TGFβ increases self-renewal is blocked by γ-secretase inhibition, indicative of concomitant Notch signaling, which is also induced by low-dose irradiation. This temporary increase in self-renewal is similar to our earlier studies showing that both high- and low LET radiation exposure primes non-malignant human epithelial cells to undergo TGFβ-dependent epithelial–mesenchymal transition (65–67). These studies underscore that even a single radiation exposure can cause phenotypic re-programing.

CANCER AND INFLAMMATION

The concept that inflammatory responses are necessary components of cancer development has recently been formalized by Mantovani et al. (68) in a two-pathway model: the intrinsic versus extrinsic. In the intrinsic pathway, genetic mutations lead to release by the transformed cells of proinflammatory factors recruiting innate immune cells. For example, oncogenic *Ras* activates the transcription of the inflammatory cytokine interleukin 8 (IL-8). Other oncogenes, such as *Bcl2*, inhibit apoptosis leading to necrotic tumor cell death and release of damage-associated molecular pattern molecules that activate innate immune cells *via* toll-like receptors (68, 69). In both circumstances, the resulting host response is a smoldering inflammation that promotes tumor growth and invasion (68, 70). In the extrinsic pathway, the chronic inflammation results from inability of the immune system to resolve an infection (e.g., hepatitis B) or from a dysregulated immune response as in autoimmune diseases (e.g., inflammatory bowel disease). The persistent inflammation cooperates with pre-existing oncogenic mutations by providing the microenvironment that promotes cancer progression, but it may also induce DNA damage resulting in the acquisition of new mutations (71, 72).

The innate immune system functions as an "interpreter" of tissue damage that not only provides a first line of defense but also translates the information to wound repair and defense systems in the body by stimulating angiogenesis and activating adaptive immunity. Therefore, it is not surprising that various types of innate immune cells have been found as part of the tumor inflammatory infiltrate. Macrophages play a central role in most solid malignancies, and most studies have found that macrophage abundance, increased microvessel density, and reduced patient survival are highly correlated (73). In fact, macrophages present within tumors are defined as tumor-associated macrophages to denote a specific phenotype that is associated with the production of several proangiogenic factors and cytokines that suppress antitumor immune responses and promote tumor growth by maintaining protumorigenic inflammation.

The application of systems biology by Balmain and colleagues uncovered a differential hub for inflammation in skin cancer (74). While a positive association exists between chronic inflammation and cancer, the innate immune system is itself a network that can be disrupted by both positive and negative stimuli. Anti-inflammatory drugs can have contradictory effects on skin tumor development (75, 76), and over-expression of proinflammatory cytokines, such as IL-1, can prevent skin tumor formation in mouse models of chemically induced skin cancer (77). In contrast, germline deletion of TNF-α, another potent proinflammatory cytokine, also confers resistance to skin tumor formation (78). The role of inflammation in cancer is, therefore, very complex, with different consequences associated with acute or chronic inflammatory conditions.

How the interplay between inflammatory cells and genetically mutated neoplastic cells promotes cancer development and progression remains a subject of intense investigation. Several important pathways have been identified. Among them, IL-6 signaling pathways play a major role (79). Macrophages are the main source of IL-6 during acute inflammation and T cells during chronic inflammation. Importantly, IL-6 orchestrates the transition from acute inflammation, dominated by granulocytes, to chronic inflammation, dominated by monocytes/macrophages and regulates, together with TGFβ, the differentiation of naïve T cells to Th17 proinflammatory phenotype, thus influencing the type of adaptive immune response (80).

Seminal studies by Wright and colleagues identified non-clonal radiation induced genomic instability in hematopoietic stem cells [reviewed in Ref. (6)], which they now explain as a result of altered cell interactions. Macrophages from irradiated mice could induce chromosomal instability in non-irradiated hematopoietic cells *via* production of TNFα and reactive oxygen and nitrogen species (81). Further studies showed that this effect was a function of mouse genotype, which affects the steady state M1 or M2 macrophage phenotype, which radiation exposure further amplifies (82). HZE particle NTE on inflammatory processes is supported by studies from Burns and colleagues who showed that chronic dietary exposure to vitamin A acetate can prevent almost all malignant and benign tumors that occur in rat skin exposed to electron radiation and most of those following ^{56}Fe ion irradiation (83). Gene expression analysis suggested that vitamin A reduced or blocked ^{56}Fe ion radiation-induced inflammation-related genes that were represented in the categories of "immune response," "response to stress," "signal transduction," and "response to biotic stress" (84).

To investigate systemic effects of HZE, the *Trp53* null mammary radiation-chimera model was irradiated with low fluences (equivalent to average dose of 11, 30, and 81 cGy) of 350 MeV/amu ^{26}Si particles and compared to contemporaneous γ-irradiated (100 cGy) and sham-irradiated mice (85). The median time to tumor detection in mice irradiated with the lowest ^{26}Si fluence or γ-radiation was similar to that in sham-irradiated mice but decreased for transplants in mice exposed to higher fluences of ^{26}Si particles. As previously reported, the growth rate of tumors arising in irradiated mice was increased compared to those arising in sham-irradiated mice but was significantly faster than high fluence Si-irradiated mice compared to γ-irradiated mice. Since the initial growth rate of tumors arising in hosts irradiated with 11-cGy ^{26}Si particles was comparable to that of tumors arising in mice irradiated with 100 cGy sparsely ionizing γ-rays, we concluded that there is an RBE of about 10 for this endpoint.

The carcinoma spectrum arising in mice exposed to ^{26}Si particles is enriched for a subclass that is ER-negative and keratin 18-positive. These tumors in Si-irradiated mice developed metastases twice as often as non-irradiated mice. As ^{26}Si irradiation of hosts primarily promotes specific ER-negative subtypes, genomic analysis of these tumors compared to a comparable group from sham-irradiated mice. Consistent with these differences, an expression profile that distinguished K18 tumors arising in ^{26}Si-irradiated compared sham-irradiated mice was enriched in MaSC, stroma, and Notch signaling genes. These data suggest that the carcinogenic effects of NTE from densely ionizing radiation compared to sparsely ionizing radiation elicit more aggressive tumors. In humans, the type, the density, and the location of immune cells within the tumor are strongly associated with prognosis (86). Together, these data support the hypothesis that radiogenic cancer risk is augmented by alterations in a network of cellular interactions, at the center of which is the innate immune system.

IMMUNE SURVEILLANCE AND SUPPRESSION

A fundamental role of the immune system is enforcing tissue homeostasis, a task accomplished by mounting inflammatory reactions that involve the coordinated activation of innate and adaptive immune cells. Radiation perturbs tissue homeostasis by activating inflammatory reactions that often do not resolve, leading to a vicious cycle of subclinical tissue damage and smoldering inflammation (87, 88). Whereas one body of work has clearly established the capacity of chronic inflammation to initiate and promote cancer (88), other studies have revealed that an intact immune system can prevent/control and shape cancer by a process best conceptualized in the "cancer immunoediting" theory (89). During initial clonal expansion, recognition of the stressed transformed cells by innate immune cells results in production of interferon-γ, a cytokine shown to play a key role in immunosurveillance against tumors (90, 91). Killing of the preneoplastic cells by natural killer cells or macrophages activated by IFN-γ to produce cytocidal reactive oxygen and nitrogen

species eventually leads to cross-presentation by dendritic cells of antigens from the dying tumor cells to T cells and activation of the adaptive immune system. The tumor-specific T cells may be able to destroy completely the incipient tumor, thus functioning as an extrinsic tumor suppressor mechanism that reduces the incidence of spontaneous and carcinogen-induced tumors, something for which there is unequivocal evidence in experimental models and supportive evidence in humans [reviewed in Ref. (39, 92)].

However, if complete elimination of transformed cells is not achieved, the immunological pressure results in selection of clones of cells that have acquired mutations or epigenetic changes conferring resistance to immune rejection, i.e., are "edited" by the immune system to select for those that are poorly immunogenic. This transition from elimination to escape can occur directly or even after a very long period of equilibrium, during which the immune response actively limits progression. The concept of equilibrium, which was initially formulated to explain clinical observations of occult tumors and tumor dormancy (93, 94), has been confirmed in experimental models showing that depletion of T cells leads to growth of occult tumors (95). Importantly, pro-tumorigenic inflammation and antitumor immunity can co-exist in the same tumor, and interventions that can alter the balance in favor of one or the other may either accelerate or hinder tumor growth (88).

We found that lymphocyte infiltrate of *Trp53* null tumors arising in the irradiated mammary chimera correlates to tumor growth rate, i.e., faster growing tumors have less lymphocytic infiltrate, and that particle irradiation elicits the most rapidly growing tumors. This observation suggests that HZE particles have a systemic impact on the immune surveillance that leads to the development of more aggressive tumors.

GENETIC MEDIATORS OF CANCER

Epidemiological and genetic studies show that there is a strong genetic component that contributes to the differences between individuals in their response to DNA damage and cancer susceptibility (96, 97). High penetrance mutations in genes, such as BRCA1/2, are responsible for a proportion of cancers that show familial aggregation (98). However, the genetic basis of susceptibility to the majority of cancers that have no obvious familial aggregation is almost completely unknown (96, 99). Most studies to identify susceptibility loci for radiation-associated cancer are limited to candidate genes involved in response to DNA damage, but there is strong evidence that other processes are important; systems genetics seeks to uncover those components that result from complex interactions between pathways and cells.

Systems genetics, unlike traditional approaches to the analysis of disease that focus on single genes or proteins in isolation, attempts to integrate the complex interaction of many kinds of genetic and biological information – genomic DNA sequence, mRNA, and protein expression, and link these to disease phenotypes. Human studies have demonstrated strong associations between polymorphic variation and regulation of gene expression (100–102). Parallel studies in mice offer many advantages for the study of the genetic basis of complex traits. The ability to control genetic background and to carry out crosses between mouse strains differing in their propensity to develop these diseases offers unprecedented opportunities to identify and investigate the primary genetic loci that control susceptibility. In addition, studies with mice allow precise exposures, standardized husbandry to control other environmental components of risk, and comprehensive analysis of phenotypes.

Applying these approaches to mouse strains with differing susceptibility to diseases identifies signaling hubs that may be important targets for therapy or prevention (103). A systems genetics approach consists of a network view of the genetic and gene expression architecture of normal host tissues that are compared after perturbation by radiation or tumor development (104, 105). An example of this strategy used gene expression profiles of skin from a population of *mus spretus* backcrossed to *mus musculus* mice to reveal the normal skin gene expression motifs associated with sensitivity to carcinogen-induced skin tumor development in contrast to those that were resistant. This analysis revealed both cell-autonomous (cell cycle and stem cell lineage) and non-cell-autonomous (inflammation and innate immunity) components that were differentially expressed in the susceptible animals. Interestingly, the highly susceptible mice exhibited increased levels of anti-inflammatory genes within the inflammation associated network, leading to the conclusion that chronic and acute inflammation are, respectively, tumor-promoting versus suppressive (106).

Multiple tumor types in mice, including thymomas, soft tissue sarcomas, and osteosarcomas, can be induced by exposure to low LET radiation, but induction is typically infrequent and tumors have long latency (i.e., survival time post-radiation). Engineered loss or misregulation of p53 increases the detection sensitivity. Radiation induces the same spectrum of tumors in p53-deficient mice that lack one or both p53 alleles; however, the survival time is dramatically reduced after a single exposure to ionizing radiation (107). Likewise, the *Trp53* null BALB/c inbred mouse strain is sensitive to mammary carcinogenesis, and radiation exposure enhances this susceptibility (108–110). The utility of this model is that tumors are diverse by all criteria, markers, histology, metastatic capacity, and genomic profiling, in a fashion that is remarkably aligned with human breast cancer (48, 111).

Recent experiments focus on the genetic contribution to NTE using the mammary chimera (112). Radioresistant SPRET/EiJ was mated to radiosensitive (BALB/c) mice, and then the progeny were backcrossed to BALB/c to generate F1 backcrossed mice (F1Bx). Our prior experiments using inbred BALB/c mice showed that host irradiation decreased *Trp53* null tumor latency, increased frequency of tumor formation at a year post-transplantation, and that tumors arising in irradiated hosts grew more rapidly (49). Consistent with our previous observations, the growth rate of *Trp53* null mammary carcinomas was greater in irradiated F1Bx host mice, a feature associated with aggressive tumors, compared to unirradiated mice. However, *Trp53* null tumor latency increased in irradiated hosts and tumor frequency was reduced by 9.6% ($p = 0.04$) at 18 months posttransplantation compared to sham-irradiated F1Bx hosts. The revelation that NTE delay rather than accelerate mammary cancers in genetically diverse hosts underscores the outcome of radiation exposure in terms of carcinogenesis depends of genetic background.

Introgression was used to determine the genetic loci that affected *Trp53* null mammary tumor latency of the radioresistant SPRET/EiJ genome using genome-wide genotyping. Only two loci were associated with tumor latency in sham-irradiated mice. Tumors in mice homozygous for the BALB/c allele at loci on chromosomes 2 and 14 appeared with a significantly shorter latency than those mice, in which one allele was from BALB/c and the other from SPRET/EiJ at these loci. Interestingly, neither of the loci affected latency in irradiated hosts. In contrast, 15 genetic loci were associated with tumor latency in irradiated mice, 11 alleles confer resistance to tumor development, and 4 alleles conferred susceptibility.

Together, the use of systems genetics with the radiation-chimera model provides new insight into the processes that mediate carcinogenic susceptibility to radiation. To further explore stromal genetic associations with cancer risk after exposure to low LET radiation, we used ingenuity pathway analysis (IPA) to identify 696 candidate genes located within the identified loci. Of these, 185 genes were within 4 loci on chromosomes 2, 11, 14, and 16 where homozygous BALB/C alleles associate with increased latency for cancer arising in irradiated mice. These genes were enriched in four pathways, γ-glutamyl cycle, leukotriene biosynthesis, alanine biosynthesis III, and glutathione biosynthesis. In contrast, 511 genes enriched for 24 pathways were within 11 regions where heterozygous SPRET/EiJ alleles associate with increased latency. Importantly, these 11 loci were enriched for genes involved in regulating the immune response including signaling pathways of natural killer cells and cytokines. Radiation-induced activation of pathways that control release of inflammatory cytokines varies among mouse strains (113, 114) and is postulated to contribute to genetic susceptibility to radiation-induced leukemia (113). Analysis of the upstream regulators of these candidate genes indicated that the TGFβ and p53 pathways might also be involved in mammary tumor susceptibility.

The observation that many more genetic loci are linked with tumor latency in the radiation-treated cohort than in the sham-irradiated cohort suggests the interesting idea that genetic contribution is actually specific to NTE, in contrast to the widely held belief that radiation exaggerates inherent susceptibility. This is exemplified by the work of Onel and colleagues who identified PRDM1 (Blimp-1), a transcriptional regulator of cell specification, with the risk of second malignancies only in those treated with radiation for childhood malignancy (115). In individuals with the homozygous protective allele, the incidence of second cancers is 3:100 by 30 years after exposure, whereas in those who were homozygous for the allele, risk is 1:3. Thus, the risk allele conferred risk comparable to BRCA1 mutation, but only in the context of radiation.

SUMMARY

Identifying mechanisms of NTE is essential to understand the biology of irradiated tissues. Two fundamental aspects of NTE in carcinogenesis warrant careful consideration for further understanding of cancer risk in irradiated populations. First is that radiation NTE may alter the shape of the dose response. Recent modeling by Cucinotta and colleagues suggest that NTE may be particularly important in the low-dose region of concern for occupational exposures. Second, NTE are targetable; the biology that ensues after exposure is persistent and may be "reset" after the fact to limit carcinogenic potential. This offers the possibility of protecting those at greatest risk, for example, children who are treated with charged particles for childhood malignancy, in which the clear benefit of dose distribution may come at the price of long-term cancer risk. Moreover, NTE will likely provide insight into the use of particles for cancer therapy as there are common microenvironment components, such as the immunoregulatory axis and the vasculature, that are likely critical to treatment outcome.

AUTHOR CONTRIBUTIONS

Dr. MHB-H outlined and wrote the manuscript. Dr. J-HM edited and contributed to this manuscript.

FUNDING

NNX13AF06G, Barcellos-Hoff, Mary Helen: 10/01/2012–01/30/2016. National Aeronautics and Space Agency: HZE radiation effects on malignant progression in human epithelial cells. Little is known about the mechanisms that underlie the greater biological effectiveness of high LET irradiation to promote solid cancer in experimental models. We hypothesize that both genetic and phenotypic changes contribute to radiation carcinogenesis. Role: P.I.

REFERENCES

1. Fry RJM, Nachtwey DS. Radiation protection guidelines for space missions. *Health Phys* (1988) 55:159–64. doi:10.1097/00004032-198808000-00006
2. Todd P. Unique biological aspects of radiation hazards – an overview. *Adv Space Res* (1983) 3:187–94. doi:10.1016/0273-1177(83)90189-8
3. Curtis SB, Letaw JR. Galactic cosmic rays and cell-hit frequencies outside the magnetosphere. *Adv Space Res* (1989) 9:292–8. doi:10.1016/0273-1177(89)90452-3
4. Blakely EA, Kronenberg A. Heavy-ion radiobiology: new approaches to delineate mechanisms underlying enhanced biological effectiveness. *Radiat Res* (1998) 150:S126–45. doi:10.2307/3579815
5. Costes S, Streuli CH, Barcellos-Hoff MH. Quantitative image analysis of laminin immunoreactivity in skin basement membrane irradiated with 1 GeV/nucleon iron particles. *Radiat Res* (2000) 154:389–97. doi:10.1667/0033-7587(2000)154[0389:QIAOLI]2.0.CO;2
6. Lorimore SA, Coates PJ, Wright EG. Radiation-induced genomic instability and bystander effects: inter-related nontargeted effects of exposure to ionizing radiation. *Oncogene* (2003) 22:7058–69. doi:10.1038/sj.onc.1207044
7. Preston DL, Ron E, Tokuoka S, Funamoto S, Nishi N, Soda M, et al. Solid cancer incidence in atomic bomb survivors: 1958-1998. *Radiat Res* (2007) 168:1–64. doi:10.1667/RR0763.1
8. Smith TR, Levine EA, Perrier ND, Miller MS, Freimanis RI, Lohman K, et al. DNA-repair genetic polymorphisms and breast cancer risk. *Cancer Epidemiol Biomarkers Prev* (2003) 12:1200–4.
9. Barcellos-Hoff MH, Adams C, Balmain A, Costes SV, Demaria S, Illa-Bochaca I, et al. Systems biology perspectives on the carcinogenic potential of radiation. *J Radiat Res* (2014) 55:i145–54. doi:10.1093/jrr/rrt211
10. Barcellos-Hoff MH, Lyden D, Wang TC. The evolution of the cancer niche during multistage carcinogenesis. *Nat Rev Cancer* (2013) 13:511–8. doi:10.1038/nrc3536
11. Bissell MJ, Radisky D, Rizki A, Weaver VM, Petersen OW. The organizing principle: microenvironmental influences in the normal and malignant breast. *Differentiation* (2002) 70:537–46. doi:10.1046/j.1432-0436.2002.700907.x
12. Barcellos-Hoff MH, Medina D. New highlights on stroma-epithelial interactions in breast cancer. *Breast Cancer Res* (2005) 7:33–6. doi:10.1186/bcr972
13. Coussens LM, Werb Z. Inflammatory cells and cancer: think different! *J Exp Med* (2001) 193:23F–6F. doi:10.1084/jem.193.6.F23
14. Mintz B, Illmensee K. Normal genetically mosaic mice produced from malignant teratocarcinoma cells. *Proc Natl Acad Sci U S A* (1975) 72:3585–9. doi:10.1073/pnas.72.9.3585
15. Pierce GB, Shikes R, Fink LM. *Cancer: A Problem of Developmental Biology*. Englewood Cliffs: Prentice-Hall, Inc. (1978).
16. Rubin H. Cancer as a dynamic developmental disorder. *Cancer Res* (1985) 45:2935–42.
17. Barcellos-Hoff MH. The potential influence of radiation-induced microenvironments in neoplastic progression. *J Mammary Gland Biol Neoplasia* (1998) 3:165–75. doi:10.1023/A:1018794806635

18. Sonnenschein C, Soto AM. Somatic mutation theory of carcinogenesis: why it should be dropped and replaced. *Mol Carcinog* (2000) 29:205–11. doi:10.1002/1098-2744(200012)29:4<205::AID-MC1002>3.0.CO;2-W
19. Bissell MJ, Radisky D. Putting tumours in context. *Nat Rev Cancer* (2001) 1:1–11. doi:10.1038/35094059
20. Wiseman BS, Werb Z. Stromal effects on mammary gland development and breast cancer. *Science* (2002) 296:1046–9. doi:10.1126/science.1067431
21. Kuperwasser C, Chavarria T, Wu M, Magrane G, Gray JW, Carey L, et al. From the cover: reconstruction of functionally normal and malignant human breast tissues in mice. *Proc Natl Acad Sci U S A* (2004) 101:4966–71. doi:10.1073/pnas.0401064101
22. Bhowmick NA, Ghiassi M, Bakin A, Aakre M, Lundquist CA, Engel ME, et al. Transforming growth factor-b1 mediates epithelial to mesenchymal transdifferentiation through a Rho-A-dependent mechanism. *Mol Biol Cell* (2001) 12:27–36. doi:10.1091/mbc.12.1.27
23. Maffini MV, Soto AM, Calabro JM, Ucci AA, Sonnenschein C. The stroma as a crucial target in rat mammary gland carcinogenesis. *J Cell Sci* (2004) 117:1495–502. doi:10.1242/jcs.01000
24. de Visser KE, Eichten A, Coussens LM. Paradoxical roles of the immune system during cancer development. *Nat Rev Cancer* (2006) 6:24–37.
25. Pitteri SJ, Faca VM, Kelly-Spratt KS, Kasarda AE, Wang H, Zhang Q, et al. Plasma proteome profiling of a mouse model of breast cancer identifies a set of up-regulated proteins in common with human breast cancer cells. *J Proteome Res* (2008) 7:1481–9. doi:10.1021/pr7007994
26. Amon LM, Pitteri SJ, Li CI, McIntosh M, Ladd JJ, Disis M, et al. Concordant release of glycolysis proteins into the plasma preceding a diagnosis of ER+ breast cancer. *Cancer Res* (2012) 72:1935–42. doi:10.1158/0008-5472.CAN-11-3266
27. Pitteri SJ, Kelly-Spratt KS, Gurley KE, Kennedy J, Buson TB, Chin A, et al. Tumor microenvironment-derived proteins dominate the plasma proteome response during breast cancer induction and progression. *Cancer Res* (2011) 71:5090–100. doi:10.1158/0008-5472.CAN-11-0568
28. Barcellos-Hoff MH. Integrative radiation carcinogenesis: interactions between cell and tissue responses to DNA damage. *Semin Cancer Biol* (2005) 15:138–48. doi:10.1016/j.semcancer.2004.08.010
29. Terzaghi M, Little JB. X-radiation-induced transformation in C3H mouse embryo-derived cell line. *Cancer Res* (1976) 36:1367–74.
30. Terzaghi M, Nettesheim P. Dynamics of neoplastic development in carcinogen-exposed tracheal mucosa. *Cancer Res* (1979) 39:3004–10.
31. Terzaghi-Howe M. Inhibition of carcinogen-altered rat tracheal epithelial cell proliferation by normal epithelial cells in vivo. *Carcinogenesis* (1986) 8:145–50. doi:10.1093/carcin/8.1.145
32. Terzaghi-Howe M. Changes in response to, and production of, transforming growth factor type b during neoplastic progression in cultured rat tracheal epithelial cells. *Carcinogenesis* (1989) 10:973–80. doi:10.1093/carcin/10.6.973
33. Terzaghi-Howe M. Interactions between cell populations influence expression of the transformed phenotype in irradiated rat tracheal epithelial cells. *Radiat Res* (1990) 121:242–7. doi:10.2307/3577772

34. Barcellos-Hoff MH, Ravani SA. Irradiated mammary gland stroma promotes the expression of tumorigenic potential by unirradiated epithelial cells. *Cancer Res* (2000) **60**:1254–60.

35. Mancuso M, Pasquali E, Leonardi S, Tanori M, Rebessi S, Di Majo V, et al. Oncogenic bystander radiation effects in patched heterozygous mouse cerebellum. *Proc Natl Acad Sci U S A* (2008) **105**:12445–50.

36. Mueller MM, Fusenig NE. Friends or foes – bipolar effects of the tumor stroma in cancer. *Nat Rev Cancer* (2004) **4**:839–49. doi:10.1038/nrc1477

37. Finak G, Bertos N, Pepin F, Sadekova S, Souleimanova M, Zhao H, et al. Stromal gene expression predicts clinical outcome in breast cancer. *Nat Med* (2008) **14**:518–27. doi:10.1038/nm1764

38. Kaplan RN, Riba RD, Zacharoulis S, Bramley AH, Vincent L, Costa C, et al. VEGFR1-positive haematopoietic bone marrow progenitors initiate the pre-metastatic niche. *Nature* (2005) **438**:820–7. doi:10.1038/nature04186

39. Dunn GP, Old LJ, Schreiber RD. The three Es of cancer immunoediting. *Annu Rev Immunol* (2004) **22**:329–60. doi:10.1146/annurev. immunol.22.012703.104803

40. Berenblum I, Shubik P. The persistence of latent tumour cells induced in the mouse's skin by a single application of 9:10-dimethyl-1:2-benzanthracene. *Br J Cancer* (1949) **3**:384–6. doi:10.1038/bjc.1949.42

41. Armitage P, Doll R. The age distribution of cancer and a multi-stage theory of carcinogenesis. *Br J Cancer* (1954) **8**:1–12. doi:10.1038/bjc.1954.1

42. Armitage P, Doll R. A two-stage theory of carcinogenesis in relation to the age distribution of human cancer. *Br J Cancer* (1957) **11**:161–9. doi:10.1038/ bjc.1957.22

43. Moolgavkar SH, Dewanji A, Venzon DJ. A stochastic two-stage model for cancer risk assessment. I. The hazard function and the probability of tumor. *Risk Anal* (1988) **8**:383–92. doi:10.1111/j.1539-6924.1988.tb00502.x

44. Moolgavkar SH, Knudson AG Jr. Mutation and cancer: a model for human carcinogenesis. *J Natl Cancer Inst* (1981) **66**:1037–52.

45. Moolgavkar SH, Luebeck G. Two-event model for carcinogenesis: biological, mathematical, and statistical considerations. *Risk Anal* (1990) **10**:323–41. doi: 10.1111/j.1539-6924.1990.tb01053.x

46. Knudson AG Jr. Mutation and cancer: statistical study of retinoblastoma. *Proc Natl Acad Sci U S A* (1971) **68**:820–3. doi:10.1073/pnas.68.4.820

47. Barcellos-Hoff MH. Cancer as an emergent phenomenon in systems radiation biology. *Radiat Env Biophys* (2007) **47**:33–8. doi:10.1007/s00411-007-0141-0

48. Medina D, Kittrell FS, Shepard A, Stephens LC, Jiang C, Lu J, et al. Biological and genetic properties of the p53 null preneoplastic mammary epithelium. *FASEB J* (2002) **16**:881–3.

49. Nguyen DH, Oketch-Rabah HA, Illa-Bochaca I, Geyer FC, Reis-Filho JS, Mao JH, et al. Radiation acts on the microenvironment to affect breast carcinogenesis by distinct mechanisms that decrease cancer latency and affect tumor type. *Cancer Cell* (2011) **19**:640–51. doi:10.1016/j.ccr.2011.03.011

50. Tang J, Fernandez-Garcia I, Vijayakumar S, Martinez-Ruiz H, Illa-Bochaca I, Nguyen DH, et al. Irradiation of juvenile, but not adult, mammary gland increases stem cell self-renewal and estrogen receptor negative tumors. *Stem Cells* (2013) **32**:649–61. doi:10.1002/stem.1533

51. Castiglioni F, Terenziani M, Carcangiu ML, Miliano R, Aiello P, Bertola L, et al. Radiation effects on development of HER2-positive breast carcinomas. *Clin Cancer Res* (2007) **13**:46–51. doi:10.1158/1078-0432.CCR-06-1490

52. Horst KC, Hancock SL, Ognibene G, Chen C, Advani RH, Rosenberg SA, et al. Histologic subtypes of breast cancer following radiotherapy for Hodgkin lymphoma. *Ann Oncol* (2014) **25**:848–51. doi:10.1093/annonc/mdu017

53. Stovall M, Smith SA, Langholz BM, Boice JD Jr, Shore RE, Andersson M, et al. Dose to the contralateral breast from radiotherapy and risk of second primary breast cancer in the WECARE study. *Int J Rad Oncol Biol Phys* (2008) **72**:1021–30. doi:10.1016/j.ijrobp.2008.02.040

54. Nguyen DH, Fredlund E, Zhao W, Perou CM, Balmain A, Mao J-H, et al. Murine microenvironment metaprofiles associate with human cancer etiology and intrinsic subtypes. *Clin Cancer Res* (2013) **19**:1353–62. doi:10.1158/1078-0432.CCR-12-3554

55. Hadj-Hamou NS, Ugolin N, Ory C, Britzen-Laurent N, Sastre-Garau X, Chevillard S, et al. A transcriptome signature distinguished sporadic from post-radiotherapy radiation-induced sarcomas. *Carcinogenesis* (2011) **32**:929–34. doi:10.1093/carcin/bgr064

56. Delys L, Detours V, Franc B, Thomas G, Bogdanova T, Tronko M, et al. Gene expression and the biological phenotype of papillary thyroid carcinomas. *Oncogene* (2007) **26**:7894–903. doi:10.1038/sj.onc.1210588

57. Clifton KH, Tanner MA, Gould MN. Assessment of radiogenic cancer initiation frequency per clonogenic rat mammary cell in vivo. *Cancer Res* (1986) **46**:2390–5.

58. Potten CS, Loeffler M. Stem cells: attributes, cycles, spirals, pitfalls and uncertainties. Lessons for and from the crypt. *Development* (1990) **110**:1001–20.

59. Smith GH, Chepko G. Mammary epithelial stem cells. *Microsc Res Tech* (2001) **52**:190–203. doi:10.1002/1097-0029(20010115)52:2<190::AID-JEMT1005> 3.0.CO;2-O

60. Reya T, Morrison SJ, Clarke MF, Weissman IL. Stem cells, cancer, and cancer stem cells. *Nature* (2001) **414**:105–11. doi:10.1038/35102167

61. Preston DL, Mattsson A, Holmberg E, Shore R, Hildreth NG, Boice JD Jr. Radiation effects on breast cancer risk: a pooled analysis of eight cohorts. *Radiat Res* (2002) **158**:220–35. doi:10.1667/0033-7587(2002)158[0220: REOBCR]2.0.CO;2

62. Welm BE, Tepera SB, Venezia T, Graubert TA, Rosen JM, Goodell MA. Sca-1(pos) cells in the mouse mammary gland represent an enriched progenitor cell population. *Dev Biol* (2002) **245**:42–56. doi:10.1006/ dbio.2002.0625

63. Visvader JE, Lindeman GJ. Mammary stem cells and mammopoiesis. *Cancer Res* (2006) **66**:9798–801. doi:10.1158/0008-5472.CAN-06-2254

64. Lim E, Wu D, Pal B, Bouras T, Asselin-Labat ML, Vaillant F, et al. Transcriptome analyses of mouse and human mammary cell subpopulations reveal multiple conserved genes and pathways. *Breast Cancer Res* (2010) **12**:R21. doi:10.1186/bcr2560

65. Andarawewa KL, Costes SV, Fernandez-Garcia I, Chou WS, Ravani SA, Park H, et al. Radiation dose and quality dependence of epithelial to mesenchymal transition (EMT) mediated by transforming growth factor β. *Int J Rad Oncol Biol Phys* (2011) **79**:1523–31. doi:10.1016/j.ijrobp.2010.11.058

66. Andarawewa KL, Erickson AC, Chou WS, Costes SV, Gascard P, Mott JD, et al. Ionizing radiation predisposes nonmalignant human mammary epithelial cells to undergo transforming growth factor beta induced epithelial to mesenchymal transition. *Cancer Res* (2007) **67**:8662–70. doi:10.1158/0008-5472.CAN-07-1294

67. Park CC, Henshall-Powell RL, Erickson AC, Talhouk R, Parvin B, Bissell MJ, et al. Ionizing radiation induces heritable disruption of epithelial cell interactions. *Proc Natl Acad Sci U S A* (2003) **100**:10728–33. doi:10.1073/ pnas.1832185100

68. Mantovani A, Allavena P, Sica A, Balkwill F. Cancer-related inflammation. *Nature* (2008) **454**:436–44. doi:10.1038/nature07205

69. Sparmann A, Bar-Sagi D. Ras-induced interleukin-8 expression plays a critical role in tumor growth and angiogenesis. *Cancer Cell* (2004) **6**:447–58. doi:10.1016/j.ccr.2004.09.028

70. Zeh HJ, Lotze MT. Addicted to death: invasive cancer and the immune response to unscheduled cell death. *J Immunother* (2005) **28**:1–9. doi:10.1097/00002371-200501000-00001

71. Guerra C, Schuhmacher AJ, Cañamero M, Grippo PJ, Verdaguer L, Pérez-Gallego L, et al. Chronic pancreatitis is essential for induction of pancreatic ductal adenocarcinoma by K-Ras oncogenes in adult mice. *Cancer Cell* (2007) **11**:291–302. doi:10.1016/j.ccr.2007.01.012

72. Farber JL, Kyle ME, Coleman JB. Mechanisms of cell injury by activated oxygen species. *Lab Invest* (1990) **62**:670–9.

73. Lewis CE, Pollard JW. Distinct role of macrophages in different tumor microenvironments. *Cancer Res* (2006) **66**:605–12. doi:10.1158/0008-5472. CAN-05-4005

74. Quigley D, To M, Kim IJ, Lin K, Albertson D, Sjolund J, et al. Network analysis of skin tumor progression identifies a rewired genetic architecture affecting inflammation and tumor susceptibility. *Genome Biol* (2011) **12**:R5. doi:10.1186/gb-2011-12-1-r5

75. Viaje A, Slaga TJ, Wigler M, Weinstein IB. Effects of antiinflammatory agents on mouse skin tumor promotion, epidermal DNA synthesis, phorbol ester-induced cellular proliferation, and production of plasminogen activator. *Cancer Res* (1977) **37**:1530–6.

76. Fischer SM, Gleason GL, Mills GD, Slaga TJ. Indomethacin enhancement of TPA tumor promotion in mice. *Cancer Lett* (1980) **10**:343–50. doi:10.1016/0304-3835(80)90052-X

77. Murphy J-E, Morales RE, Scott J, Kupper TS. IL-1{alpha}, innate immunity, and skin carcinogenesis: the effect of constitutive expression of IL-1{alpha} in epidermis on chemical carcinogenesis. *J Immunol* (2003) **170**:5697–703. doi:10.4049/jimmunol.170.11.5697

78. Moore RJ, Owens DM, Stamp G, Arnott C, Burke F, East N, et al. Mice deficient in tumor necrosis factor-[alpha] are resistant to skin carcinogenesis. *Nat Med* (1999) 5:828–31. doi:10.1038/10462

79. Naugler WE, Karin M. The wolf in sheep's clothing: the role of interleukin-6 in immunity, inflammation and cancer. *Trends Mol Med* (2008) 14:109–19. doi:10.1016/j.molmed.2007.12.007

80. Bettelli E, Carrier Y, Gao W, Korn T, Strom TB, Oukka M, et al. Reciprocal developmental pathways for the generation of pathogenic effector TH17 and regulatory T cells. *Nature* (2006) 441:235–8. doi:10.1038/nature04753

81. Lorimore SA, Chrystal JA, Robinson JI, Coates PJ, Wright EG. Chromosomal instability in unirradiated hemaopoietic cells induced by macrophages exposed in vivo to ionizing radiation. *Cancer Res* (2008) 68:8122–6. doi:10.1158/0008-5472.CAN-08-0698

82. Coates PJ, Rundle JK, Lorimore SA, Wright EG. Indirect macrophage responses to ionizing radiation: implications for genotype-dependent bystander signaling. *Cancer Res* (2008) 68:450–6. doi:10.1158/0008-5472. CAN-07-3050

83. Burns FJ, Tang MS, Frenkel K, Nádas A, Wu F, Uddin A, et al. Induction and prevention of carcinogenesis in rat skin exposed to space radiation. *Radiat Environ Biophys* (2007) 46:195–9. doi:10.1007/s00411-007-0106-3

84. Zhang R, Burns FJ, Chen H, Chen S, Wu F. Alterations in gene expression in rat skin exposed to 56Fe ions and dietary vitamin A acetate. *Radiat Res* (2006) 165:570–81. doi:10.1667/RR3556.1

85. Illa-Bochaca I, Ouyang H, Tang J, Sebastiano C, Mao J-H, Costes SV, et al. Densely ionizing radiation acts via the microenvironment to promote aggressive Trp53 null mammary carcinomas. *Cancer Res* (2014) 74:7137–48. doi:10.1158/0008-5472.CAN-14-1212

86. Bindea G, Mlecnik B, Angell HK, Galon J. The immune landscape of human tumors: implications for cancer immunotherapy. *Oncoimmunology* (2014) 3:e27456. doi:10.4161/onci.27456

87. Medzhitov R. Inflammation 2010: new adventures of an old flame. *Cell* (2010) 140:771–6. doi:10.1016/j.cell.2010.03.006

88. Grivennikov SI, Greten FR, Karin M. Immunity, inflammation, and cancer. *Cell* (2010) 140:883–99. doi:10.1016/j.cell.2010.01.025

89. Mittal D, Gubin MM, Schreiber RD, Smyth MJ. New insights into cancer immunoediting and its three component phases-elimination, equilibrium and escape. *Curr Opin Immunol* (2014) 27C:16–25. doi:10.1016/j.coi.2014.01.004

90. Street SE, Cretney E, Smyth MJ. Perforin and interferon-gamma activities independently control tumor initiation, growth, and metastasis. *Blood* (2001) 97:192–7. doi:10.1182/blood.V97.1.192

91. Dunn GP, Koebel CM, Schreiber RD. Interferons, immunity and cancer immunoediting. *Nat Rev Immunol* (2006) 6:836–48. doi:10.1038/nri1961

92. Vesely MD, Kershaw MH, Schreiber RD, Smyth MJ. Natural innate and adaptive immunity to cancer. *Annu Rev Immunol* (2011) 29:235–71. doi:10.1146/annurev-immunol-031210-101324

93. Myron Kauffman H, McBride MA, Cherikh WS, Spain PC, Marks WH, Roza AM. Transplant tumor registry: donor related malignancies. *Transplantation* (2002) 74:358–62. doi:10.1097/00007890-200208150-00011

94. MacKie RM, Reid R, Junor B. Fatal melanoma transferred in a donated kidney 16 years after melanoma surgery. *N Engl J Med* (2003) 348:567–8. doi:10.1056/NEJM200302063480620

95. Koebel CM, Vermi W, Swann JB, Zerafa N, Rodig SJ, Old LJ, et al. Adaptive immunity maintains occult cancer in an equilibrium state. *Nature* (2007) 450:903–7. doi:10.1038/nature06309

96. Ponder BAJ. Cancer genetics. *Nature* (2001) 411:336–41. doi:10.1038/35077207

97. Balmain A, Gray J, Ponder B. The genetics and genomics of cancer. *Nat Genet* (2003) 33:238–44. doi:10.1038/ng1107

98. Welcsh PL, King M-C. BRCA1 and BRCA2 and the genetics of breast and ovarian cancer. *Hum Mol Genet* (2001) 10:705–13. doi:10.1093/hmg/10.7.705

99. Peto J. Cancer epidemiology in the last century and the next decade. *Nature* (2001) 411:390–5. doi:10.1038/35077256

100. Myers AJ, Gibbs JR, Webster JA, Rohrer K, Zhao A, Marlowe L, et al. A survey of genetic human cortical gene expression. *Nat Genet* (2007) 39:1494–9. doi:10.1038/ng.2007.16

101. Emilsson V, Thorleifsson G, Zhang B, Leonardson AS, Zink F, Zhu J, et al. Genetics of gene expression and its effect on disease. *Nature* (2008) 452:423–8. doi:10.1038/nature06758

102. Morley M, Molony CM, Weber TM, Devlin JL, Ewens KG, Spielman RS, et al. Genetic analysis of genome-wide variation in human gene expression. *Nature* (2004) 430:743–7. doi:10.1038/nature02797

103. Chen Y, Zhu J, Lum PY, Yang X, Pinto S, MacNeil DJ, et al. Variations in DNA elucidate molecular networks that cause disease. *Nature* (2008) 452:429–35. doi:10.1038/nature06757

104. Mao J-H, Balmain A. Genomic approaches to identification of tumour-susceptibility genes using mouse models. *Curr Opin Genet Dev* (2003) 13:14–9. doi:10.1016/S0959-437X(03)00005-4

105. Balmain A. Cancer as a complex genetic trait: tumor susceptibility in humans and mouse models. *Cell* (2002) 108:145–52. doi:10.1016/S0092-8674(02)00622-0

106. Quigley DA, To MD, Pérez-Losada J, Pelorosso FG, Mao J-H, Nagase H, et al. Genetic architecture of murine skin inflammation and tumor susceptibility. *Nature* (2009) 458:505–8. doi:10.1038/nature07683

107. Mao J-H, Perez-losada J, Wu D, DelRosario R, Tsunematsu R, Nakayama KI, et al. Fbxw7/Cdc4 is a p53-dependent, haploinsufficient tumour suppressor gene. *Nature* (2004) 432:775–9. doi:10.1038/nature03155

108. Blackburn AC, Brown JS, Naber SP, Otis CN, Wood JT, Jerry DJ. BALB/c alleles for Prkdc and Cdkn2a interact to modify tumor susceptibility in Trp53+/- mice. *Cancer Res* (2003) 63:2364–8.

109. Okayasu R, Suetomi K, Yu Y, Silver A, Bedford JS, Cox R, et al. A deficiency in DNA repair and DNA-PKcs expression in the radiosensitive BALB/c mouse. *Cancer Res* (2000) 60:4342–5.

110. Yu Y, Okayasu R, Weil MM, Silver A, McCarthy M, Zabriskie R, et al. Elevated breast cancer risk in irradiated BALB/c mice associates with unique functional polymorphism of the Prkdc (DNA-dependent protein kinase catalytic subunit) gene. *Cancer Res* (2001) 61:1820–4.

111. Jerry DJ, Kittrell FS, Kuperwasser C, Laucirica R, Dickinson ES, Bonilla PJ, et al. A mammary-specific model demonstrates the role of the p53 tumor suppressor gene in tumor development. *Oncogene* (2000) 19:1052–8. doi:10.1038/sj.onc.1203270

112. Zhang P, Lo A, Huang Y, Huang G, Liang G, Mott J, et al. Identification of genetic loci that control mammary tumor susceptibility through the host microenvironment. *Sci Rep* (2015) 5:8919. doi:10.1038/srep08919

113. Tartakovsky B, Goldstein O, Krautghamer R, Haran-Ghera N. Low doses of radiation induce systemic production of cytokines: possible contribution to leukemogenesis. *Int J Cancer* (1993) 55:269–74. doi:10.1002/ijc.2910550217

114. Haran-Ghera N, Krautghamer R, Lapidot T, Peled A, Dominguez MG, Stanley ER. Increased circulating colony-stimulating factor-1 (CSF-1) in SJL/J mice with radiation-induced acute myeloid leukemia (AML) is associated with autocrine regulation of AML cells by CSF-1. *Blood* (1997) 89:2537–45.

115. Best T, Li D, Skol AD, Kirchhoff T, Jackson SA, Yasui Y, et al. Variants at 6q21 implicate PRDM1 in the etiology of therapy-induced second malignancies after Hodgkin's lymphoma. *Nat Med* (2011) 17:941–3. doi:10.1038/nm.2407

13

Comparison of Individual Radiosensitivity to γ-Rays and Carbon Ions

Grace Shim[1], Marie Delna Normil[1], Isabelle Testard[2], William M. Hempel[1], Michelle Ricoul[1] and Laure Sabatier[1]*

[1] Commissariat à l'Energie Atomique (CEA), DRF/PROCyTOX, Fontenay-aux-Roses, France, [2] CEA Grenoble, Laboratoire de Chimie et Biologie des Métaux, BIG, DRF, Grenoble, France

*Correspondence:
Laure Sabatier
laure.sabatier@cea.fr

Carbon ions are an up-and-coming ion species, currently being used in charged particle radiotherapy. As it is well established that there are considerable interindividual differences in radiosensitivity in the general population that can significantly influence clinical outcomes of radiotherapy, we evaluate the degree of these differences in the context of carbon ion therapy compared with conventional radiotherapy. In this study, we evaluate individual radiosensitivity following exposure to carbon-13 ions or γ-rays in peripheral blood lymphocytes of healthy individuals based on the frequency of ionizing radiation (IR)-induced DNA double strand breaks (DSBs) that was either misrepaired or left unrepaired to form chromosomal aberrations (CAs) (simply referred to here as DSBs for brevity). Levels of DSBs were estimated from the scoring of CAs visualized with telomere/centromere-fluorescence *in situ* hybridization (TC-FISH). We examine radiosensitivity at the dose of 2 Gy, a routinely administered dose during fractionated radiotherapy, and we determined that a wide range of DSBs were induced by the given dose among healthy individuals, with highly radiosensitive individuals harboring more IR-induced breaks in the genome than radioresistant individuals following exposure to the same dose. Furthermore, we determined the relative effectiveness of carbon irradiation in comparison to γ-irradiation in the induction of DSBs at each studied dose (isodose effect), a quality we term "relative dose effect" (RDE). This ratio is advantageous, as it allows for simple comparison of dose–response curves. At 2 Gy, carbon irradiation was three times more effective in inducing DSBs compared with γ-irradiation (RDE of 3); these results were confirmed using a second cytogenetic technique, multicolor-FISH. We also analyze radiosensitivity at other doses (0.2–15 Gy), to represent hypo- and hyperfractionation doses and determined that RDE is dose dependent: high ratios at low doses, and approaching 1 at high doses. These results could have clinical implications as IR-induced DNA damage and the ensuing CAs and genomic instability can have significant cellular consequences that could potentially have profound implications for long-term human health after IR exposure, such as the emergence of secondary cancers and other pathobiological conditions after radiotherapy.

Keywords: individual radiosensitivity, carbon ions, radiotherapy, relative biological effect, linear energy transfer, isodose effect

INTRODUCTION

Current radiotherapy regimens use photons or protons for the treatment of a plethora of malignancies. However, as ionizing radiation (IR) of high linear energy transfer (LET) may potentially offer radiobiological advantages over low LET IR due to their inherent physical dose distribution characteristics, cancer radiotherapy is now shifting to the use of high-LET heavier ion species (1). Low LET IR (e.g., X- and γ-rays) deposits exponentially decreasing amounts of energy, as a function of penetration depth in the target material, in a uniform pattern of distribution. High LET IR, such as heavy ions, on the other hand, are characterized by a relatively low entrance dose in the target material, followed by a pronounced sharp maximum dose near the end of their range called the Bragg peak, and energy close to 0 beyond the Bragg peak. This characteristic of high LET IR is useful especially for the treatment of deep-seated tumors in the human body, as it allows a great amount of energy to be precisely localized at the tumor site when it is placed at the Bragg peak, while minimally exposing the surrounding normal tissues (2).

Among various types of heavy ion species considered for radiotherapy, carbon ions are considered to have the most balanced and optimal properties in terms of physical dose distribution and relative biological effectiveness (RBE) along its Bragg peak curve (3). However, carbon ion radiotherapy is not yet widely used, with only a few centers worldwide (six in Asia and two in Europe) that have treated ~13,000 patients (as of December 2013), compared with ~50 active proton therapy centers worldwide that have treated over 105,000 patients (4). Though preliminary clinical data from the existing carbon ion therapy centers suggest favorable results for many of the malignancies that do poorly with conventional radiotherapy (3), further clinical research and development of more carbon ion (and other charged particles heavier than protons) therapy centers in the US and worldwide are hindered by the lack of sufficient clinical evidence of the benefit of carbon ion therapy over conventional radiotherapy that would cost-effectively justify the establishment of such expensive facilities (1). Further investigation is necessary to characterize and understand how carbon ion therapy works in comparison to conventional radiotherapy.

Clinical outcomes of radiotherapy can be significantly influenced by interindividual variations in sensitivity to IR, which is well established to exist in the general population. Highly radiosensitive patients, for instance, may develop early and/or late side effects due to radiation toxicity, while radioresistant patients may receive an insufficient dose of radiation due to dose limitations in current general radiotherapy protocols. However, current radiotherapy and radiation protection protocols do not take into account the individual variations in radiosensitivity, but rather rely on population averages of radiation responses. Refining these protocols to consider individual radiosensitivity, especially the more radiosensitive and cancer-prone, may help to alleviate the detrimental delayed effects of IR (5–7).

In this study, we evaluate individual radiosensitivity following exposure to carbon-13 ions or γ-rays in peripheral blood lymphocytes (PBL) of healthy blood donors using the telomere/centromere-fluorescence *in situ* hybridization (TC-FISH)

technique. TC-FISH, which simultaneously stains telomeres and centromeres using peptide nucleic acid (PNA) probes (8), was shown in a recent study in our laboratory (9) to be a cost-effective method that significantly simplifies and improves the "gold standard" dicentric chromosome (DC) assay, which relies on the manual scoring of DCs following Giemsa staining by trained specialists. The radiosensitivity of each analyzed individual in this analysis was ranked based on the estimation of the frequency of IR-induced DNA double strand breaks (DSBs) that either was misrepaired or left unrepaired to form chromosomal aberrations (CAs). For brevity, we refer to these misrepaired or unrepaired DSBs that generate CAs simply as "DSBs" henceforth. Levels of DSBs were estimated from the scoring of CAs visualized with TC-FISH, including dicentrics, centric and acentric rings, and acentric fragments (with 0, 2, or 4 telomeres). We demonstrated in our previous article (9) that this modified scoring technique provides improved sensitivity compared with the classical DC analyses. Additionally, as presented in this same paper, we developed a novel automated system (TCScore) that can perform these TC-FISH analyses with the same efficacy as manual scoring, but in a fraction of time; this improved, automated approach will open up new horizons for the assessment of genotoxic risk and for biological dosimetry, particularly for low doses.

We examine radiosensitivity at the dose of 2 Gy, a routinely administered dose during fractionated radiotherapy (10, 11), and at other doses (0.2–15 Gy), to represent hypo- and hyperfractionation doses. As we are particularly interested in comparing the levels of biological effect (misrepaired or unrepaired DNA DSBs generating CAs in this case) at a particular dose of carbon irradiation compared with the same dose of γ-irradiation (isodose effect), we also define a quality we term "relative dose effect" (RDE). This ratio is advantageous as it allows for simple comparison of dose–response curves.

RESULTS

Individual Radiosensitivity Following Exposure to 2 Gy of γ-Rays

Individuals in this cohort of 18 healthy blood donors were first ranked in the order of increasing radiosensitivity based on the mean number of IR-induced DSBs (i.e., misrepaired or unrepaired DSBs that generated CAs) per cell following *in vitro* exposure of isolated PBL to 2 Gy of low LET γ-rays. The mean number of DSBs per cell was calculated based on the scoring of CAs following TC-FISH staining, as described in **Figures 1A,B**, in cells undergoing first mitosis at 60 h postirradiation. As shown in **Figure 2A**, individuals were designated as Donors A through R in this order of "radioresistant" to "radiosensitive" donors. We use this ranking throughout the study as the definition of each of these donors' radiosensitivity.

Following exposure to a dose of 2 Gy of γ-irradiation, there was a range of ~1.5–2.8 DSBs per cell (1.8-fold difference), and a mean of 2.17 DSBs per cell in the PBL samples. Comparison of data obtained from samples irradiated on different dates and analyzed by different individuals showed no significant differences in the measurement of the mean number of DSBs per donor ($p > 0.05$).

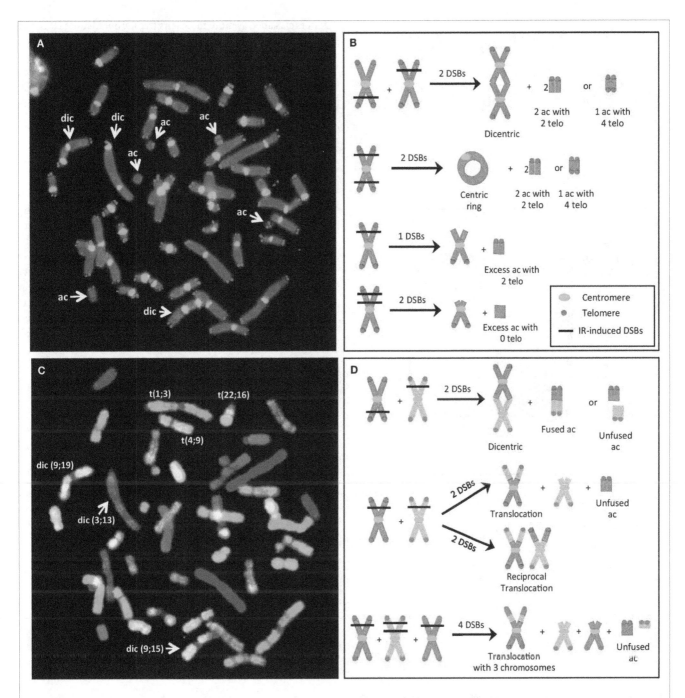

FIGURE 1 | (A) Visualization of IR-induced dicentric chromosomes (dic) and other chromosomal aberrations (CAs), such as acentric fragments (ac), using telomere/centromere-fluorescence *in situ* hybridization (TC-FISH). This image shows 3 dic and 5 ac [3 with 4 telomeres (telo), 1 with 2 telo, 1 with 0 telo]. **(B)** Examples of the method used to estimate the number of IR-induced DSBs per cell (i.e., misrepaired or unrepaired DSBs that generated CAs) using TC-FISH. A dic or a centric ring with an ac containing four telo was considered as two DSBs. Excess ac with two telomeres was considered as resulting from one DSB that failed to rejoin (terminal deletion). Excess ac with 0 telomeres were considered as resulting from 2 DSBs (interstitial deletion). Note that these sample images of chromosomes are not an analysis of **(A)**, and lines denoting DSBs from IR interactions are not necessary from traversal with the same IR track. **(C)** Visualization of IR-induced translocations using M-FISH. This image shows the same metaphase as in **(A)**. Each chromosome involved in the dic and ac can be identified. Furthermore, three additional translocations can be observed that was not able to be visualized using the TC-FISH technique. **(D)** Examples of the method used to estimate the number of IR-induced DSBs (i.e., misrepaired or unrepaired DSBs that generated CAs) using M-FISH. Dic or translocations involving two chromosomes often involve two DSBs, whereas more complex rearrangements with three chromosomes may involve four DSBs. Note that these sample images of chromosomes are not an analysis of **(C)**, and lines denoting DSBs from IR interactions are not necessary from traversal with the same IR track.

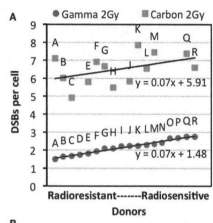

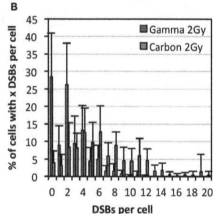

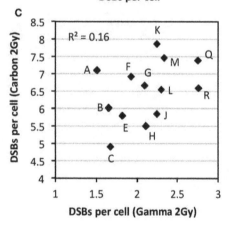

FIGURE 2 | Comparison of individual radiosensitivity following
exposure to 2 Gy of either carbon-13 ions (75 MeV/u; LET
~36.5 keV/μm at the plateau region of the Bragg peak curve) or
γ-rays. Individual radiosensitivity was evaluated in peripheral blood
lymphocytes (PBL) of healthy blood donors in cells undergoing first mitosis at
60 h postirradiation; radiosensitivity of each individual was ranked using the
TC-FISH technique based on the estimation of the frequency of IR-induced
DNA DSBs (i.e., misrepaired or unrepaired DSBs that generated CAs),
estimated as shown in **Figure 1B**. **(A)** Ranking of individual radiosensitivity to
2 Gy of carbon ions and γ-rays. Individuals were designated as Donors A
("radioresistant") through R ("radiosensitive") based on the order of increasing
radiosensitivity following γ-irradiation. **(B)** Distribution of the number of DSBs
per cell for each type of IR for all donors analyzed. **(C)** No correlations
between individual radiosensitivity following *in vitro* exposure to 2 Gy of
carbon ions and γ-rays ($R^2 = 0.16$).

Donors classified as more radiosensitive harbored more DSBs per
cell, with a wider range of distribution of DSBs per cell, compared
with the more radioresistant donors (Figure S1 in Supplementary
Material). For example, the mean of the range of DSBs per cell in
radioresistant donors (Donors A through F) was found to be 9.0
compared with 12.5 in radiosensitive donors (Donors M through
R). This indicates the presence of more IR-induced damage in
radiosensitive donors compared with radioresistant donors following exposure to a dose of 2 Gy of γ-rays.

No correlations were observed between this radiosensitivity
and levels of spontaneous or IR-induced apoptosis (0–6 Gy;
data not shown). Furthermore, no correlations were found
($R^2 = 0.045$; data not shown) between radiosensitivity to 2 Gy
of γ-irradiation and the susceptibility to IR-induced apoptosis in
the T4-EM subpopulation (measured as the slope of IR-induced
apoptosis in T4-EM lymphocytes between the doses of 0 and 6 Gy
of γ-irradiation), as previously described (12). Radiosensitivity
may be moderately correlated with interindividual variability in
the induction of global γH2AX fluorescence at 30 min postirradiation ($R^2 = 0.595$), but not at later time points postirradiation
(3–24 h); global γH2AX fluorescence data of this cohort of PBL
were previously published (13).

Individual Radiosensitivity Following Exposure to 2 Gy of Carbon Ions

Individual radiosensitivity following *in vitro* exposure to 2 Gy of
high LET carbon-13 ions (75 MeV/u; LET ~36.5 keV/μm at the
plateau region of the Bragg peak curve) was measured in PBL of
13 of the healthy blood donors analyzed for γ-irradiation above in
cells undergoing first mitosis at 60 h postirradiation.

As shown in **Figure 2A**, interindividual differences in
radiosensitivity was also observed following carbon irradiation,
a range of ~5–8 DSB per cell was measured (1.6-fold difference),
and a mean of 6.45 DSBs per cell in the PBL samples. As with
γ-irradiation, radiosensitivity was not correlated with apoptosis
and global γH2AX fluorescence (data not shown). Based on the
ranking of increasing radiosensitivity following carbon irradiation, we find that the more radiosensitive donors to carbon
irradiation harbored more DSBs per cell compared with the more
radioresistant donors (Figure S2 in Supplementary Material); for
example, the mean of the range of DSBs per cell in radioresistant
donors (Donors C, H, E, and J) was found to be 14.8 compared
with 19.8 in radiosensitive donors (Donors F, A, Q, M, and K).

No Correlations between Radiosensitivity to 2 Gy of γ-Rays and Carbon Ions

Comparison of radiosensitivity to carbon irradiation and
γ-irradiation at the dose of 2 Gy showed a different order of
increasing radiosensitivity within this cohort, as illustrated in
Figure 2A. Indeed, the order of low to high radiosensitivity as
classified according to 2 Gy of γ-irradiation did not hold for carbon irradiation following exposure to the same dose (**Figure 2A**).
This indicates that donors are not equally sensitive to different
types of IR. Interestingly, though the ranking of radiosensitivity
to carbon ions and γ-rays was different within this cohort, the
trend lines for radiosensitivity to each type of IR (plotted in the

order of increasing radiosensitivity to γ-rays) were parallel, both with a slope of 0.07. Notably, a high intracellular variability of IR-induced DSB among cells of the same donor was observed (data not shown). Intracellular variations following carbon irradiation were generally found to be larger than those following γ-irradiation. This may be expected due to the non-uniform spatial distribution of IR-induced DNA damage following heavy ion irradiation. A modest correlation was found between the dispersion of DSBs per donor (95% confidence interval) following γ- and carbon irradiation ($R^2 = 0.51$). As expected, carbon irradiation causes more dispersion in the number of DSBs induced per cell compared with γ-irradiation, with carbon ranging to up to 20 DSBs per cell and γ-rays ranging up to 12 DSBs (**Figure 2B**). This indicates that carbon irradiation causes a larger range of DSBs per cell and more IR damage that is less repaired compared with γ-rays. As shown in **Figure 2C**, we find that there are no correlations between radiosensitivity to carbon ions and γ-rays at the dose of 2 Gy ($R^2 = 0.16$).

RDE Factor of 3 after 2 Gy Irradiation Using Both TC-FISH and M-FISH Techniques

In this study, as we are particularly interested in the differences in the effectiveness of induction of DSBs (i.e., misrepaired or unrepaired DSBs that generated CAs) by carbon irradiation compared with γ-irradiation at a given dose (isodose effect), we define a new ratio, termed RDE, calculated simply by dividing the mean DSBs per cell determined using TC-FISH following exposure to carbon ions by that following exposure to the same dose of γ-rays. This ratio differs from the usual metric RBE (defined as the ratio of doses that produce an iso-effect) and is advantageous, as it allows for simple comparison of dose–response curves.

At the dose of 2 Gy, the mean number of DSBs per cell was found to be 2.17 DSB per cell after γ-irradiation (18 donors, as described in Section "Individual Radiosensitivity Following Exposure to 2 Gy of γ-Rays") and 6.45 DSB after carbon irradiation (13 donors, as described in Section "Individual Radiosensitivity Following Exposure to 2 Gy of Carbon Ions"). Therefore, the RDE of carbon ions was determined to be ~3 times that of γ-rays at the dose of 2 Gy using TC-FISH. The RBE at 2 Gy was found to be 2.6.

Relative dose effect results were confirmed using M-FISH analysis of chromosomal rearrangements, visualized as illustrated in **Figure 1C**. The number of DSBs per cell using M-FISH analysis was calculated, as illustrated in **Figure 1D**. At the dose of 2 Gy, M-FISH analyses in four donors (Donors A, C, L, and R) indicated 3.26 DSBs per cell after γ-irradiation and 9.81 DSBs per cell following carbon irradiation. As M-FISH is a more detailed analysis of chromosomal damage compared with TC-FISH (since M-FISH allows analysis of translocations, which are not visible with TC-FISH), it is expected that more DSBs per cell be calculated using M-FISH than using TC-FISH. However, as both techniques give an RDE factor of 3 at the dose of 2 Gy, the determination of RDE factor of carbon compared with γ-rays is independent of the method of scoring chromosomal damage. Thus, TC-FISH and M-FISH can be considered to be two alternative approaches for scoring chromosomal damage.

Based on these results, we propose that the TC-FISH technique is more practical for rapid assessment of genotoxic risk and for radiation dosimetry, as M-FISH is both expensive and time consuming in terms of hybridization technique and analysis compared with TC-FISH.

RDE at Other Doses: High RDE at Low Doses

To determine RDE at other doses, we compare mean DSBs per cell determined using TC-FISH following exposure to a range of doses (0.2–15 Gy) of carbon ions and γ-rays in a subset of the PBL of the healthy blood donors analyzed above. For γ-irradiation at all doses except for 2 Gy (which is the average of 18 donors; data in **Figure 2A**), the mean DSBs per cell represent the average of six donors (Donors C, F, H, J, K, and O). For carbon irradiation at all doses except for 2 Gy (which is the average of 13 donors; data in **Figure 2A**), the mean DSBs per cell represent the average of four donors (Donors G, H, K, and M).

Figure 3A shows a plot of the dose (0–5 Gy) of γ- or carbon irradiation and the mean number of DSBs per cell averaged for all donors analyzed. This plot indicated second order polynomial trends between the doses of 0 and 5 Gy for both IR types. This plot was expanded to doses of up to 15 Gy in **Figure 3B**, which shows data for the frequency of DSBs per cell (averaged for all donors analyzed) at each dose with the exact mean indicated above each bar. Error bars in **Figures 3A,B** represent the SD of the frequencies of DSBs per cell among the averaged donors, illustrating interindividual variations in radiosensitivity at various doses. RDE factors shown in **Figure 3C** were calculated by dividing the mean DSBs per cell following a dose of carbon irradiation by the mean DSBs per cell following the same dose of γ-irradiation (values shown in **Figure 3B**). The RDE factor is dose dependent, with high RDE factors at low doses (0.2 and 0.5 Gy), and an RDE factor approaching 1 at high doses (10 and 15 Gy).

DISCUSSION

In this study, we demonstrate that following *in vitro* irradiation with carbon ions or γ-rays at the dose of 2 Gy, a routinely administered dose during fractionated radiotherapy (10, 11), interindividual differences in radiosensitivity (measured in terms of misrepaired or unrepaired IR-induced DNA DSBs that led to the formation of CAs) exist in healthy individuals. In other words, a given dose of IR can induce a wide range of DNA damage among healthy individuals, with highly radiosensitive individuals harboring more IR-induced damage in the genome than radioresistant individuals following exposure to the same IR dose. These results could have important clinical implications as IR-induced DNA damage and the ensuing CAs and genomic instability can have significant cellular consequences that could potentially have profound implications for long-term human health after IR exposure, such as the emergence of secondary cancers and other pathobiological conditions after radiotherapy (14–16). A fast and reliable clinical method to measure radiosensitivity of cancer patients and/or predict radiotherapy toxicity (especially to identify hyper-radiosensitive individuals) would permit personalized

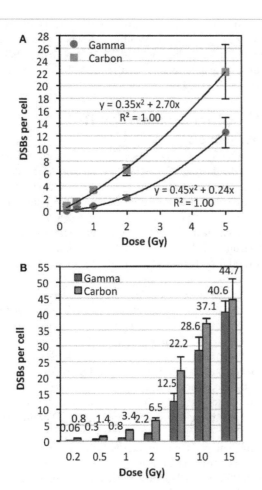

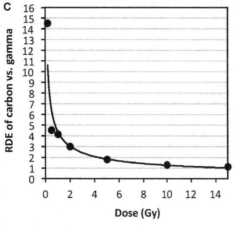

FIGURE 3 | Relative dose effect (RDE) of carbon-13 ions (75 MeV/u; LET ~36.5 keV/µm at the plateau region of the Bragg peak curve) versus γ-rays at various doses. We define RDE to be the ratio of biological effect at a given dose (isodose effect). The mean number of DSBs per cell was determined using TC-FISH as illustrated in **Figure 1B**, and dose–response curves were plotted for doses of up to **(A)** 5 Gy and **(B)** 15 Gy. The mean DSBs per cell for all donors analyzed are indicated above each bar in **(B)**. Error bars represent the SD of the frequencies of DSBs per cell among the donors. **(C)** RDE of carbon ion versus γ-rays as a function of dose.

radiotherapy treatment; however, such a method still remains to be established (17–20).

It is well established that radiosensitivity is closely linked to intrinsic, genetically determined differences in cellular responses to IR-induced damage, particularly the repair of DNA DSBs (7). In our previously published paper (13), we have demonstrated, in this same cohort of PBL from healthy individuals, a high level of interindividual variability in the induction and kinetics of γH2AX, an important DNA damage response (DDR) protein that facilitates the efficient repair of DSBs, following γ-irradiation; this variability, measured using global immunofluorescence microscopy and confirmed with flow cytometry, was found to increase with dose and diminish with repair time, in accordance with previously published observations (21–24). This finding supports the notion that these individuals vary in their DDR capacities. However, in this study, we show a moderate correlation between radiosensitivity and global γH2AX fluorescence at 30 min postirradiation ($R^2 = 0.595$), but no correlations at later time points postirradiation (3–24 h). These moderate to lack of correlations between radiosensitivity and γH2AX levels could be due to the rapid time-dependent changes in γH2AX levels postirradiation. Furthermore, the lack of correlation that we have observed between sensitivity to carbon and γ-irradiation may indicate that individuals may not be equally capable of repairing the different types of DNA damage induced by low LET and high LET IR. Indeed, high LET IR causes more *clustered* DNA DSBs and higher frequencies of complex chromosomal aberrations (CCAs) that may be less likely to be repaired correctly compared with equivalent doses of low LET IR (25–29).

Our results demonstrate that the yield of IR-induced DSBs fits a polynomial curve very close to linearity, in agreement with previous reports of upward curvature, especially following high LET IR (29, 30). We showed that RDE is dose dependent, with high RDE at low doses (0.2 and 0.5 Gy), and approaching 1 at high doses (10 and 15 Gy). This may indicate that the biological effectiveness of carbon at low doses, such as in surrounding tissue of the primary site of irradiation, may be significantly underestimated: IR exposure may be more harmful than expected. On the other hand, at very high doses per fraction, such as in hypofractionated radiotherapy schemes, biological effectiveness may be significantly overestimated. These results may be important to consider for carbon radiotherapy.

In this study, we have found that TC-FISH and M-FISH are two complementary methods for the scoring of DSBs and RDE determination at the dose of 2 Gy, as carbon ions caused three times more DSBs per cell compared with γ-irradiation with both techniques with this dose. We have recently further improved the speed of the TC-FISH technique and analysis in our laboratory with the development of a semi-automated software (TCScore) that is able to detect IR-induced CAs (dicentrics, rings, acentrics with 4, 2, 0 telomeres) with the same efficacy as manual scoring in a fraction of time (9). This software provides automated analysis of three-channel (RGB) images (red, green, and blue channels containing telomere, centromere, and

DAPI DNA staining information, respectively) split into their individual channels by any image processing software (e.g., Image J) and generates an intuitive and interactive report of CA classes that can be reviewed and corrected in batches by an investigator. This improved, automated approach will open up new horizons for the assessment of genotoxic risk for clinical uses (e.g., radiosensitivity assessment before radiotherapy) and for biological dosimetry following accidental exposure, particularly for low doses (9, 31). However, in order for these techniques to be used in the clinics for determining intrinsic individual radiosensitivity, analyses of a larger cohort of healthy individuals are needed to well establish the degree of variations within the whole human population.

Meanwhile, the M-FISH technique has been shown to be a powerful tool for detailed analyses of translocations and CCAs in the whole genome at very low to high doses of IR exposure, as it allows all chromosomal homolog pairs to be differentiated (32, 33). It was shown to be sensitive enough to detect translocations and other CAs at doses as low as 0.1 Gy of low LET IR (34). Though the long-term stability of translocations and the usefulness of this technique was recently validated (35), M-FISH analysis is laborious, time consuming (~5 days to obtain results), and expensive; standardization and automation will be key to improving the practical significance of FISH-based translocation assays. Furthermore, the frequencies of translocations at baseline and their persistence postirradiation at various doses, as well as potential interindividual variability in their levels, need to be further characterized, especially in the low dose range (36). Such data would be valuable for studying the long-term health risk of IR exposure and may generally contribute to understanding the link between CAs and human diseases and cancer (37).

In conclusion, it is evident that individual radiosensitivity exists among healthy individuals following irradiation with carbon ions and γ-rays, and individuals may not be equally sensitive to different types of IR. Furthermore, the RDE of carbon compared with γ-rays could be dose dependent, illustrating the complexity of the biological responses to IR. We propose that the calculation of IR-induced DSBs (i.e., misrepaired or unrepaired DSBs that generated CAs) using TC-FISH may be a sensitive and reliable approach to measuring individual radiosensitivity. The ability to rank and predict individual radiosensitivity has a wide range of real-world applications, as it directly impacts the formulation of cancer treatment strategies and the establishment of radiation protection guidelines. Refining radiotherapy and radiation protection protocols to consider individual radiosensitivity, especially the more radiosensitive and cancer-prone, may help to alleviate the detrimental delayed effects of IR.

MATERIALS AND METHODS

Cell Culture

Peripheral blood lymphocytes used in this study were isolated from the whole blood of 18 healthy blood donors (with negative viral status) from the Center of Blood Transfusions using the standard Ficoll isolation technique. Individuals included in this cohort were selected from a larger cohort of 63 individuals along the range of radiosensitivity measured previously based on the induction of IR-induced apoptosis (38); all analyses, however, were performed blindly. After isolation, lymphocytes were frozen in liquid nitrogen (−196°C) until use. Lymphocytes were unfrozen 24 h before irradiation and incubated at 37°C in an atmosphere of 5% CO_2 in RPMI 1640 medium (Gibco) supplemented with 20% fetal bovine serum (FBS; Eurobio) and antibiotics (penicillin/streptomycin; Gibco).

Irradiation

Peripheral blood lymphocytes were irradiated at various doses at room temperature (RT) with γ-rays from a Cesium-137 source at the CEA Fontenay-aux-Roses, France (dose-rate of 2 Gy/min).

Carbon-13 ($^{13}C^{6+}$) irradiations were performed on the Grand Accélérateur National d'Ions Lours GANIL (Caen, France) D1 high energy line (IRRABAT beam line) with energy of 75 MeV/u; details of dosimetry and other specifications were previously published (39). Lymphocytes were irradiated in small tubes with a glass wall of 2 mm thickness. Samples were irradiated at the plateau region of the Bragg peak curve; the mean LET at the sample was estimated to be ~36.5 keV/μm. The dosimetry was realized with the assistance of CIMAP–CIRIL physicists using a Faraday cup and an X-ray detector (5 μm stainless steel foil and photomultiplier). The photons emitted after traversal of the foil by the accelerated ions were counted, and a correlation at low fluences/doses was established with the real ion tracks measured on CR39 tracks detectors ($C_{12}H_{18}O_7)_n$. After exposure to the beam, the ion tracks in the CR39 were chemically etched for 8–12 min in 12 N KOH at 80°C. Several microscope fields were photographed using an Olympus Vanox-S, ×100, equipped with a Cohn Pieper FK-7512-Q video camera. The tracks were then counted using a homemade image analysis application from the Aphelion® software. X-ray detector doses were also subsequently correlated with the doses measured with an ionizing chamber (Unidos 23332 or 23344, PTW Freiburg, Germany, depending on the ion atomic number and its track length) for further verification of the dose/fluence ratio. The ionizing chamber was not used as reference dosimeter for the sample irradiations, since it was designed for measuring photon fluxes (utilized in radiotherapy).

Chromosome Preparation, Staining, and Image Acquisition

Peripheral blood lymphocytes were cultured for 60 h postirradiation, and metaphase preparations were performed using standard procedures (40). Slides with metaphase spreads were stored in −20°C until use, and were unfrozen and left at RT overnight before use.

For TC-FISH analysis, telomeres and centromeres were stained, as previously described (9) using telomere-specific Cyanine3-labeled PNA probes and centromere-specific FITC-labeled PNA probes (both from Panagene, Daejon, South Korea).

For M-FISH analysis, slides were hybridized with a 24XCyte mFISH kit (MetaSystems Altlussheim, Germany) according to the protocol recommended by the manufacturer.

After counterstaining of the DNA with 4′,6-diamidino-2-phenylindole (DAPI), slides were mounted with coverslips with PPD (1 mg/mL p-phenylenediamine-90% glycerol-10% PBS) and stored in a dark box at −4°C until automated image acquisition using the MetaSystems AutoCapt software. Images of metaphase cells were acquired with a charge-coupled device camera (Zeiss, Thornwood, NY, USA) coupled with a Zeiss Axioplan microscope. CAs were scored manually using the MetaSystems ISIS software.

Analysis of Chromosomal Aberrations

In this study, radiosensitivity was measured based on the mean number of IR-induced DSBs per cell (i.e., misrepaired or unrepaired DSBs that generated CAs) following TC-FISH staining (**Figure 1A**) in cells undergoing first mitosis at 60 h postirradiation. DSBs were calculated based on the manual scoring of CAs, as described in Ref. (9) and in **Figure 1B**. Based on the frequencies of dicentrics, centric and acentric rings, and acentric fragments (with 0, 2, or 4 telomeres), a precise estimate of the number of IR-induced DSBs that gave rise to the CA can be calculated at the studied doses, as illustrated in **Figure 1B**. Generally, a dicentric or a centric ring with an acentric fragment containing four telomeres are considered as two DSBs; excess acentric fragments with two telomeres are considered as resulting from one DSB (terminal deletion); and excess acentric fragments with 0 telomeres are considered as resulting from two DSBs (interstitial deletion).

Following M-FISH staining (**Figure 1C**), the number of DSBs per cell can be calculated based on the visualization of chromosomal rearrangements (that are not visible with TC-FISH). Examples are illustrated in **Figure 1D**; in general, dicentrics and translocations involving two chromosomes often involve two DSBs, whereas more complex rearrangements with three chromosomes may involve four DSBs.

AUTHOR CONTRIBUTIONS

GS analyzed and interpreted the data and drafted the manuscript. MN, IT, and MR worked to design, acquire, and analyze the data. WH aided in the interpretation of the data and edited the manuscript. LS directed the course of this study. All authors provided critiques for the content of the manuscript, approved of the final version of the manuscript, and attest to the accuracy and integrity of this work.

ACKNOWLEDGMENTS

The authors gratefully thank Andrea Ottolenghi for his valuable discussions.

FUNDING

This work was supported by grants from the European Community's Seventh Framework Program (EURATOM) contract Fission-2011-249689 (DOREMI) and from the CEA-NRBC.

REFERENCES

1. Schlaff CD, Krauze A, Belard A, O'Connell JJ, Camphausen KA. Bringing the heavy: carbon ion therapy in the radiobiological and clinical context. *Radiat Oncol* (2014) 9(1):88. doi:10.1186/1748-717X-9-88
2. Hall EJ. *Radiobiology for the Radiologist*. Philadelphia: Lippincott Williams & Wilkins (2006).
3. Kamada T, Tsujii H, Blakely EA, Debus J, De Neve W, Durante M, et al. Carbon ion radiotherapy in Japan: an assessment of 20 years of clinical experience. *Lancet Oncol* (2015) 16(2):e93–100. doi:10.1016/S1470-2045(14)70412-7
4. Jermann M. Particle therapy statistics in 2013. *Int J Part Ther* (2014) 1(1):40–3. doi:10.14338/IJPT.14-editorial-2.1
5. Granzotto A, Joubert A, Viau M, Devic C, Maalouf M, Thomas C, et al. [Individual response to ionising radiation: what predictive assay(s) to choose?]. *C R Biol* (2011) 334(2):140–57. doi:10.1016/j.crvi.2010.12.018
6. Joubert A, Vogin G, Devic C, Granzotto A, Viau M, Maalouf M, et al. [Radiation biology: major advances and perspectives for radiotherapy]. *Cancer Radiother* (2011) 15(5):348–54. doi:10.1016/j.canrad.2011.05.001
7. Advisory Group on Ionising Radiation. Human radiosensitivity. *Report of the Independent Advisory Group on Ionising Radiation*. Chilton: Health Protection Agency (2013).
8. Shi L, Fujioka K, Sun J, Kinomura A, Inaba T, Ikura T, et al. A modified system for analyzing ionizing radiation-induced chromosome abnormalities. *Radiat Res* (2012) 177(5):533–8. doi:10.1667/RR2849.1
9. M'Kacher R, Maalouf EE, Ricoul M, Heidingsfelder L, Laplagne E, Cuceu C, et al. New tool for biological dosimetry: reevaluation and automation of the gold standard method following telomere and centromere staining. *Mutat Res* (2014) 770(0):45–53. doi:10.1016/j.mrfmmm.2014.09.007
10. Denekamp J, Waites T, Fowler JF. Predicting realistic RBE values for clinically relevant radiotherapy schedules. *Int J Radiat Biol* (1997) 71(6):681–94. doi:10.1080/095530097143699
11. Hartel C, Nikoghosyan A, Durante M, Sommer S, Nasonova E, Fournier C, et al. Chromosomal aberrations in peripheral blood lymphocytes of prostate cancer patients treated with IMRT and carbon ions. *Radiother Oncol* (2010) 95(1):73–8. doi:10.1016/j.radonc.2009.08.031
12. Schmitz A, Bayer J, Dechamps N, Goldin L, Thomas G. Heritability of susceptibility to ionizing radiation-induced apoptosis of human lymphocyte subpopulations. *Int J Radiat Oncol Biol Phys* (2007) 68(4):1169–77. doi:10.1016/j.ijrobp.2007.03.050
13. Viau M, Testard I, Shim G, Morat L, Normil MD, Hempel WM, et al. Global quantification of gammaH2AX as a triage tool for the rapid estimation of received dose in the event of accidental radiation exposure. *Mutat Res Genet Toxicol Environ Mutagen* (2015) 793:123–31. doi:10.1016/j.mrgentox.2015.05.009
14. Sabatier L, Lebeau J, Dutrillaux B. Radiation-induced carcinogenesis: individual sensitivity and genomic instability. *Radiat Environ Biophys* (1995) 34(4):229–32. doi:10.1007/BF01209747
15. Raynaud CM, Sabatier L, Philipot O, Olaussen KA, Soria JC. Telomere length, telomeric proteins and genomic instability during the multistep carcinogenic process. *Crit Rev Oncol Hematol* (2008) 66(2):99–117. doi:10.1016/j.critrevonc.2007.11.004
16. Shim G, Ricoul M, Hempel WM, Azzam EI, Sabatier L. Crosstalk between telomere maintenance and radiation effects: a key player in the process of radiation-induced carcinogenesis. *Mutat Res Rev Mutat Res* (2014) 760:1–7. doi:10.1016/j.mrrev.2014.01.001
17. Fernet M, Hall J. Genetic biomarkers of therapeutic radiation sensitivity. *DNA Repair (Amst)* (2004) 3(8–9):1237–43. doi:10.1016/j.dnarep.2004.03.019

18. Andreassen CN, Dikomey E, Parliament M, West CM. Will SNPs be useful predictors of normal tissue radiosensitivity in the future? *Radiother Oncol* (2012) 105(3):283–8. doi:10.1016/j.radonc.2012.11.003

19. Il'yasova D, Kinev A, Melton CD, Davis FG. Donor-specific cell-based assays in studying sensitivity to low-dose radiation: a population-based perspective. *Front Public Health* (2014) 2:244. doi:10.3389/fpubh.2014.00244

20. Mirjolet C, Boidot R, Saliques S, Ghiringhelli F, Maingon P, Crehange G. The role of telomeres in predicting individual radiosensitivity of patients with cancer in the era of personalized radiotherapy. *Cancer Treat Rev* (2015) 41(4):354–60. doi:10.1016/j.ctrv.2015.02.005

21. Hamasaki K, Imai K, Nakachi K, Takahashi N, Kodama Y, Kusunoki Y. Short-term culture and gammaH2AX flow cytometry determine differences in individual radiosensitivity in human peripheral T lymphocytes. *Environ Mol Mutagen* (2007) 48(1):38–47. doi:10.1002/em.20273

22. Ismail IH, Wadhra TI, Hammarsten O. An optimized method for detecting gamma-H2AX in blood cells reveals a significant interindividual variation in the gamma-H2AX response among humans. *Nucleic Acids Res* (2007) 35(5):e36. doi:10.1093/nar/gkl1169

23. Andrievski A, Wilkins RC. The response of gamma-H2AX in human lympho-cytes and lymphocytes subsets measured in whole blood cultures. *Int J Radiat Biol* (2009) 85(4):369–76. doi:10.1080/09553000902781147

24. Horn S, Barnard S, Rothkamm K. Gamma-H2AX-based dose estimation for whole and partial body radiation exposure. *PLoS One* (2011) 6(9):e25113. doi:10.1371/journal.pone.0025113

25. Sabatier L, Al Achkar W, Hoffschir F, Luccioni C, Dutrillaux B. Qualitative study of chromosomal lesions induced by neutrons and neon ions in human lymphocytes at G0 phase. *Mutat Res* (1987) 178(1):91–7. doi:10.1016/0027-5107(87)90090-X

26. Testard I, Dutrillaux B, Sabatier L. Chromosomal aberrations induced in human lymphocytes by high-LET irradiation. *Int J Radiat Biol* (1997) 72(4):423–33. doi:10.1080/095530097143194

27. Anderson RM, Marsden SJ, Wright EG, Kadhim MA, Goodhead DT, Griffin CS. Complex chromosome aberrations in peripheral blood lympho-cytes as a potential biomarker of exposure to high-LET alpha-particles. *Int J Radiat Biol* (2000) 76(1):31–42. doi:10.1080/095530000138989

28. Testard I, Sabatier L. Assessment of DNA damage induced by high-LET ions in human lymphocytes using the comet assay. *Mutat Res* (2000) 448(1):105–15. doi:10.1016/S0027-5107(00)00006-3

29. Loucas BD, Durante M, Bailey SM, Cornforth MN. Chromosome damage in human cells by gamma rays, alpha particles and heavy ions: track inter-actions in basic dose-response relationships. *Radiat Res* (2013) 179(1):9–20. doi:10.1667/RR3089.1

30. Loucas BD, Eberle R, Bailey SM, Cornforth MN. Influence of dose rate on the induction of simple and complex chromosome exchanges by gamma rays. *Radiat Res* (2004) 162(4):339–49. doi:10.1667/RR3245

31. M'Kacher R, El Maalouf E, Terzoudi G, Ricoul M, Heidingsfelder L, Karachristou I, et al. Detection and automated scoring of dicentric chromosomes in nonstimulated lymphocyte prematurely condensed chro-mosomes after telomere and centromere staining. *Int J Radiat Oncol Biol Phys* (2015) 91(3):640–9. doi:10.1016/j.ijrobp.2014.10.048

32. Speicher MR, Gwyn Ballard S, Ward DC. Karyotyping human chromosomes by combinatorial multi-fluor FISH. *Nat Genet* (1996) 12(4):368–75. doi:10.1038/ng0496-368

33. Loucas BD, Cornforth MN. Complex chromosome exchanges induced by gamma rays in human lymphocytes: an mFISH study. *Radiat Res* (2001) 155(5):660–71. doi:10.1667/0033-7587(2001)155[0660:CCEIBG]2.0.CO;2

34. Nieri D, Berardinelli F, Antoccia A, Tanzarella C, Sgura A. Comparison between two FISH techniques in the *in vitro* study of cytogenetic markers for low-dose X-ray exposure in human primary fibroblasts. *Front Genet* (2013) 4:141. doi:10.3389/fgene.2013.00141

35. Cho MS, Lee JK, Bae KS, Han EA, Jang SJ, Ha WH, et al. Retrospective biodosimetry using translocation frequency in a stable cell of occupationally exposed to ionizing radiation. *J Radiat Res* (2015) 56(4):709–16. doi:10.1093/jrr/rrv028

36. Tucker JD. Low-dose ionizing radiation and chromosome translocations: a review of the major considerations for human biological dosimetry. *Mutat Res* (2008) 659(3):211–20. doi:10.1016/j.mrrev.2008.04.001

37. Beinke C, Meineke V. High potential for methodical improvements of FISH-based translocation analysis for retrospective radiation biodosimetry. *Health Phys* (2012) 103(2):127–32. doi:10.1097/HP.0b013e31824645fb

38. Schmitz A, Bayer J, Dechamps N, Thomas G. Intrinsic susceptibility to radiation-induced apoptosis of human lymphocyte subpopulations. *Int J Radiat Oncol Biol Phys* (2003) 57(3):769–78. doi:10.1016/S0360-3016(03)00637-0

39. Durantel F, Balanzat E, Cassimi A, Chevalier F, Ngono-Ravache Y, Madi T, et al. Dosimetry for radiobiology experiments at GANIL. *Nucl Instrum Methods Phys Res A* (2016) 816:70–7. doi:10.1016/j.nima.2016.01.052

40. International Atomic Energy Agency (IAEA). Cytogenetic dosimetry: appli-cations in preparedness for and response to radiation emergencies. *Emergency Preparedness and Response Series*. Vienna: IAEA (2011). Available from: http://www-pub.iaea.org/books/IAEABooks/8735/Cytogenetic-Dosimetry-Applications-in-Preparedness-for-and-Response-to-Radiation-Emergencies

14

Biological Effectiveness of Accelerated Protons for Chromosome Exchanges

Kerry A. George[1]*, Megumi Hada[1] and Francis A. Cucinotta[2]

[1] *Wyle Science, Technology and Engineering Group, Houston, TX, USA,* [2] *University of Nevada Las Vegas, Las Vegas, NV, USA*

*Correspondence:
Kerry A. George
kerry.a.george@nasa.gov

We have investigated chromosome exchanges induced in human cells by seven different energies of protons (5–2500 MeV) with LET values ranging from 0.2 to 8 keV/μm. Human lymphocytes were irradiated *in vitro* and chromosome damage was assessed using three-color fluorescence *in situ* hybridization chromosome painting in chemically condensed chromosomes collected during the first cell division post irradiation. The relative biological effectiveness (RBE) was calculated from the initial slope of the dose–response curve for chromosome exchanges with respect to low dose and low dose-rate γ-rays (denoted as RBE_{max}), and relative to acute doses of γ-rays (denoted as $RBE_{\gamma Acute}$). The linear dose–response term was similar for all energies of protons, suggesting that the decrease in LET with increasing proton energy was balanced by the increase in dose from the production of nuclear secondaries. Secondary particles increase slowly above energies of a few hundred megaelectronvolts. Additional studies of 50 g/cm² aluminum shielded high-energy proton beams showed minor differences compared to the unshielded protons and lower RBE values found for shielded in comparison to unshielded beams of 2 or 2.5 GeV. All energies of protons produced a much higher percentage of complex-type chromosome exchanges when compared to acute doses of γ-rays. The implications of these results for space radiation protection and proton therapy are discussed.

Keywords: chromosomal aberrations, biomarkers, protons, proton therapy, space radiation

INTRODUCTION

The study of the biological effectiveness of accelerated proton exposures is of interest for clinical treatment plans and for assessing normal tissue damage from protons of various energies that are generated outside of the Bragg peak during proton therapy (1–4). Protons are also a concern for space radiation exposures to astronauts because the space radiation flux is predominantly energetic protons or secondary protons produced in nuclear interactions (5–7). Although evidence now indicates that relative biological effectiveness (RBE) varies considerably along the proton depth-dose distribution, RBE modeling in treatment planning still involves significant uncertainties and, consequently, clinical proton therapy is usually based on the use of a generic RBE of 1.1 (4). Further experimental data are required before a consensus can be reached on weighting factors across the depth-dose profile and for different tissue effects.

Experimental studies have shown that the RBE of protons varies with biological endpoint, tissue type, dose, and energy of the protons. RBE values calculated by cell killing and mutation induction indicate that low energy protons are significantly higher than unity and values are LET dependent (8). Published data on chromosome damage have indicated that RBEs or RBE_{max} values for protons of energies above 10 MeV vary from <1 to about 2 in comparison to X-rays or γ-rays, whereas lower energy protons (<10 MeV) were significantly higher than unity and the values were LET dependent (9–11). RBEs for tumor induction were close to 1 in several studies (12, 13), and as high as 2 for Harderian gland tumors (14) and for rat mammary carcinomas (15) that were induced by 250 MeV protons. The choice of reference radiation can complicate the analysis of RBE because differences have been found for X-rays and γ-rays (16), and variability has been reported for low doses of photons and protons. In addition, high-energy protons induce nuclear spallation and other interactions that produce secondary protons, neutrons, and heavy ion fragments. Nuclear interaction cross sections generally increase with the energy of the protons (3), and the secondary particles typically have higher LET values that can increase RBE.

In the present study, we considered the induction of simple and complex-type chromosome exchanges in normal human lymphocytes. Chromosome exchanges, especially translocations, are positively correlated with many cancers, and are therefore a potential biomarker of cancer risk associated with radiation exposure (17–19). In addition, RBE factors for chromosome aberrations are similar to RBEs observed for induction of solid tumors in mice (16, 20, 21). Therefore, chromosome exchanges are a useful biomarker for cancer risk and can be compared with other biomarkers in the absence of human data for galactic cosmic rays (GCR). In earlier work (22), we considered the effects of 250 MeV protons at different dose-rates. Here, we consider several proton energies from 5 to 2500 MeV with additional studies on the effects of heavy aluminum and polyethylene shielding for the high-energy proton exposures.

MATERIALS AND METHODS

These studies were conducted in accordance with accepted ethical and humane practices, and were approved by the appropriate institutional and/or governmental committee(s) and/or organization(s).

Irradiation

Whole blood was collected from healthy volunteers and was irradiated with accelerated protons using the NASA Space Radiation Laboratory (NSRL) facility at Brookhaven National Laboratory (BNL). The same volunteer donated the blood samples for each experiment. All samples were exposed in the plateau portion of the Bragg curves and dose rates were between 0.2 and 0.5 Gy/min, depending on the dose delivered. Doses were measured at the target using ionization chambers. Samples were exposed at room temperature. Each sample received at least three pulses and no exposure lasted more than 10 min. The beam uniformity was checked using a digital beam imager and dose did not vary more than 5% over the target area. For the 2.5 and 2 GeV protons exposures, the target areas was shielded, respectively, with 50 g/cm^2 of aluminum and 50 g/cm^2 of aluminum plus 10 cm of polyethylene. At these proton energies, the dose increases as the protons pass through the shielding due to secondary radiation, and doses were normalized using BNL dosimetry to generate the same total dose to the sample as the unshielded studies.

Cell Culture

Immediately after exposure, whole-blood cultures in RPMI 1640 medium (Gibco BRL) supplemented with 20% calf serum and 1% phytohemagglutinin (Gibco, BRL) were incubated at 37°C for 48–50 h. Chemically induced PPC were collected using the method described by Durante et al. (23), which results in well-condensed chromosomes from cells in G2 and metaphase. Briefly, 50 nM calyculin A (Wako Chemicals) was added to the growth medium for the last 30 min of the incubation. Cells were then treated with hypotonic KCl (0.075M) for 15 min at 37°C and fixed in methanol:acetic acid (3:1). A 0.5 ml volume of blood from each sample was cultured with 10 μm bromodeoxyuridine (BrdU), and a differential replication staining procedure was completed on chromosomes from these samples by incubating slides in 0.5 mg/ml of Hoechst during exposure to black light (General Electric 15T8/BL bulb). Chromosomes were stained with Giemsa to visualized replication rounds, revealing the percentage of cells in first mitosis was >95% for all samples analyzed.

Fluorescence *In situ* Hybridization

Chromosomes were dropped onto clean microscope slides and hybridized *in situ* with a combination of fluorescence whole-chromosome probes for chromosomes 1, 2, and 4, or chromosome 1, 2, and 5 (Rainbow Scientific) using the procedures recommended by the manufacturer. Chromosome 1 was painted with a Texas red fluorophore, chromosome 2 was painted with FTIC, and chromosome 4 (or 5) was painted with a 1:1 combination of Texas Red and FITC that appeared yellow under the triple-band-pass filter set. Unlabeled chromosomes were always counterstained with 4′,6-diamidino-2-phenylindole (DAPI).

Chromosome Analysis

Chromosomes were analyzed on a Zeiss Axioplan fluorescence microscope. The images of all damaged cells were captured electronically using a Sensys charge-coupled device (CCD) camera (Photometrics Ltd., AZ, USA) and the Cytovision computer software. The number of cells analyzed for each sample varied, exact numbers are listed in **Table 1**. All slides analyzed in this study were coded and scored blind. Complex exchanges were scored when it was determined that an exchange involved a minimum of three breaks in two or more chromosomes (24). An exchange was defined as simple if it appeared to involve two breaks in two chromosomes, that is, dicentrics and translocations. Incomplete translocations and incomplete dicentrics were included in the category of simple exchanges, assuming that in most cases the reciprocal fragments were below the level of detection (25). Each type of exchange – dicentrics, apparently simple reciprocal exchanges, incompletes, or complex exchanges – was counted as one exchange, and values for total exchanges were derived by

TABLE 1 | Dose–response data for chromosome aberrations per 100 cells induced by 5 different energies of protons measured in first post irradiation chemically induced PCC.

Dose (Gy)	Cells scored	Simple exchanges	Complex exchanges
E = 5 MeV			
0.10	1018	2.3 ± 0.7	0 ± 0
0.20	1044	1.2 ± 0.9	0.7 ± 0.4
0.40	909	6.8 ± 1.6	1.1 ± 0.6
0.70	869	8.0 ± 1.7	2.1 ± 0.8
1.00	634	14.9 ± 2.6	4.3 ± 1.3
E = 120 MeV[a]			
0.15	1188	1.5 ± 0.6	0.4 ± 0.3
0.30	1437	2.1 ± 0.6	1.0 ± 0.4
0.50	1369	3.6 ± 0.8	2.7 ± 0.7
0.75	1136	6.1 ± 1.2	2.4 ± 0.7
1.00	825	13.8 ± 2.0	3.6 ± 1.0
1.50	357	31.2 ± 4.7	11.1 ± 2.8
2.00	203	61.0 ± 8.6	34.2 ± 6.5
E = 250 MeV			
0.25	491	1.9 ± 1.8	3.1 ± 1.3
0.50	536	2.8 ± 1.8	5.3 ± 1.6
0.80	427	5.2 ± 2.3	3.6 ± 1.5
1.20	563	7.6 ± 2.3	5.5 ± 1.6
2.00	325	29.4 ± 5.1	11.1 ± 3.0
E = 800 MeV			
0.25	330	0 ± 1.1	2.3 ± 1.4
0.50	609	0 ± 0.8	0.4 ± 0.4
0.80	655	13.8 ± 2.6	5.1 ± 1.4
1.20	561	14.0 ± 2.9	6.0 ± 1.7
2.00	263	35.2 ± 6.2	7.8 ± 2.8
E = 1000 MeV			
0.20	231	3.0 ± 2.2	0 ± 0
1.20	321	13.0 ± 3.7	4.3 ± 2.2
3.00	134	87.9 ± 15.1	38.8 ± 10.0
E = 2000 MeV			
0.25	330	0.7 ± 1.3	0.8 ± 0.8
0.50	284	9.7 ± 3.2	6.1 ± 2.3
0.80	378	13.5 ± 3.1	3.3 ± 1.5
1.20	538	9.9 ± 2.3	7.4 ± 1.8
2.00	243	46.3 ± 7.0	15.3 ± 4.0
E = 2500 MeV			
0.20	1342	1.4 ± 0.5	0.8 ± 0.4
0.40	1127	3.4 ± 0.9	2.1 ± 0.7
0.60	1635	7.6 ± 1.1	2.6 ± 0.6
0.80	218	7.1 ± 2.9	4.7 ± 2.4
1.20	304	24.7 ± 4.6	4.3 ± 1.9

Data represent whole-genome equivalent values with background subtracted. [a]150 MeV protons with 5 cm polyethylene shielding leading to residual energy of 120 MeV.

adding the yields. When two or more painted chromosomes were damaged, each was scored separately.

Statistical Analysis

The frequency of chromosomal aberrations in the painted chromosomes was evaluated as the ratio between aberrations scored and total cells analyzed. Several studies have indicated that the distribution of radiation damage among chromosomes is random, and the yield of exchanges measured within the first division after exposure is proportional to the DNA content of the chromosome analyzed, with some fluctuation of data (26). Therefore, the frequencies of exchanges in individual chromosomes can be extrapolated to whole-genome equivalents using a modified version of the Lucas et al. (27) formula, Fp = 2.05[fp(1−fp) + fp1fp2 + fp1fp3 + fp2fp3]FG. Fp is the combined frequency of exchanges in all painted chromosomes, fp is the fraction of the whole genome comprised of the painted chromosomes, fp1, fp2, and fp3 are the fractions of the genome for each individual chromosome, and FG is the whole-genome aberration frequency. Using this formula, the genomic frequency for a male donor was estimated as 2.48 times that detected in chromosomes 1, 2, and 4.

Standard errors for aberration frequencies were calculated assuming Poisson statistics. Error bars in each figure represent SEs of the mean values. The data were modeled assuming binomial errors per number of chromosomes analyzed with the frequencies of aberrations of various types extrapolated to whole-genome equivalents as described above.

A weighted linear-quadratic (LQ) or linear (L) regression model was used to fit dose–responses for each proton energy, and the γ-ray dose–responses. Using the maximum likelihood method, the linear and quadratic coefficients α and β in

$$Y = Y_0 + \alpha D + \beta D^2$$

were found for simple, complex, and total exchanges. Estimates of RBE were made from the α-coefficient from the acute response (21), denoted as $RBE_{\gamma Acute}$, and from the ratio of initial slopes for γ-rays using our previous data (28–30) of low dose and low dose-rate irradiation, denoted as RBE_{max}. For estimating a low dose and low dose-rate γ-ray component, we combined the data from our previous analysis of 0.1 Gy/h with additional data at low doses (<0.5 Gy) from the same volunteer used for the proton experiments. For complex exchanges, the low dose and dose-rate γ-rays, complex exchanges were rare and RBE_{max} estimates could not be made.

RESULTS

Tables 1 and 2 list the dose–response data for simple and complex-type chromosome exchanges for each energy of protons, and are represented as whole-genome equivalent values with background subtracted. The data, plotted in **Figure 1**, show a high degree of similarity in the dose–response for simple and complex exchanges for all proton energies considered. A weighted regression model based on the experimental errors was used to estimate α and β values with SEs for a linear-quadratic dose–response fit to the data for γ-rays and each proton energy. **Tables 3–5** show results of this analysis for total exchanges, simple exchanges, and complex exchanges respectively. Comparison of the α values for acute and low dose rate (LDR) γ-rays fits indicates a dose-rate modifier factor of 1.83 and 1.74 for total exchanges and simple exchanges, respectively.

The linear (α) coefficients from the dose–response data (**Tables 3–5**) are similar for all energies as determined by either the LQ or L weighted regression models. The α values produced from the LQ models resulted in somewhat larger SD compared to fits from the linear weighted regression model (results not shown). RBE values for simple exchanges were slightly less or more than unity using the $RBE_{\gamma Acute}$ and RBE max models, respectively.

However, a much higher frequency of complex exchanges was observed for each proton beam compared to γ-rays resulting in RBEs for complex exchanges varied from 2.1 to 4.1, and this led to a modest increase the RBEs for total exchanges. A trend toward increasing RBE_{max} values for proton energies of 1 GeV and higher was found for simple and total exchanges.

Data for the yield of chromosome exchanges in the shielded samples are listed in **Table 2** where values are represented as whole-genome equivalent with background subtracted. The 2.5 GeV protons were shielded with 50 g/cm² of aluminum, and the 2 GeV protons were shielded with 50 g/cm² of aluminum plus 10 cm polyethylene. The doses represent the values measures at the target. A comparison of shielded and unshielded data shown in **Figure 2** indicates similar dose–responses for the shielded and unshielded high-energy proton beams. However, RBE_{max} values were reduced with shielding. For example, RBE values for total exchanges induced

TABLE 2 | Dose–response data for chromosome exchanges per 100 cells induced by 2 and 2.5 GeV protons with and without shielding and measured in first post irradiation chemically induced PCC.

Dose (Gy)	Cells scored	Simple exchanges	Complex exchanges
E = 2000 MeV, no shielding			
0.25	330	0.7 ± 1.3	0.8 ± 0.8
0.50	284	9.7 ± 3.2	6.1 ± 2.3
0.80	378	13.5 ± 3.1	3.3 ± 1.5
1.20	538	9.9 ± 2.3	7.4 ± 1.8
2.00	243	46.3 ± 7.0	15.3 ± 4.0
E = 2000 MeV, 50 g/cm² Aluminum + 10 cm polyethylene			
0.25	401	1.3 ± 0.9	0.6 ± 0.6
0.5	1029	4.8 ± 1.1	2.0 ± 0.7
0.8	940	7.7 ± 1.5	1.6 ± 0.7
1.2	709	15.2 ± 2.4	4.4 ± 1.3
2.0	456	28.7 ± 4.0	3.0 ± 1.5
E = 2500 MeV, no shielding			
0.20	1342	1.4 ± 0.5	0.8 ± 0.4
0.40	1127	3.4 ± 0.9	2.1 ± 0.7
0.60	1635	7.6 ± 1.1	2.6 ± 0.6
0.80	218	7.1 ± 2.9	4.7 ± 2.4
1.20	304	24.7 ± 4.6	4.3 ± 1.9
E = 2500 MeV, 50 g/cm² aluminum			
0.20	485	1.1 ± 0.8	0.5 ± 0.5
0.40	696	2.2 ± 0.9	0.7 ± 0.5
0.60	629	9.0 ± 1.9	2.5 ± 1.0
0.80	729	8.8 ± 1.8	3.5 ± 1.1
1.2	551	19.1 ± 3.0	9.3 ± 2.1

Dose was measured at the target area for both shielded and unshielded exposures. Data represent whole-genome equivalent values with background subtracted.

TABLE 3 | Results for parameter estimates of linear-quadratic dose-response model for total exchanges, and relative biological effectiveness (RBE) factors for protons of different energies compared to acute, or low dose or low dose-rate γ-rays.

Radiation type	α (Gy⁻¹)	β (Gy⁻²)	$RBE_{γAcute}$	RBE_{max}
γ-Rays acute	0.176 ± 0.018	0.119 ± 0.038	–	–
γ-Rays LD	0.096 ± 0.01	–	–	–
Proton, 5 MeV	0.171 ± 0.018	0.043 ± 0.065	0.98 ± 0.11	1.78 ± 0.19
Proton, 120 MeV[a]	0.156 ± 0.016	0.167 ± 0.039	0.89 ± 0.09	1.62 ± 0.16
Proton, 250 MeV	0.144 ± 0.017	0.05 ± 0.032	0.82 ± 0.1	1.5 ± 0.18
Proton, 800 MeV	0.153 ± 0.036	0.114 ± 0.064	0.87 ± 0.21	1.59 ± 0.38
Proton, 1000 MeV	0.219 ± 0.037	0.12 ± 0.043	1.25 ± 0.21	2.27 ± 0.38
Proton, 2000 MeV	0.201 ± 0.033	0.093 ± 0.067	1.15 ± 0.19	2.09 ± 0.34
Proton, 2500 MeV	0.184 ± 0.006	0.105 ± 0.01	1.05 ± 0.05	1.91 ± 0.07

[a]*150 MeV protons with 5 cm polyethylene shielding leading to residual energy of 120 MeV.*

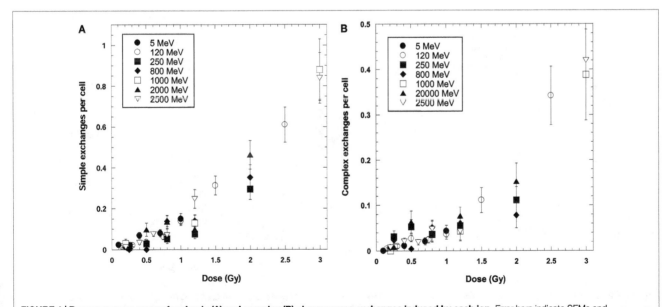

FIGURE 1 | Dose response curves for simple (A) and complex (B) chromosome exchanges induced by each ion. Error bars indicate SEMs and background values have been subtracted for all data.

by unshielded and shielded 2 GeV protons were 2.09 ± 0.34 and 1.26 ± 0.11, respectively, and values were 1.91 ± 0.67 and 1.53 ± 0.14 for unshielded and shielded 2.5 GeV protons, respectively.

DISCUSSION

The similarity in frequency of simple and complex exchanges over a wide range of proton energies found in our experiments suggests that decreases in LET with increasing proton energy is balanced by the increase in doses from secondary radiation, most notably secondary protons and neutrons (3, 31, 32). When the proton LET

decreases from about 5 keV/μm at 5 MeV to 0.24 keV/μm at the highest energy of 2.5 GeV, there is concomitant increase in the contribution from nuclear secondaries and their contribution to the biological action cross section (3). Details of the beam characteristics for the shielded and unshielded protons used in our study are given in **Table 6**. Neutrons are produced in the absorbers or tissue equivalent materials through nuclear reactions by protons and other charged particles. Low energy neutrons (<5 MeV) are known to have large RBEs for different types of biological damage, including late effects (16). For our unshielded proton experiments, neutrons produced by the small amount of absorbing material present in the NSRL beam-line and biological samples themselves are largely high energy and unlikely to have slowed down to the more biologically effective neutron energies (<5 MeV). However, our experiments comparing shielding to unshielded protons at high energies led to similar yields of chromosome exchanges per unit dose. This is consistent with previous radiobiology studies

TABLE 4 | Results for parameter estimates of linear-quadratic dose–response model for simple exchanges, and relative biological effectiveness (RBE) factors for protons of different energies compared to acute or low dose or low dose-rate γ-rays.

Radiation type	α (Gy^{-1})	β (Gy^{-2})	RBE$_{\gamma Acute}$	RBE$_{max}$
γ-Rays acute	0.157 ± 0.013	0.092 ± 0.027	–	–
γ-Rays LD	0.09 ± 0.004	–	–	–
Proton, 5 MeV	0.132 ± 0.016	0.031 ± 0.057	0.84 ± 0.1	1.5 ± 0.18
Proton, 120 MeV[a]	0.121 ± 0.015	0.137 ± 0.036	0.77 ± 0.1	1.36 ± 0.17
Proton, 250 MeV	0.088 ± 0.009	0.064 ± 0.017	0.56 ± 0.06	1.0 ± 0.1
Proton, 800 MeV	0.116 ± 0.028	0.104 ± 0.049	0.73 ± 0.18	1.3 ± 0.31
Proton, 1000 MeV	0.159 ± 0.02	0.081 ± 0.023	1.01 ± 0.13	1.79 ± 0.23
Proton, 2000 MeV	0.132 ± 0.028	0.071 ± 0.058	0.84 ± 0.19	1.49 ± 0.31
Proton, 2500 MeV	0.119 ± 0.01	0.077 ± 0.015	0.76 ± 0.07	1.35 ± 0.11

[a]150 MeV proton beam with 5 cm polyethylene shielding leading to residual energy of 120 MeV.

TABLE 5 | Results for parameter estimates of linear-quadratic dose–response model for complex exchanges, and relative biological effectiveness (RBE) factors for protons of different energies compared to acute γ-rays.

Radiation type	α (Gy^{-1})	β (Gy^{-2})	RBE$_{\gamma Acute}$
γ-Rays acute	0.015 ± 0.005	0.025 ± 0.014	–
Proton, 5 MeV	0.039 ± 0.004	0.006 ± 0.017	2.56 ± 0.85
Proton, 120 MeV[a]	0.032 ± 0.0043	0.024 ± 0.01	2.1 ± 0.28
Proton, 250 MeV	0.055 ± 0.009	0.03 ± 0.017	3.59 ± 1.3
Proton, 800 MeV	0.029 ± 0.010	0.02 ± 0.017	1.92 ± 0.87
Proton, 1000 MeV	0.06 ± 0.016	0.046 ± 0.022	3.96 ± 1.64
Proton, 2000 MeV	0.063 ± 0.009	0.028 ± 0.017	4.12 ± 1.41
Proton, 2500 MeV	0.058 ± 0.006	0.026 ± 0.01	3.81 ± 1.26

RBE$_{max}$ was not determined because low dose-rate γ-rays have very low induction of complex exchanges.

[a]150 MeV proton beam with 5 cm polyethylene shielding leading to residual energy at samples of 120 MeV.

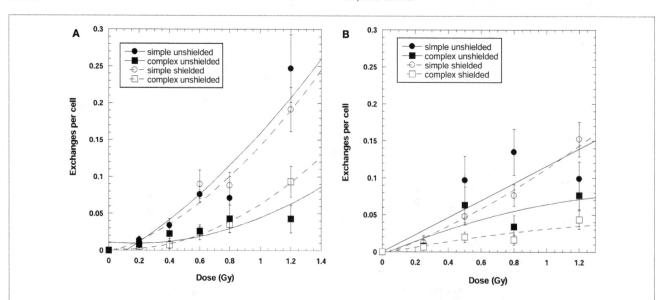

FIGURE 2 | Dose–response curves for chromosome exchanges induced by 2500 MeV protons (A) and 2000 MeV/μ protons (B). The 2000-MeV exposures were shielded with a combination of 50 g/cm² aluminum and 10 cm polyethylene. The 2500-MeV exposure were shielded with 50 g/cm² aluminum only. Error bars indicate SEMs and background values have been subtracted for all data points. Curve fit is extrapolated to the axis.

TABLE 6 | Details of protons shielding characteristics.

Energy at beam entrance (MeV)	Shielding	Energy of beam at target (MeV)	LET (keV/μm)	Percentage of dose from secondaries
5	None	–	7.80	–
120	5 cm polyethylene	42	0.64	6.4
250	None	220	0.43	17.4
800	None	770	0.24	33.1
1000	None	970	0.22	36.5
2000	None	1924	0.21	42.6
	50 g/cm^2 aluminum + 10 cm polyethylene	1624	0.21	80.0
2500	None	2470	0.21	43.7
	50 g/cm^2 aluminum	2241	0.21	78.4

Shielding from booster window, ion chambers, and binary filter contribute 1.2 g/cm^2 of aluminum equivalent shielding to all exposures (shielded or unshielded).
LET reflects values for the beam only and does not include the effect of secondary particles.

with high-energy proton beams using very thick absorbers (33) and suggests that neutrons are ineffective in producing biological damage at high energy (>100 MeV). This observation is readily predicted by the mean-free path of neutrons which is generally >10 g/cm^2 for materials of interest. Because the nuclear absorption cross sections are similar, secondary particles and target fragmentation spectrum produced by protons and neutrons are nearly identical for energies above a few hundred megaelectron-volts. Thus, high-energy protons are biologically more effective than neutrons of the same energy per unit fluence because of the proton charge state, while high-energy neutrons will have higher effectiveness per unit dose.

The NSRL beam-line and the sample holders provide a minimum of 1.2 g/cm^2 of aluminum equivalent shielding. The additional shielding used in our experiments had a minor influence on the biological effectiveness when comparing unshielded high-energy proton beams because the secondary radiation produced behind the shielding will be of similar biological effectiveness as the primary beam, while similar numbers of low energy target fragments of high-LET produced for both the primary and secondary protons and neutrons will be produced for the shielded and unshielded beams.

The α values for acute and LDR γ-rays fits indicate a dose-rate modification factor of 1.83 and 1.74 for total exchanges and simple exchanges, respectively. These values are similar to those reported for dose-rate reduction factors found by Peng et al. (34), dose and dose-rate reduction effectiveness factors (DDREF) for tumor induction in mice (21), and larger than values reported for solid tumors in the atomic bomb survivors where a DDREF of 1.3 is estimated in the BEIR VII report (35).

In the present study, we used three-color combinations of fluorescence in situ hybridization (FISH) chromosome painting probes (chromosomes 1, 2, and 4, or 1, 2, and 5) to analyze our data. Presumably complex exchanges would be underestimated with this method due to the presence of some pseudosimple-type exchanges [that is, complex patterns that are indistinguishable from those created by simple reciprocal exchanges (36)]. Although the true complexity of exchanges can be determined only by analysis of all chromosomes, a significant number of chromosome exchanges found for all proton energies in this study were determined to be complex, which were significantly increased compared to acute or low dose-rate γ-rays.

In conclusion, our study of the proton energy dependence of chromosome exchanges in human lymphocytes suggests that biological effects are similar over a wide range of proton energies (5–2500 MeV) with RBE values for total exchanges are close to unity when measured against acute γ rays, and approach 2 when measured against low dose rate γ rays due to the increased number of complex exchanges at all proton energies compared to γ-rays.

ACKNOWLEDGMENTS

The authors are grateful to the staff of the Brookhaven National Laboratory for supporting the accelerator studies. Financial support for his work was provided by National Aeronautics and Space Administration's Space Radiation Program Element (NASA contract number NAS9-02078).

REFERENCES

1. Terasawa T, Dvorak T, Ip S, Raman G, Lau J, Trikalinos TA. Systematic review: charged-particle radiation therapy for cancer. *Ann Intern Med* (2009) **151**(8):556–65. doi:10.7326/0003-4819-151-8-200910200-00145

2. Shulz-Ertner D, Tsujii H. Particle radiation therapy using proton and heavier ion beams. *J Clini Oncol* (2007) **25**:953–64. doi:10.1200/JCO.2006.09.7816

3. Cucinotta FA, Katz R, Wilson JW, Townsend LW, Shinn JL, Hajnal F. Biological effectiveness of high-energy protons: target fragmentation. *Radiat Res* (1991) **127**:130–7. doi:10.2307/3577956

4. Wouters BG, Skarsgard LD, Gerweck LE, Carabe-Fernandez A, Wong M, Durand RE, et al. Radiobiological intercomparison of the 160 MeV and 230 MeV proton therapy beams at the Harvard Cyclotron Laboratory and at Massachusetts General Hospital. *Radiat Res* (2015) **183**:174–87. doi:10.1667/RR13795.1

5. Cucinotta FA, Durante M. Cancer risk from exposure to galactic cosmic rays: implications for space exploration by human beings. *Lancet Oncol* (2006) **7**:431–5. doi:10.1016/S1470-2045(06)70695-7

6. Durante M, Cucinotta FA. Heavy ion carcinogenesis and human space exploration. *Nat Rev Cancer* (2008) **8**:465–72. doi:10.1038/nrc2391

7. NCRP. *Recommendations of Dose Limits for Low Earth Orbit*. Bethesda, MD: National Council on Radiation Protection and Measurements. NCRP Report 132 (2000).

8. Belli M, Cera F, Cherubini R, Haque AMI, Ianzini F, Moschini G, et al. Inactivation and mutation induction In V79 cells by low energy protons: re-evaluation of the results at the LNL facility. *Int J Radiat Biol* (1993) **63**:331–7. doi:10.1080/09553009314550441

9. Edwards AA, Lloyd DC, Prosser JS, Finnon P, Moquet JE. Chromosome aberrations induced by 8.7 MeV protons and 23.5 helium-3 ions. *Int J Radiat Biol* (1986) **50**:137–45. doi:10.1080/09553008614550511

10. Edwards AA, Llyod DC, Prosser JS. The induction of chromosome aberrations in human lymphocytes by accelerated particles. *Radiat Prot Dosimetry* (1985) **13**:205–9.

11. Schmid E, Roos H, Rumple G, Bauchinger M. Chromosome aberration frequencies in human lymphocytes irradiated in a multi-layer array by protons with different LET. *Int J Radiat Biol* (1998) **72**(6):661–5. doi:10.1080/095530097142816

12. Clapp NK, Darden EB Jr, Jernigan MC. Relative effects of whole-body sub-lethal doses of 60-MeV protons and 300-kVp X-rays on disease incidence in RF mice. *Radiat Res* (1974) 57:158–86. doi:10.2307/3573764

13. Weil MM, Ray FA, Genik PC, Yu Y, McCarthy M, Fallgren CM, et al. Effects of ^{28}Si ions, ^{56}Fe ions, and protons on the induction of murine acute myeloid leukemia and hepatocellular carcinoma. *PLoS One* (2014) 9(8):e104819. doi:10.1371/journal.pone.0104819

14. Alpen EL, Powers-Risius P, Curtis SB, DeGuzman R. Tumorigenic potential of high-Z, high-LET charged particle radiations. *Radiat Res* (1993) 88:132–43. doi:10.2307/3575758

15. Dicello JF, Christian A, Cucinotta FA, Gridley DS, Kathirithhamby R, Mann J, et al. *In vivo* mammary tumorigenesis in the Sprague-Dawley rat and microdosimetric correlates. *Phys Med Biol* (2004) 49:3817–30. doi:10.1088/0031-9155/49/16/024

16. ICRP. *Relative Biological Effectiveness (RBE), Quality Factor (Q), and Radiation Weighting Factor (w_R).* Pergamon: International Commission on Radiation Protection (2003). ICRP Publication 103.

17. George K, Durante M, Wu H, Willingham V, Badhwar G, Cucinotta FA. Chromosome aberrations in the blood lympho-cytes of astronauts after space flight. *Radiat Res* (2001) 156:731–8. doi:10.1667/0033-7587(2001)156[0731:CAITBL]2.0.CO;2

18. Bonassi S, Norppa H, Ceppi M, Strömberg U, Vermeulen R, Znaor A, et al. Chromosomal aberration frequency in lymphocytes predicts the risk of cancer: results from a pooled cohort study of 22 358 subjects in 11 countries. *Carcinogenesis* (2008) 29:1178–83. doi:10.1093/carcin/bgn075

19. ICRP – International Commission on Radiological Protection. Assessment of radiation exposure of astronauts in space. ICRP Publication 123. *Ann ICRP* (2013) 42(4):1–139. doi:10.1016/j.icrp.2013.05.004

20. Cucinotta FA, Kim MY, Chappell L. *Space Radiation Cancer Risk Projections and Uncertainties – 2012.* NASA TP 2013-217375 (2013). Available from: http://www.sti.nasa.gov

21. Cucinotta FAA. New approach to reduce uncertainties in space radiation can-cer risk predictions. *PLoS One* (2015) 10(3):e0120717. doi:10.1371/journal.pone.0120717

22. George K, Willingham V, Wu H, Gridley D, Nelson G, Cucinotta FA. Chromosome aberrations in human lymphocytes induced by 250 MeV pro-tons: effects of dose, dose rate and shielding. *Adv Space Res* (2002) 30:891–9. doi:10.1016/S0273-1177(02)00406-4

23. Durante M, Furusawa Y, Majima H, Kawata T, Gotoh E. Association between G2-phase block and repair of radiation-induced chromosome fragments in human lymphocytes. *Radiat Res* (1999) 151:670–6. doi:10.2307/3580205

24. Savage RK, Simpson PJ. On scoring of FISH-"painted" chromo-some-type exchange aberrations. *Mutat Res* (1994) 307:345–53. doi:10.1016/0027-5107(94)90308-5

25. Wu H, George K, Yang TC. Estimate of true incomplete exchanges using flu-orescence in situ hybridization with telomere probes. *Int J Radiat Biol* (1998) 73:521–7. doi:10.1080/095530098142068

26. Luomahaara S, Lindholm C, Mustonen R, Salomaa S. Distribution of radia-tion-induced exchange aberrations in human chromosomes 1, 2 and 4. *Int J Radiat Biol* (1999) 75:1551–6. doi:10.1080/095530099139151

27. Lucas JN, Poggensee M, Straume T. The persistence of chromosome translo-cations in a radiation worker accidentally exposed to tritium. *Cytogenet Cell Genet* (1992) 60:255–6. doi:10.1159/000133353

28. George K, Wu H, Willingham V, Furusawa Y, Kawata T, Cucinotta FA. High-and low-LET induced chromosome damage in human lymphocytes; a time course of aberrations in metaphase and interphase. *Int J Radiat Biol* (2001) 77:175–83. doi:10.1080/0955300001003760

29. George K, Cucinotta FA. The influence of shielding on the biological effective-ness of accelerated particles for the induction of chromosome damage. *Adv Space Res* (2007) 39:1076–81. doi:10.1016/j.asr.2007.01.004

30. George K, Durante M, Willingham V, Wu H, Yang TC, Cucinotta FA. Biological effectiveness of accelerated particles for the induction of chromosome damage measured in metaphase and interphase in human lymphocytes. *Radiat Res* (2003) 160:425–35. doi:10.1667/RR3064

31. Tripathi RK, Cucinotta FA, Wilson JW. Accurate universal parameterization of absorption cross sections III – light systems. *Nucl Instrum Methods Phy Res B* (1999) 155:349 56. doi:10.1016/S0168-583X(99)00479-6

32. Wilson JW, Cucinotta FA, Shinn JL, Townsend LW. *Target Fragmentation in Radiobiology.* Washington, DC (1993). NASA TM-1993-4408. Available from: http://www.sti.nasa.gov

33. Bertucci A, Durante M, Gialanella G, Grossi G, Manti L, Pugliese M, et al. Shielding of relativistic protons. *Radiat Environ Biophys* (2007) 46:107–12. doi:10.1007/s00411-006-0088-6

34. Peng Y, Hatsumi N, Warner C, Bedford JS. Genetic susceptibility: radiation effects relevant to space travel. *Health Phys* (2012) 103:607–20. doi:10.1097/HP.0b013e31826945b9

35. BEIR VII. *Health Risks from Exposure to Low Levels of Ionizing Radiation. National Academy of Sciences Committee on the Biological Effects of Radiation.* Washington, DC: National Academy of Sciences Press (2006).

36. Simpson PJ, Papworth DG, Savage JP. X-ray-induced simple, pseudosimple and complex exchanges involving two distinctly painted chromosomes. *Int J Radiat Biol* (1999) 75:11–8. doi:10.1080/095530099140753

15

Induction of Chronic Inflammation and Altered Levels of DNA Hydroxymethylation in Somatic and Germinal Tissues of CBA/CaJ Mice Exposed to ^{48}Ti Ions

Kanokporn Noy Rithidech[1]*, Witawat Jangiam[1,2], Montree Tungjai[1,3], Chris Gordon[1], Louise Honikel[1] and Elbert B. Whorton[4]

[1] Department of Pathology, Stony Brook University, Stony Brook, NY, USA, [2] Department of Chemical Engineering, Faculty of Engineering, Burapha University, Chonburi, Thailand, [3] Department of Radiologic Technology, Faculty of Associated Medical Sciences, Center of Excellence for Molecular Imaging, Chiang Mai University, Chiang Mai, Thailand, [4] StatCom, Galveston, TX, USA

*Correspondence:
Kanokporn Noy Rithidech
kanokporn.rithidech@
stonybrookmedicine.edu

Although the lung is one of the target organs at risk for cancer induction from exposure to heavy ions found in space, information is insufficient on cellular/molecular responses linked to increased cancer risk. Knowledge of such events may aid in the development of new preventive measures. Furthermore, although it is known that germinal cells are sensitive to X- or γ-rays, there is little information on the effects of heavy ions on germinal cells. Our goal was to investigate in vivo effects of 1 GeV/n ^{48}Ti ions (one of the important heavy ions found in the space environment) on somatic (lung) and germinal (testis) tissues collected at various times after a whole body irradiation of CBA/CaJ mice (0, 0.1, 0.25, or 0.5 Gy, delivered at 1 cGy/min). We hypothesized that ^{48}Ti-ion-exposure induced damage in both tissues. Lung tissue was collected from each mouse from each treatment group at 1 week, 1 month, and 6 months postirradiation. For the testis, we collected samples at 6 months postirradiation. Hence, only late-occurring effects of ^{48}Ti ions in the testis were studied. There were five mice per treatment group at each harvest time. We investigated inflammatory responses after exposure to ^{48}Ti ions by measuring the levels of activated nuclear factor kappa B and selected pro-inflammatory cytokines in both tissues of the same mouse. These measurements were coupled with the quantitation of the levels of global 5-methylcytosine (5mC) and 5-hydroxymethylcytosine (5hmC). Our data clearly showed the induction of chronic inflammation in both tissues of exposed mice. A dose-dependent reduction in global 5hmC was found in the lung at all time-points and in testes collected at 6 months postirradiation. In contrast, significant increases in global 5mC were found only in lung and testes collected at 6 months postirradiation from mice exposed to 0.5 Gy of 1 GeV/n ^{48}Ti ions. Overall, our data showed that ^{48}Ti ions may create health risks in both lung and testicular tissues.

Keywords: titanium ions, chronic inflammation, NF-κB, pro-inflammatory cytokines, lung, testes, 5-methylcytosine, 5-hydroxymethylcytosine

INTRODUCTION

Spaceflight results in unavoidable exposure of astronauts to space radiation (such as heavy ions and energetic protons) that may create potential risks for late-occurring injuries in both somatic and germinal cells/tissues. To protect astronauts, we must improve our understanding of changes at the cellular and molecular levels that are linked to increasing astronaut health risks and are valuable in developing countermeasures. In order to obtain reliable information about radiation-induced detrimental health effects, the data must be obtained using appropriate *in vivo* systems because *in vitro* systems cannot faithfully mimic the complex *in vivo* situation (1). Hence, appropriate whole-animal systems are critically important surrogates for assessment of health risks associated with exposure to space radiation.

The aim of this study was to improve our knowledge of *in vivo* biological effects of a whole body exposure to 1 GeV/n [48]Ti ions (one of the important types of heavy ions found in the space environment). We used the CBA/CaJ mouse as an experimental model to study the effects of 1 GeV/n [48]Ti ions on the lung (representing somatic tissue) and the testis (representing germinal tissue) of the same mouse, employing the inflammatory responses and DNA methylation endpoints. These two endpoints have not been used to evaluate the biological effects of 1 GeV/n [48]Ti ions in somatic and germinal cells of the same mouse, setting our approach apart from the existing reports.

It is known that the lung is a highly radiosensitive organ (2–4) and that impairment of the immune function in the lung is one of the major concerns after exposure to low LET radiation (4–7). It also has been suggested that the lung is one of the target organs at risk for cancer induction from exposure to heavy ions found in space (8). However, very little is known about the responses of the lung to space radiation. Recently, it was found that 350 MeV/n [28]Silicon ([28]Si) or [56]Iron ([56]Fe) ions, which are also important heavy ions found in the space environment, induced both histological and functional injuries in the lungs of exposed C3H/HeNCrl mice (9). Furthermore, it was reported that 1 GeV/n [56]Fe ions induced lung cancer in transgenic mice (the Kras[LA1] mice) engineered to be susceptible to lung cancer (10, 11).

With respect to testes, deleterious effects (e.g., DNA double-strand breaks, cytogenetic effects, and mutagenesis) of X or γ rays on spermatogenesis were reported several decades ago (12–19). It is known that the testis is one of the most radiosensitive organs (20) and is more sensitive to radiation exposure than female germ cells (21). Thus, male-mediated reproductive and developmental toxicology has been a concern for decades in atomic bomb survivors and in the Sellafield nuclear plant workers (22). However, very little is known about the effects of heavy ions on testes. It was found that exposure to 2.0–8.07 Gy of 0.35 GeV/n [12]Carbon (^{12}C) ions (LET = 13 keV/μm) or to 0.3–2.0 Gy of 1 GeV/n [56]Fe ions (LET = 147 keV/μm) did not increase mutation rates (assayed by the specific locus and the dominant lethal tests in Medaka fish), as compared to those exposed to 250 kVp X rays, a reference radiation (22). However, prenatal irradiation of pregnant rats to 0.1–2.0 Gy of 0.3 GeV/n ^{12}C or to 0.1–0.5 Gy of 0.4 MeV/n [20]Neon ([20]Ne) ions (LET = 30 keV/μm) caused abnormal testicular development and breeding activity of male offspring (23). Further, an increased

level of interleukin-1β, lower number of sperms, and an abnormal tubular architecture were found in testes of C57BL/6 mice flown with the Space Shuttle Discovery for 114 days, in relation to that of the corresponding sham controls (with no spaceflight) (24). Of note, it is known that the space environment is complex. Several factors (e.g., radiation, microgravity, and reactivation of herpes virus infection) may have contributed to such changes. Hence, to reduce the uncertainties in the assessment of health risks of space radiation, further ground-based studies are required to help improve our understanding of the effects of heavy ions on germinal cells and somatic cells as well.

Currently, there is no information on the *in vivo* effects of 1 GeV/n [48]Ti ions to the lung and the testes. Based upon the existing, but limited, information on responses to 1 GeV/n [48]Ti ions (25–27), we hypothesized that 1 GeV/n [48]Ti ions induced damage to these two tissues of exposed mice. To address this hypothesis, we used two biological endpoints to evaluate the effects of 1 GeV/n [48]Ti ions on lung and testicular tissues of the same mouse. These endpoints were inflammatory responses and global DNA methylation, including both 5-methylcytosine (5mC) and 5-hydroxymethylcytosine (5hmC). These two biological endpoints were chosen for analyses because they are highly relevant surrogate biomarkers for assessing health risks, but they have not previously been assessed following *in vivo* exposure to 1 GeV/n [48]Ti ions. Importantly, the induction of chronic inflammation has been reported in studies of astronauts' blood samples (28–30).

There has been increasing evidence of space-radiation-induced acute and chronic inflammation (26, 31–35), and radiation-induced aberrant DNA methylation at the global (26, 36) or specific locus levels (37–41). For the inflammatory responses, in this report, we chose to study the nuclear-factor kappa B (NF-κB) pathway because NF-κB is a key transcription factor playing a pivotal role in inflammatory responses to oxidative stress induced by several stimuli, including radiation (42). Although NF-κB is a member of the ubiquitously expressed family of the Rel-related transcription factors (43), only the activation of NF-κB/p65 was the focus of our study and referred to as NF-κB throughout the article. It also has been well recognized that NF-κB is a key transcription factor known to be part of a common network between inflammation and cancer (44–46), and that there is a close association between inflammation and cancer (44, 47–54). In addition, chronic inflammation in male germinal cells has been linked to male infertility (55–57). In addition to the levels of activated NF-κB, we measured the expression, at the protein levels, of selected NF-κB-regulated pro-inflammatory cytokines, i.e., tumor necrosis factor alpha (TNF-α), interleukin-1 beta (IL-1β), and interleukin 6 (IL-6). This is because their increased levels have been found in the liver (26) of the same exposed mice included in this present study. Furthermore, the expression of these proteins (at the gene level) was elevated in human mononuclear cells obtained from healthy adult individuals who lived near the Chernobyl Nuclear Power Plant and were chronically exposed to low-dose radiation ranging from 0.18 to 49 mSv (58).

Relating to DNA methylation, it has been well recognized that it is one of the key epigenetic events that plays a critical role in carcinogenesis, both initiation and promotion, in somatic and germinal cells (59, 60), and other untoward health outcomes (14) including male-mediated developmental toxicology (61), male infertility (62–64), and transgeneration effects (65, 66). Furthermore, a high level of 5mC (hypermethylation) has been linked to gene silencing (59, 67); while a reduction in global levels of 5hmC has been associated with cancer development (68). Since inflammatory responses and DNA methylation were analyzed in the lung and the testes of the same mouse, it is possible to investigate the differential sensitivity of these two tissues in the same mouse.

MATERIALS AND METHODS

Animals
The CBA/CaJ mice included in this study were the same cohort that were used to investigate the effects of 1 GeV/n ^{48}Ti ions on the liver previously reported (26), where the description of the CBA/CaJ mice, ^{48}Ti-irradiation, and animal husbandry were presented. The experimental design of the study was approved by both the Brookhaven National Laboratory (BNL) and the Stony Brook University (SBU) Institutional Animal Care and Use Committee (IACUC). Of note, the CBA/CaJ mouse is known to be sensitive to the development of radiation-induced myeloid leukemia (ML) (69–76), liver cancer (hepatocellular carcinoma or HCC) (70, 75), and lung cancer (70).

Irradiation of Mice
Figure 1 is a diagram of the experimental design. Mice were exposed, whole-body, to average total-body doses of 0, 0.1, 0.25, or 0.5 Gy of 1 GeV/n ^{48}Ti ions, delivered at a dose rate of 0.01 Gy/min by a 20 cm × 20 cm beam. Mice included in the sham-control group (i.e., those that were exposed to 0 Gy) were age-matched to exposed mice. Therefore, the age of mice in each treatment group would be similar at each sacrifice time. The exposure of mice was done at the National Aeronautics and Space Administration (NASA) Research Laboratory (NSRL) located at BNL. Details of the NSRL facility and irradiation procedure were previously provided (26, 34, 35, 77). We designated the first day after irradiation as day 1 after exposure. Mice were transported to the animal facility of SBU in a climate-controlled vehicle within 2 days postirradiation. Similar to the animal facility located in BNL, the animal facility of SBU, where sample collections were performed, is also approved by the Association for Assessment and Accreditation of Laboratory Animal Care (AAALAC), with the same light cycle (12 h light/12 h dark), temperature (21 ± 2°C), 10–15 hourly cycles of fresh air, and relative humidity (50 ± 10%).

Collection of the Lung and Testis
For the lung, groups of mice were used for sampling at 1 week, 1 month, and 6 months following the exposure to 1 GeV/n ^{48}Ti ions. In contrast, the collection of the testis was done at 6 months postexposure only. Hence, at 6 months postirradiation, the lung and the testis were collected from the same mouse. The rational for choosing only one harvest time for the testis was because our goal was to study the effects of ^{48}Ti ions on the stem-cell compartment of spermatogenesis. It is known that spermatogenesis is a complex biological process involving the transformation of spermatogonial stem cells (types A and B) into primary and secondary spermatocytes, round spermatids, and, eventually, spermatozoa over an extended period of time within seminiferous tubules of the testis (60, 65, 78). The duration of mouse spermatogenesis from the primitive type A$_{single}$ spermatogonial stem cells (SSCs) to mature sperms (spermatozoa) is about 52 days, but 35 days from differentiated spermatogonia to mature sperms (62, 79). Hence, the results obtained from the analyses of the testes collected at 6 months postirradiation reflect the effects of radiation on type A$_{single}$ SSCs.

From each treatment group, we collected the tissues from each mouse (five mice per dose of ^{48}Ti ions). Briefly, the lung and testicular tissues were removed, rinsed three times with 1 mL phosphate buffered saline (PBS) each time to remove external contamination (i.e., blood), snap frozen in liquid nitrogen, and stored in a −80°C freezer until needed for protein extraction and further analyses. After thawing, the total lung tissue was homogenized using a Bullet Blender Homogenizer (Next Advance Inc., Averill Park, NY, USA). Likewise, after thawing, the epididymis was removed from each testis to obtain seminiferous tubules, which were homogenized for use in protein extraction. The protocols for protein extraction from the lung and the testis suggested by the manufacturer were followed. Then, the cell lysates from each tissue of each mouse were divided into two fractions, i.e., fractions A and B. Fraction A of the tissue lysate was used to extract proteins from nuclear and cytosolic samples using the method we previously described (26, 34, 35, 80, 81). The total protein obtained from the nuclear portion of the lysate suspension of the lung or the testis was used for measuring the levels of NF-κB, while the total protein obtained from the cytosolic portion was used for the measurements of NF-κB-regulated proinflammatory cytokines, i.e., TNF-α, IL-1β, and IL-6. Protein contents in the cytosolic portion and the nuclear portion of the lung or the testis were measured by the Bradford assay using a BioPhotometer (Eppendorf, Inc., Westbury, NY, USA). Fraction B of the tissue lysate was used to isolate DNA for the measurements of global 5mC and global 5hmC.

Measurement of Activated Nuclear Factor-Kappa B
As with our previous work (26, 34, 35, 81), we used the enzyme-linked immunosorbent assay (ELISA) NF-κB kits from Active Motif North America, Inc. for measuring the levels of activated NF-κB in the nuclear portions obtained from the lung and testis lysates. The assay was performed in duplicate wells for each lung or testis sample of each treatment group. The mean value of activated NF-κB levels for the tissue of each mouse was obtained and reported. Then, the mean value of ten measurements from five mice and the SE for each treatment group were obtained.

Measurement of NF-κB-Regulated Pro-Inflammatory Cytokines, Including Tumor Necrosis Factor-α, Interleukin-1β, and Interleukin-6
Coupled with the levels of activated NF-κB, we measured the expression (at the protein levels) of NF-κB-regulated pro-inflammatory

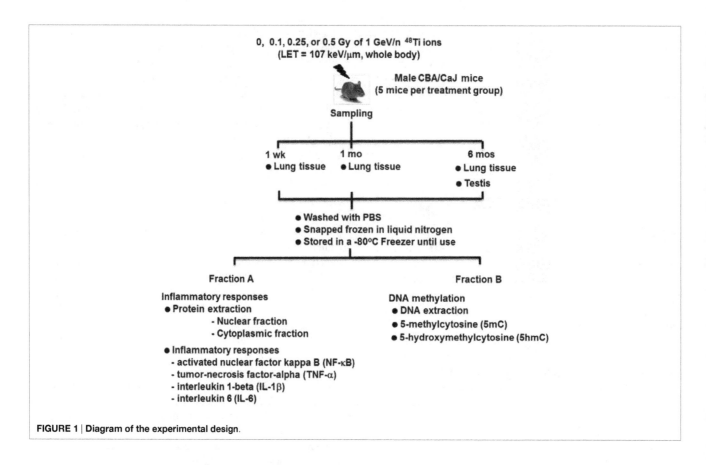

FIGURE 1 | Diagram of the experimental design.

cytokines, i.e., TNF-α, IL-1β, and IL-6. The rational for studying these pro-inflammatory cytokines has been presented in the Section "Introduction." We applied the methods routinely used in our laboratory for measuring the expression levels of these selected cytokines in lung or testicular cell suspensions (the cytosolic portions) using the specific ELISA kits for TNF-α, IL-1β, and IL-6 from Biosource (Invitrogen, Carlsbad, CA, USA) (26, 34, 35, 82). The mean value and SE of each cytokine for each treatment group were calculated from the means of five mice.

Measurement of Global 5-Methylcytosine and 5-Hydroxymethylcytosine

The methods for DNA isolation from mouse tissues have previously been presented (26, 36). Commercially available ELISA kits for the detection of global 5mC and 5hmC (Zymo Research, Inc., Irvine, CA, USA) were used to measure the percentage of global 5mC and 5hmC in the DNA samples isolated from lung or testicular tissues. The levels of global 5mC and 5hmC were measured using a microplate spectrophotometer (Molecular Devices) at 405 nm. The % 5mC and % 5hmC was calculated from a standard curve generated using the control DNA set provided by the manufacturer. The measurements of 5mC and 5hmC in the DNA sample from each tissue of each mouse were done in duplicate (using 200 ng of DNA per well). Then, the mean value of global 5mC and global 5hmC for each mouse were obtained. Finally, the mean value of ten measurements and SE of global

5mC and global 5hmC for each treatment group were calculated from the means of five mice.

Statistical Analyses

We expressed levels of each biological endpoint as mean ± SE. For each tissue, the mean value for each assay of each mouse was used as a single datum point for statistical analyses. At each harvest time, an ANOVA method appropriate for a one-factor experiment (i.e., dose of 1 GeV/n ^{48}Ti ions) was used to assess the significance of the radiation dose. Further, the Student's t-test was used, independently, to evaluate statistical differences in the mean values between each exposed group and the corresponding sham-control group. A P-value of ≤0.05 was considered as statistically significant.

RESULTS

Figures 2–7 show the effects of various doses of 1 GeV/n ^{48}Ti ions on the lung and testicular tissues of exposed CBA/CaJ mice. P values (Student's t-test) shown in each figure indicate statistically significant levels between exposed and sham-control groups. **Tables 1** and **2** show the results of the ANOVA for the lung and testicular tissues, respectively.

Activated Nuclear Factor-Kappa B

There were dose-dependent increases in the levels of activated NF-κB in lung tissues from all exposed groups (ANOVA,

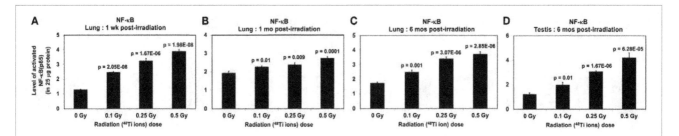

FIGURE 2 | Levels of activated NF-κB (±SE) in lung tissues collected at 1 week (A), 1 month (B), 6 months (C), and in testicular tissues collected at 6 months (D) from CBA/CaJ mice after a whole body exposure to various doses of 1 GeV/n ⁴⁸Ti ions. P values (Student's t-test) indicate significant differences in the levels of NF-κB between exposed and corresponding sham control groups.

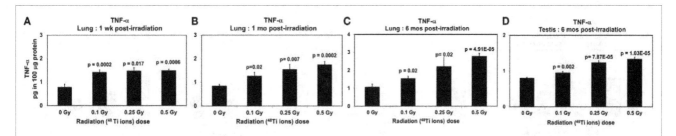

FIGURE 3 | Levels of TNF-α (±SE) in lung tissues collected at 1 week (A), 1 month (B), 6 months (C), and in testicular tissues collected at 6 months (D) from CBA/CaJ mice after a whole body exposure to various doses of 1 GeV/n ⁴⁸Ti ions. P values (Student's t-test) indicate significant differences in the levels of TNF-α between exposed and corresponding sham control groups.

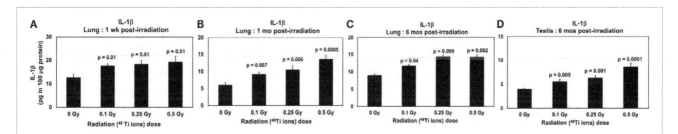

FIGURE 4 | Levels of IL-1β (±SE) in lung tissues collected at 1 week (A), 1 month (B), 6 months (C), and in testicular tissues collected at 6 months (D) from CBA/CaJ mice after a whole body exposure to various doses of 1 GeV/n ⁴⁸Ti ions. P values (Student's t-test) indicate significant differences in the levels of IL-1β between exposed and corresponding sham control groups.

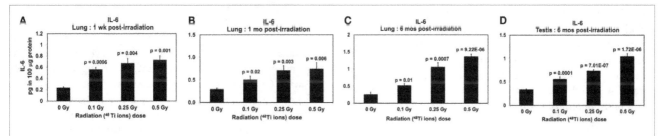

FIGURE 5 | Levels of IL-6 (±SE) in lung tissues collected at 1 week (A), 1 month (B), 6 months (C), and in testicular tissues collected at 6 months (D) from CBA/CaJ mice after a whole body exposure to various doses of 1 GeV/n ⁴⁸Ti ions. P values (Student's t-test) indicate significant differences in the levels of IL-6 between exposed and corresponding sham control groups.

$P < 0.01$), regardless of the harvest time (**Figures 2A–C**). Of note, there is a fluctuation in the levels of activated NF-κB in lung tissues collected from sham control mice (in particular in those collected at 1 month postirradiation). However, the factors contributing to this temporal change are unknown. We also detected a dose-dependent increase in the levels of activated NF-κB in the testicular tissues (ANOVA, $P < 0.01$) at 6 months postirradiation (as shown in **Figure 2D**).

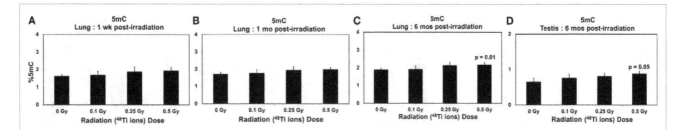

FIGURE 6 | Levels of 5mC (±SE) in lung tissues collected at 1 week (A), 1 month (B), 6 months (C), and in testicular tissues collected at 6 months (D) from CBA/CaJ mice after a whole body exposure to various doses of 1 GeV/n ⁴⁸Ti ions. *P* values (Student's *t*-test) indicate significant differences in the levels of 5mC between exposed and corresponding sham control groups.

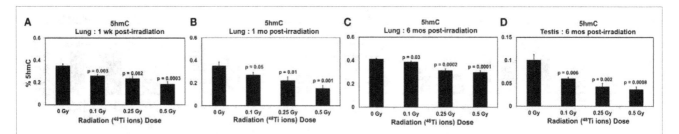

FIGURE 7 | Levels of 5hmC (±SE) in lung tissues collected at 1 week (A), 1 month (B), 6 months (C), and in testicular tissues collected at 6 months (D) from CBA/CaJ mice after a whole body exposure to various doses of 1 GeV/n ⁴⁸Ti ions. *P* values (Student's *t*-test) indicate significant differences in the levels of 5hmC between exposed and corresponding sham control groups.

Tumor Necrosis Factor-α

Similar to the levels of activated NF-κB, there were dose-dependent increases in the level of TNF-α in lung tissues collected at all time-points (ANOVA, $P < 0.01$), as shown in **Figures 3A–C**. Likewise, at 6 months postirradiation, a dose-dependent increase (ANOVA, $P < 0.01$) in the levels of IL-6 was found in testicular tissues collected at 6 months postirradiation (**Figure 3D**).

Interleukin-1β and Interleukin-6

Clearly, dose-dependent increases in the levels of IL-1β (**Figures 4A–C**) and IL-6 (**Figures 5A–C**) were observed in lung tissues collected at 1 week, 1 month, and 6 months postirradiation (ANOVA, $P < 0.01$), respectively. Of note, similar to activated NF-κB, there was a fluctuation in the levels of IL-1β in lung tissues of sham control mice, in particular in those collected at 1 month postirradiation. The cause of such fluctuation remains unidentified. Likewise, dose-dependent increases in the levels of IL-1β (**Figure 4D**) and IL-6 (**Figure 5D**) in testicular tissues collected at 6 months postirradiation (ANOVA, $P < 0.01$) were evident.

5-Methylcytosine and 5-Hydroxymethylcytosine

Figures 6A–C show the effects of ⁴⁸Ti ions on the levels of global 5mC in lung tissues of exposed mice. There was a trend of increased levels of global 5mC in the lung tissues of exposed mice, in relation to those of the corresponding sham controls. However, such increases were not statistically different, except in the lung tissues collected at 6 months from mice exposed to the highest

dose of 1 GeV/n ⁴⁸Ti ions. A similar finding was found in testicular tissues collected at 6 months postirradiation (**Figure 6D**).

In contrast, **Figures 7A–C** show significant dose-dependent decreases in the levels of 5hmC in the lungs of exposed mice (ANOVA, $P < 0.05$) at 1 week, 1 month, and 6 months, respectively. The decreases in 5hmC levels in lung tissues of exposed mice relative to the corresponding sham controls were: 1.33-, 1.48-, and 1.88-fold at 1 week postirradiation; 1.29-, 1.58-, and 2.29-fold at 1 month postirradiation; 1.06-, 1.30-, and 1.38-fold at 6 months postirradiation. Likewise, there was a dose-dependent reduction in the levels of global 5hmC in testicular tissues collected at 6 months postirradiation as shown in **Figure 7D**.

DISCUSSION

Our data are the first to report the presence of chronic inflammation and altered levels of global 5hmC in the lung and testicular tissues of CBA/CaJ mice after a whole body exposure to 1 GeV/n ⁴⁸Ti ions at low doses and a low dose-rate relevant to what is found in space, i.e., 0.1–0.5 Gy (delivered at 0.01 Gy/min). Our data also indicated that only 0.5 Gy (the highest dose used in our study) of 1 GeV/n ⁴⁸Ti ions induced significant increases in the levels of global 5mC in both tissues of the same mouse. The magnitude of the effects of ⁴⁸Ti ions on each tissue is similar. Since these two endpoints were detected in both tissues of the same mouse, it is plausible to speculate that there is a connection between chronic inflammation and altered DNA methylation. The information obtained from our study is important because these two *in vivo* endpoints are the hallmarks of cancer (52, 53, 68) and several

TABLE 1 | Analysis of variance results for lung tissues collected at 1 week, 1 month, and 6 months postirradiation, respectively (SS, sum of squares; df, degree of freedom; MS, mean of squares; *F*, *F*-statistic).

1 Week postirradiation					1 Month week postirradiation					6 Months postirradiation				
Source of variation	SS	df	MS	F	P-value	*Source of variation*	SS	df	MS	F	P-value	*Source of variation*	SS	df	MS	F	P-value

NF-κB

Source of variation	SS	df	MS	F	P-value	Source of variation	SS	df	MS	F	P-value	Source of variation	SS	df	MS	F	P-value
Between groups	18.95	3	6.32	102.1	1E-10	Between groups	1.74	3	0.58	12.6	0.0001	Between groups	12.44	3	4.15	43.86	6E-08
Within groups	0.99	16	0.06			Within groups	0.74	16	0.05			Within groups	1.51	16	0.09		
Total	19.94	19				Total	2.48	19				Total	13.95	19			

TNF-α

Between groups	1.78	3	0.59	5.25	0.01	Between groups	2.27	3	0.76	6.31	0.0049	Between groups	8.55	3	2.85	7.15	0.002
Within groups	1.81	16	0.11			Within groups	1.92	16	0.12			Within groups	6.37	16	0.40		
Total	3.59	19				Total	4.19	19				Total	14.92	19			

IL-1β

Between groups	128.91	3	42.97	2.86	0.04	Between groups	144.64	3	48.21	9.67	0.0007	Between groups	62.52	3	20.84	6.86	0.003
Within groups	240.68	16	15.04			Within groups	79.74	16	4.98			Within groups	48.58	16	3.04		
Total	369.59	19				Total	224.38	19				Total	111.09	19			

IL-6

Between groups	0.51	3	0.17	7.62	0.0029	Between groups	0.64	3	0.21	4.37	0.02	Between groups	3.50	3	1.17	29.49	2E-06
Within groups	0.31	16	0.02			Within groups	0.78	16	0.05			Within groups	0.59	16	0.04		
Total	0.82	19				Total	1.43	19				Total	111.09	19			

5mC

Between groups	0.34	3	0.11	0.49	0.68	Between groups	0.26	3	0.09	0.39	0.76	Between groups	0.61	3	0.20	1.65	0.22
Within groups	3.64	16	0.23			Within groups	3.61	16	0.23			Within groups	1.99	16	0.12		
Total	3.98	19				Total	3.87	19				Total	2.61	19			

5hmC

Between groups	0.07	3	0.02	11.38	0.0003	Between groups	0.05	3	0.02	7.29	0.003	Between groups	0.05	3	0.02	16.15	4E-05
Within groups	0.03	16	0.002			Within groups	0.01	16	0.0050			Within groups	0.01	16	0.0009		
Total	0.1	19				Total	0.06	19				Total	0.06	19			

types of male germ-cell disturbance (55–57, 62, 63, 83, 84). Hence, our findings provide an important foundation for future studies in which an association between molecular changes and the histopathological, pathological and/or functional damage in the lung and the testes, including the incidence of lung or testicular cancer, can be achieved. Of note, in future studies, it is important to measure the levels of activated NF-κB and related pro-inflammatory cytokines not only in tissues but also in plasma obtained from the same mice. The obtained information will help to determine whether there is a correlation between chronic inflammation in tissues and the levels of circulating cytokines, which should have clinical implications.

The approach we used in this study has allowed the investigation of the kinetics of effects of 1 GeV/n [48]Ti ions on the lung, not only as a function of radiation dose but also time after exposure,

since lung tissues were collected at various times up to 6 months postirradiation. We observed dose- and time-dependent increases in the levels of activated NF-κB and expression of NF-κB-related pro-inflammatory cytokines (i.e., TNF-α, IL-1β, and IL-6). Our data indicate that [48]Ti-ion-exposure induces disturbances of cytokine production, reflecting chronic inflammation and an impairment of the immune system. Relating to the kinetics of the levels of global 5mC and 5hmC in the lung, our data indicated no significant change in the levels of global 5mC, except a significant increase in lung tissues collected at 6 months postirradiation from mice exposed to 0.5 Gy of [48]Ti ions. In contrast, there were significant dose-dependent decreases in the levels of global 5hmC at all harvest time-points. Such findings were similar to those detected in the liver collected from the same mouse previously reported (26). Hence, our data suggest that the loss of global

TABLE 2 | Analysis of variance results for testicular tissues collected at 6 months postirradiation (SS, sum of squares; df, degree of freedom; MS, mean of squares; F, F-statistic).

Source of variation	SS	df	MS	F	P-value
NF-kB					
Between groups	25.70	3	8.57	27.39	1.5379E-06
Within groups	5.00	16	0.31		
Total	30.70	19			
TNF-α					
Between groups	0.91	3	0.30	29.46	9.4514E-07
Within groups	0.16	16	0.01		
Total	1.07	19			
IL1-β					
Between groups	56.46	3	18.82	14.45	8.1361E-05
Within groups	20.85	16	1.30		
Total	77.31	19			
IL-6					
Between groups	1.34	3	0.45	49.31	2.6281E-08
Within groups	0.14	16	0.01		
Total	1.48	19			
5mC					
Between groups	0.16	3	0.05	1.19	0.35
Within groups	0.72	16	0.05		
Total	0.88	19			
5hmC					
Between groups	0.01	3	0.0042	12.88	0.0001
Within groups	0.01	16	0.0003		
Total	0.02	19			

5hmC is a significant response to ^{48}Ti-ion-irradiation, regardless of tissue type. It also is reasonable to hypothesize that chronic inflammation enhances radiation-induced loss of global 5hmC and *vice versa*.

Our study is the first to report the levels of global 5hmC in the lung of mice exposed to radiation. Of note, the focus of previous studies on the effects of radiation, both low and high LET, has been on specific loci of 5mC (38, 39, 41, 85–88). We included the levels of global 5hmC because it is currently recognized that a reduction in global 5hmC is a biomarker for cancer (68). Taken together, our data suggest that a reduction in the level of global 5hmC may be a better hallmark of radiation exposure than an increased level of global 5mC. In the future, it will be important to conduct studies to determine the genome-wide profiling of 5hmC/5mC to reveal the affected regions of the genome so that, in turn, the identification of affected genes will be possible.

Regarding the testes collected at 6 months from the same mouse from which the lung tissue was collected for our study, the data clearly showed that there were dose-dependent increases in the levels of activated NF-κB and expression of NF-κB-regulated pro-inflammatory cytokines (i.e., TNF-α, IL-1β, and IL-6). These findings represent the effects of 1 GeV/n ^{48}Ti ions on the primitive type of spermatogonial stem cells (SSCs), i.e., type A$_{single}$ SSCs. The induced damage arising from exposed SSCs is highly relevant for genetic risk assessment since SSCs are capable of self-renewal and differentiation into spermatocytes and mature sperm. Hence, any induced damage in the SSC compartment, if not repaired, will be carried onto the next generation and will

adversely impact self-renewal, proliferation, and differentiation. In contrast, the damage that is induced in other male germ cell stages (e.g., spermatocytes, where cell divisions, both in meiosis and mitosis, take place) will affect progenies that are conceived shortly after irradiation. Our new data are important because it has been well recognized that SSCs are responsible for long-term effects of radiation on fertility (15, 89). Further, it was suggested that inflammation in SSCs leads to failure of testicular androgen and sperm production, resulting in infertility (90), and testicular cancer (91). Thus, exposure to 1 GeV/n ^{48}Ti ions may lead to health risks associated with the male reproductive system. At 6 months postirradiation, the effects of 1 GeV/n ^{48}Ti ions on levels of global 5mC and 5hmC in the testes of exposed mice are similar to those found in the lung of the same mouse. As mentioned previously, altered DNA methylation plays an important role in male infertility (62–64), germ cell tumors (59, 60), and transgeneration effects (65, 78). Hence, our data provide critical information for conducting further studies to investigate the potential induction of these untoward outcomes on male germinal cells from exposure to 1 GeV/n ^{48}Ti ions.

In summary, our results provide new information on *in vivo* biological responses to ^{48}Ti ions. Our new data show that 1 GeV/n ^{48}Ti ions (at doses ranging from 0.1 to 0.5 Gy, delivered at 0.01 Gy/min) can induce chronic inflammation, and a persistence of altered DNA methylation (at the global level) in lung and testicular tissues of exposed CBA/CaJ mice. Importantly, our findings provide an important foundation for further investigations on the genes/proteins involved in ^{48}Ti-ion-induced chronic inflammation and altered DNA methylation. Knowing such detailed molecular markers for health risks from exposure to heavy ions would not only greatly improve radiation protection guidance for astronauts (or cancer patients receiving heavy-ion radiation therapy) but would also provide significantly valuable insight for developing biological countermeasures.

AUTHOR CONTRIBUTIONS

KR was responsible for the study concept and design; critical revision of the manuscript for important intellectual content. WJ was responsible for acquisition of the data. MT was responsible for acquisition of the data. CG was responsible for acquisition of the data. LH was responsible for acquisition of the data. EW was responsible for statistical analyses and critical revision of the manuscript for important intellectual content.

ACKNOWLEDGMENTS

This research was supported in part by the National Aeronautics and Space Administration (NASA) Grant # NNX11AK91G and the Department of Pathology, Stony Brook University, Stony Brook, NY, USA. We thank Dr. Peter Guida and his team for logistic support, MaryAnn Petry and her staff at Brookhaven Laboratory Animal Facilities (BLAF) for their assistance in animal handling. We also thank Drs. Adam Rusek and Michael Sivertz for dosimetry support.

REFERENCES

1. Nestor C, Ottaviano R, Reinhardt D, Cruickshanks H, Mjoseng H, McPherson R, et al. Rapid reprogramming of epigenetic and transcriptional profiles in mammalian culture systems. *Genome Biol* (2015) 16(1):11. doi:10.1186/s13059-014-0576-y

2. Coggle JE, Lambert BE, Moores SR. Radiation effects in the lung. *Environ Health Perspect* (1986) 70:261–91. doi:10.1289/ehp.8670261

3. Marks LB, Yu X, Vujaskovic Z, Small W, Folz R, Anscher MS. Radiation-induced lung injury. *Semin Radiat Oncol* (2003) 13(3):333–45. doi:10.1016/S1053-4296(03)00034-1

4. Hill RP. Radiation effects on the respiratory system. *Br J Radiol* (2005) 27(Suppl 1):75–81. doi:10.1259/bjr/34124307

5. Finkelstein JN, Johnston CJ, Baggs R, Rubin P. Early alterations in extracellular matrix and transforming growth factor [beta] gene expression in mouse lung indicative of late radiation fibrosis. *Int J Radiat Oncol Biol Phys* (1994) 28(3):621–31. doi:10.1016/0360-3016(94)90187-2

6. Hong JH, Chiang CS, Tsao CY, Lin PY, McBride WH, Wu CJ. Rapid induction of cytokine gene expression in the lung after single and fractionated doses of radiation. *Int J Radiat Biol* (1999) 75(11):1421–7. doi:10.1080/095530099139287

7. Rübe CE, Wilfert F, Palm J, König J, Burdak-Rothkamm S, Liu L, et al. Irradiation induces a biphasic expression of pro-inflammatory cytokines in the lung. *Strahlenther Onkol* (2004) 180(7):442–8. doi:10.1007/s00066-004-1265-7

8. Cucinotta FA. Space radiation risks for astronauts on multiple international space station missions. *PLoS One* (2014) 9(4):e96099. doi:10.1371/journal.pone.0096099

9. Christofidou-Solomidou M, Pietrofesa RA, Arguiri E, Schweitzer KS, Berdyshev EV, McCarthy M, et al. Space radiation-associated lung injury in a murine model. *Amer J Physiol Lung Cell Mol Physiol* (2015) 308(5):L416–28. doi:10.1152/ajplung.00260.2014

10. Shay JW, Cucinotta FA, Sulzman FM, Coleman CN, Minna JD. From mice and men to earth and space: joint NASA-NCI workshop on lung cancer risk resulting from space and terrestrial radiation. *Cancer Res* (2011) 71(22):6926–9. doi:10.1158/0008-5472.CAN-11-2546

11. Kim SB, Kaisani A, Shay JW. Risk assessment of space radiation-induced invasive cancer in mouse models of lung and colorectal cancer. *J Radiat Res* (2014) 55(Suppl 1):i46–7. doi:10.1093/jrr/rrt149

12. van Buul PP. Dose-response relationship for radiation-induced translocations in somatic and germ cells of mice. *Mutat Res* (1977) 45(1):61–8. doi:10.1016/0027-5107(77)90043-4

13. Vaiserman AM, Mekhova LV, Koshel NM, Voitenko VP. Cancer incidence and mortality after low-dosage radiation exposure: epidemiological aspects. *Biophysics* (2011) 56(2):371–80. doi:10.1134/S000635091102031X

14. Vaiserman AM. Epigenetic programming by early-life stress: evidence from human populations. *Dev Dyn* (2015) 244(3):254–65. doi:10.1002/dvdy.24211

15. Hacker-Klom U. Long term effects of ionizing radiation on mouse spermatogenesis. *Acta Radiol Oncol* (1985) 24(4):363–7. doi:10.3109/02841868509136066

16. Hamer G, Roepers-Gajadien HL, van Duyn-Goedhart A, Gademan IS, Kal HB, van Buul PPW, et al. DNA double-strand breaks and γ-H2AX signaling in the testis. *Biol Reprod* (2003) 68(2):628–34. doi:10.1095/biolreprod.102.008672

17. Cordelli E, Eleuteri P, Grollino MG, Benassi B, Blandino G, Bartoleschi C, et al. Direct and delayed X-ray-induced DNA damage in male mouse germ cells. *Environ Mol Mutagen* (2012) 53(6):429–39. doi:10.1002/em.21703

18. Spalding JF, Wellnitz JM, Schweitzer WH. Effects of rapid massive doses of gamma-rays on the testes and germ cells of the rat. *Radiat Res* (1957) 7(1):65–70. doi:10.2307/3570555

19. Generoso WM, Cain KT, Cacheiro NL, Cornett CV, Gossle DG. Response of mouse spermatogonial stem cells to X-ray induction of heritable reciprocal translocations. *Mutat Res* (1984) 126(2):177–87. doi:10.1016/0027-5107(84)90060-5

20. Ory C, Ugolin N, Hofman P, Schlumberger M, Likhtarev IA, Chevillard S. Comparison of transcriptomic signature of post-chernobyl and postradiotherapy thyroid tumors. *Thyroid* (2013) 23(11):1390–400. doi:10.1089/thy.2012.0318

21. Hall EJ, editor. *Radiobiology for the Radiologist*. 2000 ed. Philadelphia: Lippincott Williams & Wilkins (2000).

22. Shimada A, Shima A, Nojima K, Seino Y, Setlow RB. Germ cell mutagenesis in medaka fish after exposures to high-energy cosmic ray nuclei: a human model. *Proc Natl Acad Sci U S A* (2005) 102(17):6063–7. doi:10.1073/pnas.0500895102

23. Verdelli C, Forno I, Vaira V, Corbetta S. Epigenetic alterations in human parathyroid tumors. *Endocrine* (2015) 49(2):324–32. doi:10.1007/s12020-015-0555-4

24. Masini MA, Albi E, Barmo C, Bonfiglio T, Bruni L, Canesi L, et al. The impact of long-term exposure to space environment on adult mammalian organisms: a study on mouse thyroid and testis. *PLoS One* (2012) 7(4):e35418. doi:10.1371/journal.pone.0035418

25. Jain MR, Li M, Chen W, Liu T, de Toledo SM, Pandey BN, et al. In vivo space radiation-induced non-targeted responses: late effects on molecular signaling in mitochondria. *Curr Mol Pharmacol* (2011) 4(2):106–14. doi:10.2174/1874467211104020106

26. Jangiam W, Tungjai M, Rithidech K. Induction of chronic oxidative stress, chronic inflammation and aberrant patterns of DNA methylation in the liver of titanium-exposed CBA/CaJ mice. *Int J Radiat Biol* (2015) 91(5):389–98. doi:10.3109/09553002.2015.1001882

27. Rabin BM, Shukitt-Hale B, Joseph JA, Carrihill-Knoll KL, Carey AN, Cheng V. Relative effectiveness of different particles and energies in disrupting behavioral performance. *Radiat Environ Biophys* (2007) 46(2):173–7. doi:10.1007/s00411-006-0071-2

28. Crucian BE, Stowe RP, Pierson DL, Sams CF. Immune system dysregulation following short- vs long-duration spaceflight. *Aviat Space Environ Med* (2008) 79(9):835–43. doi:10.3357/ASEM.2276.2008

29. Sonnenfeld G, Shearer W. Immune function during space flight. *Nutrition* (2002) 18(10):899–903. doi:10.1016/S0899-9007(02)00903-6

30. Crucian B, Stowe RP, Mehta S, Quiriarte H, Pierson D, Sams C. Alterations in adaptive immunity persist during long-duration spaceflight. *NPJ Microgravity* (2015) 1:15013. doi:10.1038/npjmgrav.2015.13

31. Gridley DS, Miller GM, Pecaut MJ. Radiation and primary response to lipopolysaccharide: bone marrow-derived cells and susceptible organs. *In Vivo* (2007) 21(3):453–61.

32. Gridley DS, Pecaut MJ, Nelson GA. Total-body irradiation with high-LET particles: acute and chronic effects on the immune system. *Amer J Physiol Regul Integr Comp Physiol* (2002) 282(3):R677–88. doi:10.1152/ajpregu.00435.2001

33. Gridley DS, Rizvi A, Makinde AY, Luo-Owen X, Mao XW, Tian J, et al. Space-relevant radiation modifies cytokine profiles, signaling proteins and Foxp3+ T cells. *Int J Radiat Biol* (2013) 89(1):26–35. doi:10.3109/09553002.2012.715792

34. Rithidech K, Reungpatthanaphong P, Honikel L, Rusek A, Simon S. Dose-rate effects of protons on in vivo activation of nuclear factor-kappa B and cytokines in mouse bone marrow cells. *Radiat Environ Biophys* (2010) 49:405–19. doi:10.1007/s00411-010-0295-z

35. Tungjai M, Whorton E, Rithidech K. Persistence of apoptosis and inflammatory responses in the heart and bone marrow of mice following whole-body exposure to 28Silicon (28Si) ions. *Radiat Environ Biophys* (2013) 52(3):339–50. doi:10.1007/s00411-013-0479-4

36. Rithidech KN, Honikle LM, Reungpatthanaphong P, Tungjai M, Jangiam W, Whorton EB. Late-occurring chromosome aberrations and global DNA methylation in hematopoietic stem/progenitor cells of CBA/CaJ mice exposed to silicon (28Si) ions. *Mutat Res* (2015) 781:22–31. doi:10.1016/j.mrfmmm.2015.09.001

37. Götze S, Schumacher EC, Kordes C, Häussinger D. Epigenetic changes during hepatic stellate cell activation. *PLoS One* (2015) 10(6):e0128745. doi:10.1371/journal.pone.0128745

38. Lima F, Ding D, Goetz W, Yang AJ, Baulch JE. High LET 56Fe ion irradiation induces tissue-specific changes in DNA methylation in the mouse. *Environ Mol Mutagen* (2014) 55(3):266–77. doi:10.1002/em.21832

39. Nzabarushimana E, Miousse IR, Shao L, Chang J, Allen AR, Turner J, et al. Long-term epigenetic effects of exposure to low doses of 56Fe in the mouse lung. *J Radiat Res* (2014) 55(4):823–8. doi:10.1093/jrr/rru010

40. Aypar U, Morgan WF, Baulch JE. Radiation-induced epigenetic alterations after low and high LET irradiations. *Mutat Res* (2011) 707(1–2):24–33. doi:10.1016/j.mrfmmm.2010.12.003

41. Miousse IR, Shao L, Chang J, Feng W, Wang Y, Allen AR, et al. Exposure to low-dose 56Fe-ion radiation induces long-term epigenetic alterations in mouse

bone marrow hematopoietic progenitor and stem cells. *Radiat Res* (2014) 182(1):92–101. doi:10.1667/RR13580.1

42. Li N, Karin M. Is NF-kappa B the sensor of oxidative stress? *FASEB J* (1999) 13(10):1137–43.

43. Verma IM, Stevenson JK, Schwarz EM, Van Antwerp D, Miyamoto S. Rel/NF-kappa B/I kappa B family: intimate tales of association and dissociation. *Genes Develop* (1995) 9(22):2723–35. doi:10.1101/gad.9.22.2723

44. Karin M, Greten FR. NF-[kappa]B: linking inflammation and immunity to cancer development and progression. *Nat Rev Immunol* (2005) 5(10):749–59. doi:10.1038/nri1703

45. Pikarsky E, Porat RM, Stein I, Abramovitch R, Amit S, Kasem S, et al. NF-[kappa]B functions as a tumour promoter in inflammation-associated cancer. *Nature* (2004) 431(7007):461–6. doi:10.1038/nature02924

46. Dolcet X, Llobet D, Pallares J, Matias-Guiu X. NF-kB in development and progression of human cancer. *Virchows Archiv* (2005) 446(5):475–82. doi:10.1007/s00428-005-1264-9

47. Coussens LM, Werb Z. Inflammation and cancer. *Nature* (2002) 420(6917):860–7. doi:10.1038/nature01322

48. Takahashi H, Ogata H, Nishigaki R, Broide DH, Karin M. Tobacco smoke promotes lung tumorigenesis by triggering IKK[beta] and JNK1-dependent inflammation. *Cancer Cell* (2010) 17(1):89–97. doi:10.1016/j.ccr.2009.12.008

49. Grivennikov SI, Greten FR, Karin M. Immunity, inflammation, and cancer. *Cell* (2010) 140(6):883–99. doi:10.1016/j.cell.2010.01.025

50. Schetter AJ, Heegaard NHH, Harris CC. Inflammation and cancer: interweaving microRNA, free radical, cytokine and p53 pathways. *Carcinogenesis* (2010) 31(1):37–49. doi:10.1093/carcin/bgp272

51. Li Q, Withoff S, Verma IM. Inflammation-associated cancer: NF-[kappa]B is the lynchpin. *Trends Immunol* (2005) 26(6):318–25. doi:10.1016/j.it.2005.04.003

52. Colotta F, Allavena P, Sica A, Garlanda C, Mantovani A. Cancer-related inflammation, the seventh hallmark of cancer: links to genetic instability. *Carcinogenesis* (2009) 30(7):1073–81. doi:10.1093/carcin/bgp127

53. Hanahan D, Weinberg Robert A. Hallmarks of cancer: the next generation. *Cell* (2011) 144(5):646–74. doi:10.1016/j.cell.2011.02.013

54. Lee JM, Yanagawa J, Peebles KA, Sharma S, Mao JT, Dubinett SM. Inflammation in lung carcinogenesis: new targets for lung cancer chemoprevention and treatment. *Crit Rev Oncol Hematol* (2008) 66(3):208–17. doi:10.1016/j.critrevonc.2008.01.004

55. Eggert-Kruse W, Boit R, Rohr G, Aufenanger J, Hund M, Strowitzki T. Relationship of seminal plasma interleukin (IL)-8 and IL-6 with semen quality. *Hum Reprod* (2001) 16(3):517–28. doi:10.1093/humrep/16.3.517

56. Haidl F, Haidl G, Oltermann I, Allam JP. Seminal parameters of chronic male genital inflammation are associated with disturbed sperm DNA integrity. *Andrologia* (2015) 47(4):464–9. doi:10.1111/and.12408

57. Schuppe HC, Meinhardt A, Allam JP, Bergmann M, Weidner W, Haidl G. Chronic orchitis: a neglected cause of male infertility? *Andrologia* (2008) 40(2):84–91. doi:10.1111/j.1439-0272.2008.00837.x

58. Albanese J, Martens K, Karkanitsa LV, Schreyer SK, Dainiak N. Multivariate analysis of low-dose radiation-associated changes in cytokine gene expression profiles using microarray technology. *Exp Hematol* (2007) 35(4 Suppl 1):47–54. doi:10.1016/j.exphem.2007.01.012

59. Feinberg AP, Ohlsson R, Henikoff S. The epigenetic progenitor origin of human cancer. *Nat Rev Genet* (2006) 7(1):21–33. doi:10.1038/nrg1748

60. Rijlaarsdam MA, Tax DMJ, Gillis AJM, Dorssers LCJ, Koestler DC, de Ridder J, et al. Genome wide DNA methylation profiles provide clues to the origin and pathogenesis of germ cell tumors. *PLoS One* (2015) 10(4):e0122146. doi:10.1371/journal.pone.0122146

61. Anderson D, Schmid TE, Baumgartner A. Male-mediated developmental toxicity. *Asian J Androl* (2014) 16(1):81–8. doi:10.4103/1008-682X.122342

62. Cisneros FJ. DNA methylation and male infertility. *Front Biosci* (2004) 1(9):1189–200. doi:10.2741/1332

63. Rajender S, Avery K, Agarwal A. Epigenetics, spermatogenesis and male infertility. *Mutat Res* (2011) 727(3):62–71. doi:10.1016/j.mrrev.2011.04.002

64. Wang X-X, Sun B-F, Jiao J, Chong Z-C, Chen Y-S, Wang X-L, et al. Genome-wide 5-hydroxymethylcytosine modification pattern is a novel epigenetic feature of globozoospermia. *Oncotarget* (2015) 6(9):6535–43. doi:10.18632/oncotarget.3163

65. Soubry A, Hoyo C, Jirtle RL, Murphy SK. A paternal environmental legacy: evidence for epigenetic inheritance through the male germ line. *Bioessays* (2014) 36(4):359–71. doi:10.1002/bies.201300113

66. Siklenka K, Erkek S, Godmann M, Lambrot R, McGraw S, Lafleur C, et al. Disruption of histone methylation in developing sperm impairs offspring health transgenerationally. *Science* (2015) 350(6261):aab2006. doi:10.1126/science.aab2006

67. Bird A. DNA methylation patterns and epigenetic memory. *Genes Dev* (2002) 16:6–12. doi:10.1101/gad.947102

68. Pfeifer G, Kadam S, Jin S-G. 5-Hydroxymethylcytosine and its potential roles in development and cancer. *Epigenet Chromatin* (2013) 6(1):631–41. doi:10.1186/1756-8935-6-10

69. Bouffler SD, Breckon G, Cox R. Chromosomal mechanisms in murine radiation acute myeloid leukaemogenesis. *Carcinogenesis* (1996) 17(4):655–9. doi:10.1093/carcin/17.4.655

70. Cronkite EP, Bond VP. *Radiation Leukemic-Prediction of Low Dose Effects*. Upton: NCI Report, Contract Y01-CO 10712 (1988).

71. Peng Y, Brown N, Finnon R, Warner CL, Liu X, Genik PC, et al. Radiation leukemogenesis in mice: loss of PU.1 on chromosome 2 in CBA and C57BL/6 mice after irradiation with 1 GeV/nucleon ⁵⁶Fe ions, X rays or γ rays. Part I. Experimental observations. *Radiat Res* (2009) 171(4):474–83. doi:10.1667/RR1547.1

72. Rithidech K, Bond VP, Cronkite EP, Thompson MH, Bullis JE. Hypermutability of mouse chromosome 2 during the development of x-ray-induced murine myeloid leukemia. *Proc Natl Acad Sci U S A* (1995) 92(4):1152–6. doi:10.1073/pnas.92.4.1152

73. Rithidech K, Dunn JJ, Roe BA, Gordon CR, Cronkite EP. Evidence for two commonly deleted regions on mouse chromosome 2 in gamma ray-induced acute myeloid leukemic cells. *Exp Hematol* (2002) 30(6):564–70. doi:10.1016/S0301-472X(02)00799-3

74. Rithidech KN, Cronkite EP, Bond VP. Advantages of the CBA mouse in leukemogenesis research. *Blood Cells Mol Dis* (1999) 25(1):38–45. doi:10.1006/bcmd.1999.0225

75. Weil MM, Bedford JS, Bielefeldt-Ohmann H, Ray FA, Genik PC, Ehrhart EJ, et al. Incidence of acute myeloid leukemia and hepatocellular carcinoma in mice irradiated with 1 GeV/nucleon ⁵⁶Fe ions. *Radiat Res* (2009) 172(2):213–9. doi:10.1667/RR1648.1

76. Verbiest T, Bouffler S, Nutt SL, Badie C. PU.1 downregulation in murine radiation-induced acute myeloid leukaemia (AML): from molecular mechanism to human AML. *Carcinogenesis* (2015) 36(4):413–9. doi:10.1093/carcin/bgv016

77. Rithidech KN, Honikel LM, Reungpatthanaphong P, Tungjai M, Golightly M, Whorton EB. Effects of 100 MeV protons delivered at 0.5 or 1 cGy/min on the in vivo induction of early and delayed chromosomal damage. *Mutat Res* (2013) 756(1–2):127–40. doi:10.1016/j.mrgentox.2013.06.001

78. Kanherkar RR, Bhatia-Dey N, Csoka AB. Epigenetics across the human lifespan. *Front Cell Dev Biol* (2014) 2:49. doi:10.3389/fcell.2014.00049

79. Baulch JE, Aypar U, Waters KM, Yang AJ, Morgan WF. Genetic and epigenetic changes in chromosomally stable and unstable progeny of irradiated cells. *PLoS One* (2014) 9(9):e107722. doi:10.1371/journal.pone.0107722

80. Rithidech K, Tungjai M, Arbab E, Simon SR. Activation of NF-kappa B in bone marrow cells of BALB/cJ mice following exposure in vivo to low doses of 137Cs gamma rays. *Radiat Environ Biophys* (2005) 44(2):139–43. doi:10.1007/s00411-005-0004-5

81. Rithidech KN, Tungjai M, Reungpatthanaphong P, Honikel L, Simon SR. Attenuation of oxidative damage and inflammatory responses by apigenin given to mice after irradiation. *Mutat Res* (2012) 749(1–2):29–38. doi:10.1016/j.mrgentox.2012.08.001

82. Rithidech K, Tungjai M, Reungpatthanaphong P, Honikel L, Sanford SR. Attenuation of oxidative damage and inflammatory responses by apigenin given to mice after irradiation. *Mutat Res* (2012) 749(1–2):29–38. doi:10.1016/j.mrgentox.2012.08.001

83. Curley JP, Mashoodh R, Champagne FA. Epigenetics and the origins of paternal effects. *Horm Behav* (2011) 59(3):306–14. doi:10.1016/j.yhbeh.2010.06.018

84. Aston KI, Uren PJ, Jenkins TG, Horsager A, Cairns BR, Smith AD, et al. Aberrant sperm DNA methylation predicts male fertility status and embryo quality. *Fertil Steril* (2015) 104(6):1388–97.e5. doi:10.1016/j.fertnstert.2015.08.019

85. Goetz W, Morgan MNM, Baulch JE. The effect of radiation quality on genomic DNA methylation profiles in irradiated human cell lines. *Radiat Res* (2011) 175(5):575–87. doi:10.1667/RR2390.1

86. Koturbash I, Pogribny I, Kovalchuk O. Stable loss of global DNA methylation in the radiation-target tissue – a possible mechanism contributing to radiation carcinogenesis? *Biochem Biophys Res Commun* (2005) 337(2):526–33. doi:10.1016/j.bbrc.2005.09.084

87. Kovalchuk O, Burke P, Besplug J, Slovack M, Filkowski J, Pogribny I. Methylation changes in muscle and liver tissues of male and female mice exposed to acute and chronic low-dose X-ray-irradiation. *Mutat Res* (2004) 548(1–2):75–84. doi:10.1016/j.mrfmmm.2003.12.016

88. Pogribny I, Raiche J, Slovack M, Kovalchuk O. Dose-dependence, sex- and tissue-specificity, and persistence of radiation-induced genomic DNA methylation changes. *Biochem Biophys Res Commun* (2004) 320(4):1253–61. doi:10.1016/j.bbrc.2004.06.081

89. Meistrich ML. Effects of chemotherapy and radiotherapy on spermatogenesis in humans. *Fertil Steril* (2013) 100(5):1180–6. doi:10.1016/j.fertnstert.2013.08.010

90. Hedger MP. Toll-like receptors and signalling in spermatogenesis and testicular responses to inflammation – a perspective. *J Reprod Immunol* (2011) 88(2):130–41. doi:10.1016/j.jri.2011.01.010

91. Singh SR, Burnicka-Turek O, Chauhan C, Hou SX. Spermatogonial stem cells, infertility and testicular cancer. *J Cell Mol Med* (2011) 15(3):468–83. doi:10.1111/j.1582-4934.2010.01242.x

16

Decreased RXRα is Associated with Increased βββ-Catenin/TCF4 in ⁵⁶Fe-Induced Intestinal Tumors

Shubhankar Suman[1], Santosh Kumar[1], Albert J. Fornace Jr.[1,2] and Kamal Datta[1]*

[1] Department of Biochemistry and Molecular and Cellular Biology, Lombardi Comprehensive Cancer Center, Georgetown University, Washington, DC, USA, [2] Center of Excellence in Genomic Medicine Research (CEGMR), King Abdulaziz University, Jeddah, Saudi Arabia

*Correspondence:
Kamal Datta,
Department of Biochemistry and
Molecular and Cellular Biology,
Georgetown University, Research
Building, Room E518, 3970 Reservoir
Road, NW, Washington, DC 20057,
USA
kd257@georgetown.edu

Although it is known that accumulation of oncogenic β-catenin is critical for intestinal tumorigenesis, the underlying mechanisms have not yet been fully explored. Post-translational β-catenin level is regulated via the adenomatous polyposis coli (APC)-dependent as well as the APC-independent ubiquitin–proteasome pathway (UPP). Employing an APC-mutant mouse model (APC^Min/+) the present study aimed to investigate the status of RXRα, an APC-independent factor involved in targeting β-catenin to UPP for degradation, in tumor-bearing and tumor-free areas of intestine after exposure to energetic ⁵⁶Fe ions. APC^Min/+ mice were exposed to energetic ⁵⁶Fe ions (4 or 1.6 Gy) and intestinal tumor samples and tumor-free normal intestinal samples were collected 100–110 days after exposure. The status of TCF4, β-catenin, cyclin D1, and RXRα was examined using immunohistochemistry and immunoblots. We observed increased accumulation of the transcription factor TCF4 and its co-activator β-catenin as well as their downstream oncogenic target protein cyclin-D1 in ⁵⁶Fe ion-induced intestinal tumors. Further, decreased expression of RXRα in tumors as well as in adjacent normal epithelium was indicative of perturbations in β-catenin proteasomal-targeting machinery. This indicates that decreased UPP targeting of β-catenin due to downregulation of RXRα can contribute to further accumulation of β-catenin and to ⁵⁶Fe-induced tumorigenesis.

Keywords: APC^Min/+, intestinal tumor, space radiation, heavy ion radiation, tumorigenesis, proteasome, β-catenin

Introduction

Heavy ion charged particle (HZE) radiation, such as ⁵⁶Fe ions, is prevalent in deep space, and is a major concern for astronauts' health (1). Recently, using APC^Min/+ mice, a well-accepted mouse model for human colorectal cancer (CRC), we found increased risk of CRC development accompanied by increased nuclear accumulation of oncogenic β-catenin and activation of its downstream signaling after exposure to ⁵⁶Fe ions (2–5). However, the mechanisms behind the accumulation of oncogenic β-catenin are not yet fully understood.

Cellular levels of free β-catenin are tightly regulated via the ubiquitin–proteasome pathway (UPP). Targeting of β-catenin to the proteasome and its subsequent degradation involves two adenomatous polyposis coli (APC)-dependent (i.e., APC/GSK3β/AXIN and APC/Siah1) and one APC-independent (RXRα-mediated) mechanisms (6). In gastrointestinal (GI) tumors, genes involved in APC-dependent (APC, Siah1, and Axin) targeting of β-catenin are often mutated (7–11), and similarly in APC^Min/+ mice, tumor formation is mostly driven through inactivation of the wild type

APC allele (12). Thus, APC-dependent proteasomal targeting of β-catenin is eventually disabled in these tumors. In the absence of proteasomal targeting, β-catenin accumulates and interacts with T-cell factor transcription factors (TCF4) in the nucleus leading to activation of oncogenic signaling pathways (13). In view of the known perturbations in APC-dependent proteasomal targeting of β-catenin early in the GI tumorigenesis process, only the APC-independent (RXRα-dependent) pathway would remain to control its accumulation. However, the status of the APC-independent proteasomal targeting of the β-catenin in heavy ion radiation-induced intestinal tumors has not been explored. In this study, using the APC$^{Min/+}$ intestinal tumor mouse model (14), we demonstrated downregulation of RXRα expression, which may complement the disabled APC-dependent proteasomal degradation pathway to increase β-catenin accumulation in ^{56}Fe-induced tumors. Downregulation of RXRα observed in this study could potentially play a crucial role in heavy ion radiation-induced increased risk of intestinal tumorigenesis and would warrant further investigation.

Materials and Methods

Mice and Genotyping

Male APC$^{Min/+}$ mice (The Jackson Laboratory, Bar Harbor, ME, USA) were bred with female C57BL/6J mice at the Georgetown University (GU)'s animal facility. Genotyping using tail DNA samples were done using reverse-transcription polymerase chain reaction (RT-PCR) to identify heterozygous offspring as per the Jackson Laboratory protocol. The mouse colony was maintained on standard certified rodent diet and filtered water in a humidity and temperature-controlled room with 12 h dark/light cycle. All experimental procedures were performed in compliance with the protocols approved by the Institutional Animal Care and Use Committee (IACUC) at GU and Brookhaven National Laboratory (BNL). Both the facilities are Association for Assessment and Accreditation of Laboratory and Animal Care International (AAALACI) accredited facilities and we followed The Guide for the Care and Use of Laboratory Animals.

Irradiation and Sample Collection

APC$^{Min/+}$ female mice (6–8-weeks old) were placed in well-ventilated transparent plastic boxes (1 mouse/box) allowing easy movement and irradiated with 4 or 1.6 Gy whole body ^{56}Fe radiation (energy: 1000 MeV/n; LET: 148 keV/μm; dose rate: 1 Gy/min) at the NASA Space Radiation Laboratory (NSRL) at BNL. These two doses were used in our previously published tumorigenesis experiments and samples collected during that study were used for molecular analysis in this study. For ^{56}Fe exposure, both control and treatment groups were shipped to BNL for irradiation and brought back to GU after irradiation in a temperature-controlled vehicle for a same day delivery to minimize stress to the animals. Age-matched ^{56}Fe-irradiated and control mice were euthanized by CO_2 asphyxiation between 100 and 110 days after radiation exposure. The small intestinal tract was surgically removed, washed with phosphate-buffered saline (PBS), and cut open longitudinally at room temperature. A dissecting scope (Leica MZ6, Buffalo Grove, IL, USA) was used

to visualize and dissect tumors, which were then flash frozen in liquid nitrogen and stored at −80°C for further use. Also, intestinal samples (~3 cm) with tumor-bearing and surrounding tumor-free area were fixed overnight in 10% buffered formalin, embedded in paraffin, and 4 μm-thick sections were obtained for immunohistochemistry staining.

Immunohistochemistry

Intestinal sections ($n = 5$ mice per group) were used for immunohistochemistry with a protocol described earlier (3). Briefly, immunostaining for active-β-catenin (Cat#05-665, Millipore, Billerica, MA, USA; dilution: 1:100), TCF4 (Cat#05-511, Millipore; dilution: 1:100), RXRα (Cat#sc-553, Santa Cruz Biotechnology, Dallas, TX, USA; dilution: 1:40), and cyclin D1 (Cat#04-1151; Millipore; dilution: 1:150) were performed by soaking slides in antigen retrieval citrate buffer (pH 6.0; Dako, Carpinteria, CA, USA) and heating at 100°C for 15 min in a microwave oven. Further, endogenous peroxidase activity was quenched using 3% hydrogen peroxide in methanol followed by incubation in blocking buffer (5% bovine serum albumin in PBS) for 30 min. After blocking sections were incubated overnight at 4°C with the respective primary antibody. Signal detection and color development was done using SuperPicture 3rd Gen IHC detection kit (Cat#87-9673; Invitrogen, Carlsbad, CA, USA). Sections were counterstained using hematoxylin and images were acquired using bright field microscopy at a magnification of 20×. At least 10 randomly chosen images from the tumor-bearing as well as from the tumor-free areas were acquired from each mouse and a representative image from each group is shown in the results. Images were analyzed using color deconvolution and image-based tool for counting nuclei (ITCN) plug-ins of ImageJ v1.45 software (National Institutes of Health, Bethesda, MD, USA). Quantification data were statistically analyzed using two-tailed paired Student's t-test and difference between control and irradiated group was considered significant when p-value was <0.05. Error bars represent mean $\pm$ SEM.

Immunoblots

Frozen intestinal tumor samples ($n = 5$ mice per group) were pooled and used for immunoblot analysis of RXRα level with a protocol described previously (3). Briefly, samples were homogenized in ice-cold lysis buffer, centrifuged, and supernatant collected. Protein was estimated in supernatant and equal amount of protein was used for sodium dodecyl sulfate-polyacrylamide gel electrophoresis (SDS-PAGE). Protein was transferred to PVDF membrane, incubated with RXRα antibody, and protein detected using horseradish peroxidase (HRP) conjugated secondary antibody and enhanced chemiluminescence (ECL) detection system (Cat# 34080, Thermo Fisher Scientific, Rockford, IL, USA) and representative images shown in the results.

Results

Increased β-Catenin and TCF4 Levels in ^{56}Fe-Induced Intestinal Tumor

Intestinal tumors stained for β-catenin showed increased level in 4 Gy ^{56}Fe-irradiated samples relative to control tumors from sham-irradiated mice (**Figures 1A,B**) and this is consistent with our previous results after 1.6 Gy [56]Fe irradiation (3). Higher levels were also observed for TCF4 in [56]Fe-irradiated intestinal tumors relative to controls (**Figures 1C,D**). Transcription factor TCF4 along with the transcriptional co-activator β-catenin are involved in transcribing pro-proliferative factors, such as cyclin D1, and increased cyclin D1 was observed in the current study (**Figures 1E,F**) as well.

Reduced Expression of RXRα in Tumor-Bearing and Tumor-Free Areas of APC^Min/+ Mice After Exposure to [56]Fe Radiation

Immunohistochemistry in tumor samples demonstrated that expression of RXRα was reduced after 4 Gy (**Figure 2A**). Quantification and statistical analysis of stained sections from five mice showed that RXRα was significantly lowered in [56]Fe-irradiated

tumors relative to sham-irradiated tumors (**Figure 2B**). Intestinal tumors from 1.6 Gy [56]Fe-irradiated mice also showed decreased RXRα staining (**Figure 2C**) and quantification and statistical analysis showed that the staining in irradiated samples were significantly lower compared to controls (**Figure 2D**). However, quantification did not show significant difference in RXRα staining between two radiation doses. Immunoblots of 4 Gy (**Figure 2E**) and 1.6 Gy (**Figure 2F**) intestinal tumor samples also showed decreased RXRα. We also performed immunohistochemistry for RXRα on tumor-free intestinal sections from APC^Min/+ mice exposed to either 1.6 or 4 Gy [56]Fe ions. Staining of tumor-free intestinal section showed lower expression of RXRα after 4 Gy [56]Fe relative to corresponding controls (**Figure 3A**). Decreased RXRα after 4 Gy [56]Fe was statistically significant compared to sham-irradiated controls (**Figure 3B**). Conversely, we also observed downregulation of RXRα in 1.6 Gy irradiated samples

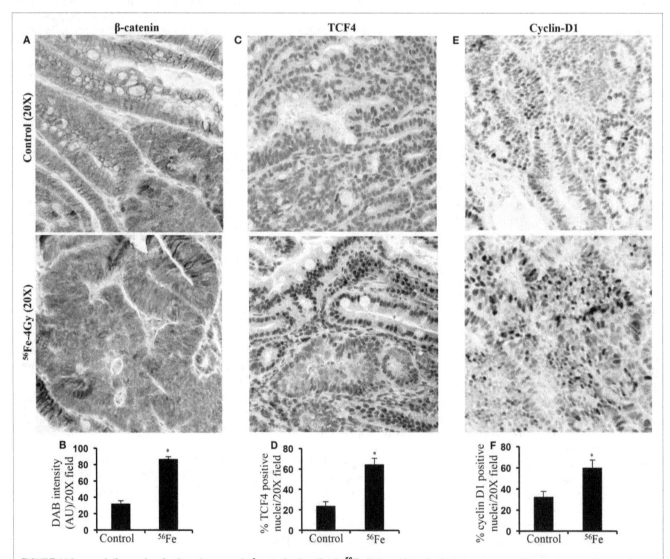

FIGURE 1 | Accumulation and activation of oncogenic β-catenin signaling in [56]Fe-induced intestinal tumors compared to spontaneous tumors from sham-irradiated mice (control). **(A)** Immunohistochemical detection of active-β-catenin in [56]Fe-induced intestinal tumors. **(B)** Quantification of β-catenin expression in intestinal tumors. **(C)** Immunohistochemical detection of β-catenin transcriptional regulator TCF4 in [56]Fe-induced intestinal tumors. **(D)** Quantification of TCF4 positive nuclei in intestinal tumors. **(E)** Immunohistochemical detection of β-catenin/TCF4 oncogenic target cyclin-D1 in [56]Fe-induced intestinal tumors. **(F)** Quantification of cyclin-D1 positive nuclei in intestinal tumors. Error bars represent mean ± SEM and $p < 0.05$ was considered significant. AU – Arbitrary Unit.

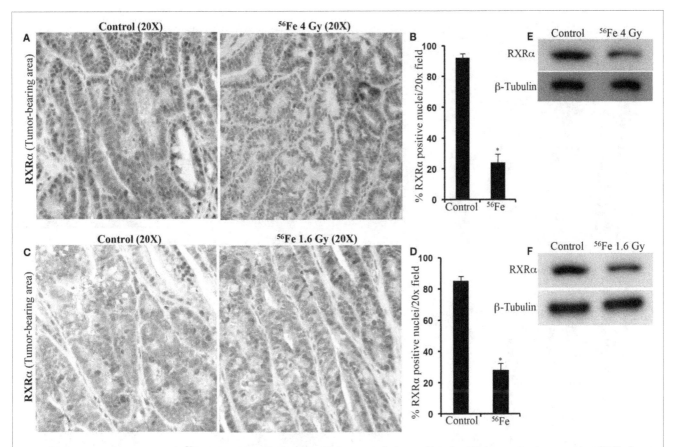

FIGURE 2 | Lower RXRα expression in [56]Fe-induced intestinal tumors. (A) Representative immunohistochemistry images showing expression of RXRα in spontaneous and 4 Gy [56]Fe-induced intestinal tumors. (B) Quantification of RXRα in spontaneous and 4 Gy [56]Fe-induced intestinal tumors. (C) Expression of RXRα in spontaneous and 1.6 Gy [56]Fe-induced intestinal tumors. (D) Quantification of RXRα in spontaneous and 1.6 Gy [56]Fe-induced intestinal tumors. (E) Immunoblots of RXRα in spontaneous and 4 Gy [56]Fe-induced intestinal tumors. (F) Immunoblots of RXRα in spontaneous and 1.6 Gy [56]Fe-induced intestinal tumors. Error bars represent mean ± SEM and $p < 0.05$ was considered significant.

compared to controls (**Figure 3C**) and quantification showed statistically significant difference between irradiated and sham-irradiated samples (**Figure 3D**).

Discussion

The carcinogenic potential of ionizing radiation is well known and using animal models it has been established that high LET heavy ion radiation has higher carcinogenic potential compared to low-LET radiation (15). Increased frequencies of site-specific cancer following heavy ion exposure have been reported in various rodent models with upregulation of oncogenic signaling mediated through genetic, epigenetic, and/or physiological changes (3, 15–17). Earlier studies conducted in APC[Min/+] mice revealed increased tumor induction and a higher number of adenocarcinomas, which was associated with greater upregulation of β-catenin signaling after [56]Fe exposure relative to γ radiation; this is indicative of perturbations in the molecular events upstream of β-catenin (3). The purpose of the current study was to develop mechanistic insight into greater tumorigenesis observed in our previous work in APC[Min/+] mice after two doses of [56]Fe radiation relative to γ radiation. While pathways can be investigated in the wild-type mice, they are resistant to intestinal

tumorigenesis. Therefore, we used APC-mutant mice not only to quantitatively assess tumor frequency but also to understand molecular pathway alterations, which may have contributed to tumor development after radiation exposure. While we reported previously that two doses of [56]Fe caused higher tumor frequency, we are yet to fully understand molecular characteristics of the tumors and tumor-adjacent normal tissues after [56]Fe irradiation. To this end, the results presented in the current study explain in part potential underlying mechanisms contributing to increased tumor frequency after [56]Fe irradiation. We have focused on the APC-independent mechanism of β-catenin degradation via UPP. In APC-deficient adenoma, accumulation of β-catenin complexed with nuclear TCF4 results in the increased expression of its oncogenic target genes, such as cyclin-D1 that promotes intestinal cell proliferation and polyp formation (18). In agreement with our published reports in APC[Min/+] mice exposed to 1.6 Gy of [56]Fe ion, the current study also observed similar activation of β-catenin at 4 Gy of [56]Fe ion along with increased TCF4 and cyclin-D1. Significant loss of RXRα was evident in tumors as well as in tumor-free areas of intestine after [56]Fe radiation and this could contribute to decreased proteasomal targeting of β-catenin, therefore enhancing cell survival and proliferation through β-catenin/TCF4 signaling. Notably, RXRα was downregulated in

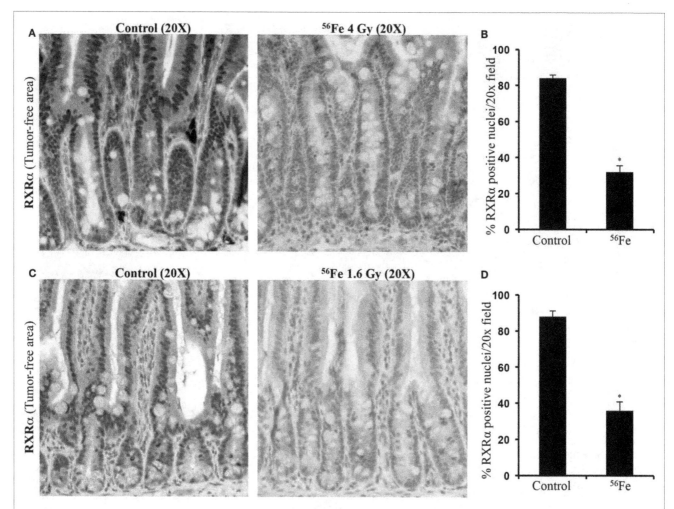

FIGURE 3 | Downregulation of RXRα was observed in tumor-free areas of intestinal samples from APC^Min/+ mice. (A) Decreased RXRα expression after 4 Gy ⁵⁶Fe radiation. **(B)** Quantification of immunohistochemistry images showed significant decrease in RXRα after 4 Gy ⁵⁶Fe. **(C)** Decreased RXRα expression after 1.6 Gy ⁵⁶Fe radiation. **(D)** Quantification of immunohistochemistry images showed significant decrease in RXRα after 1.6 Gy ⁵⁶Fe. Error bars represent mean ± SEM and $p < 0.05$ was considered significant.

both the radiation doses tested suggesting that the effect is independent of radiation dose and that the lower dose may have a proportionately greater effect relative to the higher dose. We recognize that the mean absorbed doses of energetic ⁵⁶Fe ions used in the current study are higher than the doses astronauts are expected to receive during prolonged space missions. These high doses of energetic ⁵⁶Fe ions were used as a proof of principle in our initial studies for establishing the differential effects, quantitatively and qualitatively, of space compared to γ radiation.

Loss of the remaining wild type APC allele has often been implicated as the primary mechanism for increased β-catenin signaling leading to tumor development in APC^Min/+ mice (12, 19, 20). In addition to APC, the β-catenin cellular level is also regulated through a direct proteasomal targeting mediated by RXRα (21) and downregulation of RXRα in human and rodent colonic tumors has been reported previously (22). Considering that protein turnover is critical for cellular homeostasis, availability of multiple independent pathways for protein degradation ensures that the potentially pro-carcinogenic β-catenin level

remains within physiologic limits to limit cancer initiation and progression. Downregulation of RXRα in our model system may have played a role in ⁵⁶Fe radiation-induced more aggressive tumorigenesis reported earlier (3). Apart from driving proteasomal degradation of β-catenin, RXRα also functions to suppress β-catenin-mediated upregulation of oncogenes through direct protein–protein interaction (23) in colon cancer cells. Thus, loss of RXRα expression could further stabilize β-catenin signaling in tumor cells, leading to greater cell proliferation and higher number of invasive cancers associated with ⁵⁶Fe relative to γ radiation.

Nuclear receptor RXRα is known to heterodimerize with a host of other nuclear receptors, such as the vitamin D receptor (VDR) and retinoid acid receptor (RAR), and is involved through transactivation of target genes, such as p21, in regulating normal growth and development (23, 24). Consequently, loss of RXRα is expected to cause disordered cellular proliferation, and indeed, downregulation of RXRα has been widely reported in a number of cancers including CRC (21–26). Our result demonstrates for the first time that RXRα is downregulated in tumor-free areas

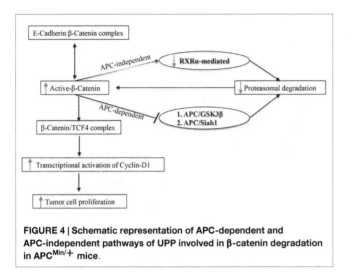

FIGURE 4 | Schematic representation of APC-dependent and APC-independent pathways of UPP involved in β-catenin degradation in APC$^{Min/+}$ mice.

of APC$^{Min/+}$ intestine ~100 days after radiation exposure. Considering that a significant number of intestinal adenomas has also been reported to arise without the loss of heterozygosity of the APC gene and these adenomas are often polyclonal (8, 20, 27), our results supports an APC-independent mechanism of β-catenin stabilization during ^{56}Fe-irradiated tumorigenesis. We believe that decreased RXRα expression in tumor-free areas of the intestine may be a reflection of the RXRα status in other areas of the GI tract and that this molecular event may be preceding intestinal tumorigenesis in APC$^{Min/+}$ mice. Furthermore, RXRα signaling is also linked to cellular redox regulation and it has been demonstrated that RXRα activation protects cell from oxidative stress and inhibition promotes ROS production (28, 29). Downregulation of RXRα observed ~100 days post-exposure in the current study aligns with our previous studies demonstrating chronic oxidative stress even 1 year after exposure to energetic ^{56}Fe ions (30). Although we observed persistent oxidative stress after γ radiation, it was less pronounced relative to equitoxic doses of ^{56}Fe radiation. Additionally, intestinal tumor frequency and grade was also higher after ^{56}Fe relative to equitoxic doses of

γ radiation. Considering that γ radiation responses were consistently lower relative to ^{56}Fe, in the current study, we have analyzed and presented ^{56}Fe-induced alterations of an alternate pathway involved in β-catenin regulation via RXRα. Our data, previous and current, demonstrate that effects of radiation on redox balance, carcinogenesis, and related molecular pathways are dependent on radiation quality and energy deposition characteristics. However, further in depth studies will be required to dissect the link between heavy ion radiation exposure and long-term molecular alterations, such as oxidative stress and RXRα downregulation. In summary, our results show that energetic heavy ion radiation is capable of lowering RXRα in tumor as well as non-tumor intestinal epithelial cells. Due to its roles in multiple cellular processes, continuous downregulation of RXRα, we believe, will have major ramifications for intestinal cellular homeostasis with implications for carcinogenesis including colorectal carcinogenesis (**Figure 4**).

Author Contributions

Conceived and designed the experiments: SS and KD. Performed the experiments: SS and SK. Analyzed the data: SS, SK, and KD. Contributed reagents/materials/analysis tools: AF and KD. Wrote the paper: SS, AF, and KD. All authors read and approved this manuscript.

Acknowledgments

This study is supported in part by NASA grants NNX13AD58G and NNX09AU95G. We are very much thankful to the members of the NASA Space Radiation Laboratory (NSRL), especially to Drs. Peter Guida and Adam Rusek from Brookhaven National Laboratory for their excellent support in conducting heavy ion radiation exposures. We are also thankful to Steve Strawn and Pelagie Ake for administrative and animal facility supports. We acknowledge the Histopathology and Tissue Shared Resources at the Georgetown University supported by Award Number P30CA051008 from the National Cancer Institute.

References

1. Cucinotta FA, Kim MH, Chappell LJ, Huff JL. How safe is safe enough? Radiation risk for a human mission to Mars. *PLoS One* (2013) 8:e74988. doi:10.1371/journal.pone.0074988

2. Trani D, Datta K, Doiron K, Kallakury B, Fornace AJJ. Enhanced intestinal tumor multiplicity and grade in vivo after HZE exposure: mouse models for space radiation risk estimates. *Radiat Environ Biophys* (2010) 49:389–96. doi:10.1007/s00411-010-0292-2

3. Datta K, Suman S, Kallakury BV, Fornace AJJ. Heavy ion radiation exposure triggered higher intestinal tumor frequency and greater beta-catenin activation than gamma radiation in APC(Min/+) mice. *PLoS One* (2013) 8:e59295. doi:10.1371/journal.pone.0059295

4. Cucinotta FA. Space radiation risks for astronauts on multiple International Space Station missions. *PLoS One* (2014) 9:e96099. doi:10.1371/journal.pone.0096099

5. Trani D, Nelson SA, Moon BH, Swedlow JJ, Williams EM, Strawn SJ, et al. High-energy particle-induced tumorigenesis throughout the gastrointestinal tract. *Radiat Res* (2014) 181:162–71. doi:10.1667/RR13502.1

6. Xiao JH, Ghosn C, Hinchman C, Forbes C, Wang J, Snider N, et al. Adenomatous polyposis coli (APC)-independent regulation of beta-catenin degradation

via a retinoid X receptor-mediated pathway. *J Biol Chem* (2003) 278:29954–62. doi:10.1074/jbc.M304761200

7. Kim CJ, Cho YG, Park CH, Jeong SW, Nam SW, Kim SY, et al. Inactivating mutations of the Siah-1 gene in gastric cancer. *Oncogene* (2004) 23:8591–6. doi:10.1038/sj.onc.1208113

8. Segditsas S, Tomlinson I. Colorectal cancer and genetic alterations in the Wnt pathway. *Oncogene* (2006) 25:7531–7. doi:10.1038/sj.onc.1210059

9. Russo A, Bazan V, Iacopetta B, Kerr D, Soussi T, Gebbia N. The TP53 colorectal cancer international collaborative study on the prognostic and predictive significance of p53 mutation: influence of tumor site, type of mutation, and adjuvant treatment. *J Clin Oncol* (2005) 23:7518–28. doi:10.1200/JCO.2005.00.471

10. Hegde MR, Roa BB. Detecting mutations in the APC gene in familial adenomatous polyposis (FAP). *Curr Protoc Hum Genet* (2006) **Chapter 10**:Unit10.8. doi:10.1002/0471142905.hg1008s50

11. Satoh S, Daigo Y, Furukawa Y, Kato T, Miwa N, Nishiwaki T, et al. AXIN1 mutations in hepatocellular carcinomas, and growth suppression in cancer cells by virus-mediated transfer of AXIN1. *Nat Genet* (2000) 24:245–50. doi:10.1038/73448

12. Levy DB, Smith KJ, Beazer-Barclay Y, Hamilton SR, Vogelstein B, Kinzler KW. Inactivation of both APC alleles in human and mouse tumors. *Cancer Res* (1994) 54:5953–8.

13. Wei W, Chua MS, Grepper S, So S. Small molecule antagonists of Tcf4/beta-catenin complex inhibit the growth of HCC cells in vitro and in vivo. *Int J Cancer* (2010) **126**:2426–36. doi:10.1002/ijc.24810

14. Suman S, Fornace AJJ, Datta K. Animal models of colorectal cancer in chemoprevention and therapeutics development. In: Ettarh R, editor. *Colorectal Cancer – From Prevention to Patient Care*. Rijeka: InTech (2012). p. 277–300. doi:10.5772/28497

15. Bielefeldt-Ohmann H, Genik PC, Fallgren CM, Ullrich RL, Weil MM. Animal studies of charged particle-induced carcinogenesis. *Health Phys* (2012) **103**:568–76. doi:10.1097/HP.0b013e318265a257

16. Peng Y, Brown N, Finnon R, Warner CL, Liu X, Genik PC, et al. Radiation leukemogenesis in mice: loss of PU.1 on chromosome 2 in CBA and C57BL/6 mice after irradiation with 1 GeV/nucleon 56Fe ions, X rays or gamma rays. Part I. Experimental observations. *Radiat Res* (2009) **171**:474–83. doi:10.1667/RR1547.1

17. Weil MM, Bedford JS, Bielefeldt-Ohmann H, Ray FA, Genik PC, Ehrhart EJ, et al. Incidence of acute myeloid leukemia and hepatocellular carcinoma in mice irradiated with 1 GeV/nucleon (56)Fe ions. *Radiat Res* (2009) **172**:213–9. doi:10.1667/RR1648.1

18. Barker N, Morin PJ, Clevers H. The Yin-Yang of TCF/beta-catenin signaling. *Adv Cancer Res* (2000) **77**:1–24. doi:10.1016/S0065-230X(08)60783-6

19. Luongo C, Dove WF. Somatic genetic events linked to the Apc locus in intestinal adenomas of the Min mouse. *Genes Chromosomes Cancer* (1996) **17**: 194–8. doi:10.1002/1098-2264(199611)17:3<194::AID-GCC2870170302>3.0. CO;2-E

20. Bienz M, Clevers H. Linking colorectal cancer to Wnt signaling. *Cell* (2000) **103**:311–20. doi:10.1016/S0092-8674(00)00122-7

21. Dillard AC, Lane MA. Retinol increases beta-catenin-RXRalpha binding leading to the increased proteasomal degradation of beta-catenin and RXRalpha. *Nutr Cancer* (2008) **60**:97–108. doi:10.1080/01635580701586754

22. Janakiram NB, Mohammed A, Qian L, Choi CI, Steele VE, Rao CV. Chemopreventive effects of RXR-selective rexinoid bexarotene on intestinal neoplasia of Apc(Min/+) mice. *Neoplasia* (2012) **14**:159–68. doi:10.1593/neo.111440

23. Han A, Tong C, Hu D, Bi X, Yang W. A direct protein-protein interaction is involved in the suppression of beta-catenin transcription by retinoid X receptor alpha in colorectal cancer cells. *Cancer Biol Ther* (2008) **7**:454–9. doi:10.4161/cbt.7.3.5455

24. Shimizu M, Shirakami Y, Imai K, Takai K, Moriwaki H. Acyclic retinoid in chemoprevention of hepatocellular carcinoma: targeting phosphorylated retinoid X receptor-α for prevention of liver carcinogenesis. *J Carcinog* (2012) **11**:11. doi:10.4103/1477-3163.100398

25. Yamazaki K, Shimizu M, Okuno M, Matsushima-Nishiwaki R, Kanemura N, Araki H, et al. Synergistic effects of RXR alpha and PPAR gamma ligands to inhibit growth in human colon cancer cells – phosphorylated RXR alpha is a critical target for colon cancer management. *Gut* (2007) **56**:1557–63. doi:10.1136/gut.2007.129858

26. Zhang F, Meng F, Li H, Dong Y, Yang W, Han A. Suppression of retinoid X receptor alpha and aberrant β-catenin expression significantly associates with progression of colorectal carcinoma. *Eur J Cancer* (2011) **47**:2060–7. doi:10.1016/j.ejca.2011.04.010

27. Merritt AJ, Gould KA, Dove WF. Polyclonal structure of intestinal adenomas in ApcMin/+ mice with concomitant loss of Apc+ from all tumor lineages. *Proc Natl Acad Sci U S A* (1997) **94**:13927–31. doi:10.1073/pnas.94.25.13927

28. Shan P, Pu J, Yuan A, Shen L, Shen L, Chai D, et al. RXR agonists inhibit oxidative stress-induced apoptosis in H9c2 rat ventricular cells. *Biochem Biophys Res Commun* (2008) **375**:628–33. doi:10.1016/j.bbrc.2008.08.074

29. Ning RB, Zhu J, Chai DJ, Xu CS, Xie H, Lin XY, et al. RXR agonists inhibit high glucose-induced upregulation of inflammation by suppressing activation of the NADPH oxidase-nuclear factor-κB pathway in human endothelial cells. *Genet Mol Res* (2013) **12**:6692–707. doi:10.4238/2013.December.13.3

30. Datta K, Suman S, Kallakury BV, Fornace AJJ. Exposure to heavy ion radiation induces persistent oxidative stress in mouse intestine. *PLoS One* (2012) **7**:e42224. doi:10.1371/journal.pone.0042224

17

The Effect of X-Ray and Heavy Ions Radiations on Chemotherapy Refractory Tumor Cells

Zhan Yu[1,2]*, Carola Hartel[1], Diana Pignalosa[1], Wilma Kraft-Weyrather[1], Guo-Liang Jiang[2,3], David Diaz-Carballo[4] and Marco Durante[1,5]

[1] Department of Biophysics, GSI Helmholtzzentrum für Schwerionenforschung, Darmstadt, Germany, [2] Department of Radiation Oncology, Shanghai Proton and Heavy Ion Center, Shanghai, China, [3] Department of Oncology, Shanghai Medical College, Fudan University, Shanghai, China, [4] Institute of Molecular Oncology and Experimental Therapeutics, Marienhospital Herne, Ruhr University of Bochum Medical School, Herne, Germany, [5] Institute of Condense Matter Physics, Darmstadt University of Technology, Darmstadt, Germany

*Correspondence:
Zhan Yu
zhan.yu@sphic.org.cn

Purpose: The purpose of this study is to link both numeric and structural chromosomal aberrations to the effectiveness of radiotherapy in chemotherapy refractory tumor cells.

Materials and methods: Neuroblastoma (LAN-1) and 79HF6 glioblastoma cells derived from patients and their chemoresistant sublines were artificially cultured as neurospheres and irradiated by X-rays and heavy ions sources. All the cell lines were irradiated by Carbon-SIS with LET of 100 keV/μm. However, 79HF6 cells and LAN-1 cells were also irradiated by Carbon-UNILAC with LET of 168 keV/μm and Nickel ions with LET of 174 keV/μm, respectively. The effect of radiation on the survival and proliferation of cells was addressed by standard clonogenic assays. In order to analyze cell karyotype standard Giemsa staining, multicolor fluorescence in situ hybridization (mFISH) and multicolor banding (mBAND) techniques were applied.

Results: Relative biological effectiveness values of heavy ion beams relative to X-rays at the D_{10} values were found between 2.3 and 2.6 with Carbon-SIS and Nickel for LAN-1 and between 2.5 and 3.4 with Carbon-SIS and Carbon-UNILAC for 79HF6 cells. Chemorefractory LAN-1[RETO] cells were found more radioresistant than untreated LAN-1[WT] cells. 79HF6[RETO] glioblastoma cells were found more radiosensitive than cytostatic sensitive cells 79HF6[WT]. Sphere formation assay showed that LAN-1[RETO] cells were able to form spheres in serum-free culture, whereas 79HF6 cells could not. Most of 79HF6[WT] cells revealed a number of 71–90 chromosomes, whereas 79HF6[RETO] revealed a number of 52–83 chromosomes. The majority of LAN-1[WT] cells revealed a number of 40–44 chromosomes. mFISH analysis showed some stable aberrations, especially on chromosome 10 as judged by the impossibility to label this region with specific probes. This was corroborated using mBAND analysis.

Conclusion: Heavy ion irradiation was more effective than X-ray in both cytostatic naive cancer and chemoresistant cell lines. LAN-1[RETO] chemoresistant neuroblastoma cells were found to be more radioresistant than the cytostatic naive cells (LAN-1[WT]), whereas this effect was not found in 79HF6 cells.

Keywords: chemoresistance, X-ray and heavy ion irradiation, relative biological effectiveness, neuroblastoma, glioblastoma

INTRODUCTION

There is convincing evidence that many solid and hematological malignancies are organized hierarchically and contain a small population of cancer stem cells (CSCs) that possess the capacity to self-renew and to cause the heterogeneous lineages of cells that form the tumor (1). Consequently, cell heterogeneity of tumors may play an important role in tumor persistence and metastasis formation. Additionally, there is growing evidence that CSCs are inherently resistant to radiation and perhaps other conventional anticancer treatments, i.e., chemotherapy (2–4). These intrinsic mechanisms of resistance are responsible for a significant number of tumor recurrences (2, 3). Consequently, an effective anticancer treatment can only be achieved if this population is eliminated.

Chemotherapy has the advantage over radiotherapy in fighting the disseminated metastatic situation but at higher costs for the organism as a whole. Contrary to that, radiotherapy is a more localized treatment, but it is less applicable once the cancer has spread to several regions. Contemporaneous studies have consistently shown that CSC phenotypes are triggered after chemotherapy courses with an accompanied radioresistance of cancer cells both *in vitro* and *in vivo* probably by preferential activation of the DNA damage response (5). This indicates the urgent necessity for reevaluation of conventional therapies and searching for new ones that focus on CSCs to enhance the efficacy of cancer treatments.

Neuroblastoma is one of the most common extracranial pediatric tumors with a wide spectrum of clinical forms. The long-term survival of children with a high-risk clinical phenotype is <40% (especially those with MYCN amplification) (6). Glioblastoma is the most aggressive brain tumor in adults. In spite of multimodal therapy, the median survival is only around 14 months with early recurrences (and infiltrative events) in the brain (7). The existence (and local spread) of CSCs may be an important reason for the treatment failure due to its resistance to conventional therapy, which leads to a poor prognosis.

Culturing cancer cells in the presence of a low dose of chemotherapeutic agents is one of the approaches to enrich subpopulations with CSC-like phenotypes and related physiology. Etoposide is a topoisomerase inhibitor and causes DNA breaks enforcing apoptosis in dividing cancer cells. It is used as a standard chemotherapy in many tumors, such as neuroblastoma. However, etoposide is also known as an inducing agent of multidrug-resistant cancer phenotypes. In this study, low dose of etoposide was used to enrich CSCs fraction in glioblastoma and neuroblastoma cell lines.

Particle radiotherapy is becoming more widely used because proton and heavy ions have a favorable depth–dose distribution and a higher relative biological effectiveness (RBE) compared with photon. Once cancer cells are exposed to this therapy, they suffer a complex and clustered DNA damage, which is unable to be repaired by cellular mechanisms independent of the reactive oxygen species formed after exposing cells to charged particles. Consequently, malignant cells are less radioresistance because the mechanisms responsible for DNA reparation work less effective (8).

Our works aimed at studying the survival of chemoresistant cells compared with their wild-type parentals after being exposed to X-rays and heavy ions. We also addressed the question if the karyotype and chromosomal number deviations are related to the survival.

MATERIALS AND METHODS

Cell Lines and Culture Conditions

Two parental and their subtypes highly chemotherapy refractory cell lines LAN-1^{WT}, LAN-1^{RETO} neuroblastoma and 79HF6^{WT}, 79HF6^{RETO} glioblastoma multiforme derived from human tumors were used in this investigation. The LAN-1 cells were isolated from a bone marrow metastasis of a 2-year-old boy with neuroblastoma (clinical Stage IV), and the 79HF6 cells were isolated from a female adult patient. The etoposide-resistant sublines usyed in this work exhibit CSC features among a set of CSC markers, broad spectrum of cross-resistance to several cytostatics, and radioresistance. The phenotype characteristics and the CSC features were published previously (5). Cells were cultured in Dulbecco's modified Eagle medium (DMEM), supplemented with 10% fetal calf serum (FCS) and 1% penicillin/streptomycin (all purchased from Biochrom AG, Berlin, Germany), and kept in a humidified atmosphere of 5% CO_2 at 37°C. Resistant to ETOposide (RETO) cells were constantly cultured in the medium containing 4 µg/ml etoposide (Teva, Germany). The cell doubling time (t_D) was determined in the exponential phase of the growth with the GSI in house program gd (©M. Krämer, 2003).

Clonogenic Assay

Clonogenic assay was performed to determine both clonogenic behavior and cell survival rates after irradiation. Cells were seeded in T25 flask containing around 100 viable colonies after irradiation. LAN-1^{WT} and LAN-1^{RETO} cells were incubated for 9 days. 79HF6^{WT} cells were incubated for 11 days, whereas 79HF6^{RETO} cells were incubated for 25 days. Colonies were fixed and stained with methylene blue. Colonies containing more than 50 cells were defined as survivors.

Sphere Formation Assay

Cells were cultured in serum-free neurobasal A medium (Gibco, Life Technologies, Germany) supplemented with B27 (Gibco, Life Technologies, Germany), 10 ng/ml human fibroblast growth factor-basic (Biochrom, Germany), 20 ng/ml human epidermal growth factor (Biochrom, Germany), and 0.1% bovine serum albumin fraction V (Roche Diagnostics, Germany) to observe the formation of neurospheres (9).

Karyotyping

For chromosome preparations, cells were seeded 48 h in T75 culture flasks with 10 ml medium before the experiment in order to allow stabile attachment. One hundred microliters of colcemid (Roche Deutschland Holding GmbH, Germany) with the concentration of 10 µg/ml were added to the cultures. After 3.5 h of incubation for LAN-1 and 79HF6^{WT} and 4 h for 79HF6^{RETO}, cells were trypsinized and harvested. Cell suspension was pelleted and carefully treated with prewarmed (37°C) 0.075M potassium chloride solution for 8 min and then fixed with 3:1 ratio of MeOH:glacial acetic acid for 30 min at room temperature. After washing, cells were resuspended in proper volume of the mentioned fixative and dropped on wet slides. The slides were then air-dried for 24 h. The slides were stained with 5% Giemsa (Merck, Germany) solution for 10 min, washed with distilled water, and dried overnight.

Multicolor Fluorescence *In Situ* Hybridization Technique and Multicolor Banding Technique

For multicolor fluorescence *in situ* hybridization (mFISH) analysis, the slides were hybridized using the 24XCyte mFISH kit (Metasystems, Altlussheim, Germany) according to the protocol recommended by the manufacturer. In brief, the slides were first subjected to a denaturation followed by dehydration. An appropriate volume of DNA denatured probe was incubated in a humidified chamber at 37°C in the dark for 2 days. Afterward, the remaining hybridization probe was washed off. Finally, all DNA material was counterstained using DAPI/antifade (250 ng/ml), and the slide was covered. The chromosomal dispersal was analyzed using fluorescence microscopy Imager Z1 (Zeiss, Germany). Probes labeled with FITC, Orange, Texas Red®, Aqua, Cy™5 (Cy5), and 4′,6-diamidino-2-phenylindol (DAPI) fluorochromes were used to visualize chromosomal segments. Karyotypes were (re)constructed using the Isis/mFISH software (Metasystems). The procedure of multicolor banding (mBAND) is similar to that of mFISH, performed with the mBAND kit (Metasystems, Altlussheim, Germany), as previously described.

Ionizing Irradiation

All the irradiations were performed in GSI. The X-ray irradiation was carried out using an Isovolt DS1 X-ray machine (Seifert, Ahrensberg, Germany), exposing cells to 250 kVp and 16 mA.

Ion irradiation was performed in a synchrotron machine of the GSI. For irradiation at Carbon-SIS facility, cells were cultured in T12.5 culture flasks and were completely filled with culture medium before irradiation. The cells were irradiated with 10 mm spread out Bragg peak (SOBP) with LET of 100 keV/μm. All the cell lines were irradiated by Carbon-SIS. For experiments using a Carbon-UNILAC, 79HF6 cells were cultured in 3 cm Petri dishes and placed into compatible Petri dish magazines for irradiation. The carbon ions had a primary energy of 11.4 MeV/u and the energy decreased to 9.9 MeV/u when stopping on target with the corresponding LET of 168 keV/μm (10). After irradiation, the inner border of Petri dish was cleaned using sterile cotton to remove unirradiated medium accumulated at the bottom of the inner border, because dishes were irradiated in a vertical position. As survival of cells is related to the LET of the beam, we use those two carbon beams with different LETs. LAN-1 cells were also irradiated by Nickel ions with energy of 1 GeV/u and LET of 174 keV/μm, because the beam time is limited in GSI and we got the chance of irradiated by Nickel ions with similar LET to Carbon-UNILAC, which is a higher LET beam compared with Carbon-SIS.

Samples in triplicate were subjected to irradiation sections for each dose with X-ray, heavy ions, and repeated at least three times. The irradiation doses for LAN-1^{WT} were fixed from 0 to 7 Gy for X-ray, from 0 to 2 Gy for Carbon, and from 0 to 2 Gy for Nickel. However, the doses for LAN-1^{RETO} were from 0 to 9 Gy for X-ray, 0 to 3.2 Gy for Carbon, and 0 to 2 Gy for Nickel. The doses for 79HF6^{WT} and 79HF6^{RETO} were applied from 0 to 10 Gy for X-ray, 0 to 5 Gy for Carbon-SIS, and 0 to 2.72 Gy for Carbon-Unilac.

Cell survival curves of X-ray were fitted with the linear-quadratic model (Eq. 1):

$$S = e^{\left(-\alpha D - \beta D^2\right)} \qquad (1)$$

Cell survival curves of heavy ions were fitted with a pure exponential equation (Eq. 2):

$$S = e^{(-\alpha D)} \qquad (2)$$

RBE$_{10}$ values were calculated at 10% of survival level according to Eq. 3:

$$RBE_{10} = D_{10} \ X\text{-}ray \ / \ D_{10} \ ions \qquad (3)$$

All of the fitting was performed with the GSI in house program gd (©M. Krämer, 2003).

Statistical Analysis

Experiments were performed at least in triplicate, and the survival fraction of cells was given as mean ± SD. Karyotype and mBAND figures were descriptive and therefore not statistically analyzed.

RESULTS

Differential Growth Patterns of LAN-1 Neuroblastoma and Glioblastoma 79HF6 Cell Lines

All four cell lines, both wild type and resistant, grew adherently. The growth kinetic for all cells shows differential pattern as jugged by their doubling times. In this regard, the replication of LAN-1^{WT}, LAN-1^{RETO}, 79HF6^{WT}, and 79HF6^{RETO} was observed at 21.7 ± 0.7, 16.9 ± 0.8, 21.6 ± 0.3, and 56.7 ± 5.2 h, respectively. LAN-1^{WT} could form spheres when cultured in serum-free neurobasal A medium, whereas the other tumor cells lines were not able to form neurospheres once cultured under this condition (**Figure 1**). LAN-1^{RETO} and 79HF6^{RETO} chemotherapy refractory cells are able to stably grow in the medium containing low concentrations of etoposide. The growth kinetic of LAN-1^{RETO} cells showed a faster cell replication than the wild-type parentals. Contrary to that, 79HF6^{RETO} cells grew slower than 79HF6^{WT}. These dissimilar growth patterns are in part a consequence of the development of chemoresistance of both tumor entities, which are biochemically dissimilar.

Effectiveness of Heavy Ion Irradiation in Comparison to X-Ray

As previously published by our group and others, resistance to etoposide induces radioresistance in both LAN-1 neuroblastoma

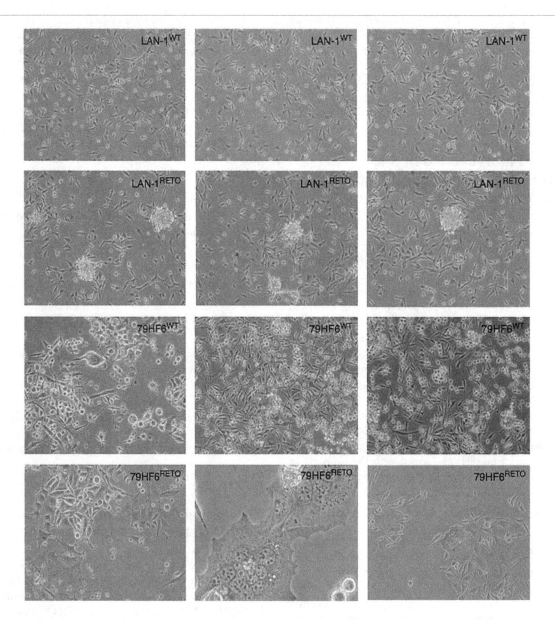

FIGURE 1 | Neurosphere-forming cells. LAN-1^WT/RETO neuroblastoma cells and 79HF6^WT/RETO glioblastoma cells have shown different morphology in serum-free neurobasal A medium. Resistant LAN-1 subline showed the capacity to form neurospheres, whereas their wild-type parental cells are not able to form spheres. 79HF6^WT/RETO cells did not alter their growth pattern once incubated in this defined condition. Magnification: LAN-1, 10×; 79HF6^WT, 10×; 79HF6^RETO, 10×; central picture, 20×. Pictures are representative for different experiments.

and glioblastoma 79HF6 cell lines (5). To explore how heavy ion irradiation has advantages over the conventional X-ray exposures, we monitored the cell survival of these cells exposure to Carbon and Nickel ion irradiation.

The survival curves showed that heavy ion irradiation was more effective than X-ray in all four cell lines (**Figures 2** and **3**). The RBE values of heavy ions beam relative to X-rays at the D_{10} values were from 2.3 to 2.6 for LAN-1 cells and 2.5 to 3.4 for 79HF6 cells (**Table 1**). For LAN-1 cells, the etoposide-resistant subtypes (cultured in the presence of etoposide) were found to be more radioresistant than WT cells (cultured without etoposide)

after X-ray and heavy ion irradiation (**Figure 2**), but for 79HF6 cells, RETO cells are more sensitive than WT cells after X-ray and heavy ion irradiation (**Figure 3**).

Chromosomal Aberrations Found in LAN-1 Neuroblastoma and Glioblastoma 79HF6 Cell Lines

In order to search for the cause of radioresistance, we analyzed the karyotype of all cells used in our study. Most of LAN^− cells had 40–44 chromosomes, and mFISH showed some stable aberrations, especially on chromosome 10 with an unstained region (**Figure 4**), and mBAND showed the unstained region located on 10p (**Figure 5**).

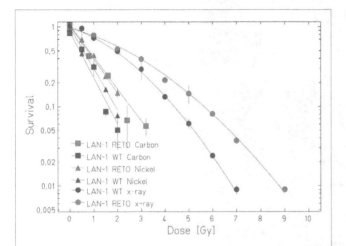

FIGURE 2 | Survival of LAN-1 neuroblastoma cells after ionizing irradiation. LAN-1[WT/RETO] cells were irradiated with X-ray, Nickel (174 keV/µm), and Carbon-SIS (100 keV/µm). Graphic depicts the results of three independent experiments. Points, the mean survival fractions; bars, SD.

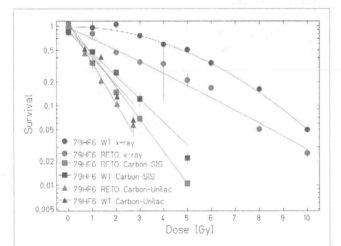

FIGURE 3 | Survival of 79HF6 glioblastoma cells after ionizing irradiation. 79HF6[WT/RETO] cells were irradiated with X-ray, Carbon-SIS (100 keV/µm), and Carbon-Unilac (168 keV/µm). Graphic depicts the results of three independent experiments. Points, the mean survival fractions; bars, SD.

The chromosomal number in 79HF6 glioblastoma cells enormously differed in the resistant subline. Most of the 79HF6[WT] cells revealed a number of 71–90 chromosomes, whereas 79HF6[WT] cells reflected 52–83 chromosomes. The chromosomal number of 79HF6[RETO] revealed two peaks (**Figure 6**). It indicated that when cells were exposed to etoposide, the chromosome had the tendency to decrease to its relative normal ploidy. This phenomenon could be explained as the effort of tumor cells on maintaining gene stability. Diploid chromosomal distribution is more stable compared with polyploidy numbers, especially when tumor cells suffer the injury of chemical agents or other stressors. Tumors cells carrying a polyploidy derived a subgroup with a more stable karyotype in order to maintain the gene stability.

DISCUSSION

Cancer stem cells show continuous self-renewal, extensive parenchymal migration/infiltration, and potential for full or partial differentiation in all cell types, which constitute a tumor. To explore how LAN-1 neuroblastoma and glioblastoma 79HF6 cell lines growth, we cultured these cells under optimal conditions for propagation in serum-free neurobasal A medium. It is known that under these conditions, cells displayed profound biological differences in growth patterns and were enforced to grow as non-adherent, multicellular spheres, inducing CSC-like populations (9).

Every cell type obviously showed different morphologies, as they were cultured in serum-free medium or serum-contained medium. Sphere formation assay (11, 12) performed to select CSC phenotypes from both cell types revealed that LAN-1[RETO] cells were able to form neurospheres after culturing them in serum-free medium, instead LAN-1[WT], 79HF6[WT], and 79HF6[RETO] cells were not capable to form neurospheres under the same conditions. CSCs may have the competence of durable self-renew, the capacity to develop and maintain tumor-related cell heterogeneity, differentiation, as well as the ability of both radioresistance and chemoresistance. To confirm the existence of CSC features, cells were transplanted to hosts and expected to induce tumor and maintain the features of parental tumor cells (13, 14). Studies in the past (5) have shown that both cell lines have CSC-like features, including chemoresistance and radioresistance to X-ray.

Our studies revealed that heavy ions had higher cell killing efficiency in both neuroblastoma and glioblastoma cell lines, despite its chemoresistance and chromosomal normality status. 79HF6[WT] cells were very resistant to X-ray. The survival rates of these cells were nearly not affected with 1 or 2 Gy of exposure to X-ray and were still around 5% with 10 Gy. This could explain why

TABLE 1 | Relative biological effectiveness values of heavy ions in LAN-1 neuroblastoma and 79HF6 glioblastoma cells.

Cell line	Carbon	Carbon-SIS	Carbon-Unilac	Nickel
LAN-1[WT]	2.60 ± 0.20	–	–	2.30 ± 0.20
LAN-1[RETO]	2.28 ± 0.09	–	–	2.42 ± 0.04
79HF6[WT]	–	2.50 ± 0.10	2.90 ± 0.20	–
79HF6[RETO]	–	2.70 ± 0.50	3.40 ± 0.20	–

The relative biological effectiveness (RBE) values of heavy ions beam relative to X-rays at the D_{10} values were found between 2.3 and 2.6 for LAN-1 and 2.5 and 3.4 for 79HF6 cells, respectively.

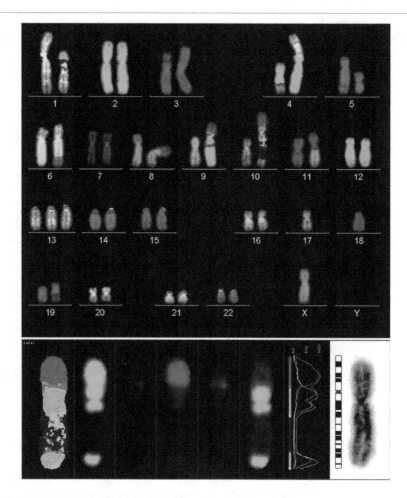

FIGURE 4 | Karyotype of LAN-1 neuroblastoma cells analyzed by mFISH. LAN-1 cells revealed a range of 40–44 chromosomes per cell. Besides the segmental exchange between chromosomes, the most prominent observation in this cell line was an unstained region in chromosome 10. Structurally, chromosome 10 appeared to be intact (lower picture) once stained with Giemsa, but lower arms were not able to hybridize with the corresponding probes. Picture is representative for several cells analyzed under the same conditions. Magnification 100×.

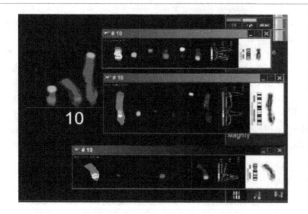

FIGURE 5 | mBAND analysis of chromosome 10 of LAN-1 neuroblastoma cells. As detected in the karyotype, LAN-1 cells showed an unstained region that was localized on 10p. This arm was not able to hybridize with the corresponding probes directed toward this region. Picture is representative for several cells analyzed under the same conditions. Magnification 100×.

glioblastoma is so hard to be treated in clinic with conventional X-ray. However, RBE_{10} was 2.5–2.9, which indicates that heavy ions had notable advantages in killing radioresistant tumors as glioblastoma.

Our studies also revealed that LAN-1[RETO] cells were found more radioresistant to X-ray than LAN-1[WT]. Contrary to that, 79HF6[RETO] glioblastoma cells were less radioresistant than its wild-type parentals. The probable reason for this difference could be the different growth rates or the chromosomal number (15, 16). 79HF6[RETO] revealed a high variation in number of chromosomes in comparison to the wild-type cells that are more homogeneous. Thus, cells with a chromosomal abnormality in number are more sensible to ion irradiation. Although LAN-1[RETO] cells were made more resistant to radiation and were able to form neurospheres after exposure to etoposide, the opposite was true for 79HF6[RETO]. This may imply the higher level point that general CSC features are enhanced by etoposide in LAN-1 and CSC features may be reduced by etoposide in 79HF6. This difference could be caused by the inherent biological difference of neuroblastoma and glioblastoma. It may also be related to the

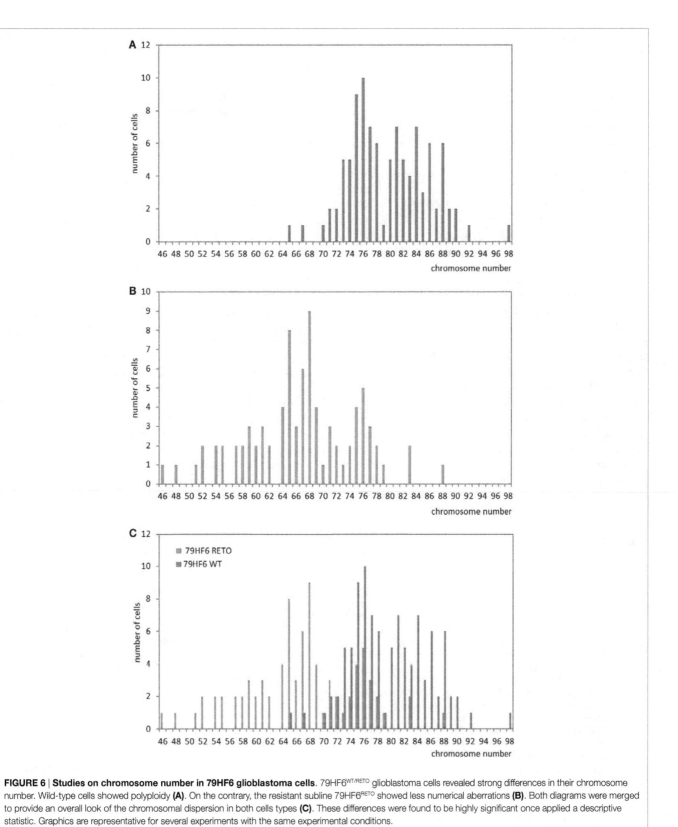

FIGURE 6 | Studies on chromosome number in 79HF6 glioblastoma cells. 79HF6^WT/RETO glioblastoma cells revealed strong differences in their chromosome number. Wild-type cells showed polyploidy (**A**). On the contrary, the resistant subline 79HF6^RETO showed less numerical aberrations (**B**). Both diagrams were merged to provide an overall look of the chromosomal dispersion in both cells types (**C**). These differences were found to be highly significant once applied a descriptive statistic. Graphics are representative for several experiments with the same experimental conditions.

concentration of etoposide. When the concentration is different, the results could change. Clearly, more work is needed to find the reason.

The biological hallmark of neuroblastomas is the complexity of the genetic abnormalities developed by the tumor cells, which are powerful prognostic markers. The most consistent abnormalities found in this tumor entity include ploidy changes, deletions of chromosome arms, amplification of the MYCN oncogene, and most frequently gains of chromosome arm 17q (6). There was a region in LAN-1 cells, which could not be stained by any fluorescence after mFISH procedure on chromosome no. 10. The analysis of mBAND corroborated that the unstained region was located on chromosome arm 10p. Homogeneously staining regions (HSRs) were localized on chromosome arm 10p and 10q of neuroblastoma cells with G-banding technique (17). HSR was cytogenetic evidence of a probable gene amplification. The unstained region of mFISH and mBAND of LAN-1[WT] cells was probably caused by repeated gene amplification or very short gene sequences. When gene segments are shorter than the probes of mFISH and mBAND, the fluorescently labeled probes could not properly anneal with the complementary sequences. Because of this, chromosome arm 10p showed an unlabeled region.

Recurrent loss of genetic material is normally found on chromosome arms 3p, 10p, 10q, 16q, and 20q in the hereditary neuroblastomas, in addition to regions usually deleted in sporadic neuroblastomas (1p36 and 11q) (18). These chromosomal sites may harbor tumor suppressor genes. Furthermore, loss of heterozygosis (LOH) at chromosome 10 is found exclusively at 10p11.23–p15.1 and consequently associated with MYCN-amplified Stage IV tumors in neuroblastoma tumors (19). LOH could induce different changes in one pair of alleles on certain gene and loss of part or even whole gene sequence of the allele. Usually, LOH is commonly related to the deficiency of tumor suppressor genes, i.e., p53. In the case where two alleles exist, the tumor suppressor gene will suppress the generation of tumors. In normal cells, when one allele is abnormal or lost, this defective

suppression drive cells to immortalization. Thus, chromosome 10p probably encloses certain tumor suppressor genes. In our study, chromosome 17 reflects a deletion. Considering that p53 gene is located on this chromosome, the lack of p53 gene due to LOH induces a defeat of tumor suppressor functions in these cells. Previous studies showed that tumor suppressor genes, i.e., p53 and so on, could regulate cell survival and death (20, 21). Chromosomal aberrations in these cells subsequently affecting tumor suppressor gene expressing could influence the survival of cells.

In summary, heavy ion irradiation is more effective than X-ray for both untreated and chemoresistant tumor cell lines. For LAN-1 cells, the chemoresistant subpopulation LAN-1[RETO] is definitely more radioresistant than untreated cells (WT), while this effect was not found in 79HF6 cells.

AUTHOR CONTRIBUTIONS

ZY: substantial contributions to the conception of the work, performing the experiments, analysis, and interpretation of data for the work and drafting the work. CH: substantial contributions to the conception of the work, performing the experiments, analysis. DP: substantial contributions to performing the experiments, analysis. WK-W: substantial contributions to the conception of the work, revising it critically for important intellectual content. G-LJ: substantial contributions to the conception of the work, revising it critically for important intellectual content. DD-C: substantial contributions to the conception of the work, revising it critically for important intellectual content. MD: substantial contributions to the conception of the work, revising it critically for important intellectual content.

REFERENCES

1. Vermeulen L, de Sousa e Melo F, Richel DJ, Medema JP. The developing cancer stem-cell model: clinical challenges and opportunities. *Lancet Oncol* (2012) **13**(2):e83–9. doi:10.1016/S1470-2045(11)70257-1

2. Singh A, Settleman J. EMT, cancer stem cells and drug resistance: an emerging axis of evil in the war on cancer. *Oncogene* (2010) **29**(34):4741–51. doi:10.1038/onc.2010.215

3. Creighton CJ, Li X, Landis M, Dixon JM, Neumeister VM, Sjolund A, et al. Residual breast cancers after conventional therapy display mesenchymal as well as tumor-initiating features. *Proc Natl Acad Sci U S A* (2009) **106**(33):13820–5. doi:10.1073/pnas.0905718106

4. Buck E, Eyzaguirre A, Barr S, Thompson S, Sennello R, Young D, et al. Loss of homotypic cell adhesion by epithelial-mesenchymal transition or mutation limits sensitivity to epidermal growth factor receptor inhibition. *Mol Cancer Ther* (2007) **6**(2):532–41. doi:10.1158/1535-7163.MCT-06-0462

5. Díaz-Carballo D, Gustmann S, Jastrow H, Acikelli AH, Dammann P, Klein J, et al. Atypical cell populations associated with acquired resistance to cytostatics and cancer stem cell features: the role of mitochondria in nuclear encapsulation. *DNA Cell Biol* (2014) **33**(11):749–74. doi:10.1089/dna.2014.2375

6. Maris JM, Hogarty MD, Bagatell R, Cohn SL. Neuroblastoma. *Lancet* (2007) **369**(9579):2106–20. doi:10.1016/S0140-6736(07)60983-0

7. Evers P, Lee PP, DeMarco J, Agazaryan N, Sayre JW, Selch M, et al. Irradiation of the potential cancer stem cell niches in the adult brain improves progression-free survival of patients with malignant glioma. *BMC Cancer* (2010) **10**:384. doi:10.1186/1471-2407-10-384

8. Pignalosa D, Durante M. Overcoming resistance of cancer stem cells. *Lancet Oncol* (2012) **13**(5):e187–8. doi:10.1016/S1470-2045(12)70196-1

9. Barrantes-Freer A, Kim E, Bielanska J, Giese A, Mortensen LS, Schulz-Schaeffer WJ, et al. Human glioma-initiating cells show a distinct immature phenotype resembling but not identical to NG2 glia. *J Neuropathol Exp Neurol* (2013) **72**(4):307–24. doi:10.1097/NEN.0b013e31828afdbd

10. Kraft G, Daues H, Fischer B, Kopf U, Liebold HP, Quis D, et al. Irradiation chamber and sample changes for biological samples. *Nucl Instrum Methods* (1980) **168**:175–9. doi:10.1016/0029-554X(80)91249-5

11. Reynolds BA, Tetzlaff W, Weiss S. A multipotent EGF-responsive striatal embryonic progenitor cell produces neurons and astrocytes. *J Neurosci* (1992) **12**(11):4565–74.

12. Reynolds BA, Weiss S. Generation of neurons and astrocytes from isolated cells of the adult mammalian central nervous system. *Science* (1992) **255**(5052):1707–10. doi:10.1126/science.1553558

13. Cho RW, Clarke MF. Recent advances in cancer stem cells. *Curr Opin Genet Dev* (2008) **18**:48–53. doi:10.1016/j.gde.2008.01.017

14. Lobo NA, Shimono Y, Qian D, Clarke MF. The biology of cancer stem cells. *Annu Rev Cell Dev Biol* (2007) **23**:675–99. doi:10.1146/annurev.cellbio.22.010305.104154

15. Yang X, Darling JL, McMillan TJ, Peacock JH, Steel GG. Heterogeneity of radiosensitivity in a human glioma cell line. *Int J Radiat Oncol Biol Phys* (1992) **22**(1):103–8. doi:10.1016/0360-3016(92)90988-T

16. Till JE. Radiosensitivity and chromosome numbers in strain L mouse cells in tissue culture. *Radiat Res* (1961) **15**:400–9. doi:10.2307/3571245

17. Sawyer JR, Miller JP, Roloson GJ. A novel reciprocal translocation (14;15) (q11;q24) in a congenital mesoblastic nephroma. *Cancer Genet Cytogenet* (1996) **88**(1):39–42. doi:10.1016/0165-4608(95)00302-9

18. Altura RA, Maris JM, Li H, Boyett JM, Brodeur GM, Look AT. Novel regions of chromosomal loss in familial neuroblastoma by comparative genomic hybridization. *Genes Chromosomes Cancer* (1997) **19**(3):176–84. doi:10.1002/(SICI)1098-2264(199707)19:3<176::AID-GCC7>3.0. CO;2-V

19. Mora J, Cheung NK, Oplanich S, Chen L, Gerald WL. Novel regions of allelic imbalance identified by genome-wide analysis of neuroblastoma. *Cancer Res* (2002) **62**(6):1761–7.

20. Wee KB, Aguda BD. Akt versus p53 in a network of oncogenes and tumor suppressor genes regulating cell survival and death. *Biophys J* (2006) **91**(3):857–65. doi:10.1529/biophysj.105.077693

21. Tarunina M, Alger L, Chu G, Munger K, Gudkov A, Jat PS. Functional genetic screen for genes involved in senescence: role of Tid1, a homologue of the *Drosophila* tumor suppressor l(2)tid, in senescence and cell survival. *Mol Cell Biol* (2004) **24**(24):10792–801. doi:10.1128/ MCB.24.24.10792-10801.2004

18

Three-Color Chromosome Painting as Seen through the Eyes of mFISH: Another Look at Radiation-Induced Exchanges and their Conversion to Whole-Genome Equivalency

Bradford D. Loucas[1], Igor Shuryak[2] and Michael N. Cornforth[1]*

[1] Department of Radiation Oncology, University of Texas Medical Branch, Galveston, TX, USA, [2] Center for Radiological Research, Columbia University, New York, NY, USA

*Correspondence:
Michael N. Cornforth
mcornfor@utmb.edu

Whole-chromosome painting (WCP) typically involves the fluorescent staining of a small number of chromosomes. Consequently, it is capable of detecting only a fraction of exchanges that occur among the full complement of chromosomes in a genome. Mathematical corrections are commonly applied to WCP data in order to extrapolate the frequency of exchanges occurring in the entire genome [whole-genome equivalency (WGE)]. However, the reliability of WCP to WGE extrapolations depends on underlying assumptions whose conditions are seldom met in actual experimental situations, in particular the presumed absence of complex exchanges. Using multi-fluor fluorescence in situ hybridization (mFISH), we analyzed the induction of simple exchanges produced by graded doses of ^{137}Cs gamma rays (0–4 Gy), and also 1.1 GeV ^{56}Fe ions (0–1.5 Gy). In order to represent cytogenetic damage *as it would have appeared to the observer* following standard three-color WCP, all mFISH information pertaining to exchanges that did not specifically involve chromosomes 1, 2, or 4 was ignored. This allowed us to reconstruct dose–responses for three-color *apparently simple* (AS) exchanges. Using extrapolation methods similar to those derived elsewhere, these were expressed in terms of WGE for comparison to mFISH data. Based on AS events, the extrapolated frequencies systematically overestimated those actually observed by mFISH. For gamma rays, these errors were practically independent of dose. When constrained to a relatively narrow range of doses, the WGE corrections applied to both ^{56}Fe and gamma rays predicted genome-equivalent damage with a level of accuracy likely sufficient for most applications. However, the apparent accuracy associated with WCP to WGE corrections is both fortuitous and misleading. This is because (in normal practice) such corrections can only be applied to AS exchanges, which are known to include complex aberrations in the form of pseudosimple exchanges. When WCP to WGE corrections are applied to *true simple exchanges*, the results are less than satisfactory, leading to extrapolated values that *underestimate* the true WGE response by unacceptably large margins. Likely explanations for these results are discussed, as well as their implications for radiation protection. Thus, in seeming contradiction to notion that complex aberrations be avoided altogether in WGE corrections – and in violation of assumptions upon which these corrections are based – their inadvertent inclusion in three-color WCP data is *actually required* in order for them to yield even marginally acceptable results.

Keywords: chromosome painting, mFISH, radiation biomarkers

INTRODUCTION

Whole-chromosome painting (WCP) involves the labeling of a few select chromosomes of the genome, thereby producing discrete changes in fluorescent color patterns that accompany the junctions of exchange breakpoints. These include junctions between the painted and unpainted chromosomes, and between the painted chromosomes themselves.

Whole-chromosome painting data can be extrapolated in order to approximate the total number of exchanges that *would have been detected* if all homologous chromosome pairs *would have been painted* a unique color, as in the combinatorial painting technologies of multi-fluor fluorescence *in situ* hybridization (mFISH) (1) or spectral karyotyping (SKY) (2). Converting WCP data to that of whole-genome equivalency (WGE) provided by mFISH or SKY makes use of relationships similar to that developed by Lucas and colleagues (3). These consider exchanges between painted and unpainted (counterstained) chromosomes, adjusting for unseen exchanges presumed to have occurred between unpainted chromosomes. After three-color WCP was introduced, subsequent refinements were made to accommodate exchanges occurring among the individually painted chromosomes as well (4, 5).

There are two central assumptions common to these mathematical extrapolations. First, that exchange breakpoints are produced *randomly* throughout the genome, in direct proportion to the size of chromosomes participating in an exchange. Second, these corrections (extrapolations) are derived solely in consideration of simple reciprocal interchange events (dicentrics and translocations). Complex exchanges, which involve rejoining among multiple chromosomes, are ignored. For that reason, corrections are usually restricted to data associated with low to moderate doses of X- or gamma rays, where the incidence of complex exchanges is assumed to be minimal. Earlier work provided support for the soundness of the basic approach and whole-genome corrections soon became routinely applied to WCP (3, 6–8) data. However, papers began to appear shortly thereafter questioning the first of the aforementioned assumptions (9–11).

More recently, and with basic intent similar to ours, Braselmann and colleagues compared genome-corrected three-color WCP data with experimental data derived independently using mFISH and SKY (4). When applied to three-color WCP data, they found that modification to the original Lucas formula (3) produced results comparable to that of mFISH or SKY. Attached to this conclusion, however, was a cautionary note about the influence of pseudosimple exchanges – aberrations that appear to be simple pairwise interchanges by WCP, but that are actually complex, involving three or more exchange breakpoints distributed among multiple chromosomes (12–14).

In this paper, we reconsider the issue in detail by comparing 24-color mFISH data to 3-color data retrospectively extracted from mFISH images. This method was used to assess the accuracy with which a commonly used mathematical formalism can be applied 3-color WCP data in order to extrapolate full 24-color genome equivalency for simple chromosome interchanges. It involves experimental conditions under which WCP extrapolations are ostensibly valid, such as low to moderate doses of gamma rays. Unlike previous reports, however, it also includes situations where the validity of such extrapolation is dubious: higher doses of gamma rays and exposure to heavy ions, both of which are well known to favor the production of complex exchanges (5, 15–22).

MATERIALS AND METHODS

Irradiations and Culture Conditions

Methods pertaining to the exposure of lymphocytes to gamma rays have been detailed elsewhere (22, 23). Whole venous blood from two healthy consenting male volunteers was exposed to graded doses of ^{137}Cs γ-rays at a rate of 1.3 Gy/min using a J.L. Shepherd Mark I cesium irradiator located at the University of Texas Medical Branch (UTMB), following procedures approved by UTMB's Institutional Review Board (IRB). 0.4 ml aliquots of blood were cultured in RPMI-1640 (Gibco) medium containing 0.1 ml phytothemagglutinin (PHA; Murix, Dartford, UK) and supplemented with 15% fetal bovine serum. Colcemid (GIBCO), to a final concentration of 0.1 µg/ml, was added 45 h later, and cultures were harvested for metaphase analysis at 48 h.

Heavy ion irradiations took place at Brookhaven National Laboratory (BNL; Upton, NY, USA) within the NASA Space Radiation Laboratory (NSRL). Procedures followed those of BNL's IRB. Whole blood was suspended in RPMI-1640 medium, supplemented with 20% fetal bovine serum. From this suspension, approximately 2×10^6 cells were loaded into custom-made Lucite holders and irradiated at room temperature with graded doses of 1.1 GeV/amu ^{56}Fe ions. The dose average LET of this beam was 147 keV/µm. Immediately after exposure, lymphocytes were aspirated from the holder and transferred into 25 cm^2 tissue culture flasks containing 10 ml of RPMI-1640 medium supplemented with 1% phytohemagglutinin (PHA; Gibco). Cultures were incubated at 37°C for 46 h before Colcemid (Gibco) was added (0.2 µg/ml final concentration) 2 h prior to the harvest of mitotic cells. Calyculin-A (50 nM final concentration) was added to Colcemid-blocked cultures to induce premature chromosome condensation (PCC) in G$_2$-phase cells (24). As a result, mitotic figures contained a mixture of metaphase chromosomes and G$_2$-phase PCC. Cells were fixed in a 3:1 mixture of methanol to acetic acid and transported to the University of Texas Medical Branch at Galveston for further processing and subsequent analysis.

mFISH Hybridization and Image Capture

Following fixation in methanol/acetic acid, lymphocytes were spread onto glass microscope slides by standard cytogenetic procedures. Slides were then treated with acetone, RNase A, and proteinase K before another fixation in 3.7% formaldehyde. Slides were dehydrated through an ethanol series (70, 85, and 100%) and air dried. In order to denature chromosomal DNA, they were next incubated in 70% formamide (72°C) in 2× SSC (0.3 M NaCl, 0.03 M sodium citrate) for 2 min. After dehydration through another ethanol series, 10 µl of denatured (10 min at 72°C) SpectraVision 24-color mFISH Assay probe (Vysis) was applied to each slide. Slides were covered with a 22 mm × 22 mm glass cover slip, sealed into position with rubber cement. Samples were allowed to hybridize for 48 h in a 37°C incubator. Following hybridization, cover slips were removed and the slides were washed for 2 min in 0.4× SSC containing IGEPAL (0.3%) non-ionic detergent at 72°C. This was followed by a 30-s wash in 2× SSC (0.1% IGEPAL) at room temperature.

Prior to image capture, 15 µl of DAPI (0.14 µg/ml) dissolved in anti-fade mounting medium (Vectashield; Vector Laboratories) was applied to each slide and covered with a 24 mm × 40 mm cover slip. Images of chromosome spreads were captured using a Zeiss Axiophot epifluorescence microscope interfaced with a SensSys black-and-white CCD camera. Karyotypes were constructed from good-quality chromosome spreads using Power-Gene image analysis software (23).

24-Color Analysis

We conducted a retrospective examination of a large 24-color mFISH data base that contained detailed information on aberrations produced in human cells by graded doses radiations of different ionization densities (22, 23). Metaphase cells were analyzed by procedures previously established (23). Briefly, mPAINT descriptors were assigned to chromosomes involved in each rearrangement. Next, each rearrangement was brought to "pattern closure" by grouping elements in the most conservative way possible, minimizing the number of breakpoints required to reconstruct the exchange (25). Reciprocal pairwise rejoinings between one chromosome (rings and interstitial deletions) or two chromosomes (translocations and dicentrics) were scored as simple exchanges. Exchanges involving three or more breakpoints were regarded as complex. This classification was also applied to incomplete exchanges where one or more elements failed to rejoin, as well as the so-called "one-way" exchanges where one or more translocated segments appeared to be missing, presumably because they were too small to be resolved by chromosome painting. The large majority of one-way staining patterns are known to be complete exchanges (26). And since we lacked the ability to simultaneously visualize telomere signals in mFISH preparations, such rearrangements were treated as being complete for the purpose of achieving pattern closure.

Retrospective Three-Color Analysis

We focused on chromosomes 1, 2, and 4, since this represents one of the more commonly used three-color painting schemes. On a cell-by-cell basis, we stripped from the full 24-color mFISH profile all information concerning exchanges except that pertaining to the three painted chromosomes. In other words, from a full 24-color karyotype, we imagined what the microscopist would have observed if, instead of mFISH, three-color WCP had been applied to the samples. From this information, we used a mathematical correction of the form described by Braselmann et al. (4) to scale WCP data back to full genome equivalency originally provided by mFISH. The correction we used applies only to simple reciprocal interchanges involving exactly two chromosomes (translocations and dicentrics). Neither mFISH nor WCP analysis specifically considered intrachanges: rings, interstitial deletions, inversions; nor were terminal deletions considered. To be clear then, the

term "exchange" (as used hereafter) refers only to interchanges. One-way exchanges were handled in a manner similar to that for mFISH.

Extraction of Three-Color Data from mFISH Images

Figure 1 depicts the process used in rendering 24-color mFISH images in order to produce 3-color WCP data. It is also meant to illustrate some of the problems inherent to WCP for aberration analysis. The figure shows various staining protocols applied to a metaphase cell that had previously been exposed in G_0 phase to 4 Gy of ^{137}Cs gamma rays. The cell is replete with various chromosome rearrangements whose complexity becomes increasingly apparent as different chromosomes are painted. Panels A, B, and C derive from an mFISH image that was rendered to exclude painting information from all chromosomes except chromosomes 1, 2, and 1 + 2 + 4, respectively.

Figure 1A is of a cell probed for chromosome 1 that contains an apparently simple (AS) translocation between chromosome 1 and an anonymous blue (DAPI-counterstained) chromosome. The cell also contains an AS dicentric involving the other homolog of chromosome 1. [In this case, the accompanying compound acentric fragment shows a "one-way" staining pattern, and is therefore assumed joined with a submicroscopic counterstained segment (26–29)]. **Figure 1B** shows the same cell, as it would appear if probed for chromosome 2 instead. Here, an AS translocation has occurred. **Figure 1C** simulates the three-color painting patterns of the same cell that derive from mFISH data, rendered so as to include data for chromosomes 1, 2, and 4 simultaneously. The full extent of complexity is revealed by mFISH in **Figure 1D**. Actually, the cell in question is shown to harbor three rearrangements. It contains a simple dicentric between chromosome 1 and the X (red arrows). This exchange would be correctly identified given the staining patterns shown in **Figures 1A,C**. Judging by staining patterns of **Figure 1A**, it also contains a simple translocation involving the homologous chromosome 1. In reality, the exchange is pseudosimple. mFISH reveals the chromosome to be part of a large complex exchange involving five other chromosomes marked by white arrows. Likewise, the AS translocation involving chromosome 2 is also pseudosimple, since mFISH shows it to be part of the same large complex exchange (white arrows).

The three-color rendering shown in **Figures 1C** represents the type of WCP data to which the CF corrections of equation (8) (shown below) were applied in order to calculate WGE. In this particular cell, three-color painting was able to detect the occurrence of the complex exchange. However, from the three-color staining pattern alone, one may conclude only that the complex involved a minimum of three chromosomes: 1, 2, and an anonymous third DAPI-stained chromosome, when six chromosomes were actually involved (**Figure 1D**). In fact, there are many instances where three-color painting fails to detect the occurrence of complex exchanges altogether. The misidentification of complex exchanges as being simple is of concern to mathematical extrapolations applied to three-color data, because it violates a central assumption that only simple exchanges be considered, a point made repeatedly in this paper.

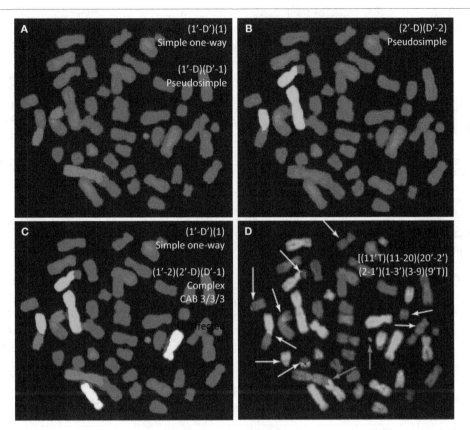

FIGURE 1 | Whole-chromosome paints applied to a human metaphase spread from a cell previously exposed to gamma rays. The same spread is shown following WCP applied to chromosomes 1 and 2 [**(A,B)**, respectively]. **(C)** The same spread following simultaneous painting with the same two probes. In **(D)**, mFISH reveals the full extent of exchange complexity. mPAINT nomenclature is used to describe the various visible rearrangements (25).

Extrapolation to Whole-Genome Equivalency

Over the years, various modifications to the original Lucas formula (3) have been used to estimate the fraction of total interchanges visible by WCP. The extrapolation we used follows closely that of Braselmann and colleagues (4). It considers exchanges between painted and unpainted (counterstained) chromosomes, as well as exchanges taking place among the uniquely painted chromosomes. It also makes provisions for the fact that dicentrics involving homologous chromosomes are detectable by mFISH, whereas translocations are not. Values for the genomic content of chromosomes used in the following derivation are from Mendelsohn et al. (30) as cited by Morton (31). Its derivation, as applied to our particular experimental system, is as follows.

Let f_p represent the fractional sum of the genome covered by the individual chromosomes 1, 2, and 4, where $f_1 = 0.0821$; $f_2 = 0.0804$; $f_4 = 0.0635$

$$f_p = (f_1 + f_2 + f_4) = 0.226. \tag{1}$$

The unpainted (DAPI-counterstained) fraction then becomes

$$(1 - f_p) = 0.774 \tag{2}$$

For WCP, the frequency of visible interchanges in the genome that can occur between painted and unpainted chromosomes

(F_P) is given by the cross product of the binomial expansion $(p + q)^2 = p^2 + 2pq + q^2$ – namely $2pq$ – where $p = (f_p)$ and $q = 1 - (f_p)$. Substituting values in Eq. (2) gives the following expression.

$$F_P = 2pq = 2f_p (1 - f_p) = 0.350 \tag{3}$$

If, as is the case here, the individual painted chromosomes can be distinguished from one another, then Eq. (3) can be expanded to include exchanges that now become visible among the three possible pairs of uniquely colored chromosomes (4, 32).

$$F_P = 2 [f_p (1 - f_p) + f_1 f_2 + f_1 f_4 + f_2 f_4] = 0.384 \tag{4}$$

Thus, three-color WCP is theoretically capable of detecting 38.4% of the interchanges occurring throughout the whole genome. However, in the context of this paper, three-color WCP frequencies are to be compared to those detected by mFISH and it should be recognized that the latter is not capable of detecting all interchanges. The frequency of all mFISH-detectable interchanges (F_{mFISH}), including translocations and dicentrics, is proportional to the sum of all products (f_i) x (f_j) representing the fractional DNA content of chromosomes i and j. But because mFISH cannot reliably detect events that occur between homologous chromosomes, an additional stipulation is that $i \neq j$. For a human karyotype containing 23 individually identifiable types of chromosomes, this can be represented by the following expression (4).

$$F_{mFISH} = 1 - \sum_{i=1}^{23} f_i^2 = 0.948 \qquad (5)$$

The numerical value resulting from Eq. (5) is essentially a constant for a given diploid species. We note that our calculated value of 0.948 (for human males) is virtually identical to the number 0.949 reported by Braselmann et al. for females (4).

A final point to consider is that mFISH typically allows for the detection of asymmetrical exchanges (dicentrics) involving homologous chromosomes, but not their symmetrical counterpart (translocations). In that sense, Eq. (5) "overcorrects" for undetectable exchanges between homologs. If we make the usual assumption that symmetrical and asymmetrical exchanges, as measured by mFISH, occur with approximately equal frequency (23), then half the deviation from unity shown in Eq. (5) no longer applies. Thus, the true frequency of interchanges visible by mFISH – to include dicentrics between homologs (but not translocations) – is given by Eq. (6).

$$F_{mFISH} = 0.948 + \left(\frac{1 - 0.948}{2} \right) = 0.974 \qquad (6)$$

In order to calculate the detection efficiency of WCP, we compare this value to the theoretical frequency of interchanges detectable by three-color FISH, F_P of Eq. (4). As compared to the frequency of interchanges visible by 24-color mFISH, the WGE for such detection by three-color WCP becomes:

$$F_{mFISH}^{3\ color} = \left(\frac{2}{0.974} \right) [f_p (1 - f_p) + f_1 f_2 + f_1 f_4 + f_2 f_4]$$
$$= 2.053 [f_p (1 - f_p) + f_1 f_2 + f_1 f_4 + f_2 f_4] = 0.394 \qquad (7)$$

Thus, by covering 23% of the genome [Eq. (1)], three-color FISH is capable of detecting 39% of the interchanges seen by mFISH. In theory, three-color WCP frequencies can be multiplied by the following correction factor CF in order to achieve full 24-color mFISH equivalency.

$$F_{WCP} \times CF = F_{mFISH}$$
$$CF = \frac{1}{0.394} = 2.54 \qquad (8)$$

This value differs from the CF of 2.9 reported by Braselmann and colleagues, mainly because the three chromosomes we have chosen to analyze (1, 2, and 4) constitute a larger proportion of the genome than the chromosome 1–4–12 triplet used by these authors. Hereafter, the derivation of Eq. (8) will be referred to as the CF *derived from first principles.*

Dose Dependency

As discussed later, correction factors derived from Eq. (8) are of limited value if they display dose dependency. In other words, the transformation of three-color data to WGE is based on the tacit assumption that the two dose–responses can be scaled to match each other (made superimposable) *over a range of doses* through use of a single multiplier, i.e., the constant CF of Eq. (8). It should be intuitively obvious that this is not possible unless certain conditions are met, foremost is that the two dose–responses share the same functional form – a comparison of two linear dose responses would be a trivial example here. However, this alone is insufficient for the general case, as demonstrated for the familiar linear-quadratic formalism of Eq. (9) below. It will be used to describe each of the underlying dose–responses considered in this paper. Let $F_{(D)}$ represent the dose-dependent frequency for simple exchanges, as given by the second-order polynomial where α, $\beta \geq 0$.

$$F_{1(D)} = \alpha_1 D + \beta_1 D^2 \qquad (9)$$

Assume that Eq. (9) represents exchanges as measured by mFISH, and that a similar expression $F_{2(D)}$ describes the dose–response as measured by three-color WCP.

$$F_{2(D)} = \alpha_2 D + \beta_2 D^2 \qquad (10)$$

The ratio of Eqs. (9) and (10) defines CF as a function of D, which hereafter is referred to as the *empirically derived* CF.

$$CF = \frac{F_{1(D)}}{F_{2(D)}} = \frac{\alpha_1 D + \beta_1 D^2}{\alpha_2 D + \beta_2 D^2} \qquad (11)$$

If we let the proportionality constant (k) hold the place of CF, then

$$\alpha_1 D + \beta_1 D^2 = k \left(\alpha_2 D + \beta_2 D^2 \right). \qquad (12)$$

Equivalently,

$$D \left(\alpha_1 - k\alpha_2 \right) + D^2 \left(\beta_1 - k\beta_2 \right) = 0. \qquad (13)$$

For our purposes, corrections must be applicable over a *range of doses* (interval of D). It follows that if either of the polynomial coefficients in Eq. (13) is non-zero, then the equation is either linear or quadratic, and can therefore have at most two solutions. Therefore Eq. (13) cannot hold over an interval of dose with k fixed unless both its coefficients are 0. In this case, the following relationships are satisfied which, as required, are invariant of dose:

$$\alpha_1 = k\alpha_2$$
$$\beta_1 = k\beta_2 \qquad (14)$$

It then follows that

$$\frac{\alpha_1}{\beta_1} = \frac{\alpha_2}{\beta_2}. \qquad (15)$$

Thus, formally speaking, the concept of a single CF can be applied to a pair of second-order polynomials only when α/β ratios of the two are equal. In principle, the validity of Eq. (15) can be used to ascertain the appropriateness of using a single CF to convert a three-color WCP data set to full genome equivalency. In practice, we found that designing a statistical test for this purpose to be problematic, largely because AS and TR frequencies are actually subsets mFISH data and, therefore, cannot be considered independent measurements. Thus, whereas testing the identity of ratios in Eq. (15) is conceptually sound (and useful in the discussion that follows) an alternative statistical approach was required to ascertain dose dependency. We used the approach described below, which models the *proportions* of AS interchanges among all interchanges (pAS = AS/mFISH) and true simple (TR) exchanges among AS exchanges (pTR = TR/AS).

Statistical Analysis

If pAS is constant and independent of radiation dose, then a multiplicative CF can be used to predict the total number of simple exchanges (interchanges) in all chromosomes (mFISH) based on the number of AS exchanges in chromosomes 1, 2, and 4. The same applies to pTR. Alternatively, if either pAS or pTR depend on dose, their dose responses will have slopes statistically different from 0.

We used logistic regression to model the potential dose dependences of pAS and pTR. Using matrix notation, the model structure is summarized as follows, where $\mathrm{logit}(x) = 1/[1 + \exp(-x)]$:

$$\mathrm{logit}\ (o)\ =\ \varphi \times V + \varepsilon \tag{16}$$

Here, o is a vector of outcome variables: predicted pAS and pTR. V is a vector of radiation doses, φ is a vector of regression coefficients, and ε is a vector of errors.

Three types of radiation dose dependences for pAS and pTR were assessed using this approach:

(a) a dose–response with intercept (the predicted value of pAS or pTR at zero dose) and slope (the predicted rate of change of pAS or pTR per unit dose), with quasi-binomial error distribution;
(b) intercept plus slope with a binomial error distribution; and
(c) intercept only (with slope effectively set to 0 and not counted as an adjustable parameter) having a binomial error distribution. We performed these analyses separately on γ-ray and Fe ion data. Model fitting was performed using R software (version 3.2.0).

According to the binomial distribution, the variance is not an independent parameter, whereas the quasi-binomial option allows the variance to be adjustable (33). Consequently, comparison of binomial and quasi-binomial model fits to the same data (i.e., options a and b), using the X^2 (Chi-squared) test on residual deviances, provides information on whether or not there is evidence of "overdispersion" in the data – in other words, whether or not the variance of the data is larger than what would be expected from the binomial distribution.

Comparison of the slope plus intercept versus intercept-only models (i.e., options b and c) on the same data provides information on whether or not the data are consistent with being represented by a constant dose-independent term (intercept-only), or if there is evidence for dose dependence (slope). This assessment was performed using the sample-size corrected Akaike information criterion (AICc). AICc is an information theoretic criterion that quantifies relative support from the data for the compared models, taking into account the sample size (number of data points) and the number of adjustable parameters in each model.

Goodness of fit (GOF) was assessed for the models under the assumption that the residual deviance follows the X^2 distribution. The null hypothesis was that the model provides an adequate fit to the data, and small p-values were interpreted to mean that the null hypothesis has poor support.

RESULTS

There are two separate issues to consider when determining how well multiplicative correction factors predict the mFISH dose–responses from three-color data. The overarching first issue is whether such a multiplicative factor *even exits* that can bring three-color data into registry with mFISH data over a range of relevant doses. Obviously, this necessitates that CFs not exhibit dose dependency. That is, assuming a linear-quadratic model for the dose responses that Eq. (15) is not violated.

The analysis of frequencies of AS and TR, as function of dose for both types of radiation (γ-rays and Fe ions) is shown in **Figure 2**, which derives from data shown in **Table 1**. For the densely ionizing Fe ions, there was no evidence for dose dependence for the proportion of AS exchanges among all exchanges (pAS), or for the proportion of TR exchanges among AS ones (pTR). This conclusion was reinforced by the finding that AICc for the intercept-only dose–response model was lower (suggesting higher support from the data), than the AICc for the intercept plus slope model. The best-fit values for pAS and pTR at all doses were 0.420 (95% CI: 0.365, 0.477) and 0.593 (0.505, 0.677), respectively. For sparsely ionizing γ-rays, pAS was also consistent with dose-independence with a best-fit value of 0.426 (0.382, 0.471).

However, the pattern was altogether different for TR exchanges. The γ-ray-induced pTR decreased with dose with a best-fit logistic slope coefficient of -0.3416 (SE: 0.1806, $p = 0.0585$) Gy^{-1}. Although the p-value for this coefficient was marginally higher than the commonly used significance threshold of 0.05, the intercept and slope model had higher support (by 1.87 AICc units) than the intercept-only model. This favors a response model containing a slope parameter over the intercept-only model having no dose dependence: the strength of evidence for the first model over the second is $\exp(1.87/2) = 2.54$. In other words, although the strength of statistical evidence falls short of being overwhelming, the data suggest that pTR decreases with radiation dose for γ-rays (**Figure 2**).

From a dose-dependency standpoint, these results show that the response for AS exchange frequencies for gamma rays and ^{56}Fe ions are *theoretically* capable of being transformed to match that from mFISH data using a simple multiplicative CF; the same for TR exchanges induced by iron ions. Unfortunately, the same cannot be said for TR exchanges produced by gamma rays, due to the aforementioned dose dependency.

Findings concerning dose dependency, however, say nothing about the inherent accuracy of the transformation constant itself, which depends entirely on the assumptions underlying the derivation of Eq. (8). This is the second issue that determines how well a particular CF applied to three-color data predict genome-equivalent frequencies. **Figures 3** and **4** are introduced to help visualize the added influence this aspect brings to whole-genome correction. The figures are not intended to imply any sort of rigorous statistical analysis, but to illustrate the overall effect of applying CFs to both AS and TR exchanges. Here, we performed least-squares regression on the data using the linear-quadratic dose–response model [Eqs. (9) and (10)]. The parameters derived from this procedure (**Table 1**) were used to generate the dose–responses for simple exchanges shown in **Figures 3** and **4**. The response in lymphocytes exposed to gamma rays is shown in **Figure 3**. The uppermost solid curve shows a regression to

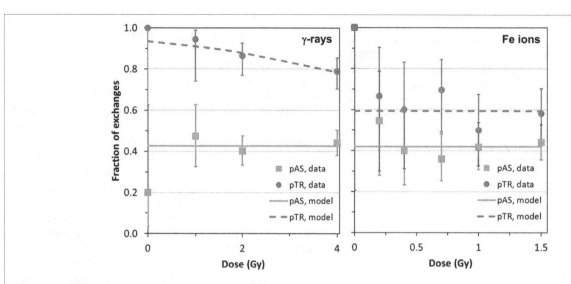

FIGURE 2 | Data (symbols) and model predictions (curves) for the proportion of apparently simple exchanges among all exchanges (pAS) and for the proportion of true simple exchanges among apparently simple exchanges (pTR). Error bars represent 95% confidence intervals (CIs) from the binomial distribution. Details are described in the main text.

TABLE 1 | Chromosome exchange data and fit parameters.

IR	Dose (Gy)	No. Cells	[a]AS (3-color)	[b]True (3-color)	[c]mFISH (24-color)	pAS = AS/mFISH	pTR = True/AS
[137]Cs γ-rays	0.0	365	1	1	5	0.200 (0.036, 0.624)[f]	1.000 (0.207, 1.000)
	1.0	238	18	17	38	0.474 (0.325, 0.627)	0.944 (0.742, 0.990)
	2.0	342	74	64	184	0.402 (0.334, 0.474)	0.865 (0.769, 0.925)
	4.0	179	109	86	247	0.441 (0.381, 0.504)	0.789 (0.703, 0.855)
	Σ	1124	202	168	474		
Parameters		[d]α	0.05 ± 0.01	0.06 ± 0.01	0.13 ± 0.05		
		[e]β	0.03 ± 0.00	0.02 ± 0.00	0.06 ± 0.02		
		α/β	2.20 ± 0.01	3.89 ± 0.01	2.27 ± 0.05		
1.1 GeV [56]Fe Ions	0.0	98	1	1	1	1.000 (0.207, 1.000)	1.000 (0.207, 1.000)
	0.2	191	6	4	11	0.545 (0.280, 0.787)	0.667 (0.300, 0.903)
	0.4	179	10	6	25	0.400 (0.234, 0.593)	0.600 (0.313, 0.832)
	0.7	197	23	16	64	0.359 (0.253, 0.482)	0.696 (0.491, 0.844)
	1.0	189	28	14	67	0.418 (0.307, 0.537)	0.500 (0.326, 0.674)
	1.5	218	55	32	125	0.440 (0.356, 0.528)	0.582 (0.450, 0.703)
	Σ	1072	123	73	293		
Parameters		α	0.14 ± 0.03	0.09 ± 0.03	0.36 ± 0.07		
		β	0.02 ± 0.03	0.00 ± 0.03	0.02 ± 0.06		
		α/β	9.53 ± 0.43	105 ± 82.4	17.6 ± 3.16		

[a]Apparently simple exchanges; chromosomes 1/2/4; [b]True simple exchanges; chromosomes 1/2/4; [c]True simple exchanges; all chromosomes, mFISH; [d,e]Linear and quadratic coefficients; $Y = \alpha D + \beta D^2$; [f]Parentheses indicate 95% confidence intervals (CIs).

the data (filled circles) for all simple reciprocal exchanges measured by mFISH. These are truly simple exchanges and represent WGE of Eq. (9) having the fitted parameters shown in the table. The open symbols of the figure represent three-color data that was extracted from this dose–response. Open circles show the response for simple exchanges as they would appear to the observer using three-color WCP; see Eq. (10). These are labeled "AS" because (as revealed by mFISH) they are partly comprised of pseudosimple exchanges.

The CF of Eq. (8) was applied to the (extracted) AS data in order to convert them to WGE (i.e., mFISH frequencies). The resultant dose–responses are shown by the two dashed-line curves of the figure. Since pseudosimple exchanges are (by definition) hidden

to three-color analysis, CFs can only be applied to AS exchanges during actual three-color painting. The resulting AS to WGE extrapolation (long-dashed curve) is symbolized by the vertical arrowed bracket of the figure labeled "apparent." As shown in the figure, the extrapolated genome-equivalent dose–response based on three-color WCP systematically *overestimates* the total frequency of simple exchanges measured by mFISH. Nevertheless, as a first approximation for gamma rays, WGE corrections produce results whose accuracy is probably adequate for many purposes, even if only marginally so at higher doses.

A noteworthy aspect of our retrospective analysis is that it also allows the extraction of TR exchanges from the three-color data, as shown by the triangles of the lowermost curve. This represents the

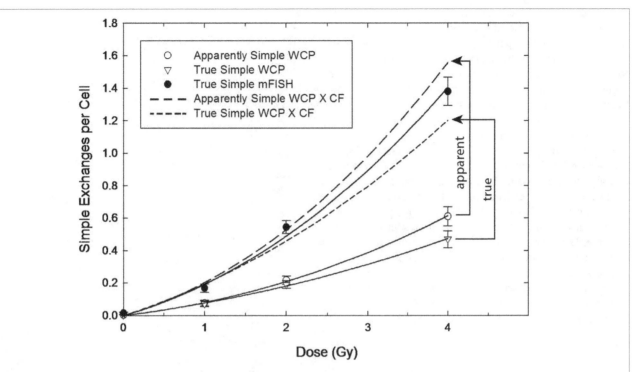

FIGURE 3 | Gamma ray dose–responses for apparently simple (AS) and true simple (TR) exchanges (open circle and triangle symbols, respectively) as reconstructed from mFISH data. Arrowed brackets show the predicted dose responses following the application of the CF from Equation (8), which can be compared to the actual whole-genome frequencies for simple exchanges measured by mFISH (solid circles).

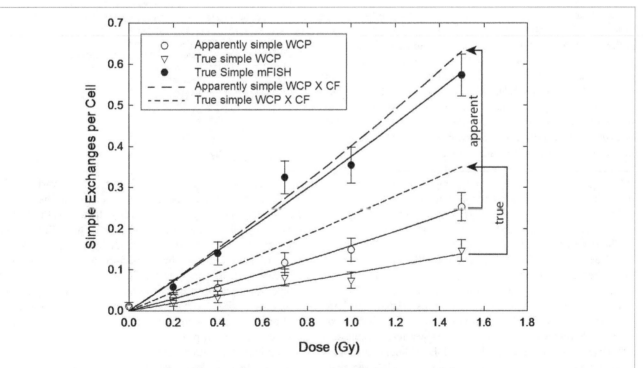

FIGURE 4 | Dose–responses for apparently simple (AS) and true simple (TR) exchanges (open circle and triangle symbols, respectively) following exposure to ^{56}Fe ions. Arrowed brackets project the dose–responses following the application of the CF from Equation (8). Solid circles are actual whole-genome frequencies for simple exchanges, as measured by mFISH.

dose–response for TR exchanges involving the three painted chromosomes, whose associated fit parameters appear in **Table 1**. The result of corrections applied to TR *exchanges* is symbolized by the vertical bracket of the figure labeled "true"; it is associated with the dose–response shown by the short-dashed curve. It should be noted that, in this case, extrapolation *underestimates* the frequencies of the mFISH dose–response.

The difference between CFs applied to AS versus TR exchanges is magnified when we consider exposure to 1.1 MeV ^{56}Fe ions, as shown in **Figure 4**. The solid symbols represent full genome equivalence for TR exchanges (mFISH). The open circles and triangles are for AS and TR exchanges, respectively, and represent 3-color data rendered from 24-color mFISH images. As with gamma rays, CFs applied to AS exchanges produced rather good results, although they tended to overestimate the mFISH response. However, the same corrections applied to TRs *grossly underestimated* WGE across the full range of doses examined.

The situation is graphically represented in **Figure 5**, which compares the results of actual (empirically derived) CFs of Eq. (11) to those derived from first principles of Eq. (8), as expressed by the following Eq. (17).

$$\% \text{ Deviation} = \left[\frac{CF(\alpha_{3\ color} + \beta_{3\ color}D)}{\alpha_{mFISH} + \beta_{mFISH}D} - 1 \right] \times 100 \quad (17)$$

The figure shows errors associated with CFs as a function of dose applied to both AS and TR exchanges. The upper portion of the **Figure 4** shows deviations as applied to AS exchanges. The errors are positive for both radiation types, meaning that the CF of Eq. (8) *over estimates* the WGE mFISH response. For gamma rays, the deviations are relatively small (~10%) and (as we have shown statistically) are practically invariant of dose. Plotted this way, errors for ^{56}Fe ions increase with dose, although as shown in a previous section, this increase could not be validated on the basis of our statistical tests. Rather unexpectedly, errors are practically nil at doses approaching 0, before climbing to about 8% at the highest dose of 1.5 Gy. When extrapolated beyond this dose (extended dashed curve) errors continue to rise in a near-linear fashion, crossing that for gamma rays at ~1.8 Gy, the significance of which is discussed in the following section.

The lower portion of the **Figure 5** refers to corrections applied to TR exchanges. Here, extrapolation to WGE badly *underestimates* the true frequency for both types of radiation, as indicated by negative percentage values shown in the figure.

For gamma rays, the (absolute) errors associated with lower doses exceed 50%. Consistent with our statistical analysis, errors decrease sharply with dose, but even at 4 Gy, values are still some 30% lower than those measured by mFISH. Although unsubstantiated by our statistical tests, for ^{56}Fe ions there is a seemingly linear increase in relative error with dose, from about 35% at doses approaching 0, to roughly 40% at 1.5 Gy, the highest dose used in these experiments. The response extrapolated to 4 Gy is shown by the dotted line, based on fitted parameters of **Table 1**.

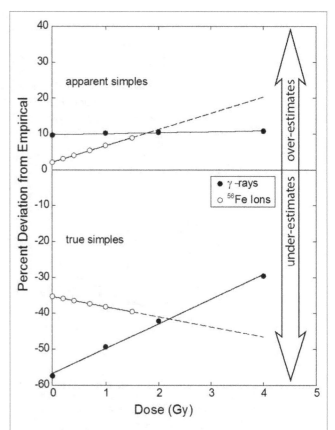

FIGURE 5 | **Percentage errors as a function of dose that result from the application of the CF to AS (upper panel) and TR exchanges (lower panel) for gamma rays and iron ions.** Symbols mark dose points where raw data (**Table 1**) was collected and whose ordinate values derive from Eq. (17). Errors for AS exchanges induced by gamma rays are invariant of dose. Dose dependency is apparent for the three remaining responses, a result statistically supported for TR exchanges induced by gamma rays. A perfect correction would be represented by a flat dose–response that is centered on 0%. See text for full explanation.

DISCUSSION

We feel compelled to point out – after attending to various tedious details specific to our experimental system – that the 2.053 constant appearing in Eq. (7) is practically identical to the 2.05 value originally published by Lucas et al. (3). Actually, we find it amusing that ignoring all such adjustments made subsequent to Eq. (4) leads to a mere 2.5% error by comparison to Eq. (7), which is small compared to the errors shown in **Figure 5**, and which we imagine would be sufficiently accurate for most experimental purposes.

Clearly, mFISH is capable of providing more cytogenetic information than three-color WCP, including the ability to distinguish TR exchanges from psuedosimples. It is also considerably more demanding of resources and, in many cases, yields data superfluous to the investigator. Presupposing that the two approaches produce quantitatively comparable results, WCP would be the method of choice in instances where less detailed information is an acceptable compromise given its lower expense, rapidity of data acquisition, and ease of analysis.

Regarding the study of whole-genome corrections, there are a couple of points in favor of our retrospective mFISH approach. Unlike earlier studies that sought to establish correlations between mFISH and multi-color data, we establish a proper *correspondence*. In other words, for each and every "three-color cell," there is a corresponding cell for which 24-color data are obtained. Most WCP studies are vexed by the very prospect of pseudosimple exchanges. For that reason, they are limited to experimental doses and radiation types for which one can reasonably assume the frequency of complex aberrations is minimal, namely low doses of sparsely ionizing radiation. The ability to cull psuedosimples from AS exchanges allows us to analyze full dose–response relationships for TR exchanges, irrespective of dose and radiation quality. Later in this section, we consider the theoretical implications of WGE corrections applied to TR exchanges (TR). But first we discuss the more practical aspects of WGE corrections, which involve their application to AS exchanges.

Apparently Simple Exchanges

As routinely practiced, WCP to WGE corrections are confined to AS events, simply because WCP is incapable of distinguishing TRs from pseudosimple exchanges. Looking to **Figure 3**, we find basic agreement with conclusions of Braselmann (4) and others (3, 7, 8) that biophysically based corrections do a reasonably good job of predicting WGE for gamma rays. Applying a multiplicative CF of Eq. (8) to three-color data overestimates mFISH frequencies for simple exchanges, but only by about 10%. Equally important is that the 10% error is essentially constant over the dose interval examined. This is a direct consequence of α/β ratios for mFISH and AS dose–responses being equal, and is reflected in the flat dose–response shown in the leftmost panel (blue-coded data) of **Figure 2**, and the upper panel of **Figure 5** for gamma rays. Thus, reducing the CF of 2.54 in Eq. (8) by 10% would lead to a near perfect match across the full range of doses examined for AS versus mFISH dose–responses shown in **Figure 3**.

Although not detected with confidence by our statistical methods (**Figure 2**), α/β ratios for ^{56}Fe ions (WCP data versus that of mFISH) are probably not precisely equivalent. This would explain the apparent sloped dose–response shown in the upper panel of **Figure 5**. If true, then there is no interval of dose over which Eq. (11) is stable enough to be represented by a constant. That being said, the Figure shows that the errors are not large. Across the range of ^{56}Fe ion doses studied, they deviate from the empirically derived CF by less than 10%, and actually *diminish* with dose. Said differently, we suspect that Eq. (15) has been violated by some small degree, but as a practical matter, this produces a CF that would be deemed acceptable for many purposes. At first glance, these results seem counterintuitive, since high LET radiations are known to produce copious quantities of complex aberrations that are cryptically embedded in the AS data as pseudosimples. However, they are entirely consistent with the interpretation that, to a first approximation, all effects from high LET radiation are "intratrack." Consequently, there would be the same fixed fraction of aberrations (of any kind, including complex exchanges) per unit dose of Fe ions.

Chromosome aberrations are a viable surrogate endpoint for mutations and cancer, and have long been the *de facto* "gold standard" for biodosimetry (34). WCP to WGE corrections, therefore, have implications for radiation protection, where concerns over the biological effects of very low doses are paramount. At issue is the concept of relative biological effectiveness (RBE), which for the present work, involves a comparison between the effects of gamma rays and heavy ions. Here, WCP finds a place because of cost and sample throughput considerations related to the need to score many cells.

As shown graphically in **Figure 5**, it is debatable whether a common CF can be assigned to *both types* of radiation that is valid over a range of doses. It was previously mentioned that the upper portion of the Figure shows that AS errors for both radiations intersect at about 2 Gy. A common CF is valid for both radiations only at this dose, which is far too large to be of practical use as regards issues of radiation risk. At more relevant lower doses, the two curves diverge sharply. This significantly complicates RBE calculations, which are made on the basis of the ratio of doses for a given isoeffect. For RBEs other than unity, the isoeffective doses will differ, meaning that separate CFs would need to be applied to each type of radiation. Moreover, in the case of 1.1 GeV ^{56}Fe ions used in these studies, CFs will also change depending on the chosen level of isoeffect. That said, and as a practical matter, **Figure 4** indicates these errors are capable of altering RBE values for ^{56}Fe ions by about 8% at very low doses. Whereas these errors do not seem particularly large in an experimental setting, in the context of RBE-related radiation protection issues, they probably should not be ignored.

True Simple Exchanges

The remaining discussion focuses on TR exchanges. Recall that the presence of complex aberrations – in this case, taking the form of pseudosimple exchanges in AS data – is specifically ignored during the derivation of Eq. (8), and only simple pairwise exchanges are considered. So, in theory, one would imagine that CFs applied to TR exchanges would produce better results than CFs applied to AS exchanges. As we have seen, the opposite is true. Errors of mFISH predictions based on TR show a pronounced dose dependency for γ-rays (**Figure 2**), and underestimates of WGE for both radiation types occur (**Figures 3 and 4**). From a predictive standpoint, the errors for ^{56}Fe ions are severe enough to render such extrapolation practically useless. Ironically then, after culling pseudosimples from the data – thus satisfying a principle assumption underlying the derivation of Eq. (8) – the resulting predictions were much poorer than if CFs were applied to AS exchanges. Said differently, our data show that the "contaminating" influence of pseudo simple exchanges actually serves to *improve* the predictive ability of WGE corrections. So, to the extent that WGE corrections are considered sufficiently accurate, they owe this accuracy to the very presence of complex aberrations! While this result may be reassuring from a practical standpoint, from theoretical perspective it is disconcerting, because it implies either that the basic approach underpinning WCP-to-WGE conversion is fundamentally flawed, or that a violation of some primary assumption has taken place.

The Discrepancy for True Simples

The derivation of Eq. (8) makes the assumption of *random* pairwise interactions between primary radiogenic breaks leading to interchanges. In that case, variance/mean ratios of unity should result, consistent with the expectations of a Poisson distribution (35, 36). The total counts of chromosomal exchanges in the genome (mFISH), as well as subsets of these data – AS and TR exchanges – showed no clear evidence of overdispersion. For both γ-rays and Fe ions, the dispersion parameter in quasi-binomial fits was always in the range of 0.58–1.19, close to unity. The X^2 test for residual deviances, which compares the fits of dose–response models with binomial and quasi-binomial errors, produced p-values of 0.43–0.88, also suggesting no overdispersion. These results are largely consistent with the analysis of the raw data to which the U-test (36) was also applied to check σ^2/Y ratios for overdispersion (data not shown). By applying this latter criterion to the data for gamma rays, we found no evidence that the distribution of TR or AS exchanges deviated from that of the Poisson. For the high LET ^{56}Fe ions, significant over dispersion was detected by the U-test, but only for one of the five doses examined. From this, we conclude that systematic deviation from randomness in the distribution of exchanges per cell is not the principle cause for the failure of Eq. (8) to predict the outcomes of TR exchanges measured by mFISH.

We think a more likely explanation for the large discrepancy involves the remaining fundamental assumption attached to the derivation of Eq. (8), namely that the probability of an exchange between two chromosomes is a product of their proportional genomic content. [We hasten to make a minor point here that, strictly speaking, it is probably more accurate to consider the length of interphase chromosome arms, or chromatin fibers (the chromonema) of individual chromosomes in such interactions (37), rather than gross DNA content, although the two parameters are sufficiently related (38) that they can probably be used interchangeably in the present context.]

During interphase, it is now well established that chromosomes occupy rather distinct globular domains (39–41), which, it is reasonable to assume, severely limit the opportunity for the interaction of radiogenic breaks between different chromosomes. Consequently, models have been developed that consider interchanges constrained to boundary regions where two chromosomes abut (42), in which case interchanges would be proportional to the product of domain surface areas. For chromosome domains of spherical shape, exchange frequencies would, therefore, be proportional to [DNA content]$^{2/3}$ (43). For spherical domains of radii r, the ratio of volume to surface area varies as $r/3$. Consequently, by comparison to models based on volume, predictions based on DNA content tend to systematically overestimate exchange frequencies involving larger chromosomes (9, 44, 45). Unfortunately, this leads to a further lowering of predicted frequencies for exchanges involving the large-sized chromosomes examined here – the opposite of what is needed to bring three-color data in line with that of mFISH for TRs (**Figure 5**; lower panel). The problem is further exacerbated when one considers that chromosome domains are not actually spherical, but globular instead, because for any irregular volume the surface-to-volume ratio is larger than that of a sphere, or for that matter, any platonic solid.

One should appreciate that simple pairwise exchanges do not form in a vacuum, meaning their formation is always in potential competition with the formation of complex exchanges. Said another way, simple and complex exchanges often compete for the same radiogenic breaks. Consider a constellation of four such *proximate* breaks, defined as breaks that – by virtue of being close in time and space – are capable of freely interacting (rejoining) with one another. An obvious rejoining possibility is that the four breaks rejoin in such a way as to give two simple exchanges. But, should any other misrejoining possibility occur, a complex exchange will result, simultaneously negating the possibility of simple pairwise exchange. Crudely put, the formation of complex exchanges can be envisioned to "steal away" breaks that would otherwise be destined to become involved in forming simple exchanges (46). In this sense, complex exchanges form *at the expense* of simple exchanges, a process that is bound to be dose dependent, since it is strongly influenced by lesion density. To our knowledge, no one has formally modeled this scenario, but it most assuredly would have the overall effect of depressing the expected yields of simple exchanges.

Other explanations for our results involve the higher order organization of the mammalian cell genome (i.e., beyond that of the 30 nm chromatin fiber). Since this remains as one of the least understood aspects of cell biology, a fair amount of speculation is unavoidable. Until now, we have assumed random interaction between radiogenic breaks – either those contained within interphase chromosome domains, or those associated with their surface areas. In fact, the radial distribution of chromosomes in the nucleus is often not random, and differs among cell type and stage of cellular differentiation (47). There is some evidence that larger human chromosomes tend to be located near the periphery of the nucleus. If true, then larger chromosomes would share a proportion of their surface area with the outside nuclear boundary – regions that presumably would be unavailable for interaction with that of more interior domains (48, 49). Such is the case for chromosome 1, at least in fibroblasts (50, 51), although there is also evidence to the contrary for lymphocytes (52, 53). Such a relationship (in principle) would necessitate a higher correction factor be applied exchanges involving the large-sized chromosomes used in this study, which would have the effect of reducing CF errors shown in **Figure 5** for TRs.

The assumption of random breakage also implies a more-or-less uniform breakage per unit length of DNA or chromatin. While this is probably true for the initial radiogenic lesions (i.e., DNA double-strand breaks), there is evidence that exchanges themselves occur preferentially in G-light bands (54, 55) or at the interface between light and dark bands (56). These regions, particularly T-bands (a subset of G-light bands) have a much higher than average gene density (57). As long as these "sensitive" regions are randomly distributed among various chromosomes, this should not materially affect the underlying assumptions relating to Eq. (8). However, certain chromosomes are known to be gene-rich, on average, a case in point being chromosome 19 (41) which, perhaps not by coincidence, is thought to occupy an interior position within the nucleus (58). By this argument, gene-rich chromosomes may be subject to increased exchange involvement compared to chromosomes with lower gene density.

Additionally, if one equates gene density with transcriptional activity, then the DNA of such regions would presumably have a more "open" or diffuse structure (59, 60), and consequently be less dense in terms DNA content/surface area. In this way, increased transcription associated with gene-rich regions (or whole chromosomes) may have the secondary effect of lowering the physical density of DNA per unit volume. The opposite would be true of more gene-poor chromosomes. With respect to interactions based on surface area, larger chromosomes would then require larger CFs to compensate, again mitigating CF discrepancies shown in **Figure 5**. These ideas represent little more than a speculative attempt to explain our findings. Whether or not they help to resolve the thorny issue of dose dependency of CFs associated with violation of Eq. (15) remains to be seen.

CONCLUSION

The good news – at least from a utilitarian perspective – is that for the purpose of converting WCP data to WGE, CFs work reasonably well across the range of doses to which they are usually applied. The less welcome news is the large discrepancy between WGE-corrected TR exchange frequencies compared to those detected by mFISH, which implies problems with the biophysical underpinnings upon which the derivation CFs rely. We imagine that the fundamental assumptions underlying Eq. (8) are overly simplistic, failing to account for structural features of chromatin, and its dynamic interactions within the interphase nucleus.

Sophisticated methods are being applied to this area of study that, in principle, can provide the investigator a "snapshot" into physical relationships that exist between interphase chromosomes (61, 62), but these fall short in addressing any potential time-dependent dynamic interactions. We have known, for the better part of a century, that initial radiogenic breaks in chromosomes need to be both spatially and temporally close for exchanges to occur (63). And yet, there are almost certainly aspects of this relationship that we do not fully understand. A phrase used often by the preeminent cytogeneticist J.R.K Savage seems an appropriate closing note: "Everything is more complex than it appears at first sight."

AUTHOR CONTRIBUTIONS

BL conducted the experiments and helped analyze the data. IS provided critical statistical support and helped edit the manuscript. MC conceived of the experiment, provided financial support, and wrote most of the paper.

ACKNOWLEDGMENTS

The authors gratefully acknowledge assistance provided by Drs. Daniel Cornforth for the proof related to Equation (15), and Dudley Goodhead for valuable theoretical discussion. This work was supported by the following grants from NASA: NNX15AG74G (MC) and NNX14AC76G (BL).

REFERENCES

1. Speicher MR, Ballard SG, Ward DC. Karyotyping human chromosomes by combinatorial multi-fluor fish. *Nat Genet* (1996) **12**:368–75. doi:10.1038/ng0496-368
2. Schrock E, du Manoir S, Veldman T, Schoell B, Wienberg J, Ferguson-Smith MA, et al. Multicolor spectral karyotyping of human chromosomes. *Science* (1996) **273**:494–7. doi:10.1126/science.273.5274.494
3. Lucas JN, Awa A, Straume T, Poggensee M, Kodama Y, Nakano M, et al. Rapid translocation frequency analysis in humans decades after exposure to ionizing radiation. *Int J Radiat Biol* (1992) **62**:53–63. doi:10.1080/09553009214551821
4. Braselmann H, Kulka U, Baumgartner A, Eder C, Muller I, Figel M, et al. Sky and fish analysis of radiation-induced chromosome aberrations: a comparison of whole and partial genome analysis. *Mutat Res* (2005) **578**:124–33. doi:10.1016/j.mrfmmm.2005.04.006
5. George KA, Hada M, Jackson LJ, Elliott T, Kawata T, Pluth JM, et al. Dose response of gamma rays and iron nuclei for induction of chromosomal aberrations in normal and repair-deficient cell lines. *Radiat Res* (2009) **171**:752–63. doi:10.1667/RR1680.1
6. Tucker JD, Ramsey MJ, Lee DA, Minkler JL. Validation of chromosome painting as a biodosimeter in human peripheral lymphocytes following acute exposure to ionizing radiation in vitro. *Int J Radiat Biol* (1993) **64**:27–37. doi:10.1080/09553009314551081
7. Nakano M, Nakashima E, Pawel DJ, Kodama Y, Awa A. Frequency of reciprocal translocations and dicentrics induced in human blood lymphocytes by x-irradiation as determined by fluorescence in situ hybridization. *Int J Radiat Biol* (1993) **64**:565–9. doi:10.1080/09553009314551781
8. Finnon P, Lloyd DC, Edwards AA. Fluorescence in situ hybridization detection of chromosomal aberrations in human lymphocytes: applicability to biological dosimetry. *Int J Radiat Biol* (1995) **68**:429–35. doi:10.1080/09553009514551391
9. Knehr S, Zitzelsberger H, Braselmann H, Bauchinger M. Analysis for DNA-proportional distribution of radiation-induced chromosome aberrations in various triple combinations of human chromosomes using fluorescence

in situ hybridization. *Int J Radiat Biol* (1994) **65**:683–90. doi:10.1080/09553009414550801
10. Knehr S, Zitzelsberger H, Braselmann H, Nahrstedt U, Bauchinger M. Chromosome analysis by fluorescence in situ hybridization: further indications for a non-DNA-proportional involvement of single chromosomes in radiation-induced structural aberrations. *Int J Radiat Biol* (1996) **70**:385–92. doi:10.1080/095530096144851
11. Barquinero JF, Knehr S, Braselmann H, Figel M, Bauchinger M. DNA-proportional distribution of radiation-induced chromosome aberrations analysed by fluorescence in situ hybridization painting of all chromosomes of a human female karyotype. *Int J Radiat Biol* (1998) **74**:315–23. doi:10.1080/095530098141456
12. Brown JM, Evans JW, Kovacs MS. Mechanism of chromosome exchange formation in human fibroblasts: insights from "chromosome painting". *Environ Mol Mutagen* (1993) **22**:218–24. doi:10.1002/em.2850220407
13. Simpson PJ, Savage JR. Detecting 'hidden' exchange events within x ray induced aberrations using multicolour chromosome paints. *Chromosome Res* (1995) **3**:69–72. doi:10.1007/BF00711165
14. Simpson PJ, Papworth DG, Savage JRK. X-ray-induced simple, pseudosimple and complex exchanges involving two distinctly painted chromosomes. *Int J Radiat Biol* (1999) **75**:11–8. doi:10.1080/095530099140753
15. Griffin CS, Marsden SJ, Stevens DL, Simpson P, Savage JR. Frequencies of complex chromosome exchange aberrations induced by 238pu alpha-particles and detected by fluorescence in situ hybridization using single chromosome-specific probes. *Int J Radiat Biol* (1995) **67**:431–9. doi:10.1080/09553009514550491
16. Griffin CS, Stevens DL, Savage JR. Ultrasoft 1.5 kev aluminum k x rays are efficient producers of complex chromosome exchange aberrations as revealed by fluorescence in situ hybridization. *Radiat Res* (1996) **146**:144–50. doi:10.2307/3579586
17. Anderson RM, Marsden SJ, Wright EG, Kadhim MA, Goodhead DT, Griffin CS. Complex chromosome aberrations in peripheral blood lymphocytes as a potential biomarker of exposure to high-let alpha-particles. *Int J Radiat Biol* (2000) **76**:31–42. doi:10.1080/095530000138989

18. George K, Wu H, Willingham V, Furusawa Y, Kawata T, Cucinotta FA. High- and low-let induced chromosome damage in human lymphocytes: a time-course of aberrations in metaphase and interphase. *Int J Radiat Biol* (2001) 77:175–83. doi:10.1080/0955300001003760

19. Anderson RM, Stevens DL, Goodhead DT. M-fish analysis shows that complex chromosome aberrations induced by alpha-particle tracks are cumulative products of localized rearrangements. *Proc Natl Acad Sci U S A* (2002) 99:12167–72. doi:10.1073/pnas.182426799

20. Durante M, Ando K, Furusawa Y, Obe G, George K, Cucinotta FA. Complex chromosomal rearrangements induced in vivo by heavy ions. *Cytogenet Genome Res* (2004) 104:240–4. doi:10.1159/000077497

21. Cornforth MN. Perspectives on the formation of radiation-induced exchange aberrations. *DNA Repair* (2006) 5:1182–91. doi:10.1016/j.dnarep.2006.05.008

22. Loucas BD, Durante M, Bailey SM, Cornforth MN. Chromosome damage in human cells by rays, particles and heavy ions: track interactions in basic dose-response relationships. *Radiat Res* (2013) 179:9–20. doi:10.1667/RR3089.1

23. Loucas BD, Cornforth MN. Complex chromosome exchanges induced by gamma rays in human lymphocytes: an mFISH study. *Radiat Res* (2001) 155:660–71. doi:10.1667/0033-7587(2001)155[0660:CCEIBG]2.0.CO;2

24. Durante M, Furusawa Y, Gotoh E. A simple method for simultaneous interphase-metaphase chromosome analysis in biodosimetry. *Int J Radiat Biol* (1998) 74:457–62. doi:10.1080/095530098141320

25. Cornforth MN. Analyzing radiation-induced complex chromosome rearrangements by combinatorial painting. *Radiat Res* (2001) 155:643–59. doi:10.1667/0033-7587(2001)155[0643:ARICCR]2.0.CO;2

26. Wu H, George K, Yang TC. Estimate of true incomplete exchanges using fluorescence in situ hybridization with telomere probes. *Int J Radiat Biol* (1998) 73:521–7. doi:10.1080/095530098142068

27. Kodama Y, Nakano M, Ohtaki K, Delongchamp R, Awa AA, Nakamura N. Estimation of minimal size of translocated chromosome segments detectable by fluorescence in situ hybridization. *Int J Radiat Biol* (1997) 71:35–9. doi:10.1080/095530097144391

28. Boei JJ, Vermeulen S, Fomina J, Natarajan AT. Detection of incomplete exchanges and interstitial fragments in x-irradiated human lymphocytes using a telomeric pna probe. *Int J Radiat Biol* (1998) 73:599–603. doi:10.1080/095530098141843

29. Fomina J, Darroudi F, Boei JJ, Natarajan AT. Discrimination between complete and incomplete chromosome exchanges in x-irradiated human lymphocytes using fish with pan-centromeric and chromosome specific DNA probes in combination with telomeric pna probe. *Int J Radiat Biol* (2000) 76:807–13. doi:10.1080/09553000050028968

30. Mayall BH, Carrano AV, Moore DH II, Ashworth LK, Bennett DE, Mendelsohn ML. The DNA-based human karyotype. *Cytometry* (1984) 5:376–85. doi:10.1002/cyto.990050414

31. Morton NE. Parameters of the human genome. *Proc Natl Acad Sci U S A* (1991) 88:7474–6. doi:10.1073/pnas.88.17.7474

32. George KA, Hada M, Chappell L, Cucinotta FA. Biological effectiveness of accelerated particles for the induction of chromosome damage: track structure effects. *Radiat Res* (2013) 180:25–33. doi:10.1667/RR3291.1

33. Agresti A, Coull BA. Approximate is better than "exact" for interval estimation of binomial proportions. *Am Stat* (1998) 52:119–26. doi:10.2307/2685469

34. Pernot E, Hall J, Baatout S, Benotmane MA, Blanchardon E, Bouffler S, et al. Ionizing radiation biomarkers for potential use in epidemiological studies. *Mutat Res* (2012) 751:258–86. doi:10.1016/j.mrrev.2012.05.003

35. Virsik RP, Harder D. Statistical interpretation of the overdispersed distribution of radiation-induced dicentric chromosome aberrations at high let. *Radiat Res* (1981) 85:13–23. doi:10.2307/3575434

36. Edwards AA, Lloyd DC, Purrott RJ. Radiation induced chromosome aberrations and the poisson distribution. *Radiat Environ Biophys* (1979) 16:89–100. doi:10.1007/BF01323216

37. Savage JRK, Papworth DG. Frequency and distribution studies of asymmetrical versus symmetrical chromosome aberrations. *Mutat Res* (1982) 95:7–18. doi:10.1016/0027-5107(82)90062-8

38. Korenberg JR, Engels WR. Base ratio, DNA content, and quinacrine-brightness of human chromosomes. *Proc Natl Acad Sci U S A* (1978) 75:3382–6. doi:10.1073/pnas.75.7.3382

39. Pinkel D, Landegent J, Collins C, Fuscoe J, Segraves R, Lucas J, et al. Fluorescence in situ hybridization with human chromosome-specific libraries:

40. Cremer T, Kreth G, Koester H, Fink RH, Heintzmann R, Cremer M, et al. Chromosome territories, interchromatin domain compartment, and nuclear matrix: an integrated view of the functional nuclear architecture. *Crit Rev Eukaryot Gene Expr* (2000) 10:179–212. doi:10.1615/CritRevEukarGeneExpr.v10.i2.60

41. Cremer T, Cremer C. Chromosome territories, nuclear architecture and gene regulation in mammalian cells. *Nat Revs Genet* (2001) 2:292–301. doi:10.1038/35066075

42. Savage JR, Papworth DG. The relationship of radiation-induced dicentric yield to chromosome arm number. *Mutat Res* (1973) 19:139–43. doi:10.1016/0027-5107(73)90122-X

43. Cigarran S, Barrios L, Barquinero JF, Caballin MR, Ribas M, Egozcue J. Relationship between the DNA content of human chromosomes and their involvement in radiation-induced structural aberrations, analysed by painting. *Int J Radiat Biol* (1998) 74:449–55. doi:10.1080/095530098141311

44. Wu H, Durante M, Lucas JN. Relationship between radiation-induced aberrations in individual chromosomes and their DNA content: effects of interaction distance. *Int J Radiat Biol* (2001) 77:781–6. doi:10.1080/09553000110050227

45. Cornforth MN, Greulich-Bode KM, Loucas BD, Arsuaga J, Vazquez M, Sachs RK, et al. Chromosomes are predominantly located randomly with respect to each other in interphase human cells. *J Cell Biol* (2002) 159:237–44. doi:10.1083/jcb.200206009

46. Loucas BD, Eberle R, Bailey SM, Cornforth MN. Influence of dose rate on the induction of simple and complex chromosome exchanges by gamma rays. *Radiat Res* (2004) 162:339–49. doi:10.1667/RR3245

47. Bridger JM, Arican-Gotkas HD, Foster HA, Godwin LS, Harvey A, Kill IR, et al. The non-random repositioning of whole chromosomes and individual gene loci in interphase nuclei and its relevance in disease, infection, aging, and cancer. *Adv Exp Med Biol* (2014) 773:263–79. doi:10.1007/978-1-4899-8032-8_12

48. Foster HA, Estrada-Girona G, Themis M, Garimberti E, Hill MA, Bridger JM, et al. Relative proximity of chromosome territories influences chromosome exchange partners in radiation-induced chromosome rearrangements in primary human bronchial epithelial cells. *Mutat Res* (2013) 756:66–77. doi:10.1016/j.mrgentox.2013.06.003

49. Themis M, Garimberti E, Hill MA, Anderson RM. Reduced chromosome aberration complexity in normal human bronchial epithelial cells exposed to low-let gamma-rays and high-let alpha-particles. *Int J Radiat Biol* (2013) 89:934–43. doi:10.3109/09553002.2013.805889

50. Sun HB, Shen J, Yokota H. Size-dependent positioning of human chromosomes in interphase nuclei. *Biophys J* (2000) 79:184–90. doi:10.1016/S0006-3495(00)76282-5

51. Zeitz MJ, Mukherjee L, Bhattacharya S, Xu J, Berezney R. A probabilistic model for the arrangement of a subset of human chromosome territories in wi38 human fibroblasts. *J Cell Physiol* (2009) 221:120–9. doi:10.1002/jcp.21842

52. Boyle S, Gilchrist S, Bridger JM, Mahy NL, Ellis JA, Bickmore WA. The spatial organization of human chromosomes within the nuclei of normal and emerin-mutant cells. *Hum Mol Genet* (2001) 10:211–9. doi:10.1093/hmg/10.3.211

53. Ioannou D, Kandukuri L, Quadri A, Becerra V, Simpson JL, Tempest HG. Spatial positioning of all 24 chromosomes in the lymphocytes of six subjects: evidence of reproducible positioning and spatial repositioning following DNA damage with hydrogen peroxide and ultraviolet b. *PLoS One* (2015) 10:e0118886. doi:10.1371/journal.pone.0118886

54. Holmberg M, Jonasson J. Preferential location of x-ray induced chromosome breakage in the r-bands of human chromosomes. *Hereditas* (1973) 74:57–67. doi:10.1111/j.1601-5223.1973.tb01104.x

55. Holmberg M, Carrano AV. Neutron induced break-points in human chromosomes have a similar location as x-ray induced break-points. *Hereditas* (1978) 89:183–7. doi:10.1111/j.1601-5223.1978.tb01274.x

56. Buckton KE. Identification with g and r banding of the position of breakage points induced in human chromosomes by in vitro x-irradiation. *Int J Radiat Biol Relat Stud Phys Chem Med* (1976) 29:475–88. doi:10.1080/09553007614550571

57. Craig JM, Bickmore WA. The distribution of cpg islands in mammalian chromosomes. [erratum appears in nat genet 1994 Aug;7(4):551]. *Nat Genet* (1994) 7:376–82. doi:10.1038/ng0794-376

58. Croft JA, Bridger JM, Boyle S, Perry P, Teague P, Bickmore WA. Differences in the localization and morphology of chromosomes in the human nucleus. *J Cell Biol* (1999) **145**:1119–31. doi:10.1083/jcb.145.6.1119

59. Franke WW, Scheer U, Trendelenburg M, Zentgraf H, Spring H. Morphology of transcriptionally active chromatin. *Cold Spring Harb Symp Quant Biol* (1978) **42**:755–72. doi:10.1101/SQB.1978.042.01.076

60. Paul J, Zollner EJ, Gilmour RS, Birnie GD. Properties of transcriptionally active chromatin. *Cold Spring Harb Symp Quant Biol* (1978) **42**(Pt 1):597–603. doi:10.1101/SQB.1978.042.01.062

61. Gondor A, Ohlsson R. Chromosome crosstalk in three dimensions. *Nature* (2009) **461**:212–7. doi:10.1038/nature08453

62. Arsuaga J, Jayasinghe RG, Scharein RG, Segal MR, Stolz R, Vazquez M. Current theoretical models fail to predict the topological complexity of the human genome. *Front Mol Biosci* (2015) **2**:48. doi:10.3389/fmolb.2015.00048

63. Lea DE. *Actions of Radiations on Living Cells*. London: Cambridge University Press (1946).

19

Higher Initial DNA Damage and Persistent Cell Cycle Arrest after Carbon Ion Irradiation Compared to X-Irradiation in Prostate and Colon Cancer Cells

Annelies Suetens[1,2†], Katrien Konings[1,3†], Marjan Moreels[1]*, Roel Quintens[1], Mieke Verslegers[1], Els Soors[1], Kevin Tabury[1], Vincent Grégoire[3] and Sarah Baatout[1]

[1] Expert Group for Molecular and Cellular Biology, Radiobiology Unit, Belgian Nuclear Research Centre (SCK•CEN), Institute for Environment, Health and Safety, Mol, Belgium, [2] Radiation Oncology Department, Center for Molecular Imaging, Radiotherapy and Oncology, Institut de Recherche Expérimentale et Clinique (IREC), Université Catholique de Louvain (UCL), Bruxelles, Belgium, [3] Laboratory of Experimental Radiotherapy, Department of Oncology, KU Leuven, Leuven, Belgium

*Correspondence:
Marjan Moreels
marjan.moreels@sckcen.be

† Annelies Suetens and Katrien Konings shared first authorship and contributed equally to this work.

The use of charged-particle beams, such as carbon ions, is becoming a more and more attractive treatment option for cancer therapy. Given the precise absorbed dose-localization and an increased biological effectiveness, this form of therapy is much more advantageous compared to conventional radiotherapy, and is currently being used for treatment of specific cancer types. The high ballistic accuracy of particle beams deposits the maximal dose to the tumor, while damage to the surrounding healthy tissue is limited. In order to better understand the underlying mechanisms responsible for the increased biological effectiveness, we investigated the DNA damage and repair kinetics and cell cycle progression in two p53 mutant cell lines, more specifically a prostate (PC3) and colon (Caco-2) cancer cell line, after exposure to different radiation qualities. Cells were irradiated with various absorbed doses (0, 0.5, and 2 Gy) of accelerated ^{13}C-ions at the Grand Accélérateur National d'Ions Lourds facility (Caen, France) or with X-rays (0, 0.1, 0.5, 1, 2, and 5 Gy). Microscopic analysis of DNA double-strand breaks showed dose-dependent increases in γ-H2AX foci numbers and foci occupancy after exposure to both types of irradiation, in both cell lines. However, 24 h after exposure, residual damage was more pronounced after lower doses of carbon ion irradiation compared to X-irradiation. Flow cytometric analysis showed that carbon ion irradiation induced a permanent G2/M arrest in PC3 cells at lower doses (2 Gy) compared to X-rays (5 Gy), while in Caco-2 cells the G2/M arrest was transient after irradiation with X-rays (2 and 5 Gy) but persistent after exposure to carbon ions (2 Gy).

Keywords: carbon ion irradiation, PC3, Caco-2, cell cycle progression, DNA double-strand break damage and repair

INTRODUCTION

Over the past decades, an increase in the use of hadrontherapy has been observed (1). Hadrontherapy uses accelerated particles, such as protons or carbon ions, thereby offering a ballistic advantage during treatment. The inverted depth–dose profile and a sharp dose fall-off result in a precise dose-localization called Bragg peak (2). As such, a very specific energy deposition is focused on the tumor, while the surrounding healthy tissue is spared to a maximum. When carbon ions are used, the high-linear energy transfer (LET) also offers biological advantages compared to X-irradiation (3). From a physical point of view, low-LET photon irradiation deposits its energy in a disperse manner. This homogeneous distribution of energy in the irradiation field strongly relies on secondary ionizations (by the formation of reactive oxygen species) in the cell that will indirectly induce DNA damage homogeneously. By contrast, with particle irradiation, energy is not released in a disperse manner but rather along the track of the beam. Therefore, damage is more straightforward along the track that induces more complex and clustered DNA damage via a direct mechanism (4, 5). In view of therapeutic measures, the induction of DNA damage and specifically the double-strand break (DSB) is seen as the most prominent target in order to destroy cancer cells (6). Since DNA damage induced by high-LET radiation is more complex compared to low-LET irradiation, the relative biological effectiveness (RBE) of particle beams will be higher compared to X-rays (6). In this regard, it has been shown that hadrontherapy with carbon ions is more cytotoxic due to the higher RBE compared to photon irradiation (7, 8). However, the specific impact of carbon ion irradiation on cell cycle changes and comparison with X-irradiation in PC3 and Caco-2 cancer cells has not been investigated so far.

When DNA damage is induced, DSBs are detected in the cell by sensing molecules, such as DNA-dependent protein kinases (DNA-PK) or Ku70, which activate a signaling cascade by phosphorylating the histone H2AX (γ-H2AX) (9, 10). Another sensing molecule that is activated after DNA damage is p53, also known as the guardian of the genome (11). Repair enzymes will be attracted to the damaged site and the cell will go into cell cycle arrest to allow time for repair. It is well known that the number of γ-H2AX foci is proportional to the amount of DSBs (12–14). By immunofluorescent staining of the γ-H2AX foci, quantitative and qualitative evaluation of the damage can be performed. A previous in vitro study investigating the differential effect of high- and low-LET radiation has shown that the initial formation (as early as 15 min) of γ-H2AX foci is similar for equal doses of different beam qualities (15). However, repair kinetics (investigated at later time points) have shown a delayed or less successful repair of DSBs after high-LET radiation (16, 17). Therefore, particle irradiation can be effective in inducing cell death even in highly radioresistant cells (18). One of the factors that plays a major role in determining radiosensitivity is p53. Mutations or deletions in the p53 gene can lead to the radioresistance of cancer cells to conventional radiotherapy (19–22). By contrast, previous studies with high-LET radiation have shown that this type of radiation can induce apoptosis effectively regardless of p53 gene status (7, 23).

In vitro studies comparing the effect of particle or photon irradiation have shown a more pronounced cell cycle arrest induced by particles (24, 25). Furthermore, it has been shown that cells are more sensitive to the induction of DSBs by X-irradiation during the G2/M-phase of the cell cycle (26). Contrarily, the radiation sensitivity of cancer cells irradiated with particles is less, but not entirely, dependent on the cell cycle stage (27). Thus, particle beam therapy is more suitable to damage a heterogeneous tumor population, consisting of cells in different cell cycle stages (24).

We previously investigated the transcriptional response of PC3 and Caco-2 cells after X- and carbon ion irradiation, in which we observed more pronounced changes in gene expression after carbon ion irradiation. Genome-wide analysis in PC3 cells showed that gene sets involved in cell cycle regulation and, interestingly, also in motility processes were found to be modulated, especially after carbon ion irradiation (28). In a next step, we further investigated the changes of genes involved in motility processes. Our results showed that the magnitude of expression of these genes was time- and dose-dependent for both PC3 and Caco-2 cells, although a cell-type-specific response to X- and carbon ion irradiation was observed (29). With regard to the changes in cell cycle-related gene sets, we further aimed to investigate the acute cellular responses induced by different radiation qualities. Therefore, in this study, we examined both DNA repair kinetics and cell cycle progression in PC3 and Caco-2 cells in response to carbon ion or X-irradiation. Cells were irradiated with different doses ranging from 0.1 up to 5 Gy depending on the type of radiation. DNA damage and repair kinetics were analyzed up to 24 h after irradiation and cell cycle progression up to 72 h after irradiation. Further elucidation of the effect of different beam qualities on different cancer cell lines will contribute to a better understanding of which therapy would be most suited for these types of cancers.

MATERIALS AND METHODS

Cell Culture

Human prostate adenocarcinoma cells (PC3; ATCC® CRL-1435™) and colorectal adenocarcinoma cells (Caco-2; ATCC® HTB-37™) were obtained from the American Type Culture Collection (ATCC, Molsheim Cedex, France). PC3 cells were cultured in Kaighn's Modification of Ham's F-12 Medium (F-12K) (ATCC) supplemented with 10% fetal bovine serum (FBS) (GIBCO, Life Technologies, Ghent, Belgium), as specifically recommended by ATCC. Caco-2 cells were cultured in Dulbecco's Modified Eagle medium (DMEM) (GIBCO) supplemented with 10% FBS and 1% non-essential amino acids (GIBCO). Cell cultures were maintained in a humidified incubator (37°C; 5% CO_2). For all irradiation experiments, the same passage number of cells was used. Cell doubling time was 26 and 20 h for PC3 and Caco-2 cells, respectively (data not shown). Cell cultures were regularly tested for mycoplasma contamination (DSMZ, Braunschweig, Germany).

X-irradiation

X-irradiation experiments were performed at the irradiation facility available at SCK•CEN (Mol, Belgium). Medium was replaced prior to irradiation in a horizontal position. Cells were exposed to different doses of X-rays (0, 0.1, 0.5, 1, 2, and 5 Gy) using a Pantak HF420 RX machine (250 kV, 15 mA, 1.2 mm Aluminum equivalent, 1 mm Cu-filtered X-rays, and a calculated dose rate of 0.25 Gy/min). The beam quality of H-250 (as recommended by ISO 4037-1) was used. This beam quality was created using a tube voltage of 250 kV and 1 mm Cu additional filtration. The secondary standard for X-rays is the NE2571 0.6 cc ionization chamber SN309 connected to Keithley 6517B SN1335646 electrometer. The calibration of this chamber in terms of air Kerma (K_{air}), for H-250 beam quality, was done in 2013 at the primary standard laboratory PTB, Germany. The reference quantity is K_{air} in one point, taken as the reference position of the irradiated sample, which typically is its center. No correction is done for the extended volume and self-absorption of the sample itself and such effect is not included in the uncertainties budget either. The irradiation is based on the ISO 4037 standard. All uncertainties are the expanded uncertainties for $k = 2$ (confidence level 95%). The dose rate was measured for each distance, by using repeatedly the same distance, one relies on stability from 1 day to another and, therefore, only periodic checks of beam stability are performed at the irradiation facility.

Carbon Ion Irradiation

For our experiment, we were assigned ^{13}C beam time at the Grand Accélérateur National d'Ions Lourds (GANIL) (Caen, France). Cells were transported by car in a transportable incubator at 37°C to GANIL. For all assays, 10^5 cells were plated in 12.5 cm^2-tissue culture flasks (Falcon; VWR; Leuven, Belgium) 3 days before transport, during which all culture flasks were completely filled with medium. After arrival, medium was changed, and cells were placed overnight in a humidified incubator. Before the irradiation, culture flasks were completely filled with medium to allow irradiation in a vertical position, perpendicular to a horizontal carbon ion beam. The cells were irradiated with a ^{13}C beam with an initial energy of 75 MeV/u (LET = 33.7 keV/μm). The applied doses were 0, 0.5, 1, and 2 Gy. Carbon ion dosimetry was performed as previously described (28, 30). The RBE of carbon ions at 10% survival was 1.67 for PC3 cells and 1.83 for Caco-2 cells (29).

Immunocytochemistry for γ-H2AX

For X-irradiation experiments, cells were plated on coverslips at a density of 20,000 cells/well and grown for 2 days. Due to practical reasons, samples were irradiated in T12.5 flasks for the carbon ion irradiation (vertical position). Irradiation with both radiation qualities was then performed with a series of doses as mentioned before. At various time points after irradiation (30 min, 1, 2, 4, 8, and 24 h), cells were fixed in 4% paraformaldehyde (Merck KGaA, Darmstadt, Germany) for at least 20 min at 4°C. Afterwards, cells were washed with PBS and permeabilized in 0.25% Triton (Sigma-Aldrich Co.) in PBS for 3 min. Subsequently, cells were probed with mouse anti-γ-H2AX antibody (ab26350, Abcam, Cambridge, UK) (1:300 dilution) and incubated overnight at 4°C. Next, the cells were washed with PBS and stained with Alexa Fluor 488 goat anti-mouse (H + L)-labeled antibody (A11001, Invitrogen, Life

technologies) (1:300 dilution) for 2 h at room temperature. All antibody dilutions were prepared in 3% bovine serum albumin (BSA). Following this, three washing steps were performed with PBS after which a cover glass was mounted on the samples with Vectashield containing 4′,6-diamidino-2-phenylindole (DAPI) (Vector Laboratories, Brussels, Belgium).

Automated Fluorescence Microscopy and Image Analysis

Images were acquired with a Nikon Eclipse Ti (automated inverted wide-field epifluorescence microscope) equipped with a 40× magnification (Plan Fluor, numerical aperture 1.3) oil objective and a Nikon TE2000-E camera controlled by the NIS Elements software. The images were taken in the same orientation as the irradiation was performed, i.e., the viewer position was perpendicular to the cellular plane. Per condition a mosaic of 25 fields was acquired with a lateral spacing of 190 μm between fields (corresponding to the size of the field of view) and each field was acquired as a z-stack of nine planes axially separated by 1 μm. Images were analyzed with Fiji software (31) using the InSCyDe-02 toolbox. The software allowed to analyze each nucleus based on the DAPI signal. Within each nucleus, pixel size and intensity emitted from the Alexa 488 fluorochrome were analyzed after which the γ-H2AX foci number per nucleus and the foci occupancy are determined in a fully automatic manner. These data were then used to count the radiation-induced damage, i.e., subtract the damage of control cells from irradiated cells. As mentioned before, for carbon ion irradiation experiments, cells were seeded in T12.5 flasks (plastic surface) since these samples were irradiated in a vertical position. X-irradiated samples were seeded on glass cover slips for γ-H2AX. As a result, image quality was less good for carbon ion samples, and as a consequence Fiji software was unable to correctly count the number of spots in each nucleus for the carbon ion-irradiated samples. Therefore, we decided to count the spots manually for the carbon ion samples. At least 170 and 100 nuclei were analyzed per sample for X-ray and carbon ion irradiation, respectively.

Cell Cycle Analysis

Cells were collected at 24, 48, and 72 h after irradiation by use of trypsinization. In addition, supernatants and PBS used during wash steps were kept as well to ensure the collection of both adherent and detached cells. After collection, samples were fixed in a cold 80% EtOH solution at 4°C for at least 1 h. Fixed samples obtained in GANIL were transported back to SCK•CEN for further processing. Next, samples were washed with PBS and stained with a 500 μl propidium iodide (PI) solution (50 μg/ml PI + 1% RNase A) (Sigma-Aldrich Co. LLC; Bornem; Belgium) for 50 min at 37°C. Samples were measured immediately afterwards by flow cytometry (Accuri C6 system; BD Biosciences, Erembodegem, Belgium). PI fluorescence of a minimum of 10,000 cells was measured. Cells in G0/G1, S, and G2/M-phase were determined after filtering for doublets and aggregates. Doublets were filtered based on a FSC-A vs. FSC-H dot plot with Accuri C6 software. In addition, sub G1 cells were identified as cells with a DNA content of between half the mean value of G1 phase and the minimum value of G1 phase. Based on the histogram, we determined the peak of G1, on which the settings were placed in such a way that 90% falls within the peak. The peak of G2 needs to be 2 × G1 and also for this the settings were placed in such a way that 90% falls within the peak. Everything in-between was seen as S-phase. Everything in-between 0.5 × G1 and the beginning of G1 phase was the sub G1 peak. Re-analysis of samples was performed with ModFit LT software (Verity Software House, Topsham, ME, USA). Representative histograms are visualized in **Figure 1**.

Statistical Analysis

Cell cycle data were analyzed by two-way analysis of variance (ANOVA) with dose and time point as independent variables. Analysis of γ-H2AX foci count data was performed using Kruskal–Wallis and *post hoc* Dunn's multiple comparison tests. All analyses were performed using GraphPad Prism 5.00 software. For all tests, a value of $p < 0.05$ was considered statistically significant.

RESULTS

DNA Damage and Repair Kinetics

DNA DSBs were visualized by immunofluorescent staining for γ-H2AX foci that were analyzed at various time points (30 min, 1, 2, 4, 8, and 24 h) after irradiation. Representative images of the γ-H2AX foci for both PC3 and Caco-2 are shown in **Figure 2**. We counted both the number of radiation-induced foci, as a measure of DSBs, and the foci occupancy because H2AX

phosphorylation as well as the size of foci differs throughout the cell cycle (32). Upon irradiation, a clear dose-dependent induction in the number and nuclear occupancy of foci was observed. A significant dose-dependent increase in foci number was detected after X-irradiation in PC3 cells as early as 30 min after irradiation (**Figure 3A**). Increased foci numbers induced by irradiation were associated with a higher percentage of the area of the nucleus covered by foci as seen in the elevated foci occupancy (**Figure 3B**). A follow-up of foci number and foci occupancy over time evidenced time-dependent repair of foci (**Figures 3A,B**). Maximum foci numbers were detected 1 h after X-irradiation (**Figure 3A**), after which repair seems to have initiated. Interestingly, most γ-H2AX foci were repaired 24 h after X-irradiation with doses up to 0.5 Gy, while residual foci were still visible after exposure to higher X-ray doses (**Figures 3A,B**). For carbon ion irradiation, the number of foci was still significantly elevated at 24 h after irradiation after all doses in PC3 cells (**Figure 3C**). Maximum foci numbers were detected 1 h after irradiation with carbon ions. A similar trend was observed for the foci occupancy in PC3 cells (**Figure 3D**).

Similar results were observed for the Caco-2 cells. More specifically, a dose-dependent increase in foci number was observed as early as 30 min after X-irradiation (**Figure 4A**). This increase was accompanied by an increase in foci occupancy (**Figure 4B**). Maximum foci numbers were observed at 1 to 2 h after X-irradiation after which a time-dependent repair was evidenced (**Figure 4A**). For the Caco-2 cells, 24 h after X-irradiation residual foci were still present for doses up to 1 Gy (**Figure 4A**).

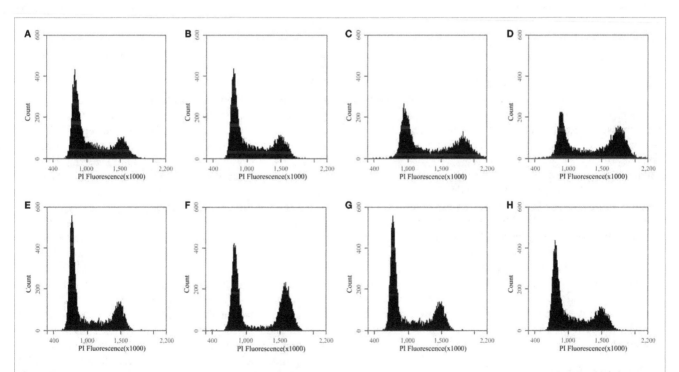

FIGURE 1 | Distribution of PC3 and Caco-2 cells in the different phases of the cell cycle. Distribution of PC3 cells in the cell cycle for control **(A)** and 2 Gy X-ray irradiated **(B)** samples 24 h after irradiation. Distribution of Caco-2 cells in the cell cycle for control **(C)** and 2 Gy X-ray-irradiated **(D)** samples 24 h after irradiation. Distribution of PC3 cells in the cell cycle for control **(E)** and 2 Gy carbon ion-irradiated **(F)** samples 24 h after irradiation. Distribution of Caco-2 cells in the cell cycle for control **(G)** and 2 Gy carbon ion-irradiated **(H)** samples 24 h after irradiation.

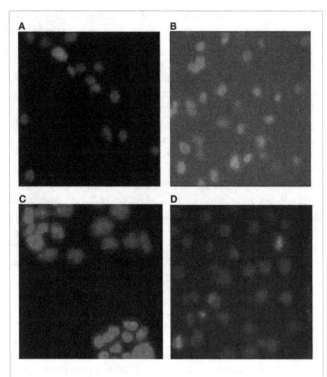

FIGURE 2 | γ-H2AX foci in PC3 and Caco-2 cells after irradiation with X-rays or carbon ions. Representative images of γ-H2AX foci in PC3 cells 1 h after 2 Gy X-irradiation **(A)** and 1 h after 2 Gy carbon ion irradiation **(B)**. Representative images of γ-H2AX foci in Caco-2 cells 1 h after 2 Gy X-irradiation **(C)** and 1 h after 2 Gy carbon ion irradiation **(D)**. Images were acquired with a Nikon Eclipse Ti (automated inverted wide-field epifluorescence microscope) equipped with a 40x magnification (Plan Fluor, numerical aperture 1.3) oil objective and a Nikon TE2000-E camera controlled by the NIS Elements software.

Similar observations were made for carbon ion-irradiated Caco-2 cells, where significantly elevated foci number were still observed 24 h after irradiation for all doses (**Figure 4C**). Maximum foci numbers were already detected 30 min after irradiation with carbon ions. Foci occupancy was also significantly elevated 24 h after 0.5 and 2 Gy of carbon ion irradiation in Caco-2 cells (**Figure 4D**).

For carbon ion experiments, we additionally correlated the number of γ-H2AX foci with the number of ion traversals (**Table 1**). This was calculated by dividing the nuclear area of the cells (PC3 or Caco-2) by the fluence (different for each dose). The higher the number of ions passing the cell nucleus, the higher the number of foci that we counted after carbon ion irradiation. In addition, the (slightly) higher number of ions that pass the cell nucleus for Caco-2 cells compared to PC3 cells correlates with the higher number of foci that were counted in Caco-2 cells compared to PC3 cells 30 min after carbon ion irradiation.

Cell Cycle Analysis

Radiation-induced cell cycle changes were analyzed by flow cytometry at 24, 48, and 72 h after X- and carbon ion irradiation

using PI staining. Representative histograms are shown in **Figure 1** for both PC3 and Caco-2 cells.

In PC3 cells, 5 Gy of X-irradiation resulted in an increase of the percentage of cells in G2 phase (~10%) at all time points at the expense of G1 cells (**Figure 5A**), suggestive of a persistent G2/M arrest. Lower doses of X-rays did not affect the cell cycle of PC3 cells. On the other hand, carbon ion irradiation of PC3 cells resulted in a significant increase of cells in G2/M-phase, 24 h after 2 Gy and 48 and 72 h after both 1 and 2 Gy (**Figure 5B**). This was combined with a decrease in cells in G1 phase at all time points both at 1 and 2 Gy. After 1 Gy carbon ion irradiation, significant changes in the fraction of S-phase cells were found after 24 and 48 h.

In Caco-2 cells, a dose of 2 and 5 Gy of X-rays increased the number of cells in G2/M-phase, although only transiently (**Figure 5C**). This was combined with a decrease in the number of cells in G1 for both doses and a decrease in cells in S-phase for 5-Gy X-irradiation. After 48 and 72 h, the G2/M arrest was resolved in Caco-2 cells irradiated with X-rays. However, a small but significant decrease (almost 4%) in G1 phase cells was found at 72 h after 5-Gy X-irradiation. Irradiation of Caco-2 cells with 2 Gy of carbon ions resulted in a persistent G2/M arrest, accompanied by a decrease of cells in G1 phase (**Figure 5D**). At the earliest time point, this could also be observed after 1 Gy carbon ion irradiation.

DISCUSSION

From a physical point of view, the rationale for the use of particle irradiation in cancer therapy has been clear for a very long time. Along with the positive patient responses observed in clinical trials using particle therapy, it has been of increasing interest to understand and unravel the underlying biological mechanisms and pathways involved by means of *in vitro* studies. Important differences between both radiation qualities in DNA damage and subsequent cell cycle arrest have been indicated (33), which explain the higher RBE induced by particle radiation. In this study, we investigated changes in DNA damage and repair kinetics of PC3 and Caco-2 cell lines exposed to carbon ion or X-irradiation. In addition, cell cycle stages in both cell lines were analyzed. We observed an increase in γ-H2AX foci number and foci occupancy after X-irradiation with some interesting differences between both cell lines. The initial induction of γ-H2AX was similar for both cell lines although foci occupancy was higher in PC3 cells than in Caco-2 cells after exposure to X-rays. One explanation for this could be the difference in radiosensitivity between both cell lines, as we previously observed (29). Exposure to carbon ions resulted in a higher initial induction of γ-H2AX foci for Caco-2 cells compared to PC3 cells. In samples exposed to X-rays relatively less residual damage after 24 h was observed in Caco-2 cells compared to PC3 cells (mean foci count after 5 Gy was 25 foci after 30 min and 20 foci after 24 h in PC3 cells, and 26 foci after 30 min and 8 foci after 24 h in Caco-2 cells). This lower residual damage observed in Caco-2 cells after X-irradiation can also be linked to a higher surviving fraction of Caco-2 cells compared to PC3 cells as we observed previously (29).

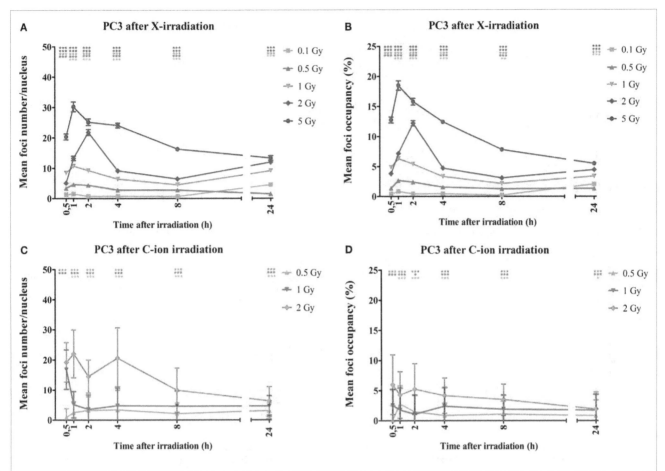

FIGURE 3 | Quantification of γ-H2AX foci number and occupancy in X- and carbon ion-irradiated PC3 cells. Dots representing mean γ-H2AX foci number per nucleus vs. time **(A)** and mean foci occupancy per nucleus vs. time **(B)** after X-irradiation in PC3 cells. Dots representing mean γ-H2AX foci number per nucleus vs. time **(C)** and mean foci occupancy per nucleus vs. time **(D)** after exposure to carbon ions. Fiji software was used to count the number of nuclei and foci occupancy in each nucleus. The number of foci in non-irradiated cells was subtracted from that of irradiated cells for each dose and time point. For X-rays, the error bars represent the SEM of three independent experiments; for carbon ion data, the error bars represent STDEV of the experiment. Statistical Kruskal–Wallis analysis with Dunn's multiple comparison tests were performed in GraphPad with $*p < 0.05$ (vs. control cells), $**p < 0.01$ (vs. control cells), and $***p < 0.001$ (vs. control cells).

We found no reports on γ-H2AX analysis of irradiated Caco-2 cells and only one for PC3 cells (34). They irradiated confluent PC3 cells with 2 Gy X-rays and visualized γ-H2AX foci after 30 min and 24 h. After 30 min, 10 foci were observed after 2 Gy of X-rays, compared to 5 foci in our PC3 cells. However 24 h after exposure we found a higher residual number of γ-H2AX foci in the PC3 cells (i.e., 7 foci observed by van Oorschot vs. 12 foci observed in our study). One explanation for this could be the different set-up of the experiment; more specifically van Oorschot et al. used a dose rate of 3 Gy/min, whereas we used a dose rate of 0.25 Gy/min. Another explanation could be a difference in the confluence of the irradiated cells, which could synchronize the cells in a certain phase making the cells more or less resistant to the effect of (X-ray) irradiation.

Our data showed that 30 min after exposure to carbon ions, a higher number of foci were induced at a therapeutic dose of 2 Gy compared to X-rays. More specifically, in PC3 cells, we observed five radiation-induced foci after irradiation with 2 Gy of X-rays compared to 19 foci after an equal dose of carbon ions. For Caco-2

cells, the number of radiation-induced foci after 2 Gy of X-rays and carbon ions was 8 and 30, respectively. This is in contrast to a study by Ghosh et al. (15) in which A549 cells were irradiated with γ-rays (1, 2, or 3 Gy) or ^{12}C ions (1 Gy, 5.2 MeV/u; LET = 290 keV/μm). They observed that equal doses of both radiation qualities induced similar numbers of foci 15 min after irradiation.

A closer look at the residual foci number (at 24 h) after 2 Gy irradiations shows that less foci are detected in carbon ion-irradiated PC3 samples compared to X-ray samples (i.e., increase of 6 foci after carbon ion irradiation; increase of 12 foci after X-rays;). However, we should note that samples exposed to carbon ions were irradiated in a vertical position, perpendicular to the irradiation beam. Since carbon ion irradiation is expected to induce more complex damage along the ionization tracks, more foci would be present behind one another along the Z-axis. This could explain why although less foci are counted in general and less are present after 24 h, the residual damage could still be more complex, which, in turn, explains the persistent G2/M arrest we observed after both 1 and 2 Gy carbon ion irradiation.

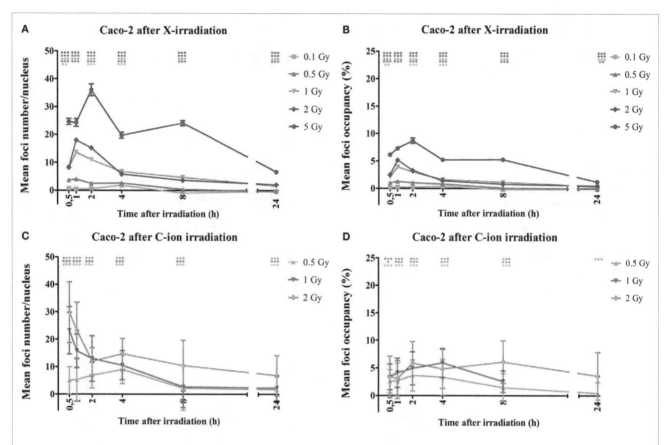

FIGURE 4 | Quantification of γ-H2AX foci number and occupancy in X- and carbon ion-irradiated Caco-2 cells. Dots representing mean γ-H2AX foci number per nucleus vs. time **(A)** and mean foci occupancy per nucleus vs. time **(B)** after X-irradiation in Caco-2 cells. Dots representing mean γ-H2AX foci number per nucleus vs. time **(C)** and mean foci occupancy per nucleus vs. time **(D)** after exposure to carbon ions. Fiji software was used to count the number of nuclei and foci occupancy in each nucleus. For X-rays, the error bars represent the SEM of three independent experiments; for carbon ion data, the error bars represent STDEV of the experiment. Statistical Kruskal–Wallis analysis with Dunn's multiple comparison tests were performed in GraphPad with **p < 0.01 (vs. control cells), ***p < 0.001 (vs. control cells).

TABLE 1 | Ion traversals per cell nucleus were calculated for PC3 and Caco-2 and compared to the results of γ-H2AX foci 30 min after carbon ion exposure.

	PC3		Caco-2	
	Number of traversals calculated	Number of foci counted after 30 min	Number of traversals calculated	Number of foci counted after 30 min
0.5 Gy	12.5	0.9	15.9	5.1
1 Gy	25.1	16.7	31.7	23.2
2 Gy	49.9	19.2	63.1	29.8

The number of traversals was calculated by dividing the nuclear area of the cells (PC3 or Caco-2) by the fluence (different for each dose). Nuclear area for PC3 cells was on average 134.7 μm and for Caco-2 cells 170.5 μm.

Additionally, because we analyzed the foci in the same direction as the position of the irradiation beam, it is possible that spots overlapped, causing the foci number to be lower than expected (35). Similar observations were made by a study of Rall et al. in which human blood-derived cells were irradiated with 2 Gy of high-LET irradiation (iron ions, LET = 155 keV/μm). Because of the higher RBE of iron ions, a higher induction of γ-H2AX

foci for iron ion-irradiated samples compared to the X-ray irradiated samples was expected, but not observed. The authors hypothesized that the formation of γ-H2AX foci along the beam track has a limited resolution, leading to lower foci numbers (12, 36, 37). In Caco-2 cells, however, we measured lower levels of residual γ-H2AX foci after 24 h in X-irradiated samples compared to carbon ions (i.e., increase of 2 foci after 2 Gy X-rays; increase of 7 foci after 2 Gy carbon ion irradiation). Also here, damage is expected to be more complex and could, therefore, be responsible for the persistent G2/M arrest induced by carbon ions, which was not observed after X-irradiation.

As could be expected, carbon ion irradiation was more potent in inducing cell cycle arrest as compared to equal doses of X-ray irradiation. A persistent G2/M arrest was observed in PC3 cells, already after a dose of 1 Gy of carbon ions. By contrast, only a dose of 5 Gy X-rays was able to induce a persistent cell cycle arrest in PC3 cells (up to 72 h post irradiation). For Caco-2 cells, 2 Gy carbon ion irradiation was capable of inducing a persistent G2/M arrest, whereas after X-radiation Caco-2 cells seemed to escape from the G2/M arrest 48 h after irradiation. These differences indicate the potency of particle radiation to induce more severe

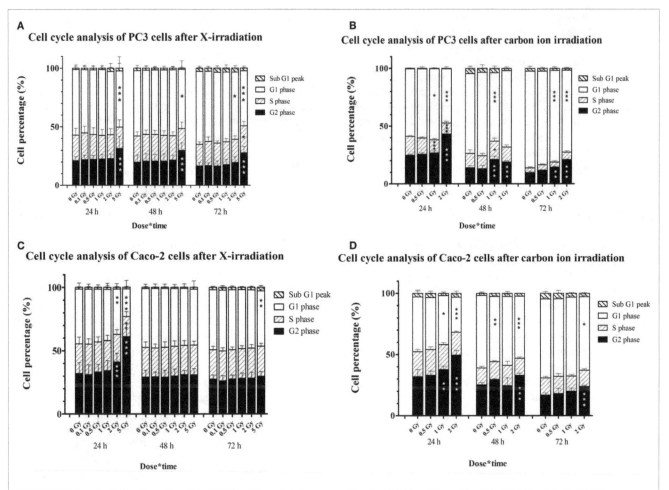

FIGURE 5 | Cell cycle distribution of irradiated PC3 and Caco-2 cells assessed by PI staining and flow cytometry. Stacked graphs representing percentages of cells per cell cycle phase in PC3 cells irradiated with X-rays **(A)** or carbon ions **(B)** and in Caco-2 cells irradiated with X-rays **(C)** or carbon ions **(D)**. Bars represent an average of three experiments for X-irradiated samples and one experiment for the carbon ion-irradiated samples. Statistical two-way ANOVA with Bonferroni *post hoc* test was performed in GraphPad Prism with *$p < 0.05$ (vs. control cells), **$p < 0.01$, and ***$p < 0.001$ (vs. control cells).

damage that can lead to (persistent) cell cycle arrest. In Caco-2 cells, a transient G2/M arrest was observed after X-irradiation; whereas in PC3 cells, this arrest persisted until 72 h after exposure. These different results could be explained by the lower residual DNA damage that we observed after 24 h in Caco-2 cells compared to PC3 cells. Another explanation could be the difference in doubling time between both cell lines, where PC3 cells have a higher doubling time compared to Caco-2 cells.

To our knowledge, no previous studies investigated the effect of particle irradiation on cell cycle progression of Caco-2 cells, while only one study investigated cell cycle changes in PC3 cells after proton irradiation (38). In their study, cells were exposed to 10, 20, or 40 Gy of either photon or proton irradiation. With regard to cell cycle changes, they observed a less pronounced and delayed G2/M arrest after photons compared to proton irradiation. This is consistent with our and previously published results comparing various cell lines irradiated with different beam qualities (25, 39–42). However, most of these studies only focused on cell cycle changes up to 24 h post irradiation. We analyzed as far as

72 h after irradiation and found that, compared to X-rays, a lower equal dose of carbon ions was sufficient to induce a permanent G2/M arrest in PC3 cells. For Caco-2 cells however, a qualitative difference in cell cycle arrest was observed. To this regard, we demonstrated that a lower dose of carbon ion particles was capable of inducing a persistent arrest that was not present after X-rays.

Differences in repair kinetics between X- and carbon ion irradiation, as we observed here, might be an indication of activation of different DNA repair pathways due to differences in the complexity of the DNA damage (37, 43, 44). In this context, it is also important to note that the genetic background of the tumor will influence the effectiveness of radiotherapy. The cell lines we used in this study do not express p53, as described in the literature (45–48) and this lack of p53 expression was confirmed for both our cell lines (data not shown). As mentioned before, p53 is normally activated in response to DNA damage and induces cell cycle arrest. Since p53 can control both G2/M and G1 cell cycle check points (49, 50), our data suggest that, at higher doses of X-rays, p53-independent mechanisms are responsible for the observed G2/M arrest. This may partly explain the radioresistance of both cell lines to X-ray therapy. Previous studies have shown that carbon ion-induced cell killing is independent of the p53 status (7, 51–53). On the other hand, the repair of γ-H2AX foci, which can be observed 24 h after exposure, also indicates that p53-independent repair mechanisms are still active within these cell lines. Importantly, our observation that the threshold for p53-independent cell cycle arrest is reached after exposure to lower doses of carbon ion irradiation, while DNA damage repair is less efficient, suggests that carbon ion radiotherapy could be more appropriate to treat radioresistant tumors with a mutated p53 status.

CONCLUSION

In the present study, we investigated the acute cellular responses after carbon ion and X-ray exposure in two p53-defective cancer cell lines. First, our results indicate that a higher amount of initial DNA damage is induced by carbon ion irradiation compared to X-irradiation, even when lower doses are used. In addition, repair kinetics of γ-H2AX foci of Caco-2 cells showed relatively more residual DNA damage at 24 h after carbon ion irradiation compared to X-irradiation. Second, cell cycle progression assays demonstrated a persistent cell cycle arrest of PC3 cells, which was induced by lower equal doses of carbon ion compared to X-irradiation. In Caco-2 cells, a persistent arrest was induced by carbon ions but not by X-irradiation. Further research is needed to better understand how different radiation qualities influence acute cellular responses, which are in part responsible for the increased biological effectiveness of particle beam irradiation.

AUTHOR CONTRIBUTIONS

AS performed experiments both at SCK•CEN and GANIL. KK performed experiments at SCK•CEN. MM designed the experimental set-up and performed experiments at GANIL. VG contributed to the design of the work. SB contributed to the design of the work, as well as with interpretation of obtained data. All co-authors critically reviewed and approved the final version to be submitted to this Journal.

ACKNOWLEDGMENTS

We would like to thank the iPAC committee of the Grand Accélérateur National d'Ions Lourds (GANIL, Caen, France) for the carbon ion beam time granted (P911-H) and the staff of the LARIA, CIRIL (GANIL) for allowing us access to and use of their facility. We also thank Bart Marlein and Ludo Melis for their continued assistance during the X-irradiations at SCK•CEN. We thank Winnok de Vos for the InSCyDe-02 toolbox used in Fiji. We are grateful to Vanessa Bol, Stefaan Vynckier and Pierre Scalliet (UCL) for their guidance in dosimetry and feedback on the experimental design.

FUNDING

This work was partly supported by the Federal Public Service in the context of the feasibility study "Application of hadrontherapy in Belgium," which is part of action 30 of the Belgian cancer plan (CO-90-2088-01), the ESA/BELSPO/Prodex IMPULSE contract (CO-90-11-2801-03). KK is a recipient of a SCK•CEN-KUL PhD grant, and AS is a recipient of a SCK•CEN-UCL PhD grant.

REFERENCES

1. Degiovanni A, Amaldi U. History of hadron therapy accelerators. *Phys Med* (2015) **31**:322–32. doi:10.1016/j.ejmp.2015.03.002
2. Karger CP, Jakel O. Current status and new developments in ion therapy. *Strahlenther Onkol* (2007) **183**:295–300. doi:10.1007/s00066-007-1645-x
3. Kramer M, Weyrather WK, Scholz M. The increased biological effectiveness of heavy charged particles: from radiobiology to treatment planning. *Technol Cancer Res Treat* (2003) **2**:427–36. doi:10.1177/153303460300200507
4. Asaithamby A, Uematsu N, Chatterjee A, Story MD, Burma S, Chen DJ. Repair of HZE-particle-induced DNA double-strand breaks in normal human fibroblasts. *Radiat Res* (2008) **169**:437–46. doi:10.1667/RR1165.1
5. Hada M, Georgakilas AG. Formation of clustered DNA damage after high-LET irradiation: a review. *J Radiat Res* (2008) **49**:203–10. doi:10.1269/jrr.07123
6. Ward JF. The complexity of DNA damage: relevance to biological consequences. *Int J Radiat Biol* (1994) **66**:427–32. doi:10.1080/09553009414551401
7. Iwadate Y, Mizoe J, Osaka Y, Yamaura A, Tsujii H. High linear energy transfer carbon radiation effectively kills cultured glioma cells with either mutant or wild-type p53. *Int J Radiat Oncol Biol Phys* (2001) **50**:803–8. doi:10.1016/S0360-3016(01)01514-0
8. Wada S, Kobayashi Y, Funayama T, Natsuhori M, Ito N, Yamamoto K. Detection of DNA damage in individual cells induced by heavy-ion irradiation with an non-denaturing comet assay. *J Radiat Res* (2002) **43**(Suppl):S153–6. doi:10.1269/jrr.43.S153
9. Kinner A, Wu W, Staudt C, Iliakis G. Gamma-H2AX in recognition and signaling of DNA double-strand breaks in the context of chromatin. *Nucleic Acids Res* (2008) **36**:5678–94. doi:10.1093/nar/gkn550

10. Rogakou EP, Pilch DR, Orr AH, Ivanova VS, Bonner WM. DNA double-stranded breaks induce histone H2AX phosphorylation on serine 139. *J Biol Chem* (1998) **273**:5858–68. doi:10.1074/jbc.273.10.5858
11. Kastan MB, Onyekwere O, Sidransky D, Vogelstein B, Craig RW. Participation of p53 protein in the cellular response to DNA damage. *Cancer Res* (1991) **51**:6304–11.
12. Costes SV, Boissiere A, Ravani S, Romano R, Parvin B, Barcellos-Hoff MH. Imaging features that discriminate between foci induced by high- and low-LET radiation in human fibroblasts. *Radiat Res* (2006) **165**:505–15. doi:10.1667/RR3538.1
13. Rothkamm K, Lobrich M. Evidence for a lack of DNA double-strand break repair in human cells exposed to very low x-ray doses. *Proc Natl Acad Sci U S A* (2003) **100**:5057–62. doi:10.1073/pnas.0830918100
14. Sedelnikova OA, Rogakou EP, Panyutin IG, Bonner WM. Quantitative detection of (125)IdU-induced DNA double-strand breaks with gamma-H2AX antibody. *Radiat Res* (2002) **158**:486–92. doi:10.1667/0033-7587(2002)158[0486:QDOIID]2.0.CO;2
15. Ghosh S, Narang H, Sarma A, Krishna M. DNA damage response signaling in lung adenocarcinoma A549 cells following gamma and carbon beam irradiation. *Mutat Res* (2011) **716**:10–9. doi:10.1016/j.mrfmmm.2011.07.015
16. Autsavapromporn N, Suzuki M, Plante I, Liu C, Uchihori Y, Hei TK, et al. Participation of gap junction communication in potentially lethal damage repair and DNA damage in human fibroblasts exposed to low- or high-LET radiation. *Mutat Res* (2013) **756**:78–85. doi:10.1016/j.mrgentox.2013.07.001
17. Rydberg B, Cooper B, Cooper PK, Holley WR, Chatterjee A. Dose-dependent misrejoining of radiation-induced DNA double-strand breaks in human fibroblasts: experimental and theoretical study for high- and low-LET radiation. *Radiat Res* (2005) **163**:526–34. doi:10.1667/RR3346

18. Hofman-Huther H, Scholz M, Rave-Frank M, Virsik-Kopp P. Induction of reproductive cell death and chromosome aberrations in radioresistant tumour cells by carbon ions. *Int J Radiat Biol* (2004) **80**:423–35. doi:10.1080/095530 00410001702319

19. Fan S, el-Deiry WS, Bae I, Freeman J, Jondle D, Bhatia K, et al. p53 gene mutations are associated with decreased sensitivity of human lymphoma cells to DNA damaging agents. *Cancer Res* (1994) **54**:5824–30.

20. McIlwrath AJ, Vasey PA, Ross GM, Brown R. Cell cycle arrests and radio-sensitivity of human tumor cell lines: dependence on wild-type p53 for radiosensitivity. *Cancer Res* (1994) **54**:3718–22.

21. O'Connor PM, Jackman J, Jondle D, Bhatia K, Magrath I, Kohn KW. Role of the p53 tumor suppressor gene in cell cycle arrest and radiosensitivity of Burkitt's lymphoma cell lines. *Cancer Res* (1993) **53**:4776–80.

22. Ribeiro JC, Barnetson AR, Fisher RJ, Mameghan H, Russell PJ. Relationship between radiation response and p53 status in human bladder cancer cells. *Int J Radiat Biol* (1997) **72**:11–20. doi:10.1080/095530097143491

23. Mori E, Takahashi A, Yamakawa N, Kirita T, Ohnishi T. High LET heavy ion radiation induces p53-independent apoptosis. *J Radiat Res* (2009) **50**:37–42. doi:10.1269/jrr.08075

24. Fournier C, Taucher-Scholz G. Radiation induced cell cycle arrest: an over-view of specific effects following high-LET exposure. *Radiother Oncol* (2004) **73**(Suppl 2):S119–22. doi:10.1016/S0167-8140(04)80031-8

25. Hu Y, Hellweg CE, Baumstark-Khan C, Reitz G, Lau P. Cell cycle delay in murine pre-osteoblasts is more pronounced after exposure to high-LET compared to low-LET radiation. *Radiat Environ Biophys* (2014) **53**:73–81. doi:10.1007/s00411-013-0499-0

26. Sinclair WK. Cyclic x-ray responses in mammalian cells in vitro. *Radiat Res* (1968) **33**:620–43. doi:10.2307/3572419

27. Linz U, editor. Ion beam therapy fundamentals, technology, clinical appli-cations. *Biological and Medical Physics, Biomedical Engineering*. Berlin, Heidelberg: Springer-Verlag (2012). XXXV, 729 p.

28. Suetens A, Moreels M, Quintens R, Chiriotti S, Tabury K, Michaux A, et al. Carbon ion irradiation of the human prostate cancer cell line PC3: a whole genome microarray study. *Int J Oncol* (2014) **44**:1056–72. doi:10.3892/ijo.2014.2287

29. Suetens A, Moreels M, Quintens R, Soors E, Buset J, Chiriotti S, et al. Dose- and time-dependent gene expression alterations in prostate and colon cancer cells after in vitro exposure to carbon ion and X-irradiation. *J Radiat Res* (2015) **56**:11–21. doi:10.1093/jrr/rru070

30. Durantel F, Balanzat E, Cassimi A, Chevalier F, Ngono-Ravache Y, Madi T, et al. Dosimetry for radiobiology experiments at GANIL. *Nucl Instrum Methods Phys Res A* (2016) **816**:70–7. doi:10.1016/j.nima.2016.01.052

31. Schindelin J, Arganda-Carreras I, Frise E, Kaynig V, Longair M, Pietzsch T, et al. Fiji: an open-source platform for biological-image analysis. *Nat Methods* (2012) **9**:676–82. doi:10.1038/nmeth.2019

32. Dieriks B, De Vos WH, Derradji H, Baatout S, Van Oostveldt P. Medium-mediated DNA repair response after ionizing radiation is correlated with the increase of specific cytokines in human fibroblasts. *Mutat Res* (2010) **687**:40–8. doi:10.1016/j.mrfmmm.2010.01.011

33. Castro JR. Results of heavy ion radiotherapy. *Radiat Environ Biophys* (1995) **34**:45–8. doi:10.1007/BF01210545

34. van Oorschot B, Hovingh SE, Rodermond H, Guclu A, Losekoot N, Geldof AA, et al. Decay of gamma-H2AX foci correlates with potentially lethal damage repair in prostate cancer cells. *Oncol Rep* (2013) **29**:2175–80. doi:10.3892/or.2013.2364

35. Nakajima NI, Brunton H, Watanabe R, Shrikhande A, Hirayama R, Matsufuji N, et al. Visualisation of gammaH2AX foci caused by heavy ion particle traversal; distinction between core track versus non-track damage. *PLoS One* (2013) **8**:e70107. doi:10.1371/journal.pone.0070107

36. Jakob B, Scholz M, Taucher-Scholz G. Biological imaging of heavy charged-particle tracks. *Radiat Res* (2003) **159**:676–84. doi:10.1667/0033-7587(2003)159[0676:BIOHCT]2.0.CO;2

37. Rall M, Kraft D, Volcic M, Cucu A, Nasonova E, Taucher-Scholz G, et al. Impact of charged particle exposure on homologous DNA double-strand break repair in human blood-derived cells. *Front Oncol* (2015) **5**:250. doi:10.3389/fonc.2015.00250

38. Di Pietro C, Piro S, Tabbi G, Ragusa M, Di Pietro V, Zimmitti V, et al. Cellular and molecular effects of protons: apoptosis induction and potential implications for cancer therapy. *Apoptosis* (2006) **11**:57–66. doi:10.1007/s10495-005-3346-1

39. Fokas E, Kraft G, An H, Engenhart-Cabillic R. Ion beam radiobiology and cancer: time to update ourselves. *Biochim Biophys Acta* (2009) **1796**:216–29. doi:10.1016/j.bbcan.2009.07.005

40. Ghorai A, Bhattacharyya NP, Sarma A, Ghosh U. Radiosensitivity and induction of apoptosis by high LET carbon ion beam and low LET gamma radiation: a comparative study. *Scientifica (Cairo)* (2014) **2014**:438030. doi:10.1155/2014/438030

41. Hamada N, Hara T, Omura-Minamisawa M, Funayama T, Sakashita T, Sora S, et al. Energetic heavy ions overcome tumor radioresistance caused by overexpression of Bcl-2. *Radiother Oncol* (2008) **89**:231–6. doi:10.1016/j.radonc.2008.02.013

42. Lucke-Huhle C, Blakely EA, Chang PY, Tobias CA. Drastic G2 arrest in mammalian cells after irradiation with heavy-ion beams. *Radiat Res* (1979) **79**:97–112. doi:10.2307/3575025

43. Gerelchuluun A, Manabe E, Ishikawa T, Sun L, Itoh K, Sakae T, et al. The major DNA repair pathway after both proton and carbon-ion radiation is NHEJ, but the HR pathway is more relevant in carbon ions. *Radiat Res* (2015) **183**:345–56. doi:10.1667/RR13904.1

44. Zafar F, Seidler SB, Kronenberg A, Schild D, Wiese C. Homologous recom-bination contributes to the repair of DNA double-strand breaks induced by high-energy iron ions. *Radiat Res* (2010) **173**:27–39. doi:10.1667/RR1910.1

45. Aryankalayil MJ, Makinde AY, Gameiro SR, Hodge JW, Rivera-Solis PP, Palayoor ST, et al. Defining molecular signature of pro-immunogenic radio-therapy targets in human prostate cancer cells. *Radiat Res* (2014) **182**:139–48. doi:10.1667/RR13731.1

46. Isaacs WB, Carter BS, Ewing CM. Wild-type p53 suppresses growth of human prostate cancer cells containing mutant p53 alleles. *Cancer Res* (1991) **51**:4716–20.

47. Liu Y, Bodmer WF. Analysis of P53 mutations and their expression in 56 colorectal cancer cell lines. *Proc Natl Acad Sci U S A* (2006) **103**:976–81. doi:10.1073/pnas.0510146103

48. Wang W, Heideman L, Chung CS, Pelling JC, Koehler KJ, Birt DF. Cell-cycle arrest at G2/M and growth inhibition by apigenin in human colon carcinoma cell lines. *Mol Carcinog* (2000) **28**:102–10. doi:10.1002/1098-2744(200006)28:2<102::AID-MC6>3.3.CO;2-U

49. Agarwal ML, Agarwal A, Taylor WR, Stark GR. p53 controls both the G2/M and the G1 cell cycle checkpoints and mediates reversible growth arrest in human fibroblasts. *Proc Natl Acad Sci U S A* (1995) **92**:8493–7. doi:10.1073/pnas.92.18.8493

50. Nayak B, Krishnegowda N, Galindo C, Meltz M, Swanson G. Synergistic effect between curcumin (diferuloylmethane) and radiation on clonogenic cell death independent of p53 in prostate cancer cells. *J Cancer Sci Ther* (2010) **2**:171–81. doi:10.4172/1948-5956.1000046

51. Amornwichet N, Oike T, Shibata A, Ogiwara H, Tsuchiya N, Yamauchi M, et al. Carbon-ion beam irradiation kills X-ray-resistant p53-null cancer cells by inducing mitotic catastrophe. *PLoS One* (2014) **9**:e115121. doi:10.1371/journal.pone.0115121

52. Takahashi A, Matsumoto H, Furusawa Y, Ohnishi K, Ishioka N, Ohnishi T. Apoptosis induced by high-LET radiations is not affected by cellular p53 gene status. *Int J Radiat Biol* (2005) **81**:581–6. doi:10.1080/09553000500280484

53. Takahashi T, Fukawa T, Hirayama R, Yoshida Y, Musha A, Furusawa Y, et al. In vitro interaction of high-LET heavy-ion irradiation and chemotherapeutic agents in two cell lines with different radiosensitivities and different p53 status. *Anticancer Res* (2010) **30**:1961–7.

20

Transcription Factors in the Cellular Response to Charged Particle Exposure

Christine E. Hellweg*, Luis F. Spitta, Bernd Henschenmacher, Sebastian Diegeler and Christa Baumstark-Khan

Cellular Biodiagnostics, Department of Radiation Biology, Institute of Aerospace Medicine, German Aerospace Centre (DLR), Cologne, Germany

Correspondence:
Christine E. Hellweg
christine.hellweg@dlr.de

Charged particles, such as carbon ions, bear the promise of a more effective cancer therapy. In human spaceflight, exposure to charged particles represents an important risk factor for chronic and late effects such as cancer. Biological effects elicited by charged particle exposure depend on their characteristics, e.g., on linear energy transfer (LET). For diverse outcomes (cell death, mutation, transformation, and cell-cycle arrest), an LET dependency of the effect size was observed. These outcomes result from activation of a complex network of signaling pathways in the DNA damage response, which result in cell-protective (DNA repair and cell-cycle arrest) or cell-destructive (cell death) reactions. Triggering of these pathways converges among others in the activation of transcription factors, such as p53, nuclear factor κB (NF-κB), activated protein 1 (AP-1), nuclear erythroid-derived 2-related factor 2 (Nrf2), and cAMP responsive element binding protein (CREB). Depending on dose, radiation quality, and tissue, p53 induces apoptosis or cell-cycle arrest. In low LET radiation therapy, p53 mutations are often associated with therapy resistance, while the outcome of carbon ion therapy seems to be independent of the tumor's p53 status. NF-κB is a central transcription factor in the immune system and exhibits pro-survival effects. Both p53 and NF-κB are activated after ionizing radiation exposure in an ataxia telangiectasia mutated (ATM)-dependent manner. The NF-κB activation was shown to strongly depend on charged particles' LET, with a maximal activation in the LET range of 90–300 keV/μm. AP-1 controls proliferation, senescence, differentiation, and apoptosis. Nrf2 can induce cellular antioxidant defense systems, CREB might also be involved in survival responses. The extent of activation of these transcription factors by charged particles and their interaction in the cellular radiation response greatly influences the destiny of the irradiated and also neighboring cells in the bystander effect.

Keywords: charged particles, p53, Nrf2, NF-κB, AP-1, Sp1, CREB, EGR-1

INTRODUCTION

Understanding the cellular radiation response is an essential prerequisite for improving cancer radiotherapy, including carbon ion therapy. The same holds true for the risk assessment of astronauts' and for effective countermeasure development.

Radiotherapy of cancer with protons and carbon ions profits from a more precise dose deposition with charged particle beams in the tumor and in the case of carbon ions, also a higher biological effectiveness in cell killing compared to conventional radiotherapy. There are hints that with carbon ions, cell killing is less dependent on factors such as oxygen concentration and alterations in cellular signaling pathways such as the p53 pathway.

Astronauts on exploration missions are subjected to not only greater amounts of natural radiation in space than they receive on Earth but also to a differing radiation quality, which can result in immediate and long-term risks. Besides protons and α-particles, heavier nuclei are part of the radiation field encountered in space. Heavy ions represent an important part of galactic cosmic rays because of their high biological effectiveness (1).

The radiation quality of energetic ions, including protons, α-particles, and heavy ions, is usually characterized by the linear energy transfer (LET) in matter which is a measure of the average energy transferred when an ionizing particle passes through matter and loses energy (2). Indirectly, it gives information about the ionization density along the particle track.

In the cellular response to radiation, several sensors detect the induced DNA damage and trigger signal transduction pathways, resulting in cell death or survival with or without mutations (3, 4). The activation of several signal transduction pathways by ionizing radiation (IR) results in altered expression of series of target genes. The promoters or enhancers of these genes may contain binding sites for one or more transcription factors, and a specific transcription factor can influence the transcription of multiple genes. A meta-analysis revealed that two p53-dependent genes, GADD45 (especially GADD45α) and CDKN1A, and genes associated with the NER pathway (e.g., XPC) are consistently upregulated by IR exposure (5). Importantly, the transcribed subset of target genes is critical for the decision between resuming normal function after cell-cycle arrest and DNA repair, entering senescence, or proceeding through apoptosis in cases of severe DNA damage (5) and thereby for the cellular destiny and for the outcome of cancer radiotherapy. The changes in gene expression induced by IR *via* transcription factors depend on dose, dose rate, time after irradiation, radiation quality, cell type, inherited or accumulated mutations in signaling pathways, cell-cycle phase, and possibly on other factors (**Table 1**). Twelve years ago, the transcription factors to be activated after exposure to clinically relevant doses of IR were summarized, resulting in the short list of p53, nuclear factor κB (NF-κB), and the specificity protein 1 (SP1)-related retinoblastoma control proteins (RCPs) (6). In this review, the role of transcription factors in the cellular response to IR is summarized with a special focus on charged particles as far as data are available.

p53

The transcription factor *TP53* (*p53*) was first described in 1979 (7), and many names have been attributed to the factor that belongs to the class of tumor suppressor genes. The transcription factor was called "an acrobat in tumorigenesis" (8), the "good and bad cop" (9), a "death star" (10), and even the "guardian of the genome" (11). p53 is involved in the regulation of cellular survival, immune responses, and inflammation, resulting in eminent importance in cancerogenesis and inflammation. Nowadays, it is known that defects in p53 are directly or indirectly involved

in the majority (>50%) of human cancers as described by the International Cancer Genome Consortium (ICGC).

The human p53 gene is located on the short arm of chromosome 17 (17p13) and the protein size is 393 amino acids (~43 kDa). It is composed of several domains: the N-terminus contains a transactivation domain for downstream gene activation (1–43). A proline rich domain follows that mediates the response to DNA damage through apoptosis (58–101). The DNA-binding region or domain (DBD) is next (102–292) followed by an oligomerization domain (320–355) that interacts with other p53 monomers (p53 is capable of tetramerize). The C-terminus (356–393) is leucine rich and contains three putative nuclear localization signals (NLS) and so-called nuclear export signals (NES). It is postulated that when oligomerization occurs, NES are masked and p53 is retained in the nucleus. The DBD is the core domain, and it is composed of a variety of structural motifs. Single mutations within this domain can cause a major conformational change. There are in total 12 isoforms of p53 in humans discovered until now (12).

p53 has been recognized as an important checkpoint protein in the DNA damage response (DDR), which transcriptionally controls target genes involved in multiple response pathways that are as diverse as cell-cycle arrest and survival or death by apoptosis (13). It is thereby important for explaining the diversity of cellular responses to IR exposure. p53 has a short half-life and is stabilized in response to a variety of cellular stresses after phosphorylation by ataxia telangiectasia mutated (ATM) (13). After exposure to IR, phosphorylation of the serine residues 15 and 20 on p53 by checkpoint kinase 2 (CHK2) reduces its binding to MDM2, which in its bound state targets p53 for degradation by the proteasome pathway (**Figure 1**). Thus, dissociation of p53 from MDM2 prolongs the half-life of p53 (14). Other proteins, such as Pin 1, Parc, and p300, and p300/CBP-associated factor (PCAF) histone acetyltransferases regulate the transactivation activity of p53 (13). For efficient repair, especially in non-dividing cells, cellular levels of deoxyribonucleotides are increased during the DDR by p53-dependent transcriptional induction of the ribonucleotide reductase RRM2B (p53R2) (15).

It is accepted that the severity of DNA damage is the critical factor in directing the signaling cascade toward reversible cell-cycle arrest or apoptosis (13, 15). As part of the signaling cascade, the abundance of p53 protein, specific posttranslational modifications, and its interaction with downstream effectors, such as GADD45α or p21, may be responsible for directing the cellular response at this decision point (14).

Recently, Gudkov and Komarova (16) proposed that after total body irradiation (TBI) of mice severe damage occurs in tissues prone to p53-dependent apoptosis [the apoptosis response of p53 after X-irradiation was already shown in murine experiments 1996 by Norimura et al. (17)], such as the hematopoietic system, hair follicles, and oligodendroblasts in the spinal cord. Other tissues, such as the vascular endothelial cells (ECs) of the small intestine react to p53 activation by cell-cycle arrest and activation of DNA repair (16). Connective tissues and epithelial cells usually respond with growth arrest to p53 activation (16). The authors conclude from animal models that p53 is the key component of the toxicity of IR or radiomimetic (DNA damaging) drugs. It

TABLE 1 | Transcription factor activation by ionizing radiation.

Experimental model	Radiation quality	Dose	Method	Effect	Reference
p53					
H1299 (originally p53 null)	X-rays	2–5 Gy	Colony-forming ability (CFA) assay, acridine orange/ethidium bromide staining, Western blot, quantitative real time RT-PCR (RT-qPCR)	Wildtype p53 cells: higher sensitivity compared to p53 null or mutated p53 cells	(172)
	^{12}C 290 MeV/u	2–5 Gy		Low LET radiation ⇒ p53-dependent apoptosis; High LET ⇒ p53-independent apoptosis	(173)
A549, AGS, and MCF-7	X-rays	0–12 Gy	RT-qPCR, Western blot, flow cytometry, luciferase reporter assay, CFA assay	miR-375 overexpression ⇒ p53 expressions ⇓	
	Etoposide	0–100 µM		Radiosensitivity ⇓	
HCT116 (colorectal cells) p53 wt and ko cells	X-rays	0–8 Gy	Viability assay (transwell co-culture), micronuclei and apoptosis evaluation, beta-galactosidase staining, RT-qPCR	Low doses: no difference between cell lines; Higher doses: significant differences, e.g., micronuclei ⇑ and apoptotic cells ⇑ in p53$^{-/-}$ cells, p53$^{+/+}$: high levels of senescence	(174)
Lung epithelial cells	α-particles (^{238}Pu), X-rays	0–1.2 Gy, 0–2.5 Gy	Flow cytometry	p53 expression levels ⇑	(175)
HCT116	^{12}C 290 MeV/u, X-rays	0–3 Gy	CFA assay, flow cytometry, immunofluorescence	X-rays ⇒ higher sensitivity and apoptosis ⇑ in p53$^{+/+}$ cells	(176)
	X-rays	0–8 Gy		C-ions ⇒ no difference of sensitivity (mitotic catastrophe ⇑ in p53$^{-/-}$ cells, apoptosis ⇑ in p53$^{+/+}$ cells)	
NF-κB					
Human, mouse, rat, hamster normal, transformed and tumor cell lines and primary cells, animal models (rat, mouse)	X-rays, γ-radiation, protons, α-particles, Fe ions, C ions, Ar ions	0.05–100 Gy	EMSA, Western blot, immunofluorescence, reporter assays, oligonucleotide enzyme-linked immunosorbent assay (ELISA)	Dose, cell line/cell type, and radiation quality-dependent activation	(70)
Nrf2					
NIH-3T3, MCF7-AREc32, Embryonic fibroblasts from wt and Nrf2 ko mice	γ-radiation ^{137}Cs source	2–8 Gy; 10 Gy	Luciferase assay, RT-qPCR, Western blot, CFA assay, ROS measurement (H$_2$DCFH-DA)	No short-term activation of Nrf2 activation; Late activation of Nrf2; Nrf2 activation after fractionated irradiation	(88)
PC3 and DU145 prostate cancer cell lines	γ-radiation ^{60}Co source	1–10 Gy	Electrophoretic mobility shift assay (EMSA), RT-qPCR	Differences in basal Nrf2 expression determine resistance to irradiation; High basal Nrf2 activity ⇒ Nrf2 activity ⇑, target gene expression ⇑ (DU145 cells) ⇒ higher radioresistance than PC3 cells	(99)
		4 and 8 Gy	Knockdown (kd) of Nrf2 and heme oxygenase-1 (HO-1) expression using short hairpin RNA (shRNA)	Knockdown of Nrf2 ⇒ cell death ⇑	
Murine T-cell lymphoma cell line EL-4	γ-radiation ^{60}Co source	4 Gy	shRNA-kd, RT-qPCR, EMSA	ERK and Nrf2 interact in radioresistance of EL-4 cells	(102)
Dermal fibroblasts from wt mice and Nrf2 and Keap1-KO mice	UV-A–UV-B radiation	10.000 mJ/cm^2	Western blot, immunofluorescence, flow cytometry	UV-A, but not UV-B, induces Nrf2 activity, cellular survival depends on Nrf2	(103)

(Continued)

TABLE 1 | Continued

Experimental model	Radiation quality	Dose	Method	Effect	Reference
C57BL/6, CD-1, and SJL/C57BL/6 CD45.1 mice	γ-radiation	6.9, 7.0, 7.1, 7.25, 7.3, 10 Gy TBI	RT-qPCR	Interplay between Nrf2 and Notch signaling, Nrf2 mediates Notch signaling and increases hematopoietic stem cell function	(106)
Mx-Cre-Keap1^flox/flox mice	[137]Cs source				
CMV/Cre-Keap1^flox/flox mice	[12]O^6+ ions	2 Gy	RT-qPCR of Nrf2 downstream genes NAD(P)H quinine oxidoreductase 1 (NQO1), HO-1, gamma-glutamyl cysteine synthetase (γ-GCS), immunofluorescence, Western blot	NQO1, HO-1, γ-GCS ⇑ in curcumin-pretreated mice	(108)
Keap1^flox/flox mice					
HCEC CT7s cells (immortalized colon epithelic cells)	γ-radiation ^{137}Cs source (cells)	4–5 Gy	Immunohistochemistry, Western blot, subcellular fractionation, immunofluorescence, assay for chromosomal aberrations at metaphase, shRNA against Nrf2, DNA fiber assay, ChIP qPCR	Nrf2 enhances DDR and reduces number of DNA DSB	(109)
C57BL/6 wt mice	X-rays (mice)	7.5–10 Gy TBI		Nrf2 ⇒ 53BP1 expression ⇑	(107)
EA.hy926 and HMVEC cells	Photons from linear accelerator	0, 0.3, 0.5, 0.7, 1 Gy	RT-qPCR, flow cytometry, Western blot, enzyme activity of glutathione peroxidase, EMSA	Non-linear activation of Nrf2 and target genes	
				Nrf2 activation prior to irradiation ⇒ cell adhesion ⇑	
				Nrf2 expression and binding to DNA lowest at 0.5 Gy	
CREB					
Human U1-Mel cell line	[60]Co γ-rays	4.5 Gy	EMSA with nuclear extracts	CREB DNA binding ⇑	(123)
Jurkat leukemic T cell line	10 MV X-rays	1.5 and 6 Gy	Western blot	CREB phosphorylation ⇑	(115)
K562 erythroleukemia cells	10 MV X-rays	1.5 and 15 Gy	Western blot	CREB phosphorylation ⇑	(119)
Chinese Hamster V79 cells	[12]C^5+ ions	0.1 and 1 Gy	Western blot	p44/42 MAPK ⇑	(125)
AG1522 human diploid skin fibroblasts	α-particles ([238]Pu source)	0.01, 0.05, and 0.10 Gy	Western blot	p38 MAPK and ERK 1/2 ⇑	(126)
AP-1					
AG1522 human diploid skin fibroblast	α-particles ([238]Pu source)	0.003 and 0.006 Gy	EMSA	AP-1 DNA-binding activity ⇑	(126)
MRC5CV1 normal human fibroblasts	[137]Cs γ-rays	20 Gy	Western blot EMSA	c-jun phosphorylation ⇑ AP-1 DNA-binding activity ⇑	(131)
ROS 17/2.8 osteoblasts	X-rays	5 Gy	EMSA with supershift	AP-1 DNA-binding activity ⇑	(132)
Spontaneously immortalized human breast epithelial cell line MCF-10F	α-particles, LET 150 keV/μm	6 and 1.2 Gy	Northern blot and immunochemical protein staining	c-jun, c-fos, FRA1 RNA, and protein expression ⇑	(135)
C57BL/6J mice	[56]Fe ions, 1000 MeV/n, LET 148 keV/μm	1.6 Gy	SOD 1/2 and catalase activity, NADPH oxidase activity assay and immunohistochemistry of p-H3	SOD 1/2, catalase, NADPH oxidase and mitogenic activity ⇑	(98)
Sp1					
Normal human diploid fibroblasts	6 MV X-rays	0.5, 2.5, 5, 10, 20, 40 Gy	Western blot	Sp1 expression and phosphorylation ⇑	(141)
U1-Mel cells	[137]Cs γ-rays	3 and 4.5 Gy	EMSA and Western blot	Sp1 DNA binding and phosphorylation ⇑	(142)

(Continued)

TABLE 1 | Continued

Experimental model	Radiation quality	Dose	Method	Effect	Reference
H1299	α-particles, LET 123 keV/μm	1 Gy	IPA upstream regulator analysis	Sp1 network involvement	(145)
Normal human fibroblasts (HFL 3)	C ions, 290 MeV/n, LET 70 keV/μm Fe ions, 500 MeV/n, LET 200 keV/μm	2 Gy	PCC assay and immunofluorescence	DNA-PKc autophosphorylation ⇑	(146)
EGR-1					
Isolated lymphocytes	Na²¹¹At α-particles	0.05–1.6 Gy	RT-qPCR	EGR-1 gene expression ⇑	(134)
Prostate cancer cells PC-3	100 kV X-rays	5 Gy	Western blot	Protein induction ⇑	(147)
Human HL 525 myeloid leukemia cells	¹³⁷Cs γ-rays	20 Gy	Western blot	Protein expression ⇑	(148)

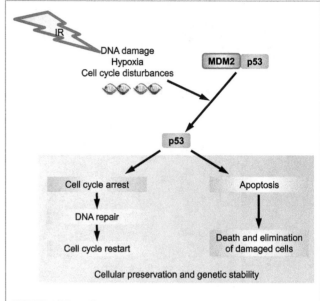

FIGURE 1 | The p53 pathway. p53 is under normal conditions inactivated by murine double minute 2 (MDM2). When, e.g., DNA damage occurs, p53 dissociates from its regulatory MDM2 complex by various pathways. In this active state, phosphorylated p53 will induce a cell-cycle arrest to permit either repair and therefore survival of the cell or induce apoptosis to eliminate a damaged cell.

thereby contributes to the hematopoietic component of the acute radiation syndrome and leads to severe adverse effects of cancer treatment (16).

p53-dependent GADD45α upregulation may play a role in apoptosis by activating the c-Jun N-terminal kinase (JNK) and/or p38 mitogen-activated protein kinase (MAPK) signaling pathways (18). Besides GADD45α, p53 regulates the expression of other proteins involved in apoptosis, including membrane-bound proteins, such as Fas/CD95, TP53 apoptosis effector related to PMP22 (PERP), and KILLER/DR5, cytoplasm-localized proteins, such as p53-inducible death domain-containing protein (PIDD) and PIGs, and mitochondrial proteins, such as BAX, NOXA, PUMA, p53Aip1, and BID (13, 14). The induction of these pro-apoptotic genes seems to be tissue specific (13). p53 also directly interacts with BAX, BCL-XL, and BCL-2 at the mitochondrial membrane (14).

So far, p53 plays a crucial role in the cellular radiation response. In future, the treatment of patients suffering from cancer will be personalized; this means that the combination of cytostatic agents and radiotherapy has to be individualized also depending on the tissue affected. For colorectal carcinoma cell lines, many tests are being performed with distinct agents where, e.g., gemcitabine, paclitaxel, or irinotecan are used in order to optimize the treatment results in combination with carbon ions. It has been already shown that after C-12 ion irradiation in cells lacking p53, paclitaxel and gemcitabine were very effective as well as irinotecan on p53 wild-type (wt) cells (19). Nevertheless, a problem with targeting the p53 pathway as a helping tool in cancer therapy by activation and thereby unleashing the protective attitudes of this pathway is that in hematological malignancies there is a low incidence of p53 mutations. Here, maybe MDM2 proteins can be addressed.

The bystander effect is a field that still needs to be understood and where experiments and the effects of a possible p53 response are barely recognized. First observations though, show that in mammalian cells lacking p53 in comparison to wt p53, the cells respond upon heavy ion exposure in the already known ways when directly irradiated (20). This fact is also to be taken into consideration when irradiation of patients is to be performed even though it does not play a major role, since the main goal is still targeting and eliminating the malignant tumors in an efficient manner.

The *tyrosine kinase c-abl* is a functional analogous to p53 in regulation of programmed cell death and DNA repair (21) interacting with p53 indirectly through modification of upstream regulators [homeodomain-interacting protein kinase 2 (HIPK2)] (22). C-abl is the ubiquitously expressed product of the cellular homolog of the transforming gene of Abelson murine leukemia virus (v-abl) shuttling between cytoplasm and nucleus of the cell (21, 23). Cytoplasmic c-abl is assumed to function in association with the F-actin cytoskeleton while nuclear c-abl participates in cell-cycle regulation, DDR, and apoptosis (23). Sparsely ionizing leads to an activation of c-abl (21, 24, 25) *via* phosphorylation by ATM at Ser-465 (26) and by DNA-dependent protein kinase (DNA-PK) (21, 23). It can function as a negative regulator of DNA repair progression, inhibiting DSB re-joining and downregulating γH2AX, decreasing the recruitment of DNA repair factors to the damage site (21), or c-abl can phosphorylate DNA PK and Rad51 to abolish their binding to DNA, thereby impeding their function (21, 25). It can also promote apoptosis with a direct influence on the p73-dependent DDR by phosphorylating the YES-associated protein (YAP). Upon phosphorylation, YAP acts together with p73 on pro-apoptotic gene targets (**Figure 2**) (21, 22).

In response to densely IR, c-abl has been surmised to partake in a p53-independent induction of apoptosis. In the model described, c-abl activates caspase 9 *via* phosphorylation at Tyr 153, initiating the cleavage of caspase 3 as a point of no return in apoptosis induction (27).

In summary, a potential role in the cellular radiation response can be attributed to c-abl as mediator of apoptosis and coordinator of DNA repair. Albeit greater focus on densely IR, such as carbon therapy, has to be introduced to fully conclude its role for this radiation quality.

NUCLEAR FACTOR κB

Although several genes induced by IR are p53-regulated, the majority are p53-independent (28–31), with the transcription factor NF-κB playing a contributing role (29, 31).

NF-κB/Rel proteins comprise a family of structurally related eukaryotic transcription factors that are involved in the control of a large number of cellular and organismal processes, such as immune system development and performance, inflammation, developmental processes, cellular growth, and apoptosis (32–35). Homo- or heterodimers of NF-κB1 (p50/p105), NF-κB2 (p52/p100), RelA (p65), RelB, or c-Rel (**Figure 3**) can be activated in response to hundreds of agents (36–38)

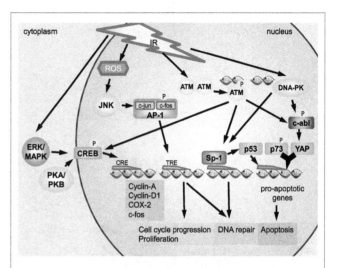

FIGURE 2 | Activation of the transcription factors CREB, AP-1, SP1, p73, and YAP upon irradiation ionizing radiation (IR) can activate protein kinase A (PKA) and B (PKB) as well as ERK/MAPK in the cytoplasm. Exposure to IR can produce reactive oxygen species (ROS) in the cytoplasm and nucleus and DNA double-strand breaks (DNA DSB) in the nucleus. PKA/PKB, ERK/MAPK, and ATM can phosphorylate CREB, which then translocates into the nucleus to bind CRE elements in order to express pro-survival proteins. ATM and DNA-PK can phosphorylate c-abl, which in turn phosphorylates YAP. Phosphorylated YAP acts together with p73 to stimulate expression of pro-apoptotic genes. ATM and DNA-PK can further induce Sp1, which can act pro-apoptotic by inducing p53 or pro-survival by regulating the DNA damage response and inducing DNA repair. IR-induced ROS can activate JNK to phosphorylate the AP-1 complex, thereby initiating DNA binding to TRE genes. Expression of TRE genes leads to induction of DNA repair and promotion of cell-cycle progression.

and thereby modulate environment-induced gene expression. Besides immune modulating agents and pathogen-derived agents (lipopolysaccharides), a variety of other cellular stress factors are able to induce this pathway, such as cytokines, phorbol esters, viruses, ultraviolet (UV) radiation, reactive oxygen species (ROS), necrotic cell products, growth factor depletion, hypoxia, heat shock, and IR (38–41).

In the inactive state, NF-κB is retained in the cytoplasm by the inhibitory *IκB proteins* (**Figure 4**), which controls nuclear translocation of NF κB by masking its NLS (42, 43). IκB proteins bind through their ankyrin repeat domain (ARD) to NF-κB. In their free state, IκB proteins are unstable and rapidly degraded, while binding to NF-κB strongly increases their stability (43). The three (NFκBIA, NFκBIB, and NFκBIE) genes code for the canonical IκB proteins, IκBα, IκBβ, and IκBε (**Figure 4**) (43). The p50:p65 heterodimer is mainly bound by IκBα. p105 and p100 proteins, which are involved in the alternative NF-κB pathway, contain the inhibitory part already in their C-terminal region in addition to the NF-κB part in the N-terminal half. Two novel IκBs (IκBζ and BCL-3) were described. BCL-3 is a non-inhibiting IκB family member that acts as transcriptional co-activator for p50:p50 and p52:p52 homodimers (44). Further novel atypical IκB proteins were recently reviewed by Arnemann et al. (45).

Upon activation, IκBα can be degraded by several proteases (46) and the released NF-κB translocates to the nucleus and

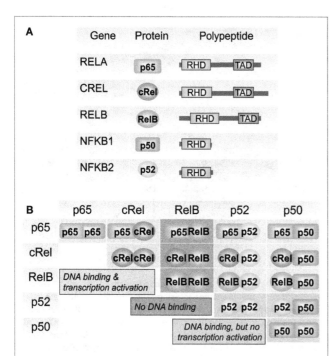

FIGURE 3 | **The members of the NF-κB family. (A)** NF-κB subunits each contain a Rel homology domain (RHD) for dimerization and DNA binding. p65 (RelA), c-Rel, and RelB bear transcriptional activation domains (TAD). **(B)** The 5 NF-κB monomers can associate to 15 potential dimers. Of these, nine can bind DNA and activate gene transcription (light gray), three (the p50 or p52 only containing dimers) bind DNA but do not activate transcription (medium gray), and three do not bind DNA (dark gray). Adapted from O'Dea and Hoffmann (43).

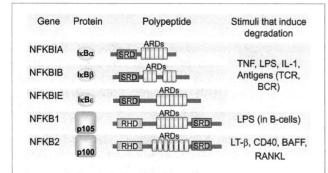

FIGURE 4 | **The members of the inhibitor of NF-κB (IκB) family.** IκB proteins contain ankyrin repeat domains (ARDs) and signal response domains (SRDs) and are degraded in response to different signals (BCR, B-cell receptor; TCR, T-cell receptor; LPS, lipopolysaccharide; LT-β, lymphotoxin-β; BAFF, B-cell-activating factor; RANKL, receptor activator of NF-κB ligand). The ARDs on p105 and p100 (which are proteolytically processed to p50 and p52 NF-κB monomers, respectively) can act to self-inhibit p50 and p52. p100 can also form a multimeric complex in which it can inhibit other latent NF-κB dimers. Adapted from O'Dea and Hoffmann (43).

binds to κB or κB-like DNA motifs [NF-κB response elements, NREs with the consensus sequence GGGRNNN(N)YCC][1] initiating gene transcription. NREs have been identified in the

[1]N, any nucleotide, R, purine, and Y, pyrimidine.

promoter or enhancer regions of more than 200 genes, including a number of IκBs, growth factors, proinflammatory cytokines (TNF-α, IL-1, IL-6) and enzymes (cyclooxygenase-2, COX-2), chemokines (IL-8/CXCL8; monocyte chemotactic cytokine 1, MCP-1/CCL2), angiogenic factors (vascular endothelial growth factor, VEGF), degradative enzymes (matrix metalloproteinases, MMPs), and adhesion molecules (intercellular adhesion molecule-1, ICAM-1; vascular cell adhesion molecule-1, VCAM-1; E-selectin). These target genes are involved in inflammation, innate immune responses, angiogenesis, tumor progression, and metastasis in various cancers and fibrosis (39, 44, 47, 48). NF-κB regulated expression of cytokines and extracellular matrix proteases after heavy ion exposure might contribute to extracellular matrix remodeling (49). Activation of NF-κB by high radiation doses (1–10 Gy) could contribute to the inflammatory response observed, e.g., in the developing brain after radiation exposure (50).

In addition, NF-κB also regulates the expression of many genes whose products are involved in the control of cell proliferation and cell death (51). In a cell culture model, it has been found that ATM plays a role in sustained activation of NF-κB in response to DNA DSB (52, 53), probably by its PI-3-kinase-like activity (54). Activation of the NF-κB pathway does not only protect cells from apoptosis after treatment with various genotoxic agents *via* expression of anti-apoptotic proteins, such as Bcl-2, GADD45β, TRAF-1, TRAF-2, cIAP-1, and cIAP-2 (55), but also gives transformed cells a growth and survival advantage and further renders tumor cells therapy resistant (56). NF-κB acts also as a transcriptional enhancer for the protective enzyme manganese superoxide dismutase (Mn-SOD) and might thereby contribute to therapy resistance. NF-κB also enhances the expression of degradative enzymes supporting the idea that it makes a major contribution to tumor progression and metastasis in various cancers (48). Therefore, NF-κB was identified quite early as potential target of innovative cancer therapies (57). Due to this anti-apoptotic effects NF-κB activation, it is an important stress response that may modulate the outcome of chemotherapy- and radiotherapy-induced toxicity.

For cells of the immune system, a misdirection of the NF-κB correlated process that normally creates immunoglobulin diversity might result in increased survivability of cells with oncogenic chromosomal translocations that prevent apoptosis and promote proliferation of pre-malignant cells. Constitutive activity of NF-κB or its over-expression has been reported for many human cancer cells (including breast cancer, colon cancer, prostate cancer, and lymphoid cancers) and can cause malignant changes in lymphoid cells in tissue culture.

NF-κB–Rel complexes can be activated and be functional in three different subpathways in different cells and tissues: the canonical or classical pathway, the alternative or non-canonical pathway, and the genotoxic stress-induced pathway (58–60).

In the *canonical or classical pathway*, the signals for activation of NF-κB are generated by cytokines, e.g., TNF-α or IL-1, by growth factors, by ligands of toll-like receptors (TLRs) or by antigens, which bind to the T-cell receptor (TCR) or the B-cell receptor (BCR). The NF-κB is mostly composed of p50:p65 and p50:c-Rel dimers.

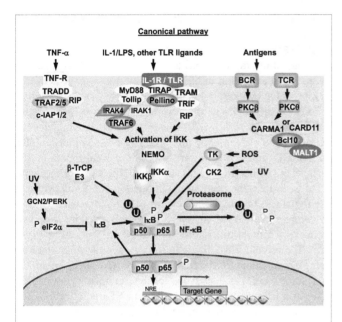

FIGURE 5 | The canonical or classical NF-κB pathway. The binding of TNF-α to TNF-R leads to a rapid recruitment of TRADD, RIP1, TRAF2, TRAF5, c-IAP1, and c-IAP2. Formation of this complex triggers TRAF2/5 and c-IAP1/2 to catalyze polyubiquitination of RIP1 and autoubiquitination of TRAF2 and/or c-IAP1 (not shown). Modified RIP1 then recruits the TAK1/TAB1/TAB2 (only TAK1 shown) and IKKα/IKKβ/NEMO complexes, leading to TAK1 activation and TAK1-mediated activation of IKKβ. Upon IL-1 stimulation of IL-1R, proteins, such as MyD88, Tollip, IRAK-1, and IRAK-4, are recruited, leading to IRAK1/4-dependent binding of TRAF6 and Pellino. TRAF6 then undergoes autoubiquitination, whereas Pellino catalyzes IRAK1 ubiquitination. Ubiquitinated TRAF6 in turn serves as a platform to recruit the TAK1/TAB1/TAB2 complex, resulting in TAK1 activation and finally IKKβ activation. TLR signaling can be MyD88 dependent or independent through TRAM, TRIF, and RIP. Activated IKK then phosphorylates IκBα, resulting in its ubiquitination and degradation. This IκBα degradation allows p50:p65 dimer to translocate to the nucleus and activate the expression of genes involved in inflammation, innate immunity, and cell survival. Ultraviolet (UV) irradiation reduces IκB levels *via* activation of GCN2 or PERK, which phosphorylate the initiation factor eIF2α, and *via* casein kinase 2 (CK2) and thymidine kinase (TK). Phosphorylated eIF2α blocks IκB synthesis. The BCR and TCR are expressed by B- and T-lymphocytes and do not act one the same cell. Adapted from O'Dea and Hoffmann (43) and Habelhah (44).

A central event in the pattern of NF-κB complex activation (**Figure 5**) is the activation of IκB kinase (IKK). This is achieved *via* a complex pathway involving several adaptor proteins, ubiquitin ligases, binding proteins, and kinases, such as receptor-interacting protein 1 (RIP1) and TNF-R-associated factor 2, 5, or 6 (TRAF2/5/6) (43, 44, 58–60), resulting in activation of IKK kinases (*IKK-K*). These kinases are responsible for phosphorylation of IKK and might be TGF-β-activated protein kinase 1 (TAK1) or MAPK kinase kinase 3 (MEKK3) after stimulation with TNF-α (44). The exact contribution of different kinases to IKK activation is not completely known, and redundancy in function may occur.

The *IKK* complex is composed of the two catalytic subunits, IKKα and IKKβ,[2] and the regulatory subunit, IKKγ/NF-κB

essential modulator (NEMO) (43). The activated IKK phosphorylates IκB at the serine residues 32 and 36 in the signal responsive domain and thereby targets IκB for ubiquitination (61). Phosphorylated IκB is polyubiquitinylated by the E3 ubiquitin ligase containing β-TrCP and subsequently degraded by the 26S proteasome (43, 58, 59). Alternatively, IκB can be phosphorylated at tyrosine 42, which has the potential to connect NF-κB directly to membrane receptor-associated tyrosine kinases (62).

Receptor signaling as described above in the canonical pathway is often dependent on the synthesis of autocrine factors, such as cytokines (64).

In response to TNF-α, IκBα is rapidly degraded, followed by NF-κB-dependent resynthesis. Persisting stimulation by binding of TNF-α to its receptor (TNF-R) results in cycles of IκBα degradation and resynthesis (43). After TNF-α stimulation, the deubiquitinases A20 (or TNF-α-induced protein 3, TNFAIP3) or CYLD (gene mutated in familial Cylindromatosis)[3] limit NF-κB activation (44, 65).

Activation of NF-κB after antigen binding to the TCR or BCR is mediated *via* activation of a phospholipase, which produces diacylglycerol, the activator of protein kinases C (PKC). PKC phosphorylates caspase recruitment domain 11 (CARD11), which then recruits other adaptor proteins – BCL-10 and MALT1 forming the CBM complex[4] with CARD11 in B-cells – leading finally to phosphorylation of IKKβ and ubiquitination of NEMO (**Figure 5**). The activated IKK complex phosphorylates IκB, leading to its degradation, as described above (65).

The *alternative or non-canonical pathway* is involved in non-inflammatory signaling, e.g., in lymph node development and osteoclastogenesis (43). It starts at membrane receptors of the TNF-R superfamily with binding of B-cell activation factor (BAFF), lymphotoxin β (LTβ), CD40 ligand (CD40L), or receptor activator of NF-κB ligand (RANKL) (**Figure 6**). BAFF is critical for B-cell survival. LTβ is involved in lymph node development. CD40L has functions in the adaptive immune response, such as B-cell proliferation and differentiation, and immunoglobulin isotype switching. RANKL is essential for osteoclast differentiation from monocytes. Receptor–ligand binding results in activation of the IKKα-containing kinase complex by NF-κB-inducing kinase (*NIK*) and sometimes of the canonical IKKβ-containing complex (43, 44). TRAF2, c-IAP1, and c-IAP2 negatively regulate NIK *via* ubiquitination- and proteasome-dependent degradation (43). In unstimulated cells, NIK is marked for degradation by the TRAF2/c-IAP1/2 complex. After receptor binding, NIK is stabilized and forms trimers that activate the IKKα complex.

In the alternative pathway, inactive NF-κB consists of a p100:RelB heterodimer. p100 in the p100:RelB complex

---

[2] "The commonly used anti-inflammatory drugs aspirin and sodium salicylate exert their effects in part by acting as competitive inhibitors of the ATP-binding site of IKKβ" (63).

[3] Mutations in the CYLD gene are very rare, affected patients develop benign tumors on the skin due to increased cell growth mediated by overactive NF-κB (66).

[4] Abnormal BCR signaling *via* CD79 and the CBM complex was observed in B-cell lymphomas (44, 65). Elevated MALT1 expression was also observed in lymphomas of mucosal-associated lymphoid tissue and might be explained in early stages by constant antigenic stimulation, and later by chromosomal translocations that position the MALT1 gene under the control of heterologous promoters (38).

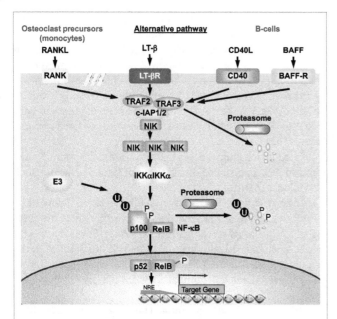

FIGURE 6 | The non-canonical or alternative NF-κB pathway. In
unstimulated cells, TRAF3 constitutively recruits NIK to the TRAF2–c-IAP1/2
complex, promoting c-IAP1/2-mediated K48-ubiquitination and degradation
of NIK. Ligation of CD40 by CD40L leads to recruitment of the TRAF3–
TRAF2–c-IAP1/2 complex to the receptor, where TRAF2 catalyzes
polyubiquitination of c-IAP1/2. It thereby promotes ubiquitin E3 ligase activity
of c-IAP1/2 toward TRAF3, leading to proteasomal degradation of the latter.
As a result, NIK can no longer be recruited to the TRAF2–c-IAP1/2 complex.
This leads to stabilization and accumulation of newly synthesized NIK and its
activation presumably via autophosphorylation, resulting in activation of the
IKKα homodimer. Activated IKKα then phosphorylates p100, leading to
proteasome-mediated processing of p100 to p52. The p52:RelB heterodimer
then translocates to the nucleus and regulates transcription of target genes.
CD40L promotes antibody isotype switching in mature B-cells, RANKL
initiates osteoclastogenesis from precursor cells, BAFF induces immune cell
survival and proliferation of B-cells, and LT-β regulates lymph node
development. The receptors represented here on one cell are therefore
restricted to distinct cell types and usually do not act in parallel. Adapted
from O'Dea and Hoffmann (43) and Habelhah (44).

is phosphorylated by the activated IKKα, which results in
polyubiquitination of p100 and proteolytic degradation of the
NF-κB-inhibiting C-terminal region of p100, releasing p52 (43).
The resulting p52:RelB dimer translocates to the nucleus where
it initiates transcription of genes involved in lymphoid organo-
genesis, immune cell survival, proliferation and maturation, and
osteoclastogenesis (44). It results in low level nuclear translocation of NF-κB for hours or days (43).

Several cross-talk mechanisms of inflammatory and developmental NF-κB signaling via the canonical and the alternative
pathway were described (43). For example, developmental
signals can also activate canonical p50:p65 dimers bound to a
dimer of p100 (called IκBδ) (43). The activated NIK as part of
the alternative pathway may amplify canonical IKK activation
(43). CD40L can activate the canonical and the alternative NF-κB
pathway (65).

Recently, a role for RelB was suggested in the therapy resistance of prostate cancer, which was explained by RelB-dependent
induction of MnSOD (67).

DNA DSB in the cell nucleus can activate the *genotoxin-induced
pathway* (68). Early studies supposed DNA-PK (69), PI3K, and
MAPK (64) as mediators of radiation-induced NF-κB activation.
In a cell culture model, it has been found that *ATM* plays a role
in sustained activation of NF-κB in response to DNA DSB (52,
53), probably by its PI-3-kinase-like activity (54). Activation of
NF-κB *via* this pathway after exposure to IR was described in
detail in a recent review (70). Briefly, DNA damage initiates the
SUMOylation of *NEMO* by the sumo ligase PIASy in a complex
with PIDD and RIP1, fostering NEMO's localization in the
nucleus (43). This nuclear SUMOylated NEMO associates with
ATM with the result of monoubiquitination of NEMO, which is
the signal for its cytoplasmic export (43). SUMOylated NEMO
in complex with ATM therefore represents the long searched
nuclear to cytoplasmic shuttle of the NF-κB activating signal
(68). The protein ELKS binds to the cytoplasmic ATM–NEMO
complex, enabling ATM-dependent activation of the canonical
IKK complex (43). As described for the canonical pathway, IKK
activation leads to IκBα degradation and NF-κB activation. The
canonical p50:p65 heterodimer initiates gene transcription in the
nucleus.

The role of the NF-κB pathway in cellular radiosensitivity was
addressed by several studies (6). In a human ovarian cancer cell
line, a human breast cancer cell line, and a murine melanoma
cell line, radiation-activated NF-κB protected the cells from
radiation-induced apoptosis (71). Inhibition of NF-κB activity can be achieved by overexpression of dominant-negative,
phosphorylation-defective IκB. This has been reported to
enhance the radiosensitivity of human fibrosarcoma cells (72),
xenografted fibrosarcomas in mice (73) and human brain tumor
cells (61, 74, 75), and to influence X-ray-induced mutations and
apoptosis in human malignant glioma cells (76). For low LET
radiation, NF-κB inhibition increased radiosensitivity of many
cancer cells (6).

As activation of the NF-κB pathway is supposed to play a role
in the negative regulation of both death receptor- and stress-
induced apoptosis (44), survival of cells with residual DNA damage might thus be favored. Also, NF-κB's role in the deregulation
of inflammatory responses contributes to its tumor-promoting
and progression-favoring characteristics (44).

Constitutive NF-κB activation is often found in human
cancers, e.g., breast, thyroid, bladder, and colon cancer (56,
77–80). It is thought to be important for maintaining survival
of the cancer cells and for angiogenesis or chemoresistance
(43, 81). The mechanisms that lead to constitutively activated
NF-κB (82) and its critical role in tumor progression are currently only partly understood for some tumors. Mutations of
the NFKBIA gene, which encodes IκBα or alterations of its
expression level, might be an explanation for the increased
NF-κB activity in tumors. In a recent study analyzing 790
human glioblastomas, deletion or low expression of NFKBIA
was associated with unfavorable outcomes (83), possibly resulting from uncontrolled NF-κB activity. In 37.5% of patients with
Hodgkin lymphoma, mutations in the NFKBIA gene in the
tumor cells were detected (84). Lake et al. (85) found NFKBIA
mutations in 3 of 20 Hodgkin lymphoma patients (15%). In
addition, a NFKBIA polymorphism (A to G variation, rs696

in the 3′ UTR)[5] was associated with colorectal cancer risk and poor treatment prognosis (86). In human adult T-cell leukemia or lymphoma associated with human T-cell leukemia virus type I, activation of the NF-κB pathway by the virus protein Tax *via* the canonical and the alternative pathway seems to be involved in the transformation process (47). Another mechanism of constitutive NF-κB activation was described in malignant melanoma cells: an elevated endogenous ROS production resulted in constitutive NF-κB translocation to the nucleus (87).

NUCLEAR ERYTHROID-DERIVED 2-RELATED FACTOR 2

Nuclear erythroid-derived 2 (NF-E2)-related factor 2 (Nrf2) that binds the antioxidant DNA response element (ARE) to induce cellular antioxidant defense systems was shown to be activated 5 days after irradiation (88). Nrf2 was identified in studies investigating the activation of detoxifying enzymes in the presence of electrophilic chemicals, such as ROS. It belongs to the cap "n" collar (CNC) family of basic leucine zipper (bZIP) transcription factors. In vertebrates, they include the p45–NF-E2 factors and the NF-E2-related factors Nrf1, Nrf2, and Nrf3. In fact, Nrf2 was first identified as a homolog of NF-E2 and was found to interact with NF-E2-binding sites (89). The natural repressor protein of Nrf2 is Kelch-like associated ECH-associated protein 1 (Keap1), also called inhibitor of Nrf2 (INrf2).

Whereas NF-E2 was found in erythroid cells, Nrf1 and Nrf2 expression was observed in many tissues (90). In humans, the Nrf2 gene is located on chromosome 2q31 and in mice on chromosome 2. Target genes of Nrf2 contain a specific binding region, the ARE or electrophilic response element (EpRE). The ARE consensus sequence is TGA(G/C)NNNGC (89). Target genes of Nrf2 include detoxifying enzymes and antioxidative enzymes, such as glutathione-*S*-transferase, superoxide dismutase (SOD), or NADPH reductase.

The Nrf2 gene consists of five exons and four introns and its promoter region contains two ARE sequences, indicating that Nrf2 controls to some extent its own expression. ARE regions are also found in the promoter regions of Keap1 and the small Maf protein MafG (91–93). The presence of an ARE sequence in the Keap1 gene suggests an auto-regulatory feedback loop between Nrf2 and Keap1 (93).

The Nrf2 protein consists of 605 amino acids in humans and 597 amino acids in mice (90, 94), and is subdivided into six domains, which are evolutionary highly conserved and are termed Nrf2–ECH homology domains, abbreviated Neh1–6. They play important roles in binding to DNA, activation and inactivation of Nrf2. Protein structure, genetics regulation, and history of discovery of Nrf2 are summarized in the in-depth reviews of Baird and Dinova-Kostova (94), Ramkissoon et al. (90), and Morita and Motohashi (89). Baird and Dinova-Kostova discuss

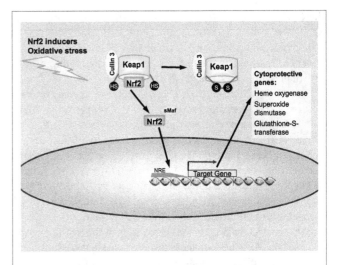

FIGURE 7 | The Nrf2–ARE pathway. Nrf2 is sequestered in the cytoplasm by Keap1 and targeted for ubiquitination by Cullin 3 and proteasomal degradation. Under conditions of oxidative stress or by chemical activators the thiol groups of cysteine residues of Keap1 are oxidized. This leads to the formation of disulfide bridges, which changes the conformation of Keap1 which is unable to bind Nrf2 now. Nrf2 is no released from Keap1 and translocates to the nucleus by forming heterodimers with sMaf proteins. In the nucleus, the Nrf2–sMaf complex binds to antioxidant responsive element (ARE) sequence in the promoter region of Nrf2 target genes, leading to the expression of antioxidative enzymes, such as heme oxygenase, superoxide dismutase, and glutathione-*S*-transferase.

several possible activation and regulation mechanisms of Nrf2, i.e., the sequester and release model, which was used in **Figure 7**, the "dissociation of Keap1 and Cullin 3 model," the "hinge and latch model," the "Keap1 nucleocytoplasmic shuttling model," and the "ubiquitination of Keap1 model," as well as some evidence suggesting that Nrf2 directly senses stressors (94). In this review, the "sequester and release model" will be featured (**Figure 7**), but it should be mentioned that it is a significant simplification of the actual mechanism underlying Nrf2 regulation within cells. What is most important from a radiation biological point of view about Nrf2 and its repressor Keap1, it is the fact that the Nrf2–ARE pathway is redox sensitive. IR induces the formation of free radicals, mainly due to radiolysis of water molecules within cells.

Reactive oxygen species form adducts with DNA, proteins, carbohydrates, and lipids. Cells are naturally exposed to ROS due to metabolic processes and by other environmental cues. Cells possess different defense mechanisms to maintain their redox equilibrium by increasing the expression of antioxidative enzymes. The activity of Nrf2 depends on the ROS level within a cell.

Nuclear erythroid-derived 2-related factor 2 is repressed by the protein Keap1 under physiological conditions. Keap1 consists of 624 amino acids and is rich in cysteine residues (25 in mice and 27 in humans) (94). Keap1 binds to Nrf2 and sequesters it in the cytoplasm and acts as a scaffold for the Cullin 3–Rbx1-E3 ubiquitin ligase, thereby promoting the proteasomal degradation of Nrf2. Under basal conditions, the half-life period of Nrf2 is thus only 10–30 min (90). As mentioned above, Keap1 possesses many cysteine residues, whose thiol groups are oxidized by ROS, leading to the formation of disulfide bridges. This changes

---

[5]UTR, untranslated region at the 3′ end of the mRNA. The reference single nucleotide polymorphism (SNP) Cluster Report rs696 is available in the National Center for Biotechnology Information (NCBI) SNP database (http://www.ncbi.nlm.nih.gov).

the conformation of Keap1, releasing Nrf2 from its binding to Keap1. Nrf2 then translocates to the nucleus together with co-transcriptional factors, such as small Mafs (also belonging to the class of bZip transcription factors). Nrf2 forms heterodimers with the small Mafs, which then bind to ARE regions.

Nuclear erythroid-derived 2-related factor 2 has many interaction partners: apart from the small Maf proteins (MafG, MafF, and MafK), another cotranscription factor is the CREB-binding protein (CBP). Nrf2 activity is downregulated by nuclear import of Keap1 where it binds Nrf2 and exports it back to the cytoplasm. Furthermore, the kinase Fyn phosphorylates the tyrosine residue 568 of Nrf2, which is a signal for the nuclear export of Nrf2 (90). Of importance is also the interaction of Nrf2 and NF-κB. NF-κB competes for CBP binding and inhibits Maf kinases (95). Keap1 was shown to contribute to the degradation of the NF-κB subunit p65 (96). ERK1/2-dependent pathways were suggested to mediate Nrf2 activation by low-dose γ-irradiation (97).

McDonald et al. (88) investigated the impact of γ-irradiation on Nrf2 activity in mouse embryonic fibroblasts derived from Nrf2 wt and knockout (ko) mice. They analyzed the expression of Nrf2 target genes by quantitative real time RT-PCR (RT-qPCR) and Nrf2 activity by a luciferase reporter system. The reporter system consisted of a plasmid where a firefly luciferase gene was fused with a promoter containing the ARE. No significant increase of either target gene expression or Nrf2 activity could be observed in this cell line 24 h after single exposure to even a high dose of up to 10 Gy of γ-radiation. Yet, 5 days after irradiation, Nrf2 activity markedly increased and this response persisted up to 8 and 15 days after irradiation. By shifting to a fractional irradiation over a time period of 5 days, a significant increase in Nrf2 target gene expression and increased reporter gene expression was observed 3 h after the end of fractionated irradiation. Additionally, they observed no effect on cellular survival of inducing Nrf2 prior to irradiation in murine fibroblasts, lymphocytes, and dendritic cells by using different chemical activators that activate Nrf2 in a brief time period of a few hours. However, immortalized fibroblasts derived from Nrf2-ko mice were more susceptible to irradiation than immortalized fibroblasts derived from Nrf2 wt mice. The increase of ROS inside cells was delayed as well with a response after 5 days. The level of ROS as measured by the fluorescence dye 2′,7′-dichlorofluorescin diacetate (DCF-DA) only increased 5 days after irradiation and was higher in Nrf2-ko fibroblasts, which moreover showed a higher basal ROS level. McDonald et al. (88) concluded from these results that Nrf2 is important for regulating long-term radiation effects and functions as a buffer system for maintaining the redox equilibrium in cells; a function than cannot be altered by exogenous chemical factors, but it is important for long-term cellular survival after radiation exposure. They speculated that long-term radiation effects may be related to an altered mitochondrial function, which results an increased production of ROS. Datta et al. (98) confirmed this for cells of the small intestine by exposing mice to γ-irradiation and accelerated iron (Fe-56, 1000 MeV/n; LET 148 keV/μm) ions. They observed a more potent induction of oxidative stress, DNA damage, and apoptosis in the small intestine of mice, which were exposed to energetic iron ions compared to mice that were γ-irradiated. Interestingly, they also observed long-term changes in the metabolism and gene expression in the intestinal tissue of mice up to 1 year after irradiation: mitochondrial function was altered and the level of ROS produced by mitochondrial metabolism increased as well as expression of NADPH oxidase, resulting in persistent elevated ROS level in the small intestine. Datta et al. (98) suspect that the induction of long-term effects after irradiation is important for the evaluation of chronic or late radiation effects.

Jayakumar et al. (99) found a connection between differences in Nrf2 expression and radiation resistance in the two different prostate cancer cell lines PC3 and DU145. Both cell lines were exposed to γ-radiation and Nrf2 content was measured prior to and after irradiation. Both cell lines differed in Nrf2 expression under basal conditions. It was found that cellular survival was higher after irradiation in the cell line DU145, which showed a higher basal Nrf2 activity. Furthermore, the level of basal and induced ROS after irradiation was higher in PC3 cells, which in contrast to DU145 exhibited a lower basal activity of Nrf2. In both cell lines, Nrf2 protein content increased after irradiation, whereas the protein level of Keap1 was reduced. Also, the expression of antioxidant enzymes increased after irradiation in both cell lines, but this response was significantly stronger in the DU145 cell line. Cellular survival was reduced in both cell lines and especially in the cell line with low basal Nrf2 expression PC3, after exposure to the chemical Nrf2 inhibitor retinoic acid. This outcome was enhanced when Nrf2 was knocked down on transcript level by transfecting both cell lines with small interfering RNA (siRNA) against Nrf2. These findings indicate that Nrf2 is important for cellular survival after exposure to IR and that radiation resistance of different cell lines, especially cancer cell lines depends upon differences in basal Nrf2 activity and upregulation of Nrf2. Examining the expression of Nrf2 in tumor tissue may therefore be important for the planning and predicting the outcome of therapeutic irradiation. Furthermore, as predominantly antioxidant enzymes were upregulated, there seems to be an association between oxidative stress and cellular survival after irradiation. Independently from radiation biological considerations, Wang et al. (100) showed that Nrf2 is antagonized by retinoic acid receptor α (RARα) in the small intestine of mice after treatment with retinoic acid, this opens the possibility to modulate Nrf2 activity chemically. Mathew et al. (101) showed that the Nrf2 activator sulforaphane (which also shows anti-cancerous effects) protects fibroblasts against IR.

In a similar setting, Patwardhan et al. (102) showed that T cell lymphoma EL-4 cells exhibit a high basal Nrf2 activity, show lower ROS levels than non-tumorigenic cells and that enhanced radiation resistance is linked to higher Nrf2 activity. siRNA against Nrf2 or treatment with all-trans retinoic acid (ATRA also called Tretinoin as a pharmaceutical) enhanced radiosensitivity of EL-4 cells.

Apart from IR, such as X-rays and γ-radiation, Nrf2 was also shown to be activated by UV radiation (103). Dermal fibroblasts showed an increased accumulation of Nrf2 in the nucleus after exposure to UV-A irradiation, but not after UV-B irradiation. Moreover, fibroblasts derived from Nrf2-ko mice exhibited a 1.7-fold increase in apoptosis after UV-A exposure compared to fibroblasts derived from wt mouse. The opposite effect was observed in Keap1-ko fibroblasts; here, the apoptosis rate was half of the rate observed in fibroblasts isolated from wt mice.

Nuclear erythroid-derived 2-related factor 2 also seems to be important for the function adult stem cells. Hochmuth et al. (104) showed that inactivation of the Nrf2 analog CncC in *Drosophila* was required for the maturation of intestinal stem cells. CncC is constitutively active in intestinal stem cells and its inactivation by Keap1 is a signal for intestinal stem cell proliferation. They observed that increased ROS levels lead to increased proliferation of intestinal stem cells, a similar effect could be observed by knocking down CncC with siRNA. This work indicates that the activation pattern of CncC is reversed in stem cells compared with differentiated cells. Whereas in differentiated cells ROS activate CncC or Nrf2, in intestinal stem cells CncC is inactivated by ROS to allow for an increased proliferation of intestinal stem cells to renew the intestinal tissue. This seems to imply an activation mode of Nrf2 that depends on cell type and developmental stage. How oxidative stress inactivates Nrf2 in intestinal stem cells remains to be investigated. Tsai et al. (105) could confirm the role of Nrf2 in controlling stem cell proliferation. They confirmed the findings of Hochmuth et al. (104) in hematopoietic stem cells. Reduced Nrf2 activity or lack of Nrf2 led to hyperproliferation of stem cells and progenitor cells. This was accompanied by a reduced self-renewal of hematopoietic stem cells and reduction of quiescence. Nrf2 proved to be a crucial factor in the regulation and function of hematopoietic stem cells. Whereas both studies did not involve radiation, Kim et al. (106) showed that Nrf2 contributes strongly to the survival of hematopoietic stem cells in a mouse model of total body γ-irradiation. Nrf2-ko mice had a lower survival and a higher impairment of hematopoietic function compared to Nrf2 wt mice. Furthermore, activation of Nrf2 prior to irradiation increased overall survival of mice after TBI. Additionally, hematopoiesis was increased in mice, which were treated with the Nrf2 activator 2-trifluoromethyl-2-methoxychalone (TMC).

Recently, Large et al. (107) investigated the role of Nrf2 in the low-dose response of ECs. Surprisingly, they found a decreased expression of Nrf2 after low-dose X-irradiation (0.5 Gy) in EA.hy926 ECs and primary human dermal microvascular ECs (HMVEC), additionally the DNA binding of Nrf2 was lowered. The expression of Nrf2 target genes and the activity of Nrf2 itself followed a non-linear pattern of expression, meaning that the observed level of mRNA increased and decreased interchangeably with increasing doses (0, 0.3, 0.5, 0.7, and 1 Gy). In all cases, the expression of glutathione peroxidase (GPx) and SOD as well as the Nrf2 binding activity were lowest after 0.5 Gy X-irradiation. This finding is interesting, as it indicates that at least in these cell lines low-dose irradiation may induce an unusual pattern of Nrf2 expression and activity and that certain doses may decrease Nrf2 activity. As they treated cells prior to irradiation with TNF-α to simulate inflammation, there might be an involvement of NF-κB, as TNF-α activates it, in the expression and activity pattern of Nrf2.

Relatively little is known about the role of Nrf2 in the cellular radiation response to heavy ion irradiation. Quite recently, Xie et al. (108) showed that curcumin (an Nrf2 activator) reduces cognitive impairment in mice after exposure carbon ions (4 Gy). They observed an upregulation of Nrf2 and Nrf2 downstream genes, NAD(P)H quinine oxidoreductase 1 (NQO1), heme oxygenase-1 (HO-1), and γ-glutamyl cysteine synthetase (γ-GCS) in the brain tissue of mice that were treated with curcumin. Kim et al. (109) found increased survival of colonic epithelial cells after exposure to iron ions (Fe-56) when Nrf2 was activated prior to radiation exposure. They focused on the interaction of Nrf2 and p53 binding protein 1 (p53BP1), as p53BP1 contains three ARE sequences. Activation of Nrf2 in colon epithelial cells prior to irradiation reduced the frequency of G1 and S/G2 chromosome aberrations. In general, the DDR was enhanced by Nrf2 activation.

The response of Nrf2 to radiation may be an important factor in tumor therapy. Mutations in Nrf2 and Keap1 are known to occur in various cancer cell lines and to confer protection to cancer cell lines toward chemo- or radiotherapy. Some cancer cell lines possess a high basal activity of Nrf2, which increases their resistance against radiation (110). In general, Nrf2 is accumulated in tumors and high levels of Nrf2 expression lead to a poor prognosis for cancer patients (111). In a lung cancer study, samples were taken from 178 lung squamous cell carcinomas (SqCCs) (112, 113) and, apart from 53BP1, most mutations were found in three genes associated with the Nrf2–ARE pathway, NFE2L2 (the gene name of Nrf2), Keap1, and Cul3 (the gene name of Cullin 3). Increased resistance to radiation therapy was linked to a high level of Nrf2.

Further studies of the function and activity of Nrf2 after exposure of cells to heavy ions, especially carbon ions, may give hints how to improve radiation therapy and will be of significance for the planning of long-term human space missions.

ROLE OF OTHER TRANSCRIPTION FACTORS IN THE CELLULAR RADIATION RESPONSE

In addition to the two key transcription factors in the cellular damage response, p53 and NF-κB, and the oxidative stress-induced Nrf2, several other transcription factors are activated in response to IR exposure (**Figure 2**). ATM-mediated phosphorylation of c-Abl appears to increase the transcription of stress response genes *via* activation of Jun kinase (15). Also, other MAPK pathways are activated, resulting, e.g., in formation of the transcription factor activated protein 1 (AP-1), which controls proliferation, senescence, differentiation, and apoptosis *via* growth factors (114). Cataldi et al. (115) propose a role for the transcription factor cyclic adenosine monophosphate (cAMP)-responsive element-binding protein (CREB) in survival responses of Jurkat T-cells after exposure to IR. The transcription factor Sp1, which is involved in cell differentiation, cell growth, apoptosis, immune responses, response to DNA damage, and chromatin remodeling, is rapidly phosphorylated in response to DNA damage, but this phosphorylation did not affect its transcriptional activity (116). The colocalization of phosphorylated Sp1 with activated ATM kinase in nuclear foci was interpreted as a sign for a role of Sp1 in DNA repair (116). A colocalization in nuclear foci was also observed for the forkhead box-O 3 (FOXO-3) transcription factor that is involved in cell-cycle control (117).

cAMP-Responsive Element-Binding Protein

cAMP-responsive element-binding protein (CREB) is a 43-kDa bZIP nuclear transcription factor involved in cAMP signaling (115). Its activation *via* phosphorylation leads to binding of the transcription factor to the cAMP-responsive element (CRE), a highly conserved sequence, inducing transcription of target genes for several cellular functions, including regulation of apoptosis and proliferation (118, 119). CREB phosphorylation is cell type and stimulus dependent. It is therefore possible for a wide range of molecules to activate the transcription factor. PKA, PKB, and ERK/MAPK phosphorylate CREB at Serine 133 (119, 120), whereas ATR and ATM phosphorylate the factor at Serine 111 and 121, respectively, in response to IR and oxidative stress (121, 122).

Sparsely IR is able to increase the binding of CREB to its consensus sequence (123). Furthermore, γ-irradiation has been shown to induce phosphorylation of CREB, thereby activating it (115, 119). Radiation-induced activation of CREB is connected with survival, as its target genes promote cellular proliferation, such as cyclin A, cyclin D1, proliferating cell nuclear antigen (PCNA), c-fos, and COX-2. In CREB knockdown studies, survival decreased (124). Co-incidental with CREB activation is low caspase-3 activity and a lack of Bax and Bcl2 level difference, further supporting an anti-apoptotic role (119).

Although an increase of ERK/MAPK expression after irradiation with carbon ions (125) and α-particles (126) was shown, no connection to CREB activation has been made. Therapeutic high LET studies lost their focus on CREB as survival factor, but it can be said that with the upcoming trend of therapeutic irradiation using heavy ions, CREB should be considered as means to increase radiosensitivity in tumor cells.

Activated Protein 1

Activated protein 1 (AP-1) is a transcription factor formed by homo- or heterodimerization of proteins of the Jun family (c-Jun, JunB, and JunD) or the Fos family (c-Fos, FosB, Fra-1, and Fra-2). Such dimers (AP-1 complexes) are able to recognize AP-1 binding sites containing the 12-O-tetradecanoylphorbol-13-acetate (TPA) response element (TRE), its DNA target sequence (127). C-jun regulates the expression of cyclin D1, a promoter of cell-cycle progression into G1-phase (128, 129). In addition to genes regulating cell-cycle progression, AP-1 controls its own expression, having a TRE in the promoter region of the c-jun gene (130).

The transcriptional activity of c-Jun can be enhanced by phosphorylation of Serine 63 and 73 by JNK. It has been shown that c-Jun is phosphorylated by JNK in the nucleus after γ-irradiation (**Figure 2**). Furthermore, the same study showed increased DNA-binding activity of AP-1 in response to sparsely IR with AP-1 complexes containing c-Jun as well as JunD and JunB (131). X-radiation has also been shown to increase DNA-binding activity of AP-1 (132). Exposure to an 18 MeV electron beam (4 Gy) activated AP-1 in HepG2 cells (133).

Elevated gene expression of c-jun and protein expression of AP-1-associated factors (c-jun, c-fos, Fra1, and JNK2)

was observed in response to α-particles exposure (134, 135). Binding activity of AP-1 increased after irradiation with very low doses of α-particles (6 mGy). This binding was inhibited by SOD indicating a response of AP-1 to oxidative stress (126). Iron ion (Fe-56, 1000 MeV/n, LET 148 keV/μm) irradiation has been associated with proliferation of intestinal epithelium cells, connecting irradiation-induced oxidative stress with activation AP-1 (98).

Reactive oxygen species and other radiation-released free radicals can stimulate JNK and AP-1 activity (23), therefore promoting cell-cycle progression, although influence in apoptosis induction has also been reported (136). Additionally, the radiation-induced activation of AP-1 was also correlated to increased levels of glutamylcysteine synthetase, which is directly associated with synthesis of glutathione, a cellular radical scavenger (133). Therefore, AP-1 might be relevant in high LET radiation therapy by enhancing the cellular defense against ROS and regulation the cellular apoptotic response to radiation.

Specificity Protein 1

The Sp1 belongs to the specificity protein/Krüppel-like factor (Sp/XKLF) family of transcription factors that contain 3 conserved Cys2His2 zinc fingers for DNA binding (137). Loss of these zinc fingers abolishes not only DNA-binding capacity but also nuclear translocation (138). Sp1 is ubiquitously expressed in all mammalian cells and regulates cellular functions, such as apoptosis, cell-cycle progression, growth/proliferation, and metabolism (137, 139). The fate of Sp1 differs greatly depending on its posttranslational modification. Many different proteins modify Sp1 through all stages of the cell cycle *via* SUMOylation, glycosylation, ubiquitination, acetylation, or phosphorylation. Overexpression of Sp1 regulates apoptosis in a p53-dependent manner after suppression of cell growth (137).

ATM can activate Sp1 *via* phosphorylation in response to X-rays and H_2O_2 (140), which is recruited to DNA DSB and can promote repair in a non-transcriptional manner (141). Sp1 acts also in a transcriptional manner upon IR, as it is associated with coordination of cellular response after treatment with γ-rays, activated by DNA-PK through phosphorylation (142). Furthermore, an increased nuclear expression of Sp1 has been observed for irradiation with 20 Gy X-rays (143) as well as increased binding activity upon γ-irradiation (123, 144).

Microarray gene expression experiments assume activation of Sp1 in cells irradiated with α-particles (LET 123 keV/μm), and its involvement in subsequent cellular responses of directly and indirectly exposed (bystander) cells (145). The Sp1-dependent gene expression profile included up- and downregulation of 16 and 6 genes, respectively, in cells directly hit by α-particles, while upregulation of a smaller subset (10 genes) dominated in bystander cells (145). As with sparsely IR, Sp1 could act in a more administrative manner upon high LET radiation, as DNA-PK is strongly activated after carbon and iron ion exposure (146).

Sp1 has various roles in the DDR, ranging from orchestrating the response, to actively regulating apoptosis or repair. For cancer treatment with carbon ions, Sp1 is well worth investigating, as there are not many distinct approaches to study this versatile transcription factor in context of high LET particle irradiation.

Early Growth Response 1

The transcription factor early growth response 1 (EGR-1) is a member of the EGR family and is suggested to act as anti-proliferative signal for tumor cells, as well as an apoptotic enhancer (147). It has been shown to be activated by X- (147) and γ-rays (148). Radiation-induced activation of EGR-1 is associated with ROS (148). Upon irradiation, EGR-1 can act p53-independently as mediator for TNF-α-induced apoptosis (147). Gene expression of EGR-1 has been found to be increased also in response to irradiation with α-particles (134). The role of EGR-1 in the cellular radiation response is pro-apoptotic and in light of heavy ion radiation therapy, it would be instructive to know the extent of its pro-apoptotic capabilities upon high LET irradiation.

INFLUENCE OF LINEAR ENERGY TRANSFER ON TRANSCRIPTION FACTOR ACTIVATION

The cellular response to high LET radiation shows quantitative and in some aspects qualitative differences compared to the low LET radiation response. For different radiation types, the biological effects, observed at the same absorbed dose, depend on their quality (sparsely or densely IR). Comparison of the biological effects of different radiation qualities is usually being performed in terms of relative biological effectiveness (RBE).[6] In radiotherapy, the RBE is not only of highest interest for cell killing but also for late effects such as cancerogenesis (149). For the various biological endpoints, the RBE can depend on many factors, such as LET, dose rate, dose fractionation, radiation dose, and type of the irradiated cells or tissues.

One of the earliest systematic studies of the dependence of RBE on LET showed that the RBE reached a maximum at an LET of 100–200 keV/μm for survival of human kidney T1 cells after irradiation with deuterium ($_1^2$H) and α-particles (151–153). Thereafter, an LET–RBE function was determined for many biological endpoints and reached a maximum at with an LET from 90 to 200 keV/μm (154–157). In these studies, the RBE for mutation induction was higher compared to inactivation for all examined LETs (154). In HEK cells, the maximal RBE for reproductive cell death was 2.5 (158). For LETs above 900 keV/μm, RBE values for reproductive cell death dropped to 1 or below 1. Stoll et al. (159) also found an RBE for inactivation by high LET lead ions (>10,000 keV/μm) far below 1 and for nickel ions (>1000 keV/μm) around 1. In a human neuronal progenitor cell line (Ntera2), the RBE$_{max}$ for apoptosis 48 h after iron ion exposure (1 GeV/n) was at least 3.4 (160). The RBE for induction

of double-strand breaks was determined to be 1.8 for iron ions compared to X-rays, as detected by immunostaining of γ-H2AX 0.5 h after radiation exposure (161), or by pulsed-field gel electrophoresis (162) or other methods such as alkaline elution (163). For α-particles (LET 27–124 keV/μm), it ranged between 1.2 and 1.4 (164).

For improvement of cancer therapy, studies with several cancer cells and with various heavy ions, especially carbon ions, had been performed. In a microarray analysis of oral SqCC cells, 84 genes were identified that were modulated by carbon and neon ion (LET ~75 keV/μm) irradiation at all doses (1, 4, and 7 Gy) (165). Among these genes, three genes (TGFBR2, SMURF2, and BMP7) were found to be involved in the transforming growth factor β signaling pathway and two genes (CCND1 and E2F3) in the cell-cycle G1/S checkpoint regulation pathway. The relevance of these results for normal tissues cells or non-cancer cell lines has to be determined. In normal skin tissue, low doses (0.01 and 1 Gy) of IR resulted in transient alterations in the expression of genes involved in DNA and tissue remodeling, cell-cycle transition, and inflammation (TNF, interleukins) (166), suggesting an involvement of the NF-κB pathway, the main inflammatory pathway, in the cellular response to IR. As exposure to accelerated argon ions (95 MeV/n Ar, LET 271 keV/μm) resulted in strong activation of NF-κB in human cells (167), the RBE for NF-κB activation by heavy ions of different LET was determined (158). NF-κB-dependent gene induction after exposure to heavy ions was detected in stably transfected human 293 reporter cells. For comparison, cells were exposed to 150 kV X-rays. The maximal biologic effect ranged between 70 and 300 keV/μm. Argon ions (271 keV/μm) had the maximal potency (RBE ~9) to activate NF-κB-dependent gene expression in HEK cells. The effect of carbon ions was less pronounced and comparable the activation observed after X-ray exposure (168). Inhibition of ATM resulted in complete abolishment of NF-κB activation by X-rays and heavy ions. Therefore, NF-κB activation in response to heavy ions is ATM dependent and seems to be mediated by a nuclear signal from the damaged DNA as described for the genotoxin-induced NF-κB subpathway.

Assuming that NF-κB activation promotes survival, it can be hypothesized that the extreme capacity of energetic heavy ions in the LET range of 70–300 keV/μm to activate NF-κB's transcriptional effects might be responsible for the lower relative effectiveness in cell killing observed in this range. Above 300 keV/μm, the overkill effect (meaning that with further increase of the deposited energy in a small volume of the cell no more biologically relevant damages can be caused) possibly results in a decrease of the RBE.

Other groups report NF-κB translocation after exposure of normal human monocytes (MM6 cells) to 0.7 Gy of ^{56}Fe ions using a DNA-binding assay (169). This clearly indicates that high LET iron ion exposure induces rapid and persistent NF-κB activation. This activation of NF-κB was shown to be mediated through phosphorylation of IκBα and the subsequent proteasome-dependent degradation pathway. The iron study only revealed binding of NF-κB to its consensus sequence of 5'-GGGGACTTTCC-3', and not transcriptional activation.

Scarce LET dependence data exist for p53 expression in human neuronal progenitor cells (160). Screening of gene expression in the nematode *Caenorhabditis elegans* suggests an LET

---

[6]The absorbed dose of a test radiation necessary to induce a defined biological endpoint and a defined severity of this endpoint (survival, cell cycle arrest, mutagenesis, chromosome aberrations, tumor induction in laboratory animals, and others) is compared to the dose of a reference radiation needed for induction of the same biological effect (150). Sparsely ionizing radiation such as γ-rays or X-rays is often used as reference radiation. In some cases, protons are applied as reference. The RBE is calculated according to the following formula:

$$RBE = \frac{\text{Absorbed dose of reference radiation inducing biologic effect (Gy)}}{\text{Absorbed dose of test radiation inducing biologic effect (Gy)}}$$

dependence or track structure dependence of the gene expression changes (170). In human lens epithelial cells, transcription and translation of CDKN1A [p21$^{CIP1/WAF1}$] are both temporally regulated after exposure to 4 Gy of high-energy accelerated iron-ion beams (~150 keV/μm) as well as to protons (~1 keV/μm) and X-rays, whereby the magnitude and kinetics of the expression enhancement seem to depend on the LET of the radiation (171).

CONCLUSION

Increased understanding of signaling pathways leading to transcription factor activation or inhibition in response to high LET radiation exposure will help to identify and make use of new targets for radiosensitization of tumor tissue and/or increasing radioresistance of surrounding normal tissue. The question which transcription factor offers a suitable target for charged particle cancer therapy is still open, as very few studies on transcription factor activation by carbon ions in tumor cells were performed. Also, not in all studies clinically relevant doses were applied, and extrapolation of the effects from high to lower doses is not constructive when the dose–response curves are unknown.

Although the role of p53 seems to be quite clear in low LET radiation therapy with increased radiosensitivity in case of functionality, this is not yet the case for charged particle therapy. Some studies suggest p53-independent cell killing by high LET which is a large advantage for treatment of tumors with p53 mutations. More studies with different cancer cell types are required. Concerning surrounding tissues, p53 inhibition might prevent precipitous apoptosis in apoptosis prone tissues. In tissues where p53-induced cell-cycle arrest dominates, p53 inhibition might impede this protective pathway and have detrimental effects.

The anti-apoptotic effects of NF-κB could support tumor cell survival during chemo- or radiotherapy; therefore, NF-κB is an interesting target for combined cancer therapies including carbon ion therapy. In several tumor cell types, inhibition of NF-κB resulted in radiosensitization. Activation of NF-κB in the normal tissue might not only limit detrimental effects by cell killing but also promote inflammation.

The activity of Nrf2 after irradiation seems to follow a complicated pattern, i.e., different time scales seem to be involved, and most striking is the occurrence of long-term effects in fibroblasts and intestinal epithelial cells. In the case of intestinal epithelial cells, the occurrence of long-term oxidative stress points to an inefficient activation of Nrf2 or a reduced oxidative stress response. It would be interesting to investigate this further. Of particular interest would be to compare differentiated cells with tissue-specific stem cells after irradiation; as in the case of intestinal stem cells, some studies suggest that oxidative stress inhibits the action of Nrf2 and that here might be differences between fully differentiated cells and stem cells in the regulation of Nrf2. Another open question is how to modulate the Nrf2 response in healthy tissue for radiation protection to reduce the side effects of radiation therapy and to mitigate radiation effects in spaces in case of manned missions. Modulating the elevated level of Nrf2 activity in cancer cells may be beneficial for cancer therapy. As described above, Nrf2 is upregulated in many cancer tissues and

a high level of Nrf2 expression corresponds to a poor prognosis for patients. In this sense, Nrf2 can serve as an indicator for the outcomes of cancer radio- and chemotherapy. So far, relatively little is known about chemicals that may inhibit Nrf2 directly (apart from retinoic acid) or upregulate Keap1, research in this direction may lead to the discovery of novel drug candidates supplementing radiation therapy. Using siRNA for therapeutic means may also be an option for those cancers that show a high expression and activity of Nrf2.

CREB, AP-1, Sp1, and EGR-1 (or up- or downstream events in these pathways) were activated by low doses of high LET α-particles and the first three were also shown to be involved in the cellular response to carbon and/or iron ions. For low LET radiation, many studies suggest a subordinate importance of these factors in cellular radiation responses compared to p53, NF-κB, and Nrf2. Nevertheless, we discuss how modification of these transcription factors may influence therapy results.

CREB itself is a factor inducing cellular survival, activated by phosphorylation due to (among others) ATM. Amorino et al. (124) detected a decreased survival of CREB-ko cells after IR exposure compared to wt cells. As also high LET irradiation stimulates ATM kinase activity, which in turn can activate CREB, a potential therapy approach is to inhibit phosphorylation of CREB or its binding to DNA in the vicinity of cancerous tissue. This can be accomplished through siRNA or other CREB-inhibiting substances, which are then applied directly to target tissue (in case of superficial tumors) or transported to the tumor via homing probes (in case of hard-to-reach tumors). After reducing the survivability of the tumor in such a way, radiation-induced apoptosis via p53-dependent and -independent mechanisms can fight the tumor more effectively.

This approach bears the problem that, with drug-induced inhibition of CREB in tumor vicinity, also non-transformed tissue may be affected and therefore more susceptible for radiation-induced cell death. In this case, the high fidelity of dose deposition in heavy ion therapy may prove advantageous.

AP-1 is a sensory factor for oxidative stress and is activated by ROS and other free radicals besides IR (low LET like X- and γ-rays as well as high LET α particles). This activation can lead to apoptosis; therefore, a supplementary approach in heavy ion therapy would be to enrich AP-1 in tumor tissue, delivered as mentioned above, so that more AP-1 is activated by high LET radiation and apoptosis is induced more effectively in tumor cells. C-abl is a negative regulator of γH2AX and can induce apoptosis in a p53-independent manner. Therefore, a supplementary strategy for heavy ion therapy is again enrichment of the protein to increase apoptotic induction and weaken repair of damaged DNA in tumor cells.

Sp1 is, besides other functions, a regulator for apoptosis and the orchestration of the DDR and can initiate repair of DNA damages. An obvious strategy to reinforce high LET radiation effects would be inhibition of Sp1. However, the transcription factor assumes many various roles within the cell, so that manipulation of Sp1 might result in unwanted side effects. Genes regulated by Sp1 might be better targets for combating tumors and their expression in tumor cells in response to heavy ion irradiation should be analyzed.

Upon activation, the transcription factor EGR-1 has various pro-apoptotic and anti-proliferative effects in tumors. Its activation has been demonstrated so far for low LET irradiation and high LET α-particles. Before considering it as target in charged particle therapy, its response to carbon ion exposure should be determined. If high LET radiation induces pro-apoptotic effects in tumors cells *via* EGR-1 as well, an artificial enrichment of the factor could be beneficial.

These various strategies are attuned to particular effects of each respective transcription factor and could be amplified *via* combination. However, cross connectivity of these factors with other signaling pathways may exert considerable influence on the therapeutic result. Furthermore, radiation-induced bystander effects, inter- and intracellular modifications in response to various signaling factors, are strongly to be considered for both tumor and healthy tissue. It is undoubtedly certain that the more we know about pathway connections among themselves, especially in respect to heavy ion therapy, the better are chances to develop more effective strategies to fight tumors.

In summary, above mentioned transcription factors and associated proteins are involved in a wide spectrum of cellular functions upon treatment with IR, ranging from regulation of cell cycle, DNA repair, cell proliferation, differentiation, adhesion, migration, and apoptosis to immune responses including inflammation. All factors show increased activity and/or expression for low and (as far as tested) high LET irradiation and are involved in the cellular radiation response.

AUTHOR CONTRIBUTIONS

CH had the idea for this review, designed it and contributed the introduction, the NF-κB chapter, the NF-κB **Figures 3–6**, and the conclusion, redesigned **Figures 1**, **2**, **7**, inserted the references, corrected and edited all other parts, especially the conclusion, and did the revision according to the reviewers' comments. LS wrote the p53 chapter, contributed the p53 input for **Table 1**, and designed **Figure 1**. BH wrote the Nrf2 chapter, contributed the Nrf2 input for **Table 1**, and designed **Figure 7**. SD wrote the chapter "other transcription factors," contributed to **Table 1**, and invented **Figure 2**. CB-K contributed to the idea and design of the review and critically reviewed and corrected the manuscript.

ACKNOWLEDGMENTS

SD and BH were supported by a scholarship of the Helmholtz Space Life Sciences Research School (SpaceLife Grant No. VH-KO-300) funded by the Helmholtz Association and the German Aerospace Center (DLR). **Figures 3–6** were designed by CH for her habilitation thesis (Freie Universität Berlin, Faculty of Veterinary Medicine), which is not publicly available.

REFERENCES

1. Durante M. Space radiation protection: destination mars. *Life Sci Space Res* (2014) 1:2–9. doi:10.1016/j.lssr.2014.01.002
2. ICRP. Glossary. In: Valentin J, editor. *The 2007 Recommendations of the International Commission on Radiological Protection. ICRP Publication 103 [Annals of the ICRP 37 (2–3)]*. Amsterdam: Elsevier (2007). p. 26.
3. Ohnishi T, Takahashi A, Ohnishi K. Studies about space radiation promote new fields in radiation biology. *J Radiat Res (Tokyo)* (2002) 43(Suppl):S7–12. doi:10.1269/jrr.43.S7
4. National Aeronautics and Space Administration (NASA). *The Vision for Space Exploration [NP-2004-01-334-HQ]*. Washington, DC: NASA Headquarters (2004).
5. Snyder AR, Morgan WF. Gene expression profiling after irradiation: clues to understanding acute and persistent responses? *Cancer Metastasis Rev* (2004) 23:259–68. doi:10.1023/B:CANC.0000031765.17886.fa
6. Criswell T, Leskov K, Miyamoto S, Luo G, Boothman DA. Transcription factors activated in mammalian cells after clinically relevant doses of ionizing radiation. *Oncogene* (2003) 22:5813–27. doi:10.1038/sj.onc.1206680
7. Crawford LV, Pim DC, Gurney EG, Goodfellow P, Taylor-Papadimitriou J. Detection of a common feature in several human tumor cell lines – a 53,000-dalton protein. *Proc Natl Acad Sci U S A* (1981) 78:41–5. doi:10.1073/pnas.78.1.41
8. Moll UM, Schramm LM. p53 – an acrobat in tumorigenesis. *Crit Rev Oral Biol Med* (1998) 9:23–37. doi:10.1177/10454411980090010101
9. Sharpless NE, DePinho RA. p53: good cop/bad cop. *Cell* (2002) 110:9–12. doi:10.1016/S0092-8674(02)00818-8
10. Vousden KH. p53: death star. *Cell* (2000) 103:691–4. doi:10.1016/S0092-8674(00)00171-9
11. Lane DP. Cancer. p53, guardian of the genome. *Nature* (1992) 358:15–6. doi:10.1038/358015a0
12. Bourdon JC, Fernandes K, Murray-Zmijewski F, Liu G, Diot A, Xirodimas DP, et al. p53 isoforms can regulate p53 transcriptional activity. *Genes Dev* (2005) 19:2122–37. doi:10.1101/gad.1339905
13. Fei P, El-Deiry WS. p53 and radiation responses. *Oncogene* (2003) 22:5774–83. doi:10.1038/sj.onc.1206677
14. Pawlik TM, Keyomarsi K. Role of cell cycle in mediating sensitivity to radiotherapy. *Int J Radiat Oncol Biol Phys* (2004) 59:928–42. doi:10.1016/j.ijrobp.2004.03.005
15. Karagiannis TC, El-Osta A. Double-strand breaks: signaling pathways and repair mechanisms. *Cell Mol Life Sci* (2004) 61:2137–47. doi:10.1007/s00018-004-4174-0
16. Gudkov AV, Komarova EA. Pathologies associated with the p53 response. *Cold Spring Harb Perspect Biol* (2010) 2:a001180. doi:10.1101/cshperspect.a001180
17. Norimura T, Nomoto S, Katsuki M, Gondo Y, Kondo S. p53-dependent apoptosis suppresses radiation-induced teratogenesis. *Nat Med* (1996) 2:577–80. doi:10.1038/nm0596-577
18. Harkin DP, Bean JM, Miklos D, Song YH, Truong VB, Englert C, et al. Induction of GADD45 and JNK/SAPK-dependent apoptosis following inducible expression of BRCA1. *Cell* (1999) 97:575–86. doi:10.1016/S0092-8674(00)80769-2
19. Adeberg S, Baris D, Habermehl D, Rieken S, Brons S, Weber KJ, et al. Evaluation of chemoradiotherapy with carbon ions and the influence of p53 mutational status in the colorectal carcinoma cell line HCT 116. *Tumori* (2014) 100:675–84. doi:10.1700/1778.19278
20. Suzuki M. [Significance of radiation-induced bystander effects in radiation therapy]. *Igaku Butsuri* (2014) 34:70–8.
21. Meltser V, Ben-Yehoyada M, Reuven N, Shaul Y. c-Abl downregulates the slow phase of double-strand break repair. *Cell Death Dis* (2010) 1:e20. doi:10.1038/cddis.2009.21
22. Reuven N, Adler J, Porat Z, Polonio-Vallon T, Hofmann TG, Shaul Y. The tyrosine kinase c-Abl promotes -interacting protein kinase 2 (HIPK2) accumulation and activation in response to DNA damage. *J Biol Chem* (2015) 290:16478–88. doi:10.1074/jbc.M114.628982
23. Van Etten RA. Cycling, stressed-out and nervous: cellular functions of c-Abl. *Trends Cell Biol* (1999) 9:179–86. doi:10.1016/S0962-8924(99)01549-4
24. Choi SY, Kim MJ, Kang CM, Bae S, Cho CK, Soh JW, et al. Activation of Bak and Bax through c-abl-protein kinase Cdelta-p38 MAPK signaling in

response to ionizing radiation in human non-small cell lung cancer cells. *J Biol Chem* (2006) **281**:7049–59. doi:10.1074/jbc.M512000200

25. Kharbanda S, Pandey P, Jin S, Inoue S, Bharti A, Yuan ZM, et al. Functional interaction between DNA-PK and c-Abl in response to DNA damage. *Nature* (1997) **386**:732–5. doi:10.1038/386732a0

26. Baskaran R, Wood LD, Whitaker LL, Canman CE, Morgan SE, Xu Y, et al. Ataxia telangiectasia mutant protein activates c-Abl tyrosine kinase in response to ionizing radiation. *Nature* (1997) **387**:516–9. doi:10.1038/387516a0

27. Mori E, Takahashi A, Yamakawa N, Kirita T, Ohnishi T. High LET heavy ion radiation induces p53-independent apoptosis. *J Radiat Res* (2009) **50**:37–42. doi:10.1269/jrr.08075

28. Amundson SA, Bittner M, Chen Y, Trent J, Meltzer P, Fornace AJ Jr. Fluorescent cDNA microarray hybridization reveals complexity and heterogeneity of cellular genotoxic stress responses. *Oncogene* (1999) **18**:3666–72. doi:10.1038/sj.onc.1202676

29. Park WY, Hwang CI, Im CN, Kang MJ, Woo JH, Kim JH, et al. Identification of radiation-specific responses from gene expression profile. *Oncogene* (2002) **21**:8521–8. doi:10.1038/sj.onc.1205977

30. Chaudhry MA, Chodosh LA, McKenna WG, Muschel RJ. Gene expression profile of human cells irradiated in G1 and G2 phases of cell cycle. *Cancer Lett* (2003) **195**:221–33. doi:10.1016/S0304-3835(03)00154-X

31. Chen X, Shen B, Xia L, Khaletzkiy A, Chu D, Wong JY, et al. Activation of nuclear factor kappaB in radioresistance of TP53-inactive human keratinocytes. *Cancer Res* (2002) **62**:1213–21.

32. Barnes PJ, Karin M. Nuclear factor-kappaB: a pivotal transcription factor in chronic inflammatory diseases. *N Engl J Med* (1997) **336**:1066–71. doi:10.1056/NEJM199704103361506

33. Schreck R, Rieber P, Baeuerle PA. Reactive oxygen intermediates as apparently widely used messengers in the activation of the NF-kappa B transcription factor and HIV-1. *EMBO J* (1991) **10**:2247–58.

34. Sonenshein GE. Rel/NF-kappa B transcription factors and the control of apoptosis. *Semin Cancer Biol* (1997) **8**:113–9. doi:10.1006/scbi.1997.0062

35. Wu M, Lee H, Bellas RE, Schauer SL, Arsura M, Katz D, et al. Inhibition of NF-kappaB/Rel induces apoptosis of murine B cells. *EMBO J* (1996) **15**:4682–90.

36. Pahl HL. Activators and target genes of Rel/NF-kappaB transcription factors. *Oncogene* (1999) **18**:6853–66. doi:10.1038/sj.onc.1203239

37. Bonizzi G, Karin M. The two NF-kappaB activation pathways and their role in innate and adaptive immunity. *Trends Immunol* (2004) **25**:280–8. doi:10.1016/j.it.2004.03.008

38. Karin M. Nuclear factor-kappaB in cancer development and progression. *Nature* (2006) **441**:431–6. doi:10.1038/nature04870

39. Ghosh S, May MJ, Kopp EB. NF-kappa B and Rel proteins: evolutionarily conserved mediators of immune responses. *Annu Rev Immunol* (1998) **16**:225–60. doi:10.1146/annurev.immunol.16.1.225

40. Li N, Karin M. Is NF-kappaB the sensor of oxidative stress? *FASEB J* (1999) **13**:1137–43.

41. Aggarwal BB, Sethi G, Nair A, Ichikawa H. Nuclear factor-kappa B: a holy grail in cancer prevention and therapy. *Curr Signal Transduct Ther* (2006) **1**:25–52. doi:10.2174/157436206775269235

42. Zabel U, Henkel T, Silva MS, Baeuerle PA. Nuclear uptake control of NF-kappa B by MAD-3, an I kappa B protein present in the nucleus. *EMBO J* (1993) **12**:201–11.

43. O'Dea E, Hoffmann A. NF-kappaB signaling. *Wiley Interdiscip Rev Syst Biol Med* (2009) **1**:107–15. doi:10.1002/wsbm.30

44. Habelhah H. Emerging complexity of protein ubiquitination in the NF-kappaB pathway. *Genes Cancer* (2010) **1**:735–47. doi:10.1177/1947601910382900

45. Annemann M, Plaza-Sirventa C, Schustera M, Katsoulis-Dimitrioua K, Kliche S, Schravena B, et al. Atypical IκB proteins in immune cell differentiation and function. *Immunol Lett* (2016) **171**:26–35. doi:10.1016/j.imlet.2016.01.006

46. Alkalay I, Yaron A, Hatzubai A, Orian A, Ciechanover A, Ben-Neriah Y. Stimulation-dependent IκBα phosphorylation marks the NF-κB inhibitor for degradation via the ubiquitin-proteasome pathway. *Proc Natl Acad Sci U S A* (1995) **92**:10599–603. doi:10.1073/pnas.92.23.10599

47. Shen HM, Tergaonkar V. NFkappaB signaling in carcinogenesis and as a potential molecular target for cancer therapy. *Apoptosis* (2009) **14**:348–63. doi:10.1007/s10495-009-0315-0

48. Duffey DC, Chen Z, Dong G, Ondrey FG, Wolf JS, Brown K, et al. Expression of a dominant-negative mutant inhibitor-kappaBalpha of nuclear factor-kappaB in human head and neck squamous cell carcinoma inhibits survival, proinflammatory cytokine expression, and tumor growth in vivo. *Cancer Res* (1999) **59**:3468–74.

49. NCRP. *Report No. 153: Information Needed to Make Radiation Protection Recommendations for Space Missions Beyond Low-Earth Orbit* (Vol. **153**). Bethesda, MD: National Council on Radiation Protection and Measurements (NCRP) (2006). p. 1–427.

50. Monje ML, Toda H, Palmer TD. Inflammatory blockade restores adult hippocampal neurogenesis. *Science* (2003) **302**:1760–5. doi:10.1126/science.1088417

51. Baichwal VR, Baeuerle PA. Activate NF-kappa B or die? *Curr Biol* (1997) **7**:R94–6. doi:10.1016/S0960-9822(06)00046-7

52. Li N, Banin S, Ouyang H, Li GC, Courtois G, Shiloh Y, et al. ATM is required for IkappaB kinase (IKKk) activation in response to DNA double strand breaks. *J Biol Chem* (2001) **276**:8898–903. doi:10.1074/jbc.M009809200

53. Piret B, Schoonbroodt S, Piette J. The ATM protein is required for sustained activation of NF-kappaB following DNA damage. *Oncogene* (1999) **18**:2261–71. doi:10.1038/sj.onc.1202541

54. Durocher D, Jackson SP. DNA-PK, ATM and ATR as sensors of DNA damage: variations on a theme? *Curr Opin Cell Biol* (2001) **13**:225–31. doi:10.1016/S0955-0674(00)00201-5

55. Wang CY, Mayo MW, Korneluk RG, Goeddel DV, Baldwin AS Jr. NF-kappaB antiapoptosis: induction of TRAF1 and TRAF2 and c-IAP1 and c-IAP2 to suppress caspase-8 activation. *Science* (1998) **281**:1680–3. doi:10.1126/science.281.5383.1680

56. Baldwin AS. Control of oncogenesis and cancer therapy resistance by the transcription factor NF-kappaB. *J Clin Invest* (2001) **107**:241–6. doi:10.1172/JCI11991

57. Waddick KG, Uckun FM. Innovative treatment programs against cancer: II. Nuclear factor-kappaB (NF-kappaB) as a molecular target. *Biochem Pharmacol* (1999) **57**:9–17. doi:10.1016/S0006-2952(98)00224-X

58. Hayden MS, Ghosh S. Signaling to NF-kappaB. *Genes Dev* (2004) **18**:2195–224. doi:10.1101/gad.1228704

59. Kulms D, Poppelmann B, Schwarz T. Ultraviolet radiation-induced interleukin 6 release in HeLa cells is mediated via membrane events in a DNA damage-independent way. *J Biol Chem* (2000) **275**:15060–6. doi:10.1074/jbc.M910113199

60. Li H, Lin X. Positive and negative signaling components involved in TNFalpha-induced NF-kappaB activation. *Cytokine* (2008) **41**:1–8. doi:10.1016/j.cyto.2007.09.016

61. Miyakoshi J, Yagi K. Inhibition of I kappaB-alpha phosphorylation at serine and tyrosine acts independently on sensitization to DNA damaging agents in human glioma cells. *Br J Cancer* (2000) **82**:28–33.

62. Imbert V, Rupec RA, Livolsi A, Pahl HL, Traenckner EB, Mueller-Dieckmann C, et al. Tyrosine phosphorylation of I kappa B-alpha activates NF-kappa B without proteolytic degradation of I kappa B-alpha. *Cell* (1996) **86**:787–98. doi:10.1016/S0092-8674(00)80153-1

63. Wong ET, Tergaonkar V. Roles of NF-kappaB in health and disease: mechanisms and therapeutic potential. *Clin Sci (Lond)* (2009) **116**:451–65. doi:10.1042/CS20080502

64. Dent P, Yacoub A, Contessa J, Caron R, Amorino G, Valerie K, et al. Stress and radiation-induced activation of multiple intracellular signaling pathways. *Radiat Res* (2003) **159**:283–300. doi:10.1667/0033-7587(2003)159[0283:SARIAO]2.0.CO;2

65. Staudt LM. Oncogenic activation of NF-kappaB. *Cold Spring Harb Perspect Biol* (2010) **2**:a000109. doi:10.1101/cshperspect.a000109

66. Netherlands Organization for Scientific Research. *Function of Cancer Genes Discovered*. ScienceDaily (2005). Available from: http://www.sciencedaily.com/releases/2005/05/050513224031.htm

67. Holley AK, Xu Y, St Clair DK, St Clair WH. RelB regulates manganese superoxide dismutase gene and resistance to ionizing radiation of prostate cancer cells. *Ann N Y Acad Sci* (2010) **1201**:129–36. doi:10.1111/j.1749-6632.2010.05613.x

68. Habraken Y, Piette J. NF-kappaB activation by double-strand breaks. *Biochem Pharmacol* (2006) **72**:1132–41. doi:10.1016/j.bcp.2006.07.015

69. Basu S, Rosenzweig KR, Youmell M, Price BD. The DNA-dependent protein kinase participates in the activation of NF kappa B following DNA damage. *Biochem Biophys Res Commun* (1998) **247**:79–83. doi:10.1006/bbrc.1998.8741

70. Hellweg CE. The nuclear factor kappaB pathway: a link to the immune system in the radiation response. *Cancer Lett* (2015) **368**:275–89. doi:10.1016/j.canlet.2015.02.019

71. Shao R, Karunagaran D, Zhou BP, Li K, Lo SS, Deng J, et al. Inhibition of nuclear factor-kappaB activity is involved in E1A-mediated sensitization of radiation-induced apoptosis. *J Biol Chem* (1997) **272**:32739–42. doi:10.1074/jbc.272.52.32739

72. Wang CY, Mayo MW, Baldwin AS Jr. TNF- and cancer therapy-induced apoptosis: potentiation by inhibition of NF-kappaB. *Science* (1996) **274**:784–7. doi:10.1126/science.274.5288.784

73. Wang CY, Cusack JC Jr, Liu R, Baldwin AS Jr. Control of inducible chemoresistance: enhanced anti-tumor therapy through increased apoptosis by inhibition of NF-kappaB. *Nat Med* (1999) **5**:412–7. doi:10.1038/10577

74. Yamagishi N, Miyakoshi J, Takebe H. Enhanced radiosensitivity by inhibition of nuclear factor kappa B activation in human malignant glioma cells. *Int J Radiat Biol* (1997) **72**:157–62. doi:10.1080/095530097143374

75. Ding GR, Honda N, Nakahara T, Tian F, Yoshida M, Hirose H, et al. Radiosensitization by inhibition of IkappaB-alpha phosphorylation in human glioma cells. *Radiat Res* (2003) **160**:232–7. doi:10.1667/RR3018

76. Ding GR, Yaguchi H, Yoshida M, Miyakoshi J. Increase in X-ray-induced mutations by exposure to magnetic field (60 Hz, 5 mT) in NF-kappaB-inhibited cells. *Biochem Biophys Res Commun* (2000) **276**:238–43. doi:10.1006/bbrc.2000.3455

77. Lee CH, Jeon YT, Kim SH, Song YS. NF-kappaB as a potential molecular target for cancer therapy. *Biofactors* (2007) **29**:19–35. doi:10.1002/biof.5520290103

78. Van Waes C. Nuclear factor-kappaB in development, prevention, and therapy of cancer. *Clin Cancer Res* (2007) **13**:1076–82. doi:10.1158/1078-0432.CCR-06-2221

79. Kim HJ, Hawke N, Baldwin AS. NF-kappaB and IKK as therapeutic targets in cancer. *Cell Death Differ* (2006) **13**:738–47. doi:10.1038/sj.cdd.4401877

80. Nakanishi C, Toi M. Nuclear factor-kappaB inhibitors as sensitizers to anticancer drugs. *Nat Rev Cancer* (2005) **5**:297–309. doi:10.1038/nrc1588

81. Dolcet X, Llobet D, Pallares J, Matias-Guiu X. NF-kB in development and progression of human cancer. *Virchows Arch* (2005) **446**:475–82. doi:10.1007/s00428-005-1264-9

82. Barkett M, Gilmore TD. Control of apoptosis by Rel/NF-kappaB transcription factors. *Oncogene* (1999) **18**:6910–24. doi:10.1038/sj.onc.1203238

83. Bredel M, Scholtens DM, Yadav AK, Alvarez AA, Renfrow JJ, Chandler JP, et al. NFKBIA deletion in glioblastomas. *N Engl J Med* (2011) **364**:627–37. doi:10.1056/NEJMoa1006312

84. Liu X, Yu H, Yang W, Zhou X, Lu H, Shi D. Mutations of NFKBIA in biopsy specimens from Hodgkin lymphoma. *Cancer Genet Cytogenet* (2010) **197**:152–7. doi:10.1016/j.cancergencyto.2009.11.005

85. Lake A, Shield LA, Cordano P, Chui DT, Osborne J, Crae S, et al. Mutations of NFKBIA, encoding IkappaB alpha, are a recurrent finding in classical Hodgkin lymphoma but are not a unifying feature of non-EBV-associated cases. *Int J Cancer* (2009) **125**:1334–42. doi:10.1002/ijc.24502

86. Gao J, Pfeifer D, He LJ, Qiao F, Zhang Z, Arbman G, et al. Association of NFKBIA polymorphism with colorectal cancer risk and prognosis in Swedish and Chinese populations. *Scand J Gastroenterol* (2007) **42**:345–50. doi:10.1080/00365520600880856

87. Brar SS, Kennedy TP, Whorton AR, Sturrock AB, Huecksteadt TP, Ghio AJ, et al. Reactive oxygen species from NAD(P)H:quinone oxidoreductase constitutively activate NF-kappaB in malignant melanoma cells. *Am J Physiol Cell Physiol* (2001) **280**:C659–76.

88. McDonald JT, Kim K, Norris AJ, Vlashi E, Phillips TM, Lagadec C, et al. Ionizing radiation activates the Nrf2 antioxidant response. *Cancer Res* (2010) **70**:8886–95. doi:10.1158/0008-5472.CAN-10-0171

89. Morita M, Motohashi M. Survival strategy and disease pathogenesis according to the Nrf2-small Maf heterodimer. In: Farooqui T, Farooqui AA, editors. *Oxidative Stress in Vertebrates and Invertebrates: Molecular Aspects of Cell Signaling.* Brisbane: Wiley (2012). p. 63–83.

90. Ramkissoon A, Shapiro AM, Loniewska MM, Wells PG. Neurodegeneration from drugs and aging-derived free radicals. In: Villamean FR, editor. *Molecular Basis of Oxidative Stress: Chemistry, Mechanisms, and Disease Pathogenesis.* Brisbane: Wiley (2013). p. 237–311.

91. Kwak MK, Itoh K, Yamamoto M, Kensler TW. Enhanced expression of the transcription factor Nrf2 by cancer chemopreventive agents: role of antioxidant response element-like sequences in the nrf2 promoter. *Mol Cell Biol* (2002) **22**:2883–92. doi:10.1128/MCB.22.9.2883-2892.2002

92. Katsuoka F, Motohashi H, Engel JD, Yamamoto M. Nrf2 transcriptionally activates the mafG gene through an antioxidant response element. *J Biol Chem* (2005) **280**:4483–90. doi:10.1074/jbc.M411451200

93. Lee OH, Jain AK, Papusha V, Jaiswal AK. An auto-regulatory loop between stress sensors INrf2 and Nrf2 controls their cellular abundance. *J Biol Chem* (2007) **282**:36412–20. doi:10.1074/jbc.M706517200

94. Baird L, Dinkova-Kostova AT. The cytoprotective role of the Keap1-Nrf2 pathway. *Arch Toxicol* (2011) **85**:241–72. doi:10.1007/s00204-011-0674-5

95. Liu GH, Qu J, Shen X. NF-kappaB/p65 antagonizes Nrf2-ARE pathway by depriving CBP from Nrf2 and facilitating recruitment of HDAC3 to MafK. *Biochim Biophys Acta* (2008) **1783**:713–27. doi:10.1016/j.bbamcr.2008.01.002

96. Yu M, Li H, Liu Q, Liu F, Tang L, Li C, et al. Nuclear factor p65 interacts with Keap1 to repress the Nrf2-ARE pathway. *Cell Signal* (2011) **23**:883–92. doi:10.1016/j.cellsig.2011.01.014

97. Tsukimoto M, Tamaishi N, Homma T, Kojima S. Low-dose gamma-ray irradiation induces translocation of Nrf2 into nuclear in mouse macrophage RAW264.7 cells. *J Radiat Res* (2010) **51**:349–53. doi:10.1269/jrr.10002

98. Datta K, Suman S, Kallakury BV, Fornace AJ Jr. Exposure to heavy ion radiation induces persistent oxidative stress in mouse intestine. *PLoS One* (2012) **7**:e42224. doi:10.1371/journal.pone.0042224

99. Jayakumar S, Kunwar A, Sandur SK, Pandey BN, Chaubey RC. Differential response of DU145 and PC3 prostate cancer cells to ionizing radiation: role of reactive oxygen species, GSH and Nrf2 in radiosensitivity. *Biochim Biophys Acta* (2014) **1840**:485–94. doi:10.1016/j.bbagen.2013.10.006

100. Wang XJ, Hayes JD, Henderson CJ, Wolf CR. Identification of retinoic acid as an inhibitor of transcription factor Nrf2 through activation of retinoic acid receptor alpha. *Proc Natl Acad Sci U S A* (2007) **104**:19589–94. doi:10.1073/pnas.0709483104

101. Mathew ST, Bergstrom P, Hammarsten O. Repeated Nrf2 stimulation using sulforaphane protects fibroblasts from ionizing radiation. *Toxicol Appl Pharmacol* (2014) **276**:188–94. doi:10.1016/j.taap.2014.02.013

102. Patwardhan RS, Checker R, Sharma D, Sandur SK, Sainis KB. Involvement of ERK-Nrf-2 signaling in ionizing radiation induced cell death in normal and tumor cells. *PLoS One* (2013) **8**:e65929. doi:10.1371/journal.pone.0065929

103. Hirota A, Kawachi Y, Itoh K, Nakamura Y, Xu X, Banno T, et al. Ultraviolet A irradiation induces NF-E2-related factor 2 activation in dermal fibroblasts: protective role in UVA-induced apoptosis. *J Invest Dermatol* (2005) **124**:825–32. doi:10.1111/j.0022-202X.2005.23670.x

104. Hochmuth CE, Biteau B, Bohmann D, Jasper H. Redox regulation by Keap1 and Nrf2 controls intestinal stem cell proliferation in *Drosophila*. *Cell Stem Cell* (2011) **8**:188–99. doi:10.1016/j.stem.2010.12.006

105. Tsai JJ, Dudakov JA, Takahashi K, Shieh JH, Velardi E, Holland AM, et al. Nrf2 regulates haematopoietic stem cell function. *Nat Cell Biol* (2013) **15**:309–16. doi:10.1038/ncb2699

106. Kim JH, Thimmulappa RK, Kumar V, Cui W, Kumar S, Kombairaju P, et al. Nrf2-mediated Notch pathway activation enhances hematopoietic reconstitution following myelosuppressive radiation. *J Clin Invest* (2014) **124**:730–41. doi:10.1172/JCI70812

107. Large M, Hehlgans S, Reichert S, Gaipl US, Fournier C, Rodel C, et al. Study of the anti-inflammatory effects of low-dose radiation: the contribution of biphasic regulation of the antioxidative system in endothelial cells. *Strahlenther Onkol* (2015) **191**:742–9. doi:10.1007/s00066-015-0848-9

108. Xie Y, Zhao QY, Li HY, Zhou X, Liu Y, Zhang H. Curcumin ameliorates cognitive deficits heavy ion irradiation-induced learning and memory deficits through enhancing of Nrf2 antioxidant signaling pathways. *Pharmacol Biochem Behav* (2014) **126**:181–6. doi:10.1016/j.pbb.2014.08.005

109. Kim SB, Pandita RK, Eskiocak U, Ly P, Kaisani A, Kumar R, et al. Targeting of Nrf2 induces DNA damage signaling and protects colonic epithelial cells from ionizing radiation. *Proc Natl Acad Sci U S A* (2012) **109**:E2949–55. doi:10.1073/pnas.1207718109

110. Shibata T, Kokubu A, Saito S, Narisawa-Saito M, Sasaki H, Aoyagi K, et al. Nrf2 mutation confers malignant potential and resistance to chemoradiation therapy in advanced esophageal squamous cancer. *Neoplasia* (2011) **13**:864–73. doi:10.1593/neo.11750

111. Jaramillo MC, Zhang DD. The emerging role of the Nrf2-Keap1 signaling pathway in cancer. *Genes Dev* (2013) **27**:2179–91. doi:10.1101/gad.225680.113

112. Abazeed M, Hammerman P, Creighton C, Adams D, Giacomelli A, Meyerson M. Nrf2 pathway activation regulates radiation resistance in lung squamous cell carcinoma. *Int J Radiat Oncol* (2012) **84**:S179–80. doi:10.1016/j.ijrobp.2012.07.465

113. Abazeed ME, Adams DJ, Hurov KE, Tamayo P, Creighton CJ, Sonkin D, et al. Integrative radiogenomic profiling of squamous cell lung cancer. *Cancer Res* (2013) **73**:6289–98. doi:10.1158/0008-5472.CAN-13-1616

114. Dent P, Yacoub A, Fisher PB, Hagan MP, Grant S. MAPK pathways in radiation responses. *Oncogene* (2003) **22**:5885–96. doi:10.1038/sj.onc.1206701

115. Cataldi A, Di Giacomo V, Rapino M, Zara S, Rana RA. Ionizing radiation induces apoptotic signal through protein kinase Cdelta (δ) and survival signal through Akt and cyclic-nucleotide response element-binding protein (CREB) in Jurkat T cells. *Biol Bull* (2009) **217**:202–12.

116. Iwahori S, Yasui Y, Kudoh A, Sato Y, Nakayama S, Murata T, et al. Identification of phosphorylation sites on transcription factor Sp1 in response to DNA damage and its accumulation at damaged sites. *Cell Signal* (2008) **20**:1795–803. doi:10.1016/j.cellsig.2008.06.007

117. Tsai WB, Chung YM, Takahashi Y, Xu Z, Hu MC. Functional interaction between FOXO3a and ATM regulates DNA damage response. *Nat Cell Biol* (2008) **10**:460–7. doi:10.1038/ncb1709

118. Choi YJ, Kim SY, Oh JM, Juhnn YS. Stimulatory heterotrimeric G protein augments gamma ray-induced apoptosis by up-regulation of Bak expression via CREB and AP-1 in H1299 human lung cancer cells. *Exp Mol Med* (2009) **41**:592–600. doi:10.3858/emm.2009.41.8.065

119. Cataldi A, di Giacomo V, Rapino M, Genovesi D, Rana RA. Cyclic nucleotide response element binding protein (CREB) activation promotes survival signal in human K562 erythroleukemia cells exposed to ionising radiation/etoposide combined treatment. *J Radiat Res* (2006) **47**:113–20. doi:10.1269/jrr.47.113

120. Zhang J, Wang Q, Zhu N, Yu M, Shen B, Xiang J, et al. Cyclic AMP inhibits JNK activation by CREB-mediated induction of c-FLIP(L) and MKP-1, thereby antagonizing UV-induced apoptosis. *Cell Death Differ* (2008) **15**:1654–62. doi:10.1038/cdd.2008.87

121. Dodson GE, Tibbetts RS. DNA replication stress-induced phosphorylation of cyclic AMP response element-binding protein mediated by ATM. *J Biol Chem* (2006) **281**:1692–7. doi:10.1074/jbc.M509577200

122. Shi Y, Venkataraman SL, Dodson GE, Mabb AM, LeBlanc S, Tibbetts RS. Direct regulation of CREB transcriptional activity by ATM in response to genotoxic stress. *Proc Natl Acad Sci U S A* (2004) **101**:5898–903. doi:10.1073/pnas.0307718101

123. Sahijdak WM, Yang CR, Zuckerman JS, Meyers M, Boothman DA. Alterations in transcription factor binding in radioresistant human melanoma cells after ionizing radiation. *Radiat Res* (1994) **138**:S47–51. doi:10.2307/3578760

124. Amorino GP, Hamilton VM, Valerie K, Dent P, Lammering G, Schmidt-Ullrich RK. Epidermal growth factor receptor dependence of radiation-induced transcription factor activation in human breast carcinoma cells. *Mol Biol Cell* (2002) **13**:2233–44. doi:10.1091/mbc.01-12-0572

125. Mitra AK, Bhat N, Sarma A, Krishna M. Alteration in the expression of signaling parameters following carbon ion irradiation. *Mol Cell Biochem* (2005) **276**:169–73. doi:10.1007/s11010-005-3903-5

126. Azzam EI, de Toledo SM, Spitz DR, Little JB. Oxidative metabolism modulates signal transduction and micronucleus formation in bystander cells from α-particle-irradiated normal human fibroblast cultures. *Cancer Res* (2002) **62**:5436–42.

127. Tanos T, Marinissen MJ, Leskow FC, Hochbaum D, Martinetto H, Gutkind JS, et al. Phosphorylation of c-Fos by members of the p38 MAPK family. Role in the AP-1 response to UV light. *J Biol Chem* (2005) **280**:18842–52. doi:10.1074/jbc.M500620200

128. Jochum W, Passegue E, Wagner EF. AP-1 in mouse development and tumorigenesis. *Oncogene* (2001) **20**:2401–12. doi:10.1038/sj.onc.1204389

129. Vermeulen K, Van Bockstaele DR, Berneman ZN. The cell cycle: a review of regulation, deregulation and therapeutic targets in cancer. *Cell Prolif* (2003) **36**:131–49. doi:10.1046/j.1365-2184.2003.00266.x

130. Marinissen MJ, Chiariello M, Gutkind JS. Regulation of gene expression by the small GTPase Rho through the ERK6 (p38 gamma) MAP kinase pathway. *Genes Dev* (2001) **15**:535–53. doi:10.1101/gad.855801

131. Lee SA, Dritschilo A, Jung M. Impaired ionizing radiation-induced activation of a nuclear signal essential for phosphorylation of c-Jun by dually phosphorylated c-Jun amino-terminal kinases in ataxia telangiectasia fibroblasts. *J Biol Chem* (1998) **273**:32889–94. doi:10.1074/jbc.273.49.32889

132. Chae HJ, Chae SW, Kang JS, Bang BG, Han JI, Moon SR, et al. Effect of ionizing radiation on the differentiation of ROS 17/2.8 osteoblasts through free radicals. *J Radiat Res* (1999) **40**:323–35. doi:10.1269/jrr.40.323

133. Morales A, Miranda M, Sanchez-Reyes A, Colell A, Biete A, Fernandez-Checa JC. Transcriptional regulation of the heavy subunit chain of gamma-glutamylcysteine synthetase by ionizing radiation. *FEBS Lett* (1998) **427**:15–20. doi:10.1016/S0014-5793(98)00381-0

134. Turtoi A, Schneeweiss FH. Effect of (211)At alpha-particle irradiation on expression of selected radiation responsive genes in human lymphocytes. *Int J Radiat Biol* (2009) **85**:403–12. doi:10.1080/09553000902838541

135. Calaf GM, Roy D, Hei TK. Immunochemical analysis of protein expression in breast epithelial cells transformed by estrogens and high linear energy transfer (LET) radiation. *Histochem Cell Biol* (2005) **124**:261–74. doi:10.1007/s00418-005-0033-9

136. Moreno-Manzano V, Ishikawa Y, Lucio-Cazana J, Kitamura M. Suppression of apoptosis by all-trans-retinoic acid. Dual intervention in the c-Jun N-terminal kinase-AP-1 pathway. *J Biol Chem* (1999) **274**:20251–8. doi:10.1074/jbc.274.29.20251

137. Chuang JY, Wu CH, Lai MD, Chang WC, Hung JJ. Overexpression of Sp1 leads to p53-dependent apoptosis in cancer cells. *Int J Cancer* (2009) **125**:2066–76. doi:10.1002/ijc.24563

138. Beishline K, Azizkhan-Clifford J. Sp1 and the 'hallmarks of cancer'. *FEBS J* (2015) **282**:224–58. doi:10.1111/febs.13148

139. Zhang JP, Zhang H, Wang HB, Li YX, Liu GH, Xing S, et al. Down-regulation of Sp1 suppresses cell proliferation, clonogenicity and the expressions of stem cell markers in nasopharyngeal carcinoma. *J Transl Med* (2014) **12**:222. doi:10.1186/s12967-014-0222-1

140. Olofsson BA, Kelly CM, Kim J, Hornsby SM, Azizkhan-Clifford J. Phosphorylation of Sp1 in response to DNA damage by ataxia telangiectasia-mutated kinase. *Mol Cancer Res* (2007) **5**:1319–30. doi:10.1158/1541-7786.MCR-07-0374

141. Beishline K, Kelly CM, Olofsson BA, Koduri S, Emrich J, Greenberg RA, et al. Sp1 facilitates DNA double-strand break repair through a nontranscriptional mechanism. *Mol Cell Biol* (2012) **32**:3790–9. doi:10.1128/MCB.00049-12

142. Yang CR, Wilson-Van PC, Planchon SM, Wuerzberger-Davis SM, Davis TW, Cuthill S, et al. Coordinate modulation of Sp1, NF-kappa B, and p53 in confluent human malignant melanoma cells after ionizing radiation. *FASEB J* (2000) **14**:379–90.

143. Nenoi M, Ichimura S, Mita K, Yukawa O, Cartwright IL. Regulation of the catalase gene promoter by Sp1, CCAAT-recognizing factors, and a WT1/Egr-related factor in hydrogen peroxide-resistant HP100 cells. *Cancer Res* (2001) **61**:5885–94.

144. Meighan-Mantha RL, Riegel AT, Suy S, Harris V, Wang FH, Lozano C, et al. Ionizing radiation stimulates octamer factor DNA binding activity in human carcinoma cells. *Mol Cell Biochem* (1999) **199**:209–15. doi:10.1023/A:1006958217143

145. Ghandhi SA, Ponnaiya B, Panigrahi SK, Hopkins KM, Cui Q, Hei TK, et al. RAD9 deficiency enhances radiation induced bystander DNA damage and transcriptomal response. *Radiat Oncol* (2014) **9**:206. doi:10.1186/1748-717X-9-206

146. Okayasu R, Okada M, Okabe A, Noguchi M, Takakura K, Takahashi S. Repair of DNA damage induced by accelerated heavy ions in mammalian cells proficient and deficient in the non-homologous end-joining pathway. *Radiat Res* (2006) **165**:59–67. doi:10.1667/RR3489.1

147. Ahmed MM, Sells SF, Venkatasubbarao K, Fruitwala SM, Muthukkumar S, Harp C, et al. Ionizing radiation-inducible apoptosis in the absence of p53 linked to transcription factor EGR-1. *J Biol Chem* (1997) **272**:33056–61. doi:10.1074/jbc.272.52.33056

148. Datta R, Taneja N, Sukhatme VP, Qureshi SA, Weichselbaum R, Kufe DW. Reactive oxygen intermediates target CC(A/T)6GG sequences to mediate activation of the early growth response 1 transcription factor gene by ionizing radiation. *Proc Natl Acad Sci U S A* (1993) **90**:2419–22. doi:10.1073/pnas.90.6.2419

149. Jäkel O. The relative biological effectiveness of proton and ion beams. *Z Med Phys* (2008) **18**:276–85. doi:10.1016/j.zemedi.2008.06.012

150. ICRP. *RBE for Deterministic Effects. ICRP Publication 58. Annals of the ICRP 20 (4).* Oxford: Pergamon Press (1989).

151. Barendsen GW, Beusker TL, Vergroesen AJ, Budke L. Effects of different radiations on human cells in tissue culture. II. Biological experiments. *Radiat Res* (1960) **13**:841–9. doi:10.2307/3570859

152. Barendsen GW, Walter HM, Fowler JF, Bewley DK. Effects of different ionizing radiations on human cells in tissue culture. III. Experiments with cyclotron-accelerated alpha-particles and deuterons. *Radiat Res* (1963) **18**:106–19. doi:10.2307/3571430

153. Skarsgard LD. Radiobiology with heavy charged particles: a historical review. *Phys Med* (1998) **14**(Suppl 1):1–19.

154. Yatagai F. Mutations induced by heavy charged particles. *Biol Sci Space* (2004) **18**:224–34. doi:10.2187/bss.18.224

155. Thacker J, Stretch A, Stephens MA. Mutation and inactivation of cultured mammalian cells exposed to beams of accelerated heavy ions. II. Chinese hamster V79 cells. *Int J Radiat Biol Relat Stud Phys Chem Med* (1979) **36**:137–48. doi:10.1080/09553007914550891

156. Ainsworth EJ, Kelly LS, Mahlmann LJ, Schooley JC, Thomas RH, Howard J, et al. Response of colony-forming units-spleen to heavy charged particles. *Radiat Res* (1983) **96**:180–97. doi:10.2307/3576177

157. Kraft G, Kraft-Weyrather W, Ritter S, Scholz M, Stanton J. Cellular and subcellular effect of heavy ions: a comparison of the induction of strand breaks and chromosomal aberration with the incidence of inactivation and mutation. *Adv Space Res* (1989) **9**:59–72. doi:10.1016/0273-1177(89)90423-7

158. Hellweg CE, Baumstark-Khan C, Schmitz C, Lau P, Meier MM, Testard I, et al. Activation of the nuclear factor kappaB pathway by heavy ion beams of different linear energy transfer. *Int J Radiat Biol* (2011) **87**:954–63. doi:10.31 09/09553002.2011.584942

159. Stoll U, Barth B, Scheerer N, Schneider E, Kiefer J. HPRT mutations in V79 Chinese hamster cells induced by accelerated Ni, Au and Pb ions. *Int J Radiat Biol* (1996) **70**:15–22. doi:10.1080/095530096145283

160. Guida P, Vazquez ME, Otto S. Cytotoxic effects of low- and high-LET radiation on human neuronal progenitor cells: induction of apoptosis and TP53 gene expression. *Radiat Res* (2005) **164**:545–51. doi:10.1667/RR3367.1

161. Whalen MK, Gurai SK, Zahed-Kargaran H, Pluth JM. Specific ATM-mediated phosphorylation dependent on radiation quality. *Radiat Res* (2008) **170**:353–64. doi:10.1667/RR1354.1

162. Löbrich M, Cooper PK, Rydberg B. Non-random distribution of DNA double-strand breaks induced by particle irradiation. *Int J Radiat Biol* (1996) **70**:493–503. doi:10.1080/095530096144680

163. Prise KM, Ahnstrom G, Belli M, Carlsson J, Frankenberg D, Kiefer J, et al. A review of dsb induction data for varying quality radiations. *Int J Radiat Biol* (1998) **74**:173–84. doi:10.1080/095530098141564

164. Frankenberg D, Brede HJ, Schrewe UJ, Steinmetz C, Frankenberg-Schwager M, Kasten G, et al. Induction of DNA double-strand breaks by 1H and 4He Ions in primary human skin fibroblasts in the LET range of 8 to 124 keV/μm. *Radiat Res* (1999) **151**:540–9. doi:10.2307/3580030

165. Fushimi K, Uzawa K, Ishigami T, Yamamoto N, Kawata T, Shibahara T, et al. Susceptible genes and molecular pathways related to heavy ion irradiation in oral squamous cell carcinoma cells. *Radiother Oncol* (2008) **89**:237–44. doi:10.1016/j.radonc.2008.04.015

166. Berglund SR, Rocke DM, Dai J, Schwietert CW, Santana A, Stern RL, et al. Transient genome-wide transcriptional response to low-dose ionizing

radiation in vivo in humans. *Int J Radiat Oncol Biol Phys* (2008) **70**:229–34. doi:10.1016/j.ijrobp.2007.09.026

167. Baumstark-Khan C, Hellweg CE, Arenz A, Meier MM. Cellular monitoring of the nuclear factor kappaB pathway for assessment of space environmental radiation. *Radiat Res* (2005) **164**:527–30. doi:10.1667/RR3397.1

168. Hellweg CE, Baumstark-Khan C, Schmitz C, Lau P, Meier MM, Testard I, et al. Carbon-ion-induced activation of the NF-kappaB pathway. *Radiat Res* (2011) **175**:424–31. doi:10.1667/RR2423.1

169. Natarajan M, Aravindan N, Meltz ML, Herman TS. Post-translational modification of I-kappa B alpha activates NF-kappa B in human monocytes exposed to ^{56}Fe ions. *Radiat Environ Biophys* (2002) **41**:139–44. doi:10.1007/s00411-002-0143-x

170. Nelson GA, Jones TA, Chesnut A, Smith AL. Radiation-induced gene expression in the nematode *Caenorhabditis elegans*. *J Radiat Res* (2002) **43**(Suppl):S199–203. doi:10.1269/jrr.43.S199

171. Chang PY, Bjornstad KA, Rosen CJ, McNamara MP, Mancini R, Goldstein LE, et al. Effects of iron ions, protons and X rays on human lens cell differentiation. *Radiat Res* (2005) **164**:531–9. doi:10.1667/RR3368.1

172. Takahashi A, Matsumoto H, Yuki K, Yasumoto J, Kajiwara A, Aoki M, et al. High-LET radiation enhanced apoptosis but not necrosis regardless of p53 status. *Int J Radiat Oncol Biol Phys* (2004) **60**:591–7. doi:10.1016/j.ijrobp.2004.05.062

173. Liu Y, Xing R, Zhang X, Dong W, Zhang J, Yan Z, et al. miR-375 targets the p53 gene to regulate cellular response to ionizing radiation and etoposide in gastric cancer cells. *DNA Repair (Amst)* (2013) **12**:741–50. doi:10.1016/j.dnarep.2013.06.002

174. Widel M, Lalik A, Krzywon A, Poleszczuk J, Fujarewicz K, Rzeszowska-Wolny J. The different radiation response and radiation-induced bystander effects in colorectal carcinoma cells differing in p53 status. *Mutat Res* (2015) **778**:61–70. doi:10.1016/j.mrfmmm.2015.06.003

175. Hickman AW, Jaramillo RJ, Lechner JF, Johnson NF. Alpha-particle-induced p53 protein expression in a rat lung epithelial cell strain. *Cancer Res* (1994) **54**:5797–800.

176. Amornwichet N, Oike T, Shibata A, Ogiwara H, Tsuchiya N, Yamauchi M, et al. Carbon-ion beam irradiation kills X-ray-resistant p53-null cancer cells by inducing mitotic catastrophe. *PLoS One* (2014) **9**:e115121. doi:10.1371/journal.pone.0115121

Permissions

The contributors of this book come from diverse backgrounds, making this book a truly international effort. This book will bring forth new frontiers with its revolutionizing research information and detailed analysis of the nascent developments around the world.

We would like to thank all the contributing authors for lending their expertise to make the book truly unique. They have played a crucial role in the development of this book. Without their invaluable contributions this book wouldn't have been possible. They have made vital efforts to compile up to date information on the varied aspects of this subject to make this book a valuable addition to the collection of many professionals and students.

This book was conceptualized with the vision of imparting up-to-date information and advanced data in this field. To ensure the same, a matchless editorial board was set up. Every individual on the board went through rigorous rounds of assessment to prove their worth. After which they invested a large part of their time researching and compiling the most relevant data for our readers.

The editorial board has been involved in producing this book since its inception. They have spent rigorous hours researching and exploring the diverse topics which have resulted in the successful publishing of this book. They have passed on their knowledge of decades through this book. To expedite this challenging task, the publisher supported the team at every step. A small team of assistant editors was also appointed to further simplify the editing procedure and attain best results for the readers.

Apart from the editorial board, the designing team has also invested a significant amount of their time in understanding the subject and creating the most relevant covers. They scrutinized every image to scout for the most suitable representation of the subject and create an appropriate cover for the book.

The publishing team has been an ardent support to the editorial, designing and production team. Their endless efforts to recruit the best for this project, has resulted in the accomplishment of this book. They are a veteran in the field of academics and their pool of knowledge is as vast as their experience in printing. Their expertise and guidance has proved useful at every step. Their uncompromising quality standards have made this book an exceptional effort. Their encouragement from time to time has been an inspiration for everyone.

The publisher and the editorial board hope that this book will prove to be a valuable piece of knowledge for researchers, students, practitioners and scholars across the globe.

List of Contributors

Stefan Walenta and Wolfgang Mueller-Klieser
Institute of Pathophysiology, University Medical Center, University of Mainz, Mainz, Germany

Melanie Rall and Lisa Wiesmüller
Department of Obstetrics and Gynaecology, Ulm University, Ulm, Germany

Daniela Kraft, Meta Volcic, Aljona Cucu, Elena Nasonova, Gisela Taucher-Scholz and Claudia Fournier
Department of Biophysics, GSI Helmholtz Center for Heavy Ion Research, Darmstadt, Germany

Halvard Bönig
German Red Cross Blood Service Baden-Wuerttemberg – Hessen, Institute for Transfusion Medicine and Immunohematology, Johann Wolfgang Goethe-University Hospital, Frankfurt, Germany

Dalong Pang, Sergey Chasovskikh and Anatoly Dritschilo
Radiation Medicine, Georgetown University Medical Center, Washington, DC, USA

James E. Rodgers
Radiation Oncology, Medstar Franklin Square Medical Center, Rosedale, MD, USA

Kathryn D. Held, Qi Liu and Henning Willers
Department of Radiation Oncology, Massachusetts General Hospital, Harvard Medical School, Boston, MA, USA

Hidemasa Kawamura
Gunma University Heavy Ion Medical Center, Gunma, Japan
Department of Radiation Oncology, Gunma University Graduate School of Medicine, Gunma, Japan

Takuya Kaminuma
Department of Radiation Oncology, Massachusetts General Hospital, Harvard Medical School, Boston, MA, USA
Gunma University Heavy Ion Medical Center, Gunma, Japan
Department of Radiation Oncology, Gunma University Graduate School of Medicine, Gunma, Japan

Athena Evalour S. Paz, Yukari Yoshida and Akihisa Takahashi
Gunma University Heavy Ion Medical Center, Gunma, Japan

Palma Simoniello, Joana Zink, Eva Thoennes and Maike Stange
Department of Biophysics, GSI Helmholtzzentrum für Schwerionenforschung, Darmstadt, Germany

Julia Wiedemann and Marco Durante
Department of Biophysics, GSI Helmholtzzentrum für Schwerionenforschung, Darmstadt, Germany
Department of Biology, Technische Universität Darmstadt, Darmstadt, Germany

Paul G. Layer
Department of Biology, Technische Universität Darmstadt, Darmstadt, Germany

Maximilian Kovacs and Maurizio Podda
Department of Dermatology, Darmstadt Hospital, Darmstadt, Germany

Claudia Fournier
Department of Biophysics, GSI Helmholtzzentrum für Schwerionenforschung, Darmstadt, Germany
Hochschule Darmstadt, Darmstadt, Germany

Ivana Dokic, Martin Niklas, Ferdinand Zimmermann, Philipp Seidel, Jürgen Debus and Amir Abdollahi
German Cancer Consortium, Translational Radiation Oncology, National Center for Tumor Diseases, German Cancer Research Center, Heidelberg University Medical School, Heidelberg, Germany
Heidelberg Ion Therapy Center, Heidelberg, Germany
Heidelberg Institute of Radiation Oncology, National Center for Radiation Research in Oncology, Heidelberg, Germany

Andrea Mairani
Heidelberg Ion Therapy Center, Heidelberg, Germany
National Center for Oncological Hadrontherapy, Pavia, Italy

Damir Krunic
Light Microscopy Facility, German Cancer Research Center, Heidelberg, Germany

Oliver Jäkel
Heidelberg Ion Therapy Center, Heidelberg, Germany
Heidelberg Institute of Radiation Oncology, National Center for Radiation Research in Oncology, Heidelberg, Germany
Division of Medical Physics in Radiation Oncology, German Cancer Research Center, Heidelberg, Germany

Steffen Greilich
Heidelberg Institute of Radiation Oncology, National Center for Radiation Research in Oncology, Heidelberg, Germany
Division of Medical Physics in Radiation Oncology, German Cancer Research Center, Heidelberg, Germany

Takahiro Oike, Hiro Sato and Shin-ei Noda
Department of Radiation Oncology, Gunma University Graduate School of Medicine, Gunma, Japan

Takashi Nakano
Department of Radiation Oncology, Gunma University Graduate School of Medicine, Gunma, Japan
Gunma University Heavy Ion Medical Center, Gunma, Japan

Nicole B. Averbeck, Jana Topsch, Michael Scholz and Wilma Kraft-Weyrather
Department of Biophysics, GSI Helmholtzzentrum für Schwerionenforschung GmbH, Darmstadt, Germany

Marco Durante and Gisela Taucher-Scholz
Department of Biophysics, GSI Helmholtzzentrum für Schwerionenforschung GmbH, Darmstadt, Germany
Technische Universität Darmstadt, Darmstadt, Germany

Christopher P. Allen, Neelam Sharma, Jingyi Nie, Cory Sicard, Maurice King III and Jac A. Nickoloff
Department of Environmental and Radiological Health Sciences, Colorado State University, Fort Collins, CO, USA

Walter Tinganelli
GSI Helmholtzzentrum für Schwerionenforschung GmbH, Darmstadt, Germany
Research Development and Support Center, National Institute of Radiological Sciences, Chiba, Japan

Francesco Natale and Marco Durante
GSI Helmholtzzentrum für Schwerionenforschung GmbH, Darmstadt, Germany

Steven B. Keysar and Antonio Jimeno
Division of Medical Oncology, University of Colorado School of Medicine, Aurora, CO, USA

Yoshiya Furusawa
Research Development and Support Center, National Institute of Radiological Sciences, Chiba, Japan
Research Center for Radiation Protection, National Institute of Radiological Sciences, Chiba, Japan

Ryuichi Okayasu and Akira Fujimori
Research Center for Charged Particle Therapy, National Institute of Radiological Sciences, Chiba, Japan

Sujatha Muralidharan, Maria A. Zuriaga and Kenneth X. Walsh
Whitaker Cardiovascular Institute, Boston University School of Medicine, Boston, MA, USA

Sharath P. Sasi
Cardiovascular Research Center, GeneSys Research Institute, Boston, MA, USA

Karen K. Hirschi
Yale Cardiovascular Research Center, Yale School of Medicine, New Haven, CT, USA

Christopher D. Porada
Wake Forest Institute for Regenerative Medicine, Wake Forest School of Medicine, Winston-Salem, NC, USA

Matthew A. Coleman
Radiation Oncology, School of Medicine, University of California Davis, Sacramento, CA, USA
Lawrence Livermore National Laboratory, Livermore, CA, USA

Xinhua Yan
Cardiovascular Research Center, GeneSys Research Institute, Boston, MA, USA
Tufts University School of Medicine, Boston, MA, USA

David A. Goukassian
Whitaker Cardiovascular Institute, Boston University School of Medicine, Boston, MA, USA
Cardiovascular Research Center, GeneSys Research Institute, Boston, MA, USA
Tufts University School of Medicine, Boston, MA, USA

Alexander Helm, Ryonfa Lee and Sylvia Ritter
Department of Biophysics, GSI Helmholtz Centre for Heavy Ion Research, Darmstadt, Germany

Marco Durante
Department of Biophysics, GSI Helmholtz Centre for Heavy Ion Research, Darmstadt, Germany
Department of Condensed Matter Physics, Technical University of Darmstadt, Darmstadt, Germany

Mary Helen Barcellos-Hoff
Department of Radiation Oncology, University of California San Francisco, San Francisco, CA, USA

Jian-Hua Mao
Lawrence Berkeley National Laboratory, Berkeley, CA, USA

Grace Shim, Marie Delna Normil, William M. Hempel, Michelle Ricoul and Laure Sabatier
Commissariat à l'Energie Atomique (CEA), DRF/PROCyTOX, Fontenay-aux-Roses, France

Isabelle Testard
CEA Grenoble, Laboratoire de Chimie et Biologie des Métaux, BIG, DRF, Grenoble, France

Kerry A. George and Megumi Hada
Wyle Science, Technology and Engineering Group, Houston, TX, USA

Francis A. Cucinotta
University of Nevada Las Vegas, Las Vegas, NV, USA

Kanokporn Noy Rithidech, Chris Gordon and Louise Honikel
Department of Pathology, Stony Brook University, Stony Brook, NY, USA

Witawat Jangiam
Department of Pathology, Stony Brook University, Stony Brook, NY, USA
Department of Chemical Engineering, Faculty of Engineering, Burapha University, Chonburi, Thailand

Montree Tungjai
Department of Pathology, Stony Brook University, Stony Brook, NY, USA
Department of Radiologic Technology, Faculty of Associated Medical Sciences, Center of Excellence for Molecular Imaging, Chiang Mai University, Chiang Mai, Thailand

Elbert B. Whorton
StatCom, Galveston, TX, USA

Shubhankar Suman, Santosh Kumar and Kamal Datta
Department of Biochemistry and Molecular and Cellular Biology, Lombardi Comprehensive Cancer Center, Georgetown University, Washington, DC, USA

Albert J. Fornace Jr.
Department of Biochemistry and Molecular and Cellular Biology, Lombardi Comprehensive Cancer Center, Georgetown University, Washington, DC, USA
Center of Excellence in Genomic Medicine Research (CEGMR), King Abdulaziz University, Jeddah, Saudi Arabia

Zhan Yu
Department of Biophysics, GSI Helmholtzzentrum für Schwerionenforschung, Darmstadt, Germany
Department of Radiation Oncology, Shanghai Proton and Heavy Ion Center, Shanghai, China

Carola Hartel, Diana Pignalosa and Wilma Kraft-Weyrather
Department of Biophysics, GSI Helmholtzzentrum für Schwerionenforschung, Darmstadt, Germany

Guo-Liang Jiang
Department of Radiation Oncology, Shanghai Proton and Heavy Ion Center, Shanghai, China
Department of Oncology, Shanghai Medical College, Fudan University, Shanghai, China

David Diaz-Carballo
Institute of Molecular Oncology and Experimental Therapeutics, Marienhospital Herne, Ruhr University of Bochum Medical School, Herne, Germany

Marco Durante
Department of Biophysics, GSI Helmholtzzentrum für Schwerionenforschung, Darmstadt, Germany
Institute of Condense Matter Physics, Darmstadt University of Technology, Darmstadt, Germany

Bradford D. Loucas and Michael N. Cornforth
Department of Radiation Oncology, University of Texas Medical Branch, Galveston, TX, USA

Igor Shuryak
Center for Radiological Research, Columbia University, New York, NY, USA

Annelies Suetens
Expert Group for Molecular and Cellular Biology, Radiobiology Unit, Belgian Nuclear Research Centre (SCK•CEN), Institute for Environment, Health and Safety, Mol, Belgium
Radiation Oncology Department, Center for Molecular Imaging, Radiotherapy and Oncology, Institut de Recherche Expérimentale et Clinique (IREC), Université Catholique de Louvain (UCL), Bruxelles, Belgium

Katrien Konings
Expert Group for Molecular and Cellular Biology, Radiobiology Unit, Belgian Nuclear Research Centre (SCK•CEN), Institute for Environment, Health and Safety, Mol, Belgium
Laboratory of Experimental Radiotherapy, Department of Oncology, KU Leuven, Leuven, Belgium

Marjan Moreels, Roel Quintens, Mieke Verslegers, Els Soors, Kevin Tabury and Sarah Baatout
Expert Group for Molecular and Cellular Biology, Radiobiology Unit, Belgian Nuclear Research Centre (SCK•CEN), Institute for Environment, Health and Safety, Mol, Belgium

Vincent Grégoire
Laboratory of Experimental Radiotherapy, Department of Oncology, KU Leuven, Leuven, Belgium

Christine E. Hellweg, Luis F. Spitta, Bernd Henschenmacher, Sebastian Diegeler and Christa Baumstark-Khan
Cellular Biodiagnostics, Department of Radiation Biology, Institute of Aerospace Medicine, German Aerospace Centre (DLR), Cologne, Germany

Index

Printed in the USA
CPSIA information can be obtained
at www.ICGtesting.com
JSHW061343201123
52413JS00005B/61